BF207
T48

Readings in

BEHAVIORAL PHARMACOLOGY

Edited by

TRAVIS THOMPSON

ROY PICKENS

RICHARD A. MEISCH

University of Minnesota

APPLETON-CENTURY-CROFTS

EDUCATIONAL DIVISION

New York   MEREDITH CORPORATION

JUL 12 '7f

161357

Copyright © 1970 by

MEREDITH CORPORATION

All rights reserved

This book, or parts thereof, must not be used or reproduced in any manner without written permission. For information address the publisher, Appleton-Century-Crofts, Educational Division, Meredith Corporation, 440 Park Avenue South, New York, N.Y. 10016.

740-1

Library of Congress Card Number: 76-118261

PRINTED IN THE UNITED STATES OF AMERICA

390-87490-6

PREFACE

An extensive and growing research literature concerned with behavioral actions of drugs poses problems for students in behavioral pharmacology. The diversity of goals, methods, and conceptual frameworks has created what appears to be an incomprehensible mountain of disparate facts. The present book is an effort to provide students with a framework within which to approach the literature. It is important to keep in mind, however, that organization *per se* may be of little value and can, in fact, be misleading. It is only when the order imposed on scientific data contributes to our understanding of the relations among arrays of independent and dependent variables that organization becomes worthwhile. The organizational framework of the present volume evolved from more than a decade of research relating behavioral actions of drugs to the variables experimentally demonstrated to control behavior. Because this approach has proved useful in generating effective drug-behavior research, and establishing meaningful relations between classes of independent and dependent behavioral variables, we believed it worthwhile to explicitly describe and illustrate the framework. Our purpose was to bring together those studies best illustrating the way in which this general framework is valuable in understanding the behavioral actions of drugs.

Our first and deepest thanks go to the authors who so kindly permitted us to reproduce their work in this volume. Their research constitutes the building blocks of knowledge in behavioral pharmacology. Some sections include few papers, while others incorporate many. This is largely due to the relative availability of good studies to illustrate our points. In some cases there were numerous excellent papers which could equally well have illustrated the kind of analysis of interest. In such cases our decision to include one paper and exclude others was often based on such practical considerations as the length of the paper, the number of figures, and the relative ease of obtaining publishing rights. We are indebted to the various publishers for their cooperation and patience in providing republication permission.

Special thanks are due to our teachers Dr. Gordon T. Heistad and Dr. William F. Crowder, and in particular to Dr. Kenneth MacCorquodale, co-editor of the Century Psychology Series. Whatever good comes of this book is as much their achievement as it is ours. The students in the Psychopharmacology Training Program at the University of Minnesota deserve a special note of gratitude, for they read and constructively criticized every paper, and played a significant role in selection. Finally, we wish to express our very great thanks to Cheryl Yano and Grace Jaeger, who so competently did all of the necessary clerical and editorial-assistant work, and to Bruce Rogers, for preparing the figures.

T.T., R.P., R.A.M.

CONTENTS

CONTRIBUTORS

	Articles
HARVEY ANCHEL	20
JAMES B. APPEL	39
HERBERT BARRY III	34
DALBIR BINDRA	11, 20
DONALD S. BLOUGH	15
JOSEPH V. BRADY	6, 14, 21
PETER L. CARLTON	25, 27
MAY-I CHOW	27
LINCOLN D. CLARK	24
ROBERT CLARK	21
LEONARD COOK	13, 41, 55
WILLIAM F. CROWDER	3
ARNOLD DAVIDSON	13
DIXON J. DAVIS	13
PETER B. DEWS	8, 18, 44, 45, 50, 51, 54
PAULINE DIDAMO	25
WILLIAM S. DOCKENS	52
JOHN L. FALK	23
CHARLES B. FERSTER	39
O. FONTAINE	47
CYRIL M. FRANKS	1
WILLIAM FRY	55
ARNOLD A. GERALL	7
STEVEN R. GOLDBERG	5

Readings in
BEHAVIORAL
PHARMACOLOGY

INTRODUCTION

Behavioral pharmacology [1] is the scientific domain concerned with the behavioral actions of drugs. It is based on an integration of principles and methods of experimental psychology with those of pharmacology. The goal of behavioral pharmacology is a description of the behavioral mechanisms by which drugs alter behavior. Realization of this goal is contingent on a thorough understanding of the environmental variables controlling behavior. This book is designed to illustrate some of the ways in which drugs can interact with variables known to control behavior. A description of these interactions in an essential first step in arriving at an understanding of the behavioral mechanisms of drug action (Thompson and Schuster, 1968).

The two key terms in this scientific enterprise are "drug" and "behavior." A *drug* can be defined as *any chemical substance which affects a biological system. Behavior* refers *to the movements of an organism or its parts within some spatially and temporally defined frame of reference, as observed by other organisms.*

In general pharmacology, the goal is to discover the mechanism(s) of drug action. The "mechanism of action" refers to any verifiable description of a drug's effects which can be shown to covary uniquely with a specific measured "response." Generally, this relation can be subsumed under some more general set of relations or principles. The term "response" is used in pharmacology to refer to any change in an organism produced by a drug, whether it is a biochemical, physiological, or behavioral change. In behavioral pharmacology, the scope is limited to *behavioral* mechanisms of action, i.e., mechanisms describable in terms of general principles used to account for behavioral events. Thus, in this book we will not be concerned with neurochemical and neurophysiological mechanisms, but rather

---

[1] The origin of this term isn't clear, though a number of investigators began establishing "behavioral pharmacology" laboratories in the mid-1950's, and the first article explicitly addressing itself to this topic was published in 1959 (see Article 9).

with mechanisms based on interactions of drugs with environmental variables controlling behavior.

As indicated above, behavior is described in terms of movements of an organism with respect to specific aspects of the environment. When some part of behavior can be shown to covary with a specific aspect of the environment, the former is called a *response* and the latter a *stimulus* (Skinner, 1938). Behavior which occurs intact on the first presentation of a stimulus is called *unconditioned*, since it requires no conditioning or training. Thus, an eyelid blinks the first time a puff of air is directed at the cornea. The eyeblink is an *unconditioned response* to the puff of air, an *unconditioned stimulus*. If, however, a tone is repeatedly presented immediately prior to the puff of air, soon the tone comes to elicit the eyeblink. The tone becomes capable of eliciting the response through conditioning, and is therefore called a *conditioned stimulus*. The establishment of conditioned reflexes by this procedure is called *respondent* or *Pavlovian conditioning* (Pavlov, 1927).

It is very important for the reader to understand that respondent conditioning is defined solely by the procedure of pairing two stimuli, with a resulting change in behavior. Conditioning is *not* defined by the kind of musculature used, the response topography, or the size of the behavioral unit under consideration. The criterion of conditioning is that a previously ineffective stimulus can be shown to produce a qualitatively comparable change in some aspect of behavior through the repeated pairing of stimuli. This procedural definition becomes particularly important in analyzing the effects of drugs on complex conditioning procedures involving two kinds of conditioned responses.

The effects of drugs on conditioned behavior controlled by its consequences will occupy the major portion of this book. When a specific aspect of behavior covaries with a part of the environment which is *produced* by the response, the response is called an *operant*. The consequence which strengthens the response that produces it is called a *reinforcer*. The procedure of strengthening behavior by presentation of a controlling consequence is called *operant conditioning* (Skinner, 1953). A thirsty animal that received water following a button press will be likely to press the button again when thirsty. The operant response of button-pressing has been strengthened by the reinforcer, water.

The foregoing two kinds of conditioned behavior will be

the dependent variables in the papers presented in this volume. Repeatedly throughout these pages the reader will find reference to studies taking the form "The Effects of Drug X on Behavior Y." All too often, after reading a paper of this sort we are inclined to ask, "Where do these findings fit into the larger scheme of things?" or, perhaps more succinctly, "So what?" Why do we ask such a question about a drug-correlated behavioral change, but would not ask it about a change in intestinal motility? A change in intestinal motility can be produced by an array of physiological and biochemical mechanisms which have undergone intensive investigation for many years. Physiologists and biochemists have provided an extensive background of information about the factors controlling this effect. Thus, when a pharmacologist introduces a drug which changes intestinal motility, he will turn to the known mechanisms and ask, "With which of these mechanisms is the drug interacting to produce the change in intestinal motility?" His research is usually designed to elucidate the mechanisms which were involved in producing the measured effect. For the most part, when it is reported that a drug increases the latency of a respondently conditioned response, or reduces rate of operant responding, we have no set of *mechanisms* to which these findings can be referred. We have a very limited body of background information into which to fit a specific experimental behavioral finding. Furthermore, experiments are very frequently designed without reference to the few basic factors which *are* known to control behavior. Thus, unless we are prepared to show some relation to a more general set of principles, the question "So what?" is legitimate. When little knowledge is available in a given area, it is often necessary to do the basic behavioral background research prior to or concurrently with the drug studies.

A functional analysis [2] of behavior reveals the mechanisms with which drugs may interact to determine a given behavioral drug-effect. Just as cholinergic nerve transmisson and afferent nerve impulses from mechanical stimulation are known to mediate control of intestinal motility, specific environmental variables have been shown to be controlling factors for behavior. These variables differ according to the defining procedures for operant and respondently condi-

---

[2] The term "functional" is used in the logical sense that A is a function of B $[A = f(B)]$ rather than the theoretical sense of, for example, an evolutionary function.

tioned responses. In respondent conditioning, the main factors controlling behavior are unconditioned and conditioned stimulus variables, and response variables. Drugs can have quite different effects on respondently conditioned response as a function of the kind or magnitude of the unconditioned stimulus, and the kind or magnitude of the conditioned stimulus. It should be obvious that not all respondently conditioned responses will be affected the same way by the same drug. A conditioned smooth muscle response would, in all likelihood, respond differently to atropine than a striate muscle response.

Operant behavior is affected by four primary classes of procedural variables: antecedent variables, current stimulus conditions, response variables, and response-consequence variables. Among the more important antecedent variables controlling operant behavior are deprivation conditions (e.g., food) and the organism's past history. Animals that have been severely food-deprived will respond differently to a given dosage of a drug than less hungry animals. Current stimulus conditions can also profoundly alter the actions of a drug. A drug may alter behavior controlled by a stimulus whose intensity is near the absolute threshold more readily than a more intense stimulus. Drugs may have stimulus properties themselves which can control the actions of the drug. The kind of response measured can determine whether a drug alters performance. The consequences of an operant response are obviously among the most important factors controlling behavior. The type of reinforcer (e.g., food, sex, shock), the magnitude of reinforcement, whether a reinforcer is effective without prior conditioning or was established as a reinforcer through conditioning, may all be significant factors determining the behavioral action of a drug. Behavior controlled by punishment rather than by negative reinforcement can be differentially affected by drugs. Finally, the specific contingencies of reinforcement may be important determinants of a drug's effect.

This book has been organized around the variables with which drugs may interact to affect behavior. Each paper in this volume has been selected because it illustrates the way in which one procedural manipulation can be used to reveal the interaction of a specific variable with the actions of a drug. Most important, these procedural variables are the basic mechanisms controlling behavior. Often other manipulations have been performed which are not germane to the point being illustrated, and interpretations outside this general framework are made by the authors. However, the procedures and data are independent of interpretation and are valuable as indications of methods of arriving at some understanding of behavioral mechanisms of drug action.

REFERENCES

Pavlov, I. P. *Conditioned reflexes: An investigation of the physiological activity of the cerebral cortex.* (Trans. and ed. by G. V. Anrep.) London: Oxford University Press, 1927.

Skinner, B. F. *The behavior of organisms.* New York: Appleton-Century-Crofts, 1938.

Skinner, B. F. *Science and human behavior.* New York: Macmillan, 1953.

Thompson, T., and Schuster, C. R. *Behavioral pharmacology.* Englewood Cliffs, N.J.: Prentice-Hall, 1968.

Part I   RESPONDENT CONDITIONING

Respondent conditioning [1] is a procedure for effecting change in the behavior of organisms. It involves the repeated pairing of two *stimuli* with the result that the response elicited by one stimulus comes to be elicited also by the other stimulus. The procedure is one by which the *reflexive* [2] behavior of the organism is most generally conditioned, although occasionally these changes are measured in terms of the organism's non-reflexive (operant) behavior.

The classic experiment in respondent conditioning is that of Pavlov, who first described the procedure. Pavlov was a Russian physiologist studying the role of salivation in digestion around the turn of the century. In his research dogs were prepared with salivary fistulas, and recordings were made of the amount of saliva produced by introducing meat powder into the hungry animal's mouth. Pavlov noted that initially only the meat powder would elicit salivation, but that after a few food presentations the *sight* or *smell* of the meat powder came to elicit salivation also. Pavlov reasoned that it was the repeated pairing of these stimuli with the food that led to the change in the organism's behavior. In order to investigate the phenomenon more carefully, dogs were placed in isolation rooms where food and other stimuli could be presented automatically. It was first demonstrated that whereas meat powder alone would elicit saliva-

---

[1] The procedure has also been called classical, Pavlovian, and Type-S conditioning.

[2] As used here, "reflexive" refers to any measurable aspect of behavior which is reliably elicited by a known stimulus.

7

tion each time it was presented, the ticking of a metronome would not. However, after the sound of the metronome had been paired several times with the presentation of food, the sound came to elicit a flow of saliva as well. Thus, a change had occurred in the behavior of the animal. Originally the dog did not salivate to the sound of the ticking metronome, but it was now doing so.

By use of this procedure, a number of other responses have since been conditioned to a variety of stimuli. Some of the responses which have been respondently conditioned include the pupillary reflex, vasomotor reactions, diuresis, knee jerk reflex, respiration rate, and previously conditioned responses. However, the most frequently used responses with humans have been the eyeblink elicited by a puff of air and the galvanic skin response elicited by a brief electric shock, and with lower animals the suppression in lever-pressing rate elicited by electric shock, leg flection elicited by electric shock, and the pharmacological effects of a drug.

For the general case, the stimulus used to elicit the behavior to be conditioned is called the *unconditioned stimulus* (US), the behavior so elicited is called the *unconditioned response* (UR), and the stimulus to be paired with the unconditioned stimulus is called the *conditioned stimulus* (CS). Thus, the basic paradigm for respondent conditioning is as follows:

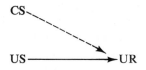

The response which the conditioned stimulus comes to elicit as a result of the pairing with the unconditioned stimulus is called the *conditioned response* (CR). The conditioned response is usually measured in terms of its magnitude and latency.

There are a number of variables known to affect respondent conditioning. Stimulus variables include the type, number, duration, and intensity of the CS and US, the temporal relationship between the CS and US (simultaneous, delayed, trace, or backward conditioning), the percent of CS presentations associated with US presentations, the CS-US interval, and the time between successive CS-US pairings. Response variables include the type, duration, and magnitude of the UR, and organismic variables include the species, age, sex, weight, and health of the animal.

Drugs have previously been considered as another type of variable affecting respondent conditioning. They were thought to exert their effects on behavior directly in the same manner as other behavioral variables. The view expressed here, however, is that for the most part a drug's effect can best be understood in terms of the effects of the drug on the *variables* which control respondent conditioning. By modulating these variables, a change in behavior is produced which is then referred to as the drug's "behavioral effect." So viewed, many of the experimental findings with drugs in respondent conditioning can be explained, rather than just determined. To explain a drug effect in this manner is not simple, however. Suppose, for example, that a drug is found to increase the speed of acquisition of a certain conditioned response. In what way might the drug have produced this effect? To answer this question, the first step would be to ascertain the behavioral variables which are known to increase the rate of acquisition of the CR. One might find that its acquisition is facilitated by increasing the US intensity, increasing the US duration, or by decreasing the CS-US interval. The next step would then be to determine on which of these variables the drug is acting. Such an answer can only come after experimentation, of course.

With this approach, experimental questions can also be proposed in other ways. For example, with some responses an inverse relationship has been found between the CS-US intertrial interval and speed of acquisition of the CR. The slower acquisition rate observed with shorter intertrial intervals has been attributed to fatigue. Drugs with anti-fatigue action (e.g., amphetamine) would therefore be expected to decrease the effects of short intertrial intervals, facilitating speed of acquisition of the CR. It is also known that the magnitude of the UR is related to speed of acquisition of the CR. Drugs which raise the threshold for stimulation (e.g., LSD) would therefore be expected to decrease acquisition rate. Within the proposed framework, many other possibilities for future experiments are also apparent.

The articles in Part I were selected to show the effects of drugs on behavioral variables known to influence respondent conditioning. Unfortunately, however, because there has been relatively little research in respondent conditioning in this country, there has also been little research dealing with the effects of drugs on this behavior. Because of this relative dearth of research reports, only seven articles have been selected for inclusion in Part I.

Section **A**   STIMULUS VARIABLES

The four papers in this section are concerned with the effects of drugs on stimulus variables. Article 1 reports the effects of several drugs on the conditioning of an eyeblink response in humans, under conditions of different percentage of US presentation (60 and 0 percent) following CS, to compare drug effects during acquisition and extinction of the CR. Article 2, which also has humans as subjects, uses a drug as a tool in the analysis of heart-rate conditioning, which is studied as a function of US intensity. In Article 3, a drug injection serves as the US, and the effects of the CS-US pairing interval on conditioning of the drug response are determined. Article 4 investigates the stimulus properties of drugs in respondent conditioning by demonstrating that a response conditioned under a drug's influence does not necessarily transfer to a non-drug state.

1

Effects of amobarbital sodium and dexamphetamine sulfate on the conditioning of the eyeblink response

CYRIL M. FRANKS and D. TROUTON

Of the numerous depressant and stimulant drugs, amobarbital sodium and amphetamine sulfate are probably among the most widely investigated in psychological experiments and the most frequently used clinically. There is evidence, chiefly from experiments on animals, to suggest that although these two drugs are by no means perfect antagonists, they have opposite effects on conditioning, the former increasing and the latter decreasing the ease with which CRs can be extinguished (e.g., 1, 3). Since in most investigations only one class of drug is used, and since both the reflex studied and the techniques of experimentation tend to vary greatly from one experiment to another, it is extremely difficult to make direct comparisons of the effects of stimulants and depressants. In particular, it cannot be safely assumed that agents which modify the performance of already established CRs will have a similar action upon the learning of new CRs. No one, as far as the present authors are aware, has made a direct comparison of the influence of stimulant and depressant drugs upon the learning of a *new* CR in man. This was therefore made the aim of the experiment which is reported here.

METHOD

SUBJECTS.   The *S*s were 80 paid volunteer graduate female students of education, ranging in age from 21 to 35 and having English as their mother tongue. They were told that they were to receive a harmless drug and that measures would be taken of how they were able to "relax in a quiet room under various conditions." All *S*s were asked not to eat anything for at least 2 hr. before coming to the hospital and to avoid taking any "tablets" or stimulant beverages for at least 12 hr. prior to the experiment. All *S*s had been given a brief medical interview beforehand to ensure that there was no contraindication to their receiving either of the drugs and also to exclude those with a history of psychiatric or neurological disorders.

PROCEDURE.   All satisfactory *S*s were allocated at random to one of four different treatment groups.[1] One *E* (C. M. F.) carried out the condi-

From *Journal of Comparative and Physiological Psychology*, 1958, **51**, 220–222. Copyright 1958 by the American Psychological Association, Washington, D.C.

[1] As a routine departmental procedure all *S*s were given a personality questionnaire

tioning; the other *E* was responsible for all other procedural and administrative details. Neither *S* nor the former *E* was aware which treatment each *S* had received. As soon as the time interval appropriate to the treatment concerned had elapsed, each *S* was brought to the conditioning laboratory and introduced to the new *E* for the first time. Contamination and suggestion effects were further reduced by restricting personal contact between *E* and *S* to a minimum before, during, and after conditioning,

Treatments. The four different treatments were 4.5 gr. of amobarbital sodium 45 min. before starting the experiment (Treatment A), placebo 45 min. beforehand (Treatment P), 10 mg. of dexamphetamine sulfate 45 min. beforehand (Treatment SD), and 10 mg. of dexamphetamine sulfate 2 hr. beforehand (Treatment LD).

It has been reported that amphetamine, especially when the dose is heavy, tends initially to produce unpredictable, and at times paradoxical, effects (e.g., 2, 13). With the knowledge at present available, it is apparently impossible to ascertain the optimum dose or time interval for eliciting any specific effect.[2] Consequently, a second amphetamine treatment group was included, having a somewhat arbitrarily chosen time interval of 2 hr.

All treatments were oral (intravenous techniques would have reduced the number of volunteers), and given in exactly similar capsules, the placebo capsule containing lactose. As reliance cannot be placed upon doses determined according to age and body weight (10, 11), a fixed dose was given to all *S*s in the same treatment group. A "no treatment" group was not included in the design since it has been shown, using the same laboratory and apparatus as in the present experiment that, as far as conditioned eyeblink responses are concerned, placebo and "no treatment" groups behave in a similar manner (8).

Conditioning. The apparatus and soundproof conditioning laboratory have been described in detail elsewhere (4, 6). The US consisted of an air puff, lasting 500 msec. and delivered at a pressure of 65 mm. of mercury into the right eye. The CS was a pure tone of frequency 1,100 cps, duration 800 msec., and intensity 65 db. above *S*'s hearing threshold, delivered to both ears through a pair of balanced headphones. The air puff began 350 msec. after the commencement of the tone, all time intervals and other physical variables being controlled electronically. The eyelid movements

---

before treatment. The findings, although not directly relevant to the present study, are of considerable theoretical interest. No relationship was obtained between eyeblink conditionability and the measure of introversion-extraversion used. Although complicated by the presence of drugs, this is contrary both to theoretical expectation and to previous experimental findings (5, 7).

[2] With certain agents, such as alcohol, there is some correlation between the blood level and the psychological effects, but determination of the blood levels of amphetamine is unlikely to be of use in this context, as it tends to disappear rapidly from the blood stream, presumably because it becomes localized in other tissues such as the brain.

in generalizing about the effects of amobarbital sodium and dexamphetamine sulphate upon reflexes other than the response studied in the present experiment.

SUMMARY

The aim of the experiment was to compare the acquistion and extinction of eyeblink CRs while under the influence of a stimulant or a depressant drug. Eighty female Ss received at random one of four treatments: amobarbital sodium, placebo, dexamphetamine sulfate 45 min. prior to conditioning, or dexamphetamine sulfate 2 hr. beforehand. It was found that the 2-hr. dexamphetamine sulfate group conditioned more readily than the placebo group, whereas the amobarbital sulfate group conditioned less readily. No significant or even apparent differences were found between the conditionability of the placebo and the 45-min. dexamphetamine groups.

REFERENCES

1. Alpern, S. B., Finkelstein, N., and Gantt, W. H. Effect of amphetamine (benzedrine) sulfate upon higher nervous activity. *Bull. Johns Hopkins Hosp.*, 1943, **73**, 287–299.
2. Carl, G. P., and Turner, W. D. The effects of benzedrine sulfate (amphetamine sulfate) on performance in a comprehensive psychometric examination, *J. Psychol.*, 1939, 8, 165–216.
3. Dworkin, S., Bourne, W., and Roginsky, B. B. Changes in conditioned responses brought about by anaesthetics and sedatives. *Can. med. Ass. J.*, 1937, **37**, 136–139.
4. Franks, C. M. The establishment of a conditioning laboratory for the investigation of personality and cortical functioning. *Nature,* 1955, **175**, 984–985.
5. Franks, C. M. Conditioning and personality. *J. abnorm. soc. Psychol.* 1956, **52**, 143–150.
6. Franks, C. M. Recidivism, psychopathy and personality. *Brit. J. Delinq.*, 1956, 6, 192–201.
7. Franks, C. M. Personality factors and the rate of conditioning. *Brit. J. Psychol.*, 1957, **48**, 119–126.
8. Franks, C. M., and Laverty, S. G. Sodium amytal and eyelid conditioning. *J. ment. Sci.*, 1955, **101**, 654–663.
9. Franks, C. M., and Withers, W. C. R. Photoelectric recording of eyelid movements. *Amer. J. Psychol.*, 1955, **68**, 467–471.
10. Goodman, L., and Gilman, A. *The pharmacological basis of therapeutics.* New York: Macmillan, 1941.
11. Laverty, S. G., and Franks, C. M. Sodium amytal and behavior in neurotic subjects. *J. Neurol. Neurosurg. Psychiat.*, 1956, **19**, 137–143.
12. Pavlov, I. P. *Lectures on conditioned reflexes.* Vol. 1. *The higher nervous activity*

(*behavior*) *of animals.* (Trans. by W. H. Gantt.) London: Laurence & Wishart, 1928.

13. Reifenstein, E. C., and Davidoff, E. The psychological effects of benzedrine sulfate. *Amer. J. Psychol.,* 1939, **52**, 56–64.

14. Settlage, P. H. The effect of sodium amytal on the formation and elicitation of conditioned reflexes. *J. comp. Psychol.,* 1936, **22**, 339–343.

2

Heart rate during conditioning in humans: Effects of UCS intensity, vagal blockade, and adrenergic block of vasomotor activity [1]

PAUL A. OBRIST, DONALD M. WOOD, and
MARIO PEREZ-REYES

The physiological basis of heart-rate changes in human Ss during classical conditioning was investigated in order to determine the influence of the vagal and sympathetic innervations of the heart and of peripherally initiated homeostatic reflexes. The heart-rate changes regarded as conditioned, i.e., those changes occurring either between CS and UCS onset or for a more sustained period following CS onset on nonreinforced trials, are in certain respects paradoxical and subject to the question of whether they are conditioned responses or only artifacts of the conditioning process. When a noxious UCS is used, such responses are reported to be either a deceleration of heart rate or a biphasic response characterized by an initial acceleration followed by a usually more sustained deceleration (Deane, 1964; Fuhrer, 1964; Geer, 1964; Lang and Hnatiow, 1962; Notterman, Schoenfeld, and Bersh, 1952; Wilson, 1964; Wood and Obrist, 1964; Zeaman, Deane, and Weger, 1954; Zeaman and Smith, 1964; Zeaman and Wegner, 1957). Recently, Wood and Obrist (1964) have demonstrated that the initial acceleratory component of the biphasic response is a respiratory artifact, which leaves only the deceleration as a possible conditioned response.

Two questions now arise. First, why is there no sympathetic acceleratory response since, under these conditions, such a sympathetic effect would be expected and was observed as measured by GSR and vasomotor responses? There is evidence that vagal inhibition, manifested as a deceleration of heart rate, is able to mask sympathetic activity (Rushmer, 1958; Samaan, 1934–35a). Therefore, the purpose of the first of two experiments to be reported was to determine whether sympathetic effects are present during conditioning but are not manifested due to the dominance of vagal restraint. For this purpose, heart-rate changes during conditioning in Ss with an intact vagus are compared to those with vagal activity pharmacologically

From *Journal of Experimental Psychology*, 1965, **70**, 32–42. Copyright 1965 by the American Psychological Association, Washington, D.C.

[1] These studies were supported principally by Research Grants M-6020-A and MH-07995, National Institutes of Health, United States Public Health Service, and by faculty grants from the University of North Carolina. The technical assistance of James Howard and Norma Thomas is gratefully acknowledged.

blocked. Additionally, two intensities of the UCS were used to determine whether sympathetic effects become more pronounced with a far more intense UCS than was previously used (Wood and Obrist, 1964). It was anticipated that a more intense UCS would result in an observable sympathetic effect even with the vagus intact, due to the possibility of greater fear or anxiety-producing qualities of the stimulus (Martin, 1961). The conditioned GSR was also evaluated to demonstrate the presence of sympathetic activity.

A second question concerned whether the deceleratory response is a conditioned response or rather is artifactual, resulting from homeostatic reflex mechanisms initiated by a conditioned pressor response. The use of a noxious UCS as well as the evidence of conditioned vasomotor responses indicate that such pressor responses may occur. Further, the presence of such reflex influences on heart rate is well documented (Neil and Heymans, 1962), but their significance during conditioning has not been determined. Therefore, the second experiment reported was to determine whether the deceleratory response was still observed once pressor responses of vasomotor origin were pharmacologically blocked. In order to evaluate the effectiveness of the pharmacological agent, direct recordings of both diastolic and systolic blood pressure were obtained.

EXPERIMENT I

METHOD.   *Subjects.*   The *S*s were 60 healthy male undergraduate students randomly selected from the introductory psychology class.

Apparatus.   Methods for measuring heart rate, respiration, and skin resistance have been previously described (Obrist, Hallman, and Wood, 1964; Wood and Obrist, 1964). Additionally, R-R interval time was measured to the nearest .001 sec. on a sequence event timer and recorder (SETAR; Welford, 1952) and recorded on punch tape for computer analysis.

Procedure.   There were four experimental conditions with *S*s assigned randomly to each. This provided a comparison of the effects of vagal and nonvagal blockade at two intensities of the UCS. Vagal blockade was achieved by an IV injection of atropine sulfate (.02 mg/kg of body weight) just prior to the first conditioning trial. The dosage was derived from pilot studies. The *S*s not given atropine received IV 5 cc of saline but were eliminated from the experiment prior to data analysis either because they could not relate correctly which CS was followed by shock, or the atropine in part or whole was administered subdermally. Therefore, the final *N* was: saline, less intense UCS, *N* = 12; vagal block, less intense UCS, *N* = 11; saline, more intense UCS, *N* = 13; and vagal block, more intense UCS, *N* = 13.

1. UCS intensity. The intensity of the UCS was adjusted for each S as follows. All Ss were given a 9-point scale extending from "just felt" to "very painful" by which to judge a series of shocks. They were then given an ascending series of 6-sec., 60-cycle shocks spaced 30 sec. apart and administered to the finger tips of the left hand through two dry 5-mm. diameter silver EEG electrodes. At random intervals, the intensity was decreased one step to determine the reliability of S's judgments. At the point where the shock was first judged as "very painful," the series was stopped. For Ss in the low-intensity UCS groups, this was the level to be used during conditioning and S was so informed. This intensity approximated the level used in the Wood and Obrist (1964) study. For Ss in the high-intensity UCS groups, E entered the S room following the "very painful" judgment and read an appeal for S to take considerably more shock, which was defined to S as "as much as you can humanly stand." Thus, an appeal was made to his masculinity in addition to offering him a substantial financial bonus. After the first five conditioning trials, these Ss were again asked to take one further increase (.3 ma.), but most refused. The average amount of current for the less and more intense conditions was 1.88 and 3.86 ma., respectively ($t = 10.61$, $p < .001$).

2. Respiratory control. Respiration was controlled throughout conditioning by requiring S to maintain his normal resting frequency and depth so as to minimize the influence of respiratory effects on heart-rate changes in Ss not receiving vagal block. These procedures are similar to those previously reported (Wood and Obrist, 1964), with one exception. Respiratory activity was paced by an auditory signal which mimicked human breathing sounds. This signal could be adjusted with respect to both inspiration and expiration time as well as the pause between each so as to follow exactly any one S's resting pattern.

3. Conditioning procedures. A 10-min. rest period, training for respiratory control, UCS intensity determination and a 10-trial adaptation series preceded, in that order, differential trace conditioning procedures. During adaptation each CS was presented five times in a fixed random order. Conditioning consisted of a series of 36 trials, with 16 reinforced, 10 test, and 10 sensitization control trials, presented in a fixed random order. Short rest periods were given after every 12 trials. Test trials were used so as to determine the heart-rate changes during the period when the UCS would normally occur, since the maximum deceleration occurs during this time (Wood and Obrist, 1964). The CS+ and CS— were dim red and blue lights with a duration of 2 sec. The 6-sec. UCS started 7 sec. after CS onset. The intertrial interval averaged 75 sec. with a range of 60 to 90 sec. These intervals were varied in a fixed random order. Except during instructions, a low-level white masking noise was used. Respiratory control was continuous except during rest periods. The Ss were instructed that only one of the lights would be followed by shock and then only some of the time.

Data quantification.   The following are data quantification procedures.

1. Heart rate. Second-by-second changes in R-R interval from a pre-CS base line for each of the 25 sec., following CS onset were averaged separately for the 5 CS+ and 5 CS— adaptation trials, 10 test, 10 sensitization control, and 6 of the UCS trials, using procedures previously described (Wood and Obrist, 1964). This period was used in order to observe long latency sympathetic effects (see Dykman and Gannt, 1959). These analyses were done for each experimental condition except adaptation. Here the saline and vagal blockade groups were combined for each level of UCS intensity since atropine had not yet been administered. This increased the N to 23 in one group and 25 in the other. As in the previous study (Wood and Obrist, 1964), heart-rate changes, either acceleratory or deceleratory, were not related to base level. Therefore, no correction for base level was used.

2. Respiration. A mean change score was calculated as a ratio of the pre-CS average respiratory amplitude to the single largest inspiration during the first 6, next 9, and last 10 sec. following CS onset. This was calculated separately for test, sensitization, and UCS trials. This method of quantification is more completely described elsewhere (Wood and Obrist, 1964).

3. GSR. Conditioned GSR activity was quantified for test and senitization control trials by first obtaining the highest resistance level (ohms) up through 2.0 sec. following CS onset and the lowest resistance level occurring between 2 and 10 sec. after CS onset. In cases where there were two or more responses having a 600-ohm or greater change and a recovery of at least 60 ohms, the lowest level was obtained by totaling the magnitude of all such responses and subtracting this from the highest level. These two levels were then averaged for each S separately for test and sensitization control trials and then converted to conductance units. The difference between these two-level scores was then obtained as the measure of GSR magnitude and then averaged for only the two experimental groups not receiving the vagal blockade, since atropine blocks GSR activity. This resulted in an N too small to correct for base-level effects by regression analysis (Lacey and Lacey, 1962).

RESULTS.   No significant differences were observed in the second-by-second heart-rate changes between the CS+ and CS— during adaptation. Therefore, the sensitization control (CS—) was used as a base line from which heart-rate changes on nonreinforced test trials and UCS trials could be evaluated. A direct comparison of the heart-rate changes between vagal blockade and nonvagal blockade groups was prohibited by the very large difference in variance between groups. Base-level heart rate is greatly elevated by vagal blockade, resulting in a reduction of responsiveness. However, since the principal effects of vagal blockade were expected to be a shift in the direction of the response, that is, from deceleration to acceleration, an evaluation of the reliability of heart-rate changes within each experimental group makes direct comparisons unnecessary.

The deceleration of heart rate during conditioning was found to be the result of an increase in vagal restraint which masked sympathetic effects. This result was most obvious with the more intense UCS condition. The high-intensity UCS group without vagal blockade showed a biphasic response. There was an initial acceleration extending from Sec. 2–6, the effect being significant on Sec. 3 and 4. This was followed by a more sustained deceleration extending from Sec. 7–15, the effect being significant on Sec. 8 and 9. On the other hand, when the vagus was blocked, only an acceleratory response was observed on test trials with the exception of the first second (see Fig. 1 and Table 1). The acceleration was significant on Sec. 4–10, peaking at the exact second that the deceleration peaked when the vagus was not blocked, i.e., Sec. 9. There was a second less pronounced acceleration which began around Sec. 16 and peaked on Sec. 21, the amplitude being significant on both Sec. 21 and 22.

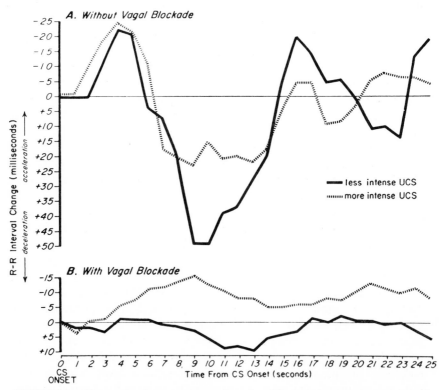

FIGURE 1.   Heart-rate changes expressed as the difference between test and sensitization control trials with and without vagal blockade at two intensities of the UCS.

TABLE 1.   Second-by-second changes in R-R interval (milliseconds) expressed as test minus sensitization control trial mean differences.

Sec. since CS Onset	Low-Intensity UCS				High-Intensity UCS			
	No Vagal Blockade $N = 12$		Vagal Blockade $N = 11$		No Vagal Blockade $N = 13$		Vagal Blockade $N = 13$	
	$\bar{x}$	t	$\bar{x}$	t	$\bar{x}$	t	$\bar{x}$	t
1	0	<1	+ 2	1.17	0	<1	+ 4	3.49**
2	0	<1	+ 2	<1	−10	1.34	− 1	<1
3	−11	<1	+ 4	1.07	−19	2.79*	− 1	<1
4	−22	1.47	− 1	<1	−24	2.54*	− 5	2.30*
5	−20	1.25	− 1	<1	−21	1.70	− 7	2.45*
6	+ 4	<1	− 1	<1	−11	1.25	−11	2.69*
7	+ 8	<1	+ 1	<1	+17	1.76	−11	2.89*
8	+21	1.46	+ 2	<1	+21	2.50*	−13	2.53*
9	+50	4.01**	+ 3	<1	+23	2.78*	−15	2.85*
10	+50	3.20**	+ 6	1.88	+16	1.38	−12	2.40*
11	+39	2.87*	+ 9	2.72*	+21	1.60	−11	2.00
12	+37	2.94*	+ 8	2.28*	+20	1.51	− 8	1.66
13	+28	2.31*	+10	3.55**	+22	1.55	− 8	1.92
14	+20	1.70	+ 6	2.58*	+18	1.15	− 5	1.32
15	− 5	<1	+ 5	2.15	+ 5	<1	− 5	1.41
16	−20	1.93	+ 4	1.92	− 4	<1	− 6	1.50
17	−14	1.34	− 1	<1	− 5	<1	− 5	1.30
18	− 4	<1	+ 1	<1	+10	1.12	− 8	1.93
19	− 5	<1	− 2	<1	+9	1.41	− 7	1.62
20	+ 1	<1	0	<1	+4	<1	−10	2.02
21	+12	<1	0	<1	−5	<1	−12	2.40*
22	+11	<1	+ 1	<1	−7	<1	−11	2.18*
23	+14	<1	+ 1	<1	−5	<1	− 9	1.62
24	−13	1.16	+ 3	<1	−6	<1	−11	1.83
25	−19	1.23	+ 6	1.23	−4	<1	− 8	1.33

Note.— + =longer R-R interval or heart-rate deceleration; − =shorter R-R interval or heart-rate acceleration.
* $p < .05$.
** $p < .01$.

The acceleration on Sec. 2–6 after CS onset observed with the high-intensity UCS with the vagus intact appears to be a momentary decrease in vagal restraint rather than a sympathetic effect. First, it has a shorter latency and peaks considerably sooner than the sympathetic effect observed with the vagus blocked. Such a latency difference has been previously proposed by Samaan (1934–35b) and Dykman and Gantt (1959). Second, this acceleration appears to be significantly influenced by uncontrolled respiratory effects. The amplitude of the acceleration is positively correlated (rho = .62, $p < .05$) with the largest single inspiration during the period of acceleration, the latter showing an 8% increase ($t = 2.02$, $p < .10$). In contrast, during vagal blockade, there was no correlation between the magnitude of the acceleration and respiratory amplitude. Therefore, even with a very intense UCS, there is little evidence that sympathetic effects are manifested when the vagal innervation is intact.

A reliable deceleratory response was also found on test trials with the less intense UCS without vagal blockade, extending from Sec. 6–14 (see

Fig. 1 and Table 1) and peaking at Sec. 9, as in the higher UCS intensity condition. In contrast, little responsiveness was observed in the lower intensity UCS condition with vagal blockade. A small deceleration, significant on Sec. 11–14, suggests that there is little sympathetic involvement at this UCS intensity, at least with respect to the heart. This latter deceleration appears due to a reduction in the amount of vagal blockade during the later test trials which allows some vagal inhibition to become manifested. An analysis of heart-rate changes was performed using only the first two test and sensitization control trials, when vagal blockade is at its maximum as measured by basal levels of heart rate. This revealed no reliable response of any kind, although the mean second-by-second effects are acceleratory from the sixth second on. This is in contrast to a large deceleratory response, which was already significant on 1 sec. in the low-UCS-intensity group without vagal blockade during the same trials.

The lower and higher UCS intensity conditions without vagal blockade were not reliably differentiated on any of the 25 sec. following CS onset (see Table 2). Only during the deceleratory phase of the response are any appreciable differences observed. But this is only a difference in degree of vagal restraint. On the other hand, when the vagus is blocked the two conditions are sharply differentiated, with the higher intensity condition having a significantly greater acceleratory response on Sec. 7–16 (see Table 2). Therefore, differences in UCS intensity result in different degrees of sympathetic activity, while having a less pronounced effect on vagal activity.

Vagal restraint was also observed to decrease the duration of the unconditioned response. In all conditions, a reliable acceleration of heart rate occurred to the UCS which was significantly greater for the more intense UCS both with and without vagal blockade. This acceleration was significant ($p < .05$ or less) with the vagus intact on 3 sec. for the less intense UCS and on 8 sec. for the more intense UCS. On the other hand, with the vagus blocked the acceleration was significant on 8 and 14 sec. for these respective conditions. Furthermore, reliable differences between the acceleratory responses to the two UCS intensities were observed on only 3 sec. with the vagus intact, but on 12 sec. with the vagus blocked.

Sympathetic activity was manifested at both UCS intensities as measured by GSR activity. A greater response on test than on sensitization control trials was observed in 11 of 12 Ss with the less intense UCS and in all Ss with the more intense UCS. There was some evidence of greater responsiveness with the more intense UCS, though no reliable differences could be demonstrated. The average number of measurable responses (i.e., those greater than 600 ohms) on the 10 test trials was 7.8 for the less intense UCS and 9.6 for the more intense UCS. Similarly, the mean response amplitude was greater with the more intense UCS, but the difference was not reliable (Mann-Whitney $U > .10$). Therefore, the failure of sym-

TABLE 2. Second-by-second difference in R-R interval (milliseconds) between the lower and higher UCS intensities determined from test minus sensitization control trial mean differences.

Sec.	Without Vagal Blockade		With Vagal Blockade	
	$\bar{x}$	t	$\bar{x}$	t
1	0	<1	− 2	<1
2	−10	<1	− 3	<1
3	− 7	<1	− 4	1.25
4	− 2	<1	− 4	1.36
5	− 1	<1	− 6	1.68
6	−15	1.07	−10	2.03
7	+ 9	<1	−12	2.49*
8	0	<1	−15	2.32*
9	−27	1.83	−18	2.80**
10	−34	1.80	−18	2.91**
11	−18	<1	−19	3.00**
12	−17	<1	−16	2.65*
13	− 6	<1	−18	3.49**
14	− 2	<1	−10	2.39*
15	+10	<1	− 9	2.22*
16	−16	1.26	− 9	2.09*
17	− 9	<1	− 4	<1
18	−14	<1	− 8	1.74
19	−14	1.56	− 6	1.08
20	+ 3	<1	−10	1.67
21	−16	1.14	−12	1.90
22	−18	1.05	−12	1.77
23	−20	1.35	− 9	1.34
24	− 8	<1	−14	1.83
25	−15	<1	−14	1.77

Note.— − = higher intensity, shorter R-R interval or faster heart rate.
* $p < .05$.
** $p < .01$.

pathetic effects to be manifested by heart rate with the less intense UCS cannot be attributed to the absence of such effects.

EXPERIMENT II

METHOD. *Subjects.* The *S*s were 11 healthy young adult male student volunteers preselected on the basis of having shown an appreciable deceleratory response during a previous conditioning session, a condition considered necessary to detect clearly the influence of homeastatic effects.

Equipment. The same equipment was used as in Exp. I in addition to a Statham 0–75 cm. Hg strain gauge for the direct recording of arterial blood pressure.

Procedure. Two conditioning sessions were required and were separated by at least 1 wk. The first was used only to preselect *S*s. During the second, pressor responses of vasomotor origin were blocked pharmacologically after the eighth test trial by an IV injection of 0.6 mg. of Hydergine-Sandoz, the maximum recommended clinical dosage. (This agent has alpha-receptor adrenergic blocking characteristics and is a combination of three ergot alkaloids.) Conditioning procedures were similar to those reported in Exp. I. The UCS was set at the less intense level. Thirteen test trials were used. Because pressor responses can also be initiated by respiratory-induced cardiac acceleration, special efforts were made to keep respiratory activity controlled in both conditioning sessions. During the second session, senitization control trials were omitted for five Ss prior to drug administration and for eight Ss following drug administration in order to expedite proceedings necessitated by the experiment. Therefore, heart-rate changes were determined for all Ss without correction for sensitization effects.

In order to evaluate the effectiveness of the adrenergic blockade, direct readings of arterial blood pressure were attempted in the last eight Ss and successfully obtained in five. Pressure was measured from the radial artery near the wrist of the right arm. The puncture was done under local anesthesia (Xylocaine) using a No. 18 cordon needle. The needle was attached to a strain guage by a catheter filled with heparin saline solution for flushing.

Data quantifications. Data were quantified as in the previous study. Both diastolic and systolic blood pressure were quantified on a second by second basis, as with heart rate. Heart rate and blood pressure changes on the first three test trials prior to drug administration were not quantified because Ss were usually less responsive on these trials. This left five test trials before, and five after drug administration to be quantified.

RESULTS.   There was no evidence to indicate that the deceleration of heart rate was the result of reflexes initiated by a pressor response. There was initially observed in all 5 Ss on whom measurements were obtained a small pressor response which had a mean peak response of 1.9 mm. Hg systolic and 1.2 mm. Hg diastolic (see Table 3). Adrenergic blockade reduced the response in all Ss, with the mean peak response being 0.3 mm. Hg, systolic and diastolic. On the other hand, a reliably large sustained deceleration of heart rate was observed both before and after adrenergic blockade (see Table 4). Based on all 11 Ss, there were clearly no reliable differences between the deceleratory responses pre- and postblockade. A comparable effect was found with the 5 Ss on whom measurements of blood pressure were obtained. However, because of the small N, the reliability of this effect was not evaluated.

The independence of pressor responses and heart-rate changes is indicated by still other aspects of the data. First, there were trials even prior to adrenergic blockade when heart rate was observed to decelerate even when no pressor response occurred. Second, in one S, the pressor response was completely suppressed following blockade but the deceleratory re-

TABLE 3.   Second-by-second mean blood pressure levels (mm. Hg) on test trials before and following adrenergic blockade ($N = 5$).

Sec.	Systolic		Diastolic	
	Preblock	Postblock	Preblock	Postblock
$\bar{x}$ Pre[a]	121.9	114.6	73.8	70.1
1	121.5	114.5	73.7	69.9
2	121.4	114.3	73.7	70.4
3	121.9	114.3	74.5	70.2
4	123.0	114.8	74.9	70.4
5	123.2	114.9	75.0	70.4
6	123.3	114.9	74.9	69.9
7	123.6	114.8	75.0	70.3
8	123.8	114.8	74.3	69.7
9	122.8	114.6	73.4	69.3
10	121.9	112.4	73.1	69.1
11	122.0	112.8	72.6	69.3
12	120.9	113.1	72.4	68.8
13	120.8	113.4	72.2	68.8
14	119.6	113.2	72.1	69.0
15	120.9	112.9	72.7	69.6

[a] $\bar{x}$ Pre = Mean of all readings in the 15 sec. before CS onset.

sponse was unaltered. Third, no correlation could be found between the amplitude of the heart-rate deceleration and the amplitude of either the systolic or the diastolic response, when these correlations were performed within Ss using responses on test trials. There was a reduction in the de-

TABLE 4.   Second-by-second changes in R-R interval (milliseconds) on test trials before and following adrenergic blockade expressed as difference from pre-CS base level ($N = 11$).

Sec.	Preblockade		Postblockade		Difference Post − Pre	
	$\bar{x}$	t	$\bar{x}$	t	$\bar{x}$	t
1	+ 6	<1	+ 7	1.37	+ 1	<1
2	+12	<1	− 4	<1	−16	<1
3	−10	<1	+ 3	<1	+13	1.20
4	+ 2	<1	+16	<1	+14	<1
5	+ 9	<1	+ 9	<1	0	<1
6	+12	1.08	+19	1.31	+ 7	<1
7	+33	3.30**	+40	2.39*	+ 7	<1
8	+41	4.24**	+59	4.00**	+18	<1
9	+45	4.43**	+65	4.84**	+20	1.24
10	+52	4.95**	+46	3.83**	− 6	<1
11	+47	4.08**	+42	2.81*	− 5	<1
12	+60	4.29**	+49	4.63**	−11	1.09
13	+43	4.66**	+38	3.91**	− 5	<1
14	+31	3.11**	+26	2.17*	− 5	<1
15	+29	3.03**	+24	2.37*	− 5	<1

Note.— + =longer R-R interval or heart-rate deceleration; − =shorter R-R interval or heart-rate acceleration.
* p <.05.
** p <.01.

celeratory response in one *S*. However, this appears attributable to the effects of *S*'s knowing when he received the adrenergic blocking agent (all *S*s had been informed of the possible postexperimental side effects of this drug, which can include hypotensively induced nausea and fainting). In this *S*, a similar reduction in the deceleratory response was observed to a saline injection on a third conditioning session. However, no reduction in the response was observed to the adrenergic blocking agent when it was then administered following the saline and when the deceleration had returned to its original amplitude.

DISCUSSION

These data indicate that the heart-rate changes observed on test trials during classical conditioning under these experimental conditions are primarily manifestations of variations in vagal activity and that sympathetic effects are only clearly manifested when a very intense UCS is used and then only when the vagal innervation is blocked. Further, the more dominant response is an increase in vagal restraint (i.e., heart-rate deceleration), especially with a less intense UCS, and this response appears to be conditioned. Considering the decelerative response as indicative of, or mediated by, some affective response such as "experimental anxiety" (Deane, 1964; Notterman *et al.*, 1952) is contraindicated by the fact that this is a vagal response. Traditionally, sympathetic activity has been at least implicitly assumed to be involved in such affective responses. This assumption is supported by the greater sympathetic involvement in the high-shock condition when the vagus is blocked, a condition which should result in a far greater affective response. On the other hand, the deceleratory response is greater under the low-shock condition, or when the least affective response might be found.

There are three other ways the decelerative heart-rate change might be viewed. First, it reflects the conditioning of homeostatic processes and as such is a type of exteroceptive-interoceptive conditioning. The UCS in this case is the pressor response to the shock while the UCS would involve CNS activity which slows heart rate. The activity of the latter is only manifested on test trials when respiratory and other effects of the UCS are minimal. This would mean that in the absence of pressor responses, as following adrenergic blockade, the CS is able to initiate anticipatory restraining activity. That such a peripheral response might be an effective UCS is suggested by data reported by Bykov (1957) where pharmacological agents were used to initiate the response. It is also reported that conditioning of this type requires from 20 to 100 reinforcements. However, in the present study, a reliable deceleratory response was observed after only four reinforcements, a fact which argues against this position.

A second explanation has been suggested by Zeaman and Smith (1964), who have observed heart-rate deceleration in anticipation of shock and both pleasant and unpleasant auditory stimuli, using a variation on standard conditioning procedures. It is proposed that this deceleration is mediated first by an attention process initiated by the CS which then initiates respiratory changes resulting in a heart-rate deceleration. However, the studies reported by Zeaman and Smith do not appear to be definitive with respect to the influence of respiration and are contrary to evidence from the Wood and Obrist (1964) study, as well as data recently reported by Deane (1964). Data from the present experiments also contraindicate any influence of respiration on the decelerative response. For example, in both experiments respiration amplitude was uncorrelated with the decelerative response and, with the exception of the more intense UCS conditions of Exp. I, remained perfectly controlled. Therefore, respiration does not appear to mediate whatever influence attention might have on cardiovascular processes.

A third possibility is suggested by some recent work of Lacey (Lacey, 1959; Lacey, Kagan, Lacey, and Moss, 1963; Lacey and Lacey, 1958) where it has been proposed that cardiovascular activity influences environmental interaction via visceral afferent control of central activity. In part, this hypothesis is based on the observation that various exteroceptive stimuli, some with clear affective value, result in both sympathetic discharge, as measured galvanically, and in cardiac deceleration (Davis and Buchwald, 1957; Lacey et al., 1963; Obrist, 1963). This deceleration of heart rate is thought to facilitate sensory intake. Therefore, the deceleration observed during conditioning could involve similar processes and have a like function. As such, it would be a conditioned response in anticipation of sensory intake (i.e., the UCS). However, there is one aspect of the conditioning data which is not consistent with this view and which, for that matter, is yet another unresolved paradox of heart-rate conditioning. This is, the deceleratory conditioned response is in the opposite direction from the UCR, which is always reported as acceleratory, a situation seemingly without parallel in the conditioning of striate and other visceral responses. Therefore, the significance of the deceleratory response is still not understood. Nonetheless, the positions of Lacey and of Zeaman and Smith appear at this time to merit further evaluation. Among other things, the peripheral and central processes involved with the UCR would appear necessary to study.

Recently, Geer (1964) has suggested that the deceleratory heart-rate change observed during conditioning is nothing more than the orienting response to the CS. This position is not supported by the present study. An assessment of such effects, based on the heart-rate response both to the first adaptation trial and to the sensitization control for the less intense UCS, reveals a significant deceleratory response which peaks at the fifth second and which has become a small nonsignificant acceleratory response by the eighth second. In contrast, the deceleratory response on test trials has a longer latency, a larger amplitude, and a longer duration with both intensities of the UCS.

Wood and Obrist (1964) have questioned the suitability of differential conditioning to assess sensitization effects and have suggested that the CS— might be significantly influenced by stimulus generalization from the CS+. Data from the present study also support this possibility. For example, there was no heart-rate change to the CS— during conditioning for the higher intensity UCS saline condition, even though a reliable deceleratory response was observed in the same condition during adaptation and to the CS— during conditioning for the less intense UCS saline condition. Respiration did not appear to be a significant factor. Also, based on the adaptation data, the magnitude of the sensitization effect (i.e., influence of UCS intensity) appears to be directly related to the magnitude of the deceleration. Stimulus generalization appears to be a possible basis for this lack of response to the CS— during conditioning since it would be expected to be greater with the more intense UCS. In part, the failure of the initial acceleratory response to differentiate on test trials between the less and more intense UCS when the vagus was intact could be attributed to the failure to assess sensitization effects.

SUMMARY

The two experiments reported here are concerned with the influence of the vagal and sympathetic innervations of the heart and of peripheral reflex mechanisms on the deceleration of heart rate observed on test trials during classical conditioning in human Ss. An increase in vagal restraint was observed to be the basis of the deceleratory response, which in turn masks the manifestation of sympathetic acceleratory effects. The latter were only observed when the vagus was pharmacologically blocked and when a very intense UCS was used. When the conditioned pressor responses were blocked pharmacologically, as evaluated by direct recordings of arterial blood pressure, the deceleratory response was not changed, indicating that the peripheral homeostatic reflex mechanisms are not the basis for this response and that it is likely a conditioned response.

REFERENCES

Bykov, K. M. *The cerebral cortex and the internal organs.* (Trans. by W. H. Gantt.) New York: Chemical Publishing, 1957.

Davis, R. C., and Buchwald, A. M. An exploration of somatic response patterns: Stimulus and sex differences. *J. comp. physiol. Psychol.*, 1957, **50**, 44–52.

Deane, G. E. Human heart rate responses during experimentally induced anxiety: A follow-up with controlled respiration. *J. exp. Psychol.,* 1964, **67**, 193–195.

Dykman, R. A., and Gantt, W. H. The parasympathetic component of unlearned and acquired cardiac responses. *J. comp. physiol.,* 1959, **52**, 163–167.

Fuhrer, M. J. Differential verbal conditioning of heart rate with minimization of changes in respiratory rate. *J. comp. physiol. Psychol.,* 1964, **58**, 283–289.

Geer, J. H. Measurement of the conditioned cardiac response. *J. comp. physiol. Psychol.,* 1964, **57**, 426–433.

Lacey, J. I. Psychophysiological approaches to the evaluation of psychotherapeutic process and outcome. In F. A. Rubenstein and M. G. Parloff (Eds.), *Research in psychotherapy.* Washington, D.C.: American Psychological Association, 1959. Pp. 160–208.

Lacey, J. I., Kagan, J., Lacey, B. C., and Moss, H. A. Situational determinants and behavioral correlates of autonomic response patterns. In P. J. Knapp (Ed.), *Expression of the emotions in man.* New York: International Univer. Press, 1963. Pp. 161–196.

Lacey, J. I., and Lacey, B. C. The relationship of resting autonomic activity to motor impulsivity. *Res. Publ. Ass. Nerv. Ment. Dis.,* 1958, **36**, 144–209.

Lacey, J. I., and Lacey, B. C. The law of initial value in the longitudinal study of autonomic constitution: Reproducibility of autonomic responses and response patterns over a four year interval. *Ann. N.Y. Acad. Sci.,* 1962, **98**, 1257–1290, 1322–1326.

Lang, P. J., and Hnatiow, M. Stimulus repetition and heart rate response. *J. comp. physiol. Psychol.,* 1962, **55**, 781–785.

Martin, B. The assessment of anxiety by physiological-behavioral measures. *Psychol. Bull.,* 1961, **58**, 234–255.

Neil, E., and Heymans, C. Cardiovascular and pulmonary reflexes. In A. A. Luisada (Ed.), *Cardiovascular functions.* New York: McGraw-Hill, 1962. Pp. 103–123.

Notterman, J., Schoenfeld, W., and Bersh, P. Conditioned heart rate responses in human beings during experimental anxiety. *J. comp. physiol. Psychol.,* 1952, **45**, 1–8.

Obrist, P. A. Cardiovascular differentiation or sensory stimuli. *Psychosom. Med.,* 1963, **25**, 450–458.

Obrist, P. A., Hallman, S. I., and Wood, D. M. Autonomic levels and lability, and performance time on a perceptual task and a sensory motor task. *Percept. mot. Skills,* 1964, **18**, 753–762.

Rushmer, R. F. Autonomic balance in cardiac control. *Amer. J. Physiol.,* 1958, **192**, 631–634.

Samaan, A. The antagonistic cardiac nerves and heart rate. *J. Physiol.,* 1934–35, **83**, 332–340. (a)

Samaan, A. Muscular work in dogs submitted to different conditions of cardiac and splanchnec innervations. *J. Physiol.,* 1934–35, **85**, 313–331. (b)

Welford, N. T. An electronic digital recording machine: The SETAR. *J. scient. Instrum.,* 1952, **29**, 1–4.

Wilson, R. S. Autonomic changes produced by noxious and innocuous stimulation. *J. comp. physiol. Psychol.,* 1964, **58**, 290–295.

Wood, D. M., and Obrist, P. A. Effects of controlled and uncontrolled respiration on the conditioned heart rate response in humans. *J. exp. Psychol.,* 1964, **68**, 221–229.

Zeaman, D., Deane, G., and Wegner, N. Amplitude and latency characteristic of the conditioned heart response. *J. Psychol.,* 1954, **38**, 234–250.

Zeaman, D., and Smith, R. W. Review and analysis of some recent findings in human cardiac conditioning. In W. F. Prokasy (Ed.), *Classical conditioning: A symposium.* New York: Appleton-Century-Crofts, 1964.

Zeaman, D., and Wegner, N. A further test of the role of drive reduction in human cardiac conditioning. *J. Psychol.,* 1957, 43, 125–133.

3

Effects of CS-US interval on conditioning of drug response, with assessment of speed of conditioning *

Roy Pickens and William F. Crowder

Although several investigators (Herrnstein, 1962; Levitt, 1964; Reiss, 1958) have shown that pharmacologic effects of drugs can be elicited by stimuli paired with drug injection, no investigation of the factors which influence such conditioning has been found. The present experiment studied the effects of several CS-US intervals on the development of a conditioned drug response. In addition, an attempt was made to demonstrate a conditioned drug response after only six CS-US pairings, as rapid conditioning of drug effects appear to be indicated (Pavlov, 1927).

EXPERIMENT 1

The purpose of this experiment was to study the effects of CS-US interval on the conditioning of amphetamine-induced locomotor activity. The CS was placement of S in an activity apparatus, and the US was an ip injection of 1.5 mg/kg d-amphetamine, an amount which preliminary dose- and time-response measures had found to produce the greatest activity increase. The CS-US pairing intervals were also selected from these measures, so that CS presentation would occur before, after, and about simultaneously with onset of drug action.

METHOD. *Subjects.* The Ss were 16 experimentally naive, 100–110 day old male albino rats of the Holtzman strain.

Apparatus. The apparatus consisted of eight stationary-type activity cages. The animal chamber of each cage was a circular alley, 15 cm high and 7.5 cm wide, with a 22.5 cm diameter inner wall and a 37.5 cm diameter outer wall. Each activity cage was enclosed in a plywood box, 50 cm wide by 75 cm long by 57.5 cm high, which was lined with plasterboard and sound-absorbing fiber glass.

The S's movements around the alley were detected by a photoelectric system. Four photocells (Clairex CL703L/2), spaced 90 degrees apart

From *Psychopharmacologia* (Berl.), 1967, 11, 88–94. Copyright 1967 by Springer-Verlag, Heidelberg, Germany.

* Preparation of this article was supported in part by USPHS Training Grant No. MH-8565 to the University of Minnesota.

around the outer wall, faced a lamp in the center of the cage. The lamp was a 6-w. 120-V clear bulb, operating at 75 V to insure against burnout. The photocell circuitry was designed to register locomotor activity only. As *S* moved by a photocell, the interruption of light falling on the photocell actuated an electromagnetic counter. Before another count could occur, *S* had to move from that photocell to an adjacent one, a distance of approximately 24 cm. Thus, successive interruptions of the same photocell, as might be produced by rearing or grooming, were not registered.

Procedure.   The *S*s were randomly assigned to four groups, with four *S*s in each group.

Acclimatization: For six days all *S*s were injected daily with 1 cc of saline solution and placed in the activity apparatus for 60 min.

Conditioning: For 63 days the schedule consisted of six conditioning days followed by one test day. On conditioning days, one group of *S*s was injected with the drug immediately before placement in the apparatus, a second group was injected 30 min before placement, and a third group, immediately after removal from the apparatus. A fourth group was injected with 1 cc of saline just before placement and with the drug 3–4 h later. Drug injections were ip, 1.5 mg/kg *d*-amphetamine sulfate in isotonic saline solution. The *S*s remained in the activity apparatus for 30 min each day.

Testing: To evaluate the effects of the CS-US intervals used during conditioning, an equal volume saline injection was substituted for the drug injection on weekly test days, but otherwise the training procedures remained the same as during conditioning.

Extinction: For seven days *S*s were extinguished. The extinction days were identical to the test days, except that a drug injection was given 3–4 h after each trial, in order to maintain *S*s at the daily drug level of conditioning.

RESULTS.   Acclimatization: The median activity rates for all *S*s combined showed a progressive decline over the six 1-h acclimatization sessions. The reduction in activity between the first three and last three sessions, however, was not significant ($t = 1.62$, $.10 < P < .20$).

Conditioning: The effect of the training procedures (CS-US intervals) on group activity levels during conditioning trials is summarized in the table. The group receiving *d*-amphetamine immediately before being placed in the apparatus (Drug Before Placement group) was most active during that period, followed by the Drug 30 Minutes Before Placement group. The Drug After Removal and Saline Before Placement groups were almost indistinguishable in their relatively low activity levels on these days. While the table shows some decline during training in the activity of the Drug Before Placement group, this decline was not a significant one.

Testing: Figure 1 shows the activity levels for the separate groups on

TABLE.   Effect of CS-US interval on group activity levels during conditioning trials.

Group	N	Median activity counts on successive three-week blocks of conditioning trials		
		1	2	3
Drug Before Placement	4	317.5	277.0	261.0
Drug 30 Minutes				
Before Placement	3[1]	230.0	221.0	225.5
Drug After Removal	4	35.0	34.5	37.0
Saline Before Placement	4	47.5	43.5	47.5

[1] One S in this group died.

the final 60 min acclimatization session, on each of the nine 30 min tests for conditioning, and on each of the seven extinction sessions. The most activity was shown by the two groups that during training had received the drug prior to placement. These two groups showed the greatest gain from acclimatization to testing and traveled further during the first 30 min test session than they did during the last 60 min acclimatization session. After this initial gain, no further increase in activity was apparent on the remaining eight test periods.

In evaluating the significance of the observed group differences in the test sessions, these nine sessions were divided into three-day blocks and, to control for initial differences in activity, S's median activity level on the last three acclimatization sessions was subtracted from that of each of

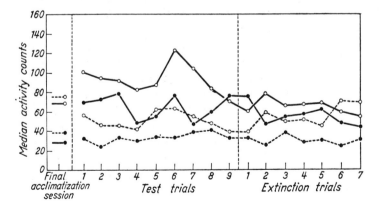

FIGURE 1.   Activity response to saline injection on last 60 min acclimatization session, on each 30 min test-for-conditioning sessions, and on the 30 min extinction session. White circles, solid line: drug before placement; black circles, solid line: drug 30 min before placement; black circles, dashed line: drug after removal; white circles, dashed line: saline before placement.

its three test blocks. Analyses of variance performed on these change-scores yielded significant group differences only for the first test block ($P < .025$); no significant group effect was found for the middle or the last block. Subsequent t tests between pairs of groups for the first test block showed that both the Drug 30 Minutes Before Placement group and Drug Before Placement group were significantly more active than the Drug After Removal group ($P < .005$ and $P < .025$, respectively) and the Saline Before Placement group ($P < .005$ and $P < .01$, respectively). No significant difference was found between the Drug 30 Minutes Before Placement group and the Drug Before Placement group, or between the Drug After Removal group and the Saline Before Placement group.

Extinction: An analysis of variance found reliable group differences in amount of decrement shown between the last three days and the last three days of extinction ($P < .025$).

EXPERIMENT 2

This experiment was an attempt to demonstrate a conditioned drug response following only six CS-US pairings. The possibility of conditioning a drug response in so few trials was suggested by the results of Experiment 1, which indicated that most of the conditioning may have occurred by the first test trial, and by other investigations (Pavlov, 1927), where rapid conditioning of drug effects have been reported, albeit in a cursory manner.

METHOD. *Subjects and apparatus.* The Ss were eight experimentally naive male Holtzman albino rats, about 175 days old. The apparatus was the same as that used in Experiment 1.

Procedure. The procedure was identical to that used in Experiment 1 with the following exceptions. Acclimatization lasted only two days, with five 1 h sessions on the first day and two half-hour sessions on the second day. Ss, paired on the basis of activity scores during the last acclimatization session, were given six training days followed by one test day. The control member of each pair was injected with saline immediately before placement in the apparatus and with the drug 3–4 h later. The experimental member was injected with the drug immediately before placement and with saline 3–4 h later. Each S received the same volume of saline as it did of drug solution.

RESULTS. On the test day, the mean activity count of the group receiving saline before placement was 61, while that of the group receiving drug before placement was 92. The difference in group means was significant ($t = 4.34, P < .025$).

DISCUSSION

In Experiment 1, the increased locomotor activity produced by d-amphetamine was conditioned to placement in an activity apparatus when the drug injection preceded placement either by a few seconds or by 30 min. No evidence of conditioning could be detected when drug injection followed removal from the apparatus either immediately or after 3–4 h. Although drug injection immediately before placement might appear to constitute backward conditioning, the effective temporal interval may be presumed to be that of short-forward conditioning, since the animal was in the apparatus well before the drug had time to significantly affect activity. No significant difference was found in the effectiveness of the drug injection immediately before, and 30 min before, placement in the apparatus. Hence, there is apparently little difference in the conditioned effect produced by onset and peak of drug action. The failure to find group differences on the middle three and last three test sessions was surprising, since the effectiveness of the drug as a US for activity did not appear to change over the course of the experiment. This failure of our animals to reflect the development of tolerance to d-amphetamine is supported by similar findings with dl-amphetamine (Torme and Lasagna, 1960).

In Experiment 2, the demonstration of a conditioned drug response after only six CS-US pairings suggests that data from animals receive drug injections repeatedly might often contain effects due to both conditioned and unconditioned factors, and that the "true" unconditioned effects of a drug might thus be inflated by a conditioned component of unknown magnitude.

Two previous studies have found apparent conditioning of the heightened activity produced by amphetamine injection to placement of S in an activity apparatus. Irwin and Armstrong (1961) found that rats receiving a single CS-US pairing were, for a two-month period, more active in the presence of the CS than those never given the drug. Such a finding could be explained in terms of inhibition of the activity-depressing effects of the strong feedback produced by running in the activity wheel. The drug, by making the animal run in the wheel, would accelerate habituation to this feedback and thus augment future running in the wheel. However, the authors mention that the majority of several attempted replications of the effect were unsuccessful.

Ross and Schnitzer (1963), while reporting conditioned activity, did not provide comparable control and experimental groups. One control group, which was given a sham injection before being placed in the activity apparatus, did not receive the drug at any time. Conceivably, the greater activity shown by the experimental group during testing was due to food deprivation resulting from the known depressant effect of the drug upon eating behavior. This conjecture is consistent with the finding that the experimental group was not more active than a second control group, which was given the drug but was not placed in the apparatus.

SUMMARY

Effects of CS-US interval on the development of a conditioned drug response was studied by pairing a 1.5 mg/kg ip d-amphetamine injection (US) with placement of S in a photocell-type locomotor activity cage (CS). Ss injected immediately before and 30 min before placement were significantly more active on saline-injection test days than were Ss injected after removal or 3–4 h later. To test for apparent rapid conditioning of drug response, Ss were given only six pairings with drug injection immediately preceding placement in the apparatus. On saline test day, these Ss were half again more active than controls, which had received saline just before placement and the drug 3–4 h later.

REFERENCES

Herrnstein, R. J. Placebo effect in the rat. *Science* 138, 677–678 (1962).

Irwin, S., and Armstrong, P. M.: Conditioned locomotor response with drug as the unconditioned stimulus: Individual differences. In E. Rothlin (Ed.), *Neuropsychopharmacology*, Vol. 2. Amsterdam: Elsevier 1961.

Levitt, R. A.: Sleep as a conditioned response. *Psychol. Sci.* 1, 273–274 (1964).

Pavlov, I. P.: *Conditioned reflexes*. London: Oxford Univ. Press 1927.

Reiss, W. J.: Conditioning of a hyperinsulin type of behavior in the white rat. *J. comp. physiol. Psychol.* 51, 301–303 (1958).

Ross, S., and Schnitzer, S. B.: Further support for a placebo effect in the rat. *Psychol. Rep.* 13, 461–462 (1963).

Torme, J., and Lasagna, L.: Relation of thyroid function to acute and chronic effects of amphetamine in the rat. *J. Pharmacol. exp. Ther.* 128, 201–209 (1960).

4

A mechanism for the effect of a tranquilizing drug on learned emotional responses *

GORDON T. HEISTAD and AURELIO A. TORRES

The rapid increase in clinical use of ataractic or "tranquilizing" drugs within recent years has not been paralleled by a proportionate increase in our understanding of the mechanisms by which these compounds influence behavior. The search for mechanisms of action for these drugs has centered primarily upon attempts to locate the brain structures that are excited or inhibited by them, or to identify the enzyme system or other biochemical locus of action. The present study departs from that tradition in attempting to identify the psychological, rather than neurophysiological or biochemical, mechanism by which an ataractic drug influences emotional behavior.

In a recent article [1] one of us (G.H.) has proposed a very simple mechanism by which drugs can influence emotional behavior within the context of well-established principles of behavior theory. Behavioral science rests firmly on the basic assumption that behavior does not occur in a chance or random fashion, but consists of responses to stimulation. A few simple stimulus-response relationships appear to be innately determined (e.g., spinal reflexes), but the vast majority of complex behavior consists of functional relationships between stimuli and responses that have been acquired or modified by the process of learning. In the process of learning, *every* aspect of the environment that is systematically associated with a response may become a part of the total stimulus complex that acquires the capacity to elicit that response on subsequent occasions. Thus, a specific change in the environment, such as the onset of a tone, may be functionally associated, by appropriate training procedures, with a specific response, such as salivation. After such learning has occurred, however, the experimentor quickly finds that many aspects of the environment in addition to the tone have become part of the stimulus for salivation. A change in pitch or intensity of the tone, a change in general noise level or illumination, the presence of different experimenters, or the use of a different laboratory will all interfere to some extent with performance of this learned response. In other words, the response had become asso-

From *Medical Bulletin, University of Minnesota,* 1959, **30,** 518–527. Copyright 1959 by Minnesota Medical Foundation, Minneapolis, Minn.

* This research was supported, in part, by a grant from the National Institute of Mental Health, U.S. Public Health Service, under Grant No. MY 2273.

ciated with all these aspects of the environment, and perhaps many more, and any change in this total stimulus complex will interfere with performance of the learned response.

In the case of emotional learning, specific emotional responses such as fighting, running away, or becoming immobile may all become functionally associated with a wide variety of stimuli in the external environment. For example, if an animal is repeatedly given a painful shock following a clicking noise, that animal will soon learn to run away when the clicker is present, or if escape is impossible, he may develop a characteristic crouching or "freezing" posture. But the onset of a clicker that has been repeatedly paired with a painful event will also elicit complex changes in the *internal* environment of the organism. This change in state of the internal environment is part of the total environmental conditions which are regularly associated with the overt emotional response; thus it has ample opportunity to become an important part of the stimulus necessary to elicit that overt response on subsequent occasions. Since the physiologic changes that accompany emotional states are mediated primarily via the autonomic, endocrine, and extrapyramidal systems, the state of function of these three systems may reasonably be expected to contribute significant stimulus properties for any behavior that is learned under conditions of emotion.

If this is true, any treatment procedure that produces a significant change in autonomic, endocrine, or extrapyramidal function would be expected to interfere with retention of emotional responses associated with the internal environmental conditions that had prevailed during the learning process. Insofar as this view is correct, such treatments would not interfere with an emotional habit (defined as a stimulus-response relationship) but rather they would bring about new (internal) stimulus conditions and thus would reduce the strength of whatever emotional responses had been associated with the old conditions of internal stimulation antedating treatment. By analogy, the effect would be the same as that obtained when an organism which has learned to respond to a specific tone is presented with some different sound to test the strength of the learned response; under these conditions, the reduction in response strength will be proportional to the amount of change in the stimulus.

Both the clinical literature and the experimental literature on tranquilizing drugs and a variety of other treatments used in psychiatry offer some support to the hypothesis that some of the behavior changes resulting from these treatments may be due to internal stimulus changes. Most, if not all, of the physiologic types of treatment employed in psychiatry have profound effects (usually referred to as "side effects") on autonomic, endocrine, and extrapyramidal function. The *direction* of these effects on the internal environment, however, is by no means the same from treatment to treatment. For example, electroshock, carbon dioxide, and some of the drugs used in psychiatric treatment result in relative sympathetic dominance of the autonomic system, while the rauwolfia alkaloids and phenothiazine derivatives generally produce some degree of parasympathetic dominance. Analysis of the effect of such treatments on endocrine and extrapyramidal function reveal definite changes, but the direction of these changes varies from one form of therapy to another. To the degree that changes in internal stimuli are responsible for the changes in behavior produced by these treatments, the effectiveness of the therapy depends upon the amount of change in these physiological functions; but the direction of change would be relatively unimportant so long as the internal stimulus conditions were made *different* from those which had been associated with the pretreatment behavior patterns.

The effects of substituting new stimulus conditions for the stimuli that prevailed during the emotional learning process might be expected to be similar for both pathologic behavior (psychiatric symptoms) and for normal or adaptive emotional responses. With the increasing use of physiologic treatments in psychiatry, numerous reports in the literature have warned of the danger of precipitating "latent psychoses" when these treatments are applied to patients who are not already psychotic. The frequency of psychotic episodes in tuberculous patients treated with iproniazid and in hypertensive patients treated with reserpine serves to illustrate the possibility of interfering with normal emotional behavior, as well as psychiatric symptoms, by the use of such treatment. Virtually all the somatic treatments employed in psychiatric therapy entail the risk of such adverse effects on normal emotional behavior. Conversely, drugs such as mescaline and lysergic acid diethylamide, which are known primarily for their ability to disrupt normal behavior in nonpsychiatric subjects, have been reported to produce at least temporary improvement in some psychiatric patients.[2] Similarly, a variety of short-acting drugs that affect the autonomic system — such as atropine, eserine, and the sympathomimetic amines — are said to produce temporary "lucid intervals" in some psychotic patients but to exert a pathological effect when given to normal subjects.[3]

Perhaps the greatest limitation on the effectiveness of tranquilizing drugs and other somatic treatments employed in psychiatry is the frequency with which symptoms reappear upon discontinuance of the treatment. The temporary character of such relief would be anticipated on the basis of the theory expressed above. For a change in stimulus cannot be expected to weaken the strength of an emotional "habit," defined as a functional relationship between a certain stimulus and a certain response. Rather, the response strength is weakened because the appropriate stimulus conditions are absent during the period when the treatment is effective in changing the internal environment. If and when the original stimulus conditions are reinstated, the original responses can be expected to recur.

Thus the temporary nature of symptomatic relief from such treatments, as well as the temporary adverse effects when these treatments are used in nonpsychiatric subjects, is fully consistent with the hypothesis that the behavior changes are mediated by a change in stimulus parameters.

But while the clinical evidence cited above appears to fit with the suggestion that many behavioral effects of tranquilizing drugs and of other somatic treatments may be due to internal stimulus changes, this evidence falls far short of conclusive proof. The hypothesis is more rigorously tested in experimental studies of the effects of such treatments on emotional behavior in laboratory animals. Naturally, great caution must be exercised in attempting to interpret changes in complex human behavior on the basis of evidence derived from studies of restricted samples of animal behavior.

The available evidence from animal experimental studies appears to be fully consistent with the hypothesis discussed above. Thus, electroshock treatment, chlorpromazine, reserpine, and a wide variety of other therapeutic procedures which alter autonomic, endocrine, and/or extrapyramidal function have been observed to be effective in interfering with specific emotional responses that were learned prior to treatment.[4-8] Such treatments differ widely in their physiologic effects, but they all share the common characteristic of changing the internal environment from what it was during the learning of these specific emotional responses.[9-11] Unpublished data from this laboratory indicate, at least in the case of electroconvulsive shock, that when an emotional response is learned under the abnormal conditions of internal environment resulting from the treatment, a change in the internal environment toward normal (i.e., physiologic recovery from the treatments) also results in a loss of the previously learned emotional response. For each of these treatments that has been investigated, the loss of the emotional responses is temporary, and the emotional response returns without additional training as soon as the drug is withdrawn or the physiologic effects of the treatment are reversed through physiologic recovery.[4, 8, 12, 13] A recent study in this laboratory [7] demonstrated that a conditioned emotional response in the rat could be attenuated by either chlorpromazine or electroconvulsive shock treatment, even though these two treatments have roughly opposite physiologic effects, at least on autonomic balance. When, however, an emotional response had already been severely weakened by electroshock, administration of chlorpromazine to counteract the autonomic effects of the electroshock treatment resulted in a significant increase or recovery of the conditioned emotional response.

Further support for this hypothesis can be found in studies of the effects of drugs on extinction of emotional responses. The process of extinction, or "unlearning," requires that the stimuli to which responses have been learned must be presented repeatedly without reinforcement. In the case of emotional behavior, this usually consists of presenting a warning signal without following it by a painful event. But, if the internal environment contributes significant stimulus properties for emotional behavior, presentation of an external warning signal, such as a clicking noise, constitutes only *part* of the total stimulus for the emotional response. Under these conditions, a change in the internal environment would be expected to interfere with the process of extinction, since the necessary conditions for extinction (nonreinforced presentations of the conditioned stimulus) cannot be entirely fulfilled. Firm evidence exists from animal experimentation that chlorpromazine and tetra-ethyl ammonium interfere with the extinction of emotional responses if the training is carried out without the drugs and extinction trials are given under medication.[13, 14]

Most of the experiments cited above were not designed to test the specific hypothesis that the behavioral effects of these treatments were due to changes in internal stimulus conditions. But the study to be reported here in detail *is* part of a systematic program designed to test this hypothesis. The general research design to be followed in this program of behavior research is: (1) to train emotional responses under several conditions of the internal environment, produced by drugs and other treatments, and (2) to test for retention of this emotional learning under conditions of the internal environment which are either (a) the same as, or (b) different from, the conditions that prevailed during the learning process. If the internal environment contributes significant stimuli for emotional learning, maximum retention of the learned emotional responses will be obtained only when retention test trials are conducted under the same conditions of internal environment as those which prevailed during the learning of those responses. In the specific case of drug-induced changes in the internal environment, a shift either from placebo to drug or from drug to placebo should interfere with retention of the emotional response if that drug changes significant aspects of the stimulus for learned emotional behavior as hypothesized above.

METHOD.   *Subjects.*   Sixty-four male albino rats of the Sprague-Dawley strain, approximately 90 days old at the beginning of the experiment, served as subjects.

Training procedures.   The learned emotional behavior investigated in this experiment is the conditioned emotional response ("anxiety") which has been described in detail by Brady and Hunt.[5] The training procedure for the entire program consists of preliminarily training the animals to press a level for an aperiodic water reward in a modified Skinner box. After a stable rate of lever pressing has been established, a clicking noise is presented to the animals during one three-minute period of their daily 9-minute run in the Skinner box. As soon as the clicking noise is terminated, a painful shock (1.5 m.a. for 0.2 seconds) is delivered to the feet of the animals through a grid floor. After several pairings of clicker and shock, a characteristic conditioned emotional response develops in the animals upon the onset of the clicker. This response consists of a crouching or "freezing" posture, defecation, piloerection, and a depression or complete cessation of lever pressing activity. The strength of this emotional response can be assessed by comparing the rate of lever pressing during the clicker with the lever pressing rate during a preceding nonclicker period.

In the present study, at the end of preliminary lever-pressing training, the experimental animals were divided into four groups matched on the basis of lever pressing rate. All animals in groups I and II received ten emotional conditioning trials (consisting of a three-minute clicker presentation followed by a brief shock) during each of their daily 9-minute trials in the Skinner box. Seven adaptation trials (no clicker or shock during the 9-minute trial) were interspersed among the emotional conditioning trials. All animals in groups III and IV received ten pseudo-emotional conditioning trials during each of which the clicker was presented for three minutes, but no shock was given, and they likewise received seven adaptation trials.

Drug treatment.   The drug selected for study was thioridazine hydrochloride (TP-21 Sandoz), a phenothiazine derivative with a piperadyl radical on the side chain. It was selected for this study on the basis of demonstrated therapeutic value in a variety of psychiatric disorders with a minimum of sedation and motor impairment.[15, 16] The relative absence of sedation and motor impairment was particularly important in our research, since these side effects often produced by other phenothiazines result in such serious interference with the lever pressing of animals during nonemotional periods that measurement of the emotional response becomes extremely difficult.

Groups I and III received their emotional training and pseudo-emotional training, respectively, under 5 mg/Kg thioridazine per day. Groups II and IV received their training under isotonic saline placebo medication. Drug and saline medications were first given three days before the first training trial and were continued throughout the training period. Injections were given intraperitoneally approximately one hour before each training trial.

Test procedure.   Following the last training trial, each of the four groups was divided into two subgroups, matched on the basis of lever pressing during the clicker as compared with an equivalent nonclicker period. Three animals in group I (emotional conditioning under thioridazine) were excluded from the study because they were observed to crouch consistently during the nonclicker as well as during the clicker periods. Half of the remaining animals in each group were then given 5 mg/Kg thioridazine per day, and the other half were given saline injections for three days and again approximately one hour before the trial test. Thus, half of the animals in each group were tested under the same internal conditions (drug or saline) as those that prevailed during the learning process, while the other half were tested under conditions that differed from the learning conditions. The retention test for all animals consisted of one 9-minute period in the Skinner box with a clicker presented during the second three-minute interval. No shock was administered during the test trial for any animal.

RESULTS.   To compare lever pressing during the clicker and during an equal period preceding the clicker, an inflection ratio, similar to that introduced by Hunt *et al.,*[17] was used ($IR = [B - A]/A$, where A equals lever presses during the three minutes before the clicker, and B equals lever presses during the three-minute clicker presentation). Complete cessation of lever pressing during the clicker (strongest emotional response) results in a ratio of -1.00, while a ratio of 0.00 or above indicates no suppression of lever pressing during the clicker and an absence of the emotional response.

At the end of ten training trials, all the remaining animals in group I, which had been given emotional training under thioridazine, had reached an inflection ratio of -1.00; and the average inflection ratio among animals in group II, which had received emotional training under saline, was almost as low ($-.97$). Both groups III and IV had average inflection ratios above 0.00 and showed no evidence of any emotional learning.

On the retention test trials, 13 out of 14 animals which had received both emotional training and testing under identical conditions of medication (drug-drug or saline-saline) showed complete retention of the emotional response. But all of the 15 animals which had been changed from drug to saline or from saline to drug showed some loss in the strength of the emotional response as indicated by an increase in inflection ratio. The Chi square for this observed difference is 22.6, which is significant beyond the 0.001 level.

Groups III and IV (pseudo-emotional training) were included in the study to determine whether or not a shift from drug to saline or from saline to drug might affect the unconditioned response to the clicking noise and, in this way, simulate a change in emotional behavior. Previous research results with chlorpromazine [7] suggested that this was a very real possibility. However, seven out of 15 animals who were given pseudo-emotional training and testing under identical conditions of medication (drug-drug or saline-saline) showed an increase in inflection ratio (comparable to a reduction in the emotional response), while the remaining eight showed no increase (comparable to complete retention of the emotional response). Among animals which received pseudo-emotional training and testing under different conditions (saline-drug or drug-saline), nine out of 15 showed an increased inflection ratio, and the remaining six showed a decrease or no change. The Chi square for this difference is 0.13, which does not approach significance. Therefore, the increased lever pressing during the clicker period which resulted from a shift from drug to saline or from saline to drug among emotionally trained animals could not have been due to a change in unconditioned behavior, and it can be described with confidence as a loss of a learned emotional response.

DISCUSSION. The present study provides the clearest evidence to date that internal stimulus conditions associated with drug or saline medication may acquire stimulus properties with respect to learned emotional responses. Administration of a tranquilizing drug (thioridazine hydrochloride) to animals which had learned an emotional response under saline resulted in a loss of the emotional response, as has been shown repeatedly for a number of such drugs. But withdrawal of the tranquilizing drug and substitution of saline medication was equally effective in interfering with an emotional response which had been acquired under conditions of thioridazine medication. While comparable data are not available for other tranquilizing drug or for a variety of somatic treatments employed in psychiatry, both clinical evidence and the results of laboratory studies support the hypothesis that a variety of these treatment procedures may interfere with previously learned emotional behavior by changing significant aspects of the internal stimuli for specific emotional responses.

REFERENCES

1. Heistad, G. T.: A biopsychological approach to somatic treatments in psychiatry, *Am. J. Psychiat.* 114:540, 1957.
2. Sandison, R. A., and Whitelaw, J. D. A.: Further studies in the therapeutic value of lysergic acid diethylamide in mental illness, *J. Ment. Sc.* 103:332, 1957.
3. Abramson, H. A., ed.: *Neuropharmacology: Transactions of the Second Conference,* New York, Josiah Macy Foundation, 1956.
4. Brady, J. V.: The assessment of drug effects on emotional behavior, *Science* 123:1033, 1956.
5. Brady, J. V., and Hunt, H. F.: A further demonstration of the effects of electroconvulsive shock on a conditioned emotional response, *J. Comp. & Physiol. Psychol.* 44:204, 1951.
6. Heistad, G. T.: An effect of electroconvulsive shock on a conditioned avoidance response, *J. Comp. & Physiol. Psychol.* 48:482, 1955.
7. Heistad, G. T.: Effects of chlorpromazine and electroconvulsive shock on a conditioned emotional response, *J. Comp. & Physiol. Psychol.* 51:209, 1958.
8. Hunt, H. F.: Some effects of meprobamate on conditioned fear and emotional behavior, *Ann. New York Acad. Sc.* 67:712, 1957.
9. Dasgupta, S. R., and Werner, G.: Inhibition of hypothalamic, medullary, and reflex vasomotor responses by chlorpromazine, *Brit. J. Pharmacol. Chemotherapy* 9:389, 1954.
10. Gellhorn, E.: *Physiological basis of neurology and psychiatry,* Minneapolis, University of Minnesota Press, 1953.

11. Kalinowski, L. B., and Hock, P. H.: *Shock treatments and other somatic treatments in psychiatry,* New York, Grune & Stratton, 1952.

12. Brady, J. V.: The effect of electroconvulsive shock on a conditioned emotional response: The permanence of the effect, *J. Comp. & Physiol. Psychol.* **44**:507, 1951.

13. Hunt, H. F.: Some effects of drugs on classical (type S) conditioning, *Ann. New York Acad. Sc.* **65**:258, 1956.

14. Davitz, J. R.: Decreased autonomic functioning and extinction of a conditioned emotional response, *J. Comp. & Physiol. Psychol.* **46**:311, 1953.

15. Fleeson, W., Glueck, B. C., Heistad, G. T., King, J. E., Lykken, D. T., Meehl, P. E., and Mena, A.: The ataraxic effect of two phenothiazine drugs, *Univ. of Minn. Med. Bull.* **29**:274, 1958.

16. Glueck, B. C., Meehl, P. E., and Heistad, G. T.: *Approaches to the quantitative assessment of clinical analysis,* Brochure accompanying a scientific exhibit, American Psychiatric Association, Philadelphia, 1959.

17. Hunt, H. F., Jemberg, P., and Lawler, W. G.: The effect of electroconvulsive shock on a conditioned emotional response: the effect of electroconvulsive shock under ether anesthesia, *J. Comp. & Physiol. Psych.* **46**:64, 1953.

Section **B**   RESPONSE VARIABLES

Articles 5–6

The two papers in this section are concerned with response variables in respondent conditioning. In Article 5 a drug is used as a US, and changes in operant response rate, heart rate, salivation, and emesis are reported to a stimulus paired with nalorphine injection in morphine-dependent monkeys. Article 6 reports the effects of drugs on different types of behavior (reflexive and operant) produced when a stimulus is paired with electric shock.

5

Conditioned suppression by a stimulus associated with nalorphine in morphine-dependent monkeys [1]

STEVEN R. GOLDBERG and CHARLES R. SCHUSTER

In morphine addicts, an abrupt and complete withdrawal of morphine is followed by an abstinence syndrome which is an indication of the addict's physical dependence on the drug. Morphine-abstinence symptoms have been described as both "non-purposive" (physiological) and "purposive" (behavioral) by Wikler (1955). Physiological changes, such as excessive salivation, body temperature changes, piloerection, muscle aching and twitching, emesis and tachycardia, involve the neuromuscular, autonomic, and endocrine systems. Behavioral changes consist of a disruption of normal ongoing behavior and a reorientation of behavior toward drug acquisition. In morphine addicts an injection of nalorphine, a potent antagonist of morphine, immediately elicits the abstinence syndrome normally associated with abrupt withdrawal of morphine. The effects of intravenously administered nalorphine are seen within seconds and last for several hours. In minimal doses, capable of producing the abstinence syndrome in morphine addicts, nalorphine has no noticeable effects on normal subjects.

Human addicts, who have been withdrawn from morphine and are no longer physically dependent upon the drug, have described the recurrence of certain withdrawal responses when they return to an environment previously associated with drug-taking behavior. Wikler (1961) has interpreted these observations as an indication that the withdrawal syndrome can be classically conditioned and that this conditioning may be a major factor in post-addicts' relapse to drug-taking. Using rats as subjects, Wikler (1965) has obtained results which indicate the occurrence of "conditioned withdrawal" produced by returning the rats to an environment previously associated with drug withdrawal.

Irwin and Seevers (1956) have provided experimental results suggesting that nalorphine-induced withdrawal can be classically conditioned. Morphine-dependent monkeys which had undergone repeated nalorphine-induced withdrawal continued to show a "withdrawal-like" response to

From *Journal of the Experimental Analysis of Behavior,* 1967, **10,** 235–242. Copyright 1967 by the Society for the Experimental Analysis of Behavior, Inc., Bloomington, Ind.

[1] This investigation was supported by USPHS research grant No. MH 08506-03.

both nalorphine and saline injections several months after they had been withdrawn from morphine. After repeated injections of saline the "withdrawal-like" response was no longer elicited.

The present experiment is the first in a series, using a procedure developed to study the conditioning of both the behavioral and physiological aspects of the morphine-withdrawal syndrome.

METHOD. *Subjects.* Experiment 1 studied an adult, male rhesus monkey weighing 5 kg and physically dependent on morphine; in Exp. 2, four adult, female rhesus monkeys weighing between 3.8 and 4.8 kg were used. The monkey in Exp. 1 and two of the monkeys (M474 and M574) in Exp. 2 had been physically dependent on morphine for approximately 18 months before these experiments. During this time they were maintained on 12 mg/kg a day of morphine sulfate, given as a subcutaneous injection of 3 mg/kg every 6 hr. The dosage for the monkey in Exp. 1 was gradually increased over a period of several months before the experiment to a final dosage of 42 mg/kg a day. The other two subjects in Exp. 2 (M2018 and M2037) were not physically dependent on morphine.

All monkeys were surgically prepared with chronic indwelling jugular catheters (Schuster and Brady, 1964). Immediately before the experiments the monkeys were reduced to 85% of free-feeding weight. They were then trained to press a lever for food reinforcement on a fixed-ratio 10 schedule (FR 10); that is, a pellet of food was delivered for every tenth response.

Apparatus. The monkeys were restrained during the experimental sessions in Foringer Primate Cockpits (Cat. #1206 M1) enclosed in isolation booths (Cat. #3011 M1). At other times they were maintained in separate cages with water available, but no food. The cockpits were equipped with mouth-operated food and water operanda (Thompson, Schuster, Dockens, and Lee, 1964). A Foringer pellet dispenser provided 0.7 g Dietrich and Gambrill monkey food pellets (Foringer Cat. #1281). Each depression of the water operandum produced 1.0 ml of water. A stimulus light panel was mounted at eye level on the door of the isolation booth. A wide-angle viewing lens allowed observation of the monkey in the booth. To mask the sounds of programming and recording equipment a white noise generator was operated continuously during all sessions. Injections were administered from outside the isolation booth by syringes connected by a polyethylene catheter (PE-100) to the implanted jugular catheter in the monkey. A 0.9% physiological saline solution was used for saline injections. Nalorphine injection solutions were prepared daily by adding the desired amount of nalorphine HCl to 0.9% physiological saline. Wound clips attached to the area of the right shoulder and left waist served as electrocardiogram leads which led from the isolation booth to an Offner Electroencephalograph. Cables connected apparatus in the isolation booth to automatic programming and recording apparatus.

General procedure. The monkey in Exp. 1 and monkeys M474 and M574 in Exp. 2 were tested for 2 hr a day, 1 to 2 hr after a morphine injection. They were conditioned initially to depress the food lever on the FR 10 schedule of reinforcement and the water operandum on an FR 1 schedule of reinforcement. After the jugular catheters were surgically implanted, the monkeys were placed on a 2-hr, three-component, chain schedule of reinforcement, which continued unchanged during all conditioning, extinction, and reconditioning sessions. The sequence of components within each 2-hr session was: 30-min FI component; 1-hr FR 10 food component; 30-min S$^\Delta$ component. Thus, the monkeys' first response on the food lever after 30 min produced a stimulus in the presence of which every tenth response was reinforced with a pellet of food. At the end of 1 hr in the FR 10 period, or after 100 reinforcements, they were advanced into a 30-min S$^\Delta$ period, in which responses had no consequences, after which they were removed from the situation. A house light was illuminated throughout the session. The discriminative stimuli during the FI period were two 6-w, 110-v blue lights; during the FR 10 food period they were two 6-w, 110-v white lights. During the 30-min S$^\Delta$ period only the house lights remained on. Water reinforcement was continuously available during the session.

After the food-lever response rate was stabilized on this schedule, an auditory stimulus (tone) was aperiodically presented every third or fourth session. The tone was presented approximately 10 min after the start of the FR 10 food component for 5 min before and after an intravenous injection of 1 cc of saline. After several sessions, neither the tone nor the injection procedure disrupted the monkeys' food-lever response rate or heart rate, thus establishing them as neutral stimuli. Following this, the tone was presented aperiodically every third or fourth session, 5 min before and after an intravenous dose of nalorphine. The subjects were intermittently observed during the session through the wide-angle viewing lens.

The two non-dependent monkeys in Exp. 2 (M2018 and M2037) were surgically prepared with chronic indwelling jugular catheters. They worked on a schedule similar to that described above, except that the present one was terminated after 80 food reinforcements or 1 hr. No tone was presented during the sessions.

For purposes of this report only the FR 10 food component is discussed.

EXPERIMENT 1.   The monkey (M4) was stabilized on the schedule without the presentation of tone-injection pairings. Several doses of nalorphine were administered during different sessions to determine a dose of the drug that immediately terminated food-lever responding for the remainder of the session. A total dose of 2 mg of nalorphine was found reliably to produce this effect. Tone-saline injection pairings (T + S) were then presented for several sessions during the FR 10 food component to establish these as neutral stimuli. After these sessions a tone-nalorphine pairing (T + N) was presented aperiodically, once every third or fourth session, during the FR 10 food component. Electrocardiogram samples were taken during all sessions. Several sessions after the third T + N session, the monkey's health declined and it was removed from the experiment.

Results.   Figure 1 shows the cumulative response records for monkey M4. Session 1 was a control session before conditioning began. It demonstrated that the stimuli associated with the injection procedure were initially neutral and produced no change in the monkey's food-lever response rate.

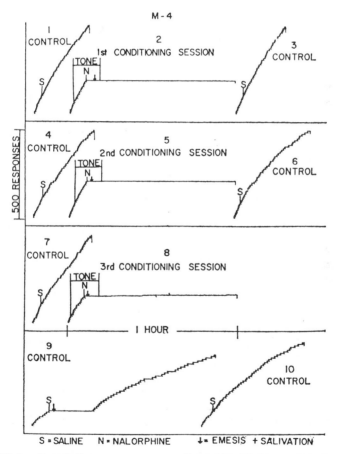

FIGURE 1. Cumulative response curves from M4. Each segment shown is the initial portion of an FR 10 food component record extracted from a 2-hr session. The numeral 1 designates a control session which established that the saline injection was a neutral stimulus; 2, 5, and 8 were conditioning sessions, and 3, 4, 6, 7, 9, and 10 were control sessions before and after conditioning sessions.

Sessions 2, 5, and 8 were conditioning sessions in which an injection of 2 mg of nalorphine was given. After injections of nalorphine the monkey's food-lever responding was completely suppressed for the remainder of the session. In addition, emesis and excessive salivation were observed and heart rate increased from an average FR 10 food period level of 180 to 190 beats per min to 240 to 250 beats per min. During control sessions 3, 4, 6, and 7 response rate and heart rate did not change after saline injections. During saline control session 9, following the third conditioning session, the saline injection completely suppressed food-lever responses and decreased heart rate to 140 to 150 beats per min. These effects lasted approximately 15 min; then, both food-lever response rate and heart rate returned to approximately the level observed before the saline injection. The monkey also showed emesis and excessive salivation, which had not occurred after the previous saline injections. In Session 10, the second control session following the third conditioning session, the saline injection no longer produced a change in food-lever response rate or heart rate. The monkey was removed from the experiment after control session 10.

Discussion.   During the sessions before the third T + N pairing, saline injections produced no change in food-lever response rate or heart rate. After the third pairing, the saline injection suppressed responses on the food lever and elicited emesis, excessive salivation, and a fall in heart rate. It should be noted that heart rate decreased after the saline injection in contrast to the increase produced by the nalorphine injections. Similar findings have been reported in studies using the conditioned emotional response paradigm with shock. The stimulus preceding shock produced a decrease in heart rate in contrast to the presentation of shock, which elicited an increase (Wilson, 1964; deToledo and Black, 1966). It appears that the stimuli associated with the injection procedure, previously neutral interoceptive stimuli, became conditioned stimuli after their association with nalorphine. This is not surprising, since the infusion of solutions into the internal jugular vein is known to have stimulus properties (Schuster and Brady, 1964). A second series of experiments was carried out to determine whether the tone preceding the injection of nalorphine could acquire the ability to suppress response rate for food and elicit salivation, emesis, and heart rate changes.

EXPERIMENT 2.   Monkeys M474 and M574 were maintained on 12 mg/kg of morphine a day. They were conditioned using 1-mg total dose of nalorphine in sessions with T + N pairings. Lower dosages of morphine and nalorphine were chosen to prevent a decline in the health of these monkeys, as occurred in M4 in Exp. 1. No saline injection was given on control days. In all other respects the schedule was the same as in Exp. 1. After the tone and injection of saline were established as neutral stimuli, five more sessions with T + S pairings were conducted. Then, 10 conditioning sessions with T + N pairings were given. The conditioning sessions were conducted every third or fourth day with control sessions interspersed. After the tenth conditioning session, extinction sessions with T + S pairings were conducted each day. Following extinction, the monkeys were reconditioned in sessions with T + N pairings. Monkeys were intermittently observed and samples of electrocardiogram records were taken during all sessions.

In the control sessions following the sixth and ninth conditioning sessions, monkey M574 exhibited what could be a trace conditioned response. At approximately the same time that the tone would have been presented, food-lever responses stopped, heart rate fell, and emesis and excessive salivation were seen. This effect lasted approximately 10 min, but disappeared by the control session on the following day and was not observed at any other time.

A control experiment was conducted with the two monkeys (M2018 and M2037) not dependent on morphine. They worked on a schedule identical to that in Exp. 2, except that it was terminated after 80 food reinforcements or 1 hr. No injections were given on control days. On test days, an injection of 1 mg of nalorphine was given. No auditory stimulus was presented.

Results.   Figure 2 shows cumulative response records of selected sessions for M574. Figure 3 shows cumulative response records of the same sessions for M474. In the control sessions before the start of conditioning, more prolonged pausing after reinforcements was exhibited than is usually seen on this type of schedule. The monkeys' performance, however, was quite stable over sessions. Session 5 was the last day of the five sessions establishing the tone and injection as neutral stimuli. The onset of the tone and the injection of saline did not disrupt the monkeys' food-lever response rate. Session 6 was the first conditioning session with a T + N pairing. The monkeys responded normally during the tone period before the injection and continued to respond for 3 to 4 food reinforcements after the nalorphine injection. Responding was then completely suppressed for the rest of the session. After nalorphine injections, emesis and excessive salivation were observed in both monkeys. Session 15 was the tenth conditioning session with a T + N pairing. This session illustrates the conditioned suppression observed in T + N sessions, 9 through 15. Before the tone in Session 15, the monkeys' performance was comparable to that on control days. With the onset of the tone, food-lever responding was immediately suppressed for the rest of the session. Emesis and excessive salivation were observed in M574 during the tone period before the injection of nalorphine and in M474 after the nalorphine injection. Session 16 was the first extinction session with a T + S pairing. The monkeys responded normally for food until the onset of the tone. Food-lever responding was then completely suppressed during the entire tone period.

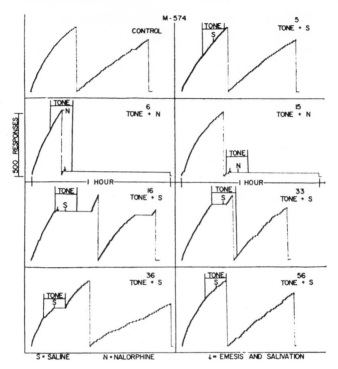

FIGURE 2.   Cumulative response curves from M574. Each segment shown is a complete FR 10 food component record extracted from a 2-hr session. A control session before tone-injection pairings is shown first; 5 was a session establishing tone and saline injection as neutral stimuli; 6 was the first conditioning session, 15 was the tenth conditioning session; 16 was the first extinction session, 33 the eighteenth, 36 the twenty-first, and 56 the forty-first extinction session. Arrows indicate observation of emesis and excessive salivation.

After the onset of the tone, emesis and excessive salivation were observed in M574. After the tone terminated, food-lever response rate was completely suppressed for 10 min in M574 and for 5 min in M474. Food-lever response rates then returned to normal. The post-tone pausing gradually disappeared during the following four extinction sessions. Emesis and excessive salivation were no longer observed in M574 during extinction after Session 25. Session 33 was the eighteenth extinction session with a T + S pairing. The monkeys responded normally for food until the onset of the tone. Food-lever response rate of M574 was completely suppressed during the tone period before the saline injection, but returned to normal in the tone period after the injection. Food-lever response rate of M474 was partially suppressed during the tone period before and after the saline injection. Session 36 was the twenty-first extinction session. The monkeys responded normally for food until the onset of the tone. After the onset of the tone, response rate of M574 was partially suppressed during the tone

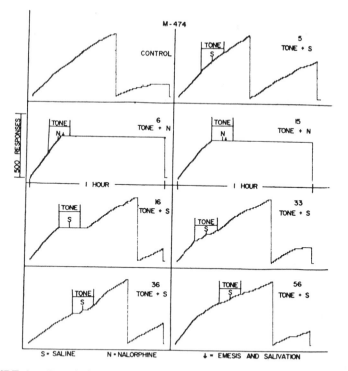

FIGURE 3. Cumulative response curves from M474. Each segment shown is a complete FR 10 food component record extracted from a 2-hr session. A control session before tone-injection pairings is shown first; 5 was a session establishing tone and saline injection as neutral stimuli; 6 was the first conditioning session, 15 was the tenth conditioning session; 16 was the first extinction session, 33 the eighteenth, 36 the twenty-first, and 56 the forty-first extinction session. Arrows indicate observation of emesis and excessive salivation.

period until the injection of saline. Immediately after the saline injection, response rate was completely suppressed until the end of the tone period. Responding by Monkey M474 was completely suppressed for about the first 3 min of the 5-min tone period before the injection. Response rate then returned to a near normal rate before the injection but was completely suppressed immediately after it and continued so for about 2 min. Response rate then returned to normal for the remainder of the tone period. Food response rate for both monkeys was normal after the tone stopped. Session 56 was one of the final extinction sessions. Both monkeys' food-lever response rate during the tone approached normal response levels observed in the initial T + S sessions. This indicates that the conditioning and extinction procedure had not interfered with the monkeys' baseline FR performance.

The percentage change in heart rate and food-lever response rate from the 5-min period preceding the tone onset to the 5-min period during the

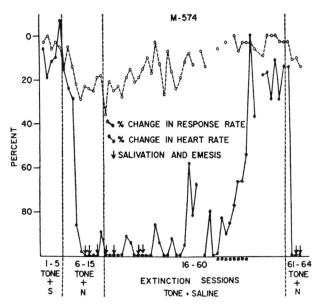

FIGURE 4. M574. Percentage change in heart rate and response rate from the 5-min period preceding the tone onset to the 5-min period during tone presentation and before injection. Numerals 1 to 5 designate sessions establishing tone and saline (S) injection as neutral stimuli; 6 to 15 were the conditioning sessions during which nalorphine (N) was administered; 16 to 60 were extinction sessions with tone + saline (S) presentations. Those marked by asterisks were sessions in which the FR requirements were reduced during the tone period; 61 to 64 were reconditioning sessions with tone + nalorphine (N) presentations. Arrows mark sessions when emesis and excessive salivation were observed in the tone period before the injection of saline or nalorphine. Breaks in the curve indicate sessions where mechanical problems prevented data collection. Each conditioning and reconditioning session was followed by 3 to 4 control sessions not indicated on the graph.

tone presentation, before the injection of nalorphine or saline, is shown in Fig. 4 for M574 and in Fig. 5 for M474.

The first five sessions established the tone and injection of saline as neutral stimuli. After Session 6, the first conditioning session, food-lever response rate during the tone decreased and was almost completely suppressed after four conditioning sessions for M574 and after six sessions for M474. Food-lever response rate remained suppressed throughout the tone period during the initial extinction sessions for both monkeys.

In conditioning sessions 9 to 15, heart rate for M574 declined during the 5-min tone period before the nalorphine injection. After the injection of nalorphine, heart rate in both monkeys rose from an average FR 10 food period level of 160 to 190 beats per min to 240 to 260 beats per min. During the initial extinction sessions, M574's heart rate continued to decline during the tone period before and after the saline injection. Emesis and excessive salivation were observed in M574 during the tone period

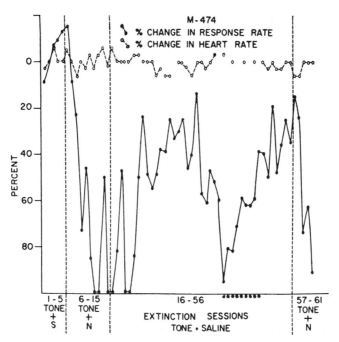

FIGURE 5.   M474. Percentage change in heart rate and response rate from the 5-min period preceding the tone onset to the 5-min period during tone presentation and before injection. Sessions 1 through 5 established tone and saline (S) injections as neutral stimuli; 6 to 15 were the conditioning sessions during which nalorphine (N) was administered; 16 to 56 were extinction sessions with tone and saline (S) presentations. Those marked by asterisks were sessions in which the FR requirements were reduced during the tone period. Sessions 57 to 61 were reconditioning sessions with tone + nalorphine (N) presentations. No emesis or excessive salivation was observed in the tone period before injection of saline or nalorphine. Breaks in the curve indicate sessions where mechanical problems prevented data collection. Each conditioning and reconditioning session was followed by 3 to 4 control sessions not indicated on the graph.

preceding the injection. This is marked on the graph with arrows. No heart rate changes, emesis or excessive salivation were observed in M474 during the tone period before the injections of nalorphine or saline.

The heart rate response of M574 during the tone was partially extinguished after 15 sessions of T + S pairings. At this time, however, the food-lever response rate remained completely suppressed during the tone and continued to be suppressed for another 13 sessions. After 10 extinction sessions, food-lever response rate of M474 approached normal baseline levels during the tone but this was not consistent and occasional suppression continued. To hasten extinction, the FR requirements were reduced during the tone period and then gradually returned to FR 10 over the next 8 to 9 sessions. These sessions are marked in Fig. 4 and 5 with asterisks. Response rates during the tone increased over these sessions to a value approximating that observed in the initial T + S sessions (1 to 5). Reconditioning sessions with T + N pairings were then conducted and results closely paralleled those in the initial conditioning sessions. Additional reconditioning sessions were not conducted because the health of both animals declined.

Figure 6 shows cumulative response records for the two monkeys (M2018 and M2037) not dependent on morphine. Sessions 1 and 3 were control sessions before and after the sessions in which nalorphine was administered. During Session 2 an injection of 1 mg of nalorphine was given after approximately 10 reinforcements. The nalorphine injections produced no change in the monkeys' FR food responding, compared to control sessions. Observation of these animals after the nalorphine injection failed to reveal any emesis or excessive salivation. It was not possible to record heart rate.

GENERAL DISCUSSION.   The results of Exp. 1 and 2 demonstrate that the intravenous administration of nalorphine to morphine-dependent monkeys abruptly terminated food-reinforced, fixed-ratio behavior for the remainder of the session. Further, these subjects showed a marked incre-

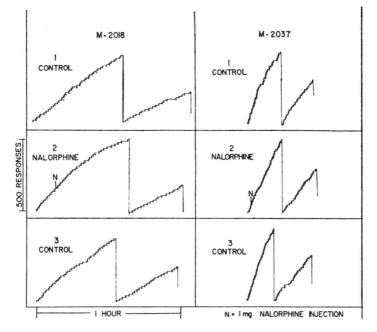

FIGURE 6. Cumulative response curves from M2037 and M2018. Each session shown is a complete FR 10 food component record. Sessions 1 and 3 are control sessions, before and after Session 2 during which nalorphine was administered.

ment in heart rate, excessive salivation, and emesis within several minutes after the injection of nalorphine. In contrast, monkeys M2018 and M2037, which were not dependent upon morphine, showed no disruption in their fixed-ratio behavior or any observable salivation or emesis after nalorphine was administered. This indicates that the behavioral disruption and physiological changes induced by nalorphine do not occur in non-dependent monkeys, but rather are effects based upon nalorphine's ability to antagonize certain actions of morphine. This is in accord with the well established fact that nalorphine can produce the withdrawal syndrome in morphine-dependent organisms at doses which have little pharmacological action in normals.

The results of Exp. 1 suggest that stimuli associated with the injection of nalorphine could acquire the ability to produce both physiological and behavioral changes. This was more definitely established in Exp. 2 where the tone preceding nalorphine administration acquired the ability to produce a complete suppression of the monkeys' fixed-ratio behavior. This suppression was rapidly established for both monkeys in both the initial conditioning sessions and in reconditioning following the extinction sessions. For M574 the tone also acquired the ability to produce emesis and excessive salivation and a marked decrement in heart rate. One possible explanation for this decrease in heart rate would be that it is due to the suppression of food-lever response rate. This explanation is not tenable, however, since we have observed sessions, before test sessions with saline or nalorphine injections, during which a monkey would not respond for food in the FR 10 food component, yet the heart rate remained at a level of 170 to 190 beats per min. Also, if a decrement in response rate were the explanation for the fall in heart rate, M474 would also have shown this effect during conditioning and extinction sessions when food responding was suppressed. This would suggest that the tone had become a conditioned stimulus capable of eliciting some of the physiological changes elicited by nalorphine in physically dependent monkeys. This may well be the explanation for the suppression of the animals' fixed-ratio behavior during the tone. That is, if the tone acquires the ability to elicit certain aspects of the withdrawal syndrome these physiological changes may in turn disrupt the animals' food-reinforced, fixed-ratio behavior. This analysis of the mechanism underlying the conditioned suppression is weakened by the fact that the conditioned physiological changes were not observed in M474. It should be noted, however, that the conditioned suppression in this subject was more variable and less resistant to extinction. Further, the failure to observe physiological changes in M474 may be a reflection of the crudeness of the present observations rather than an absence of these changes. We are currently adapting for use in this procedure certain physiological techniques which measure gastro-intestinal motility, salivation, and respiration rate. This will allow the detection of more subtle changes elicited by nalorphine and their possible conditioning to stimuli associated with nalorphine administration. In this way it may be possible to determine whether the classical conditioning of these physiological changes in a necessary pre-requisite for the conditioned suppression of the ongoing food-reinforced operant behavior.

SUMMARY.   Three rhesus monkeys, physically dependent on morphine, were trained to press a lever for food on a fixed ratio of 10 responses. A tone, initially a neutral stimulus, was aperiodically presented every third or fourth session, 5 min before and after the intravenous injection of nalor-phine, a morphine antagonist which produces an immediate withdrawal syndrome in morphine-dependent monkeys. After several sessions, condi-tioned suppression of food-lever response rate was observed. Conditioned bradycardia, emesis, and excessive salivation also occurred. In 40 to 45 sessions the conditioned suppression of food-lever response rate and the conditioned autonomic changes were extinguished by presenting pairings of a tone and saline injection. The monkeys were then reconditioned by presenting the tone aperiodically, every third or fourth session, 5 min be-fore and after the intravenous injection of nalorphine. Results were similar to the initial conditioning sessions. Two rhesus monkeys not dependent on morphine were stabilized on a food schedule similar to that used for the first three monkeys. These monkeys showed no change in food-lever re-sponse rate during or after nalorphine injections.

REFERENCES

deToledo, Leyla, and Black, A. H. Heart rate changes during conditioned suppression in rats. *Science,* 1966, **152,** 1404–1406.

Irwin, S., and Seevers, M. H. Altered responses to drugs in the post-addict (*Macaca Mulatta*). *J. Pharm. exp. Therap.,* 1956, **116,** 31–32.

Schuster, C. R., and Brady, J. V. The discriminative control of a food reinforced operant by interoceptive stimulation. *Pavlov J. higher nervous Activity,* 1964, **14,** 448–458.

Thompson, T., Schuster, C. R., Dockens, W., and Lee, R. Mouth-operated food and water manipulanda for use with monkeys. *J. exp. Anal. Behav.,* 1964, **7,** 171–172.

Wikler, A. Rationale of the diagnosis and treatment of addictions. *Conn. State med. J.,* 1955, **19,** 560.

Wikler, A. On the nature of addiction and habituation. *Brit. J. Addiction,* 1961, **57,** 73–79.

Wikler, A. Conditioning factors in opiate addiction and relapse. In D. M. Wilner and G. G. Kassebaum (Ed.), *Narcotics.* New York: McGraw-Hill, 1965, pp. 85–100.

Wilson, R. S. Autonomic changes produced by noxious and innocuous stimuli. *J. comp. physiol. Psychol.,* 1964, **58,** 290–295.

9

Assessment of drug effects on emotional behavior

JOSEPH V. BRADY

Recent developments in the use of chemicotherapeutic agents for clinical psychopathology have stimulated renewed interest in laboratory-testing methods for assessing behavioral changes associated with such drug administration. Animal-conditioning experiments promise to provide the behavioral control techniques that are basic to such an approach, although the selective assessment of specific emotional or affective responses that are of primary interest in this area has continued to present both methodological and theoretical problems. The purpose of the present report is to describe a method, based on earlier animal experimental work (1), for producing and selectively measuring emotional behavior in experimental animals and to present some data that illustrate the use of this method for investigating the behavioral effects of amphetamine and reserpine (2).

Rats and monkeys that had been deprived of solid food and liquids for 24 hours or more were trained to press a bar for a reward of water (rats) or sugared orange juice (monkeys). Initially, the animals received a drop of the liquid reward every time they pressed the lever (continuous reinforcement), although they were rapidly shifted to a schedule on which the bar-press produced the reward only occasionally (average, once in 60 seconds). When the response rates had stabilized on this variable-interval reinforcement schedule during experimental sessions that lasted several hours or more, a conditioned emotional response of the "fear" or "anxiety" type was superimposed upon the lever-pressing behavior (3). Briefly, this conditioned "anxiety" response consisted of suppression of lever pressing, crouching, defecation, and immobility upon presentation of a clicking noise that had previously been paired with a painful electric shock to the feet. In the present study, the clicking noise was presented at 7-minute intervals during the experimental session and continued for 3 minutes before termination with the grid shock (approximately 1.5 ma) to the feet. Programming of the experimental procedure and recording of the animals' behavior were accomplished automatically by timers, magnetic counters, cumulative-work recorders, and associated relay circuits.

The behavior pattern that develops as a consequence of this procedure is illustrated for one of the rats by the cumulative-response record in the top ("saline"-control) section of Fig. 1. A marked depression in lever-pressing rate is apparent during the 3-minute clicker periods, which are

From *Science,* 1956, **123**, 1033–1034.

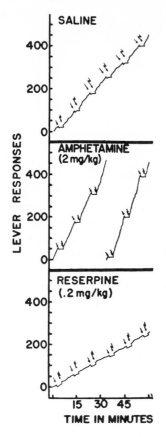

FIGURE 1. Sample cumulative-response curves for rat AA-26 showing the effect of amphetamine and reserpine on lever pressing and on the conditioned emotional response. The oblique solid arrows indicate the onset of the conditioned auditory stimulus, and the oblique broken arrows indicate the termination of the conditioned stimulus contiguously with the brief, unconditioned grid-shock stimulus to the feet.

indicated by the short offset sections of the cumulative curve between the straight ("clicker") and broken ("shock") arrows, although the stable lever-pressing rate is maintained throughout the 7-minute intervals between emotional-conditioning trials. After establishment of this pattern, the ratio of the number of lever responses during the clicker periods to the number of lever responses during the nonclicker periods has been found to remain stable (showing no consistent trend) during more than 80 to 100 experimental hours.

The center section of Fig. 1 illustrates the effects of a relatively large dose of amphetamine administered intraperitoneally to the same animal 1 hour prior to this behavior sample. The total number of lever responses during this 1-hour period shows more than a 100-percent increase over the saline-control session, although the rate increase is accounted for completely by increased lever pressing in the 7-minute periods between emotional conditioning trials. The number of lever responses during the 3-minute clicker periods is actually seen to decrease under the influence of the drug.

In contrast, daily intraperitoneal injections of 0.2 mg/kg of reserpine were found, after 4 days, to produce a decrease of more than 50 percent in the total number of lever responses during the 1-hour session for this same animal, although the conditioned suppression of responding during the 3-minute clicker periods was virtually eliminated. The lower section of Fig. 1 shows that, despite the over-all depression in lever pressing, the animal, under the influence of this drug, continued to respond throughout the 3-minute clicker presentations at the same rate as during the 7-minute intervals between conditioning trials, even though the pain shock continued to be paired with termination of the clicker.

The results obtained with this technique have been replicated with several animals (rats and monkeys). It is clear, however, that the method described does provide an approach to the selective assessment of specific drug-behavior relationships in the affective sphere while providing a control for the general behavioral and motor disturbances that frequently develop as nonspecific side effects of such drug administration.

REFERENCES AND NOTES

1. W. K. Estes and B. F. Skinner, *J. Exptl. Psychol.* **29**, 390 (1941); J. V. Brady and H. F. Hunt, *J. Psychol.* **40**, 313 (1955).
2. The author gratefully acknowledges the technical assistance of Irving Geller and Donald Conrad in the conduct of these experiments.
3. H. F. Hunt and J. V. Brady, *J. Comp. Physiol. Psychol.* **44**, 88 (1951).

Section **C**   ORGANISMIC VARIABLES

Article 7

In Article 7, a drug serves as an organismic variable, a
state or condition under which acquisition and extinction of
a conditioned pupillary dilation response are studied.

7

Classical conditioning of the pupillary dilation response of normal and curarized cats [1]

ARNOLD A. GERALL and PAUL A. OBRIST

In an earlier study (Gerall, Sampson, and Boslov, 1957) conditioning of the pupillary dilation response (PDR) was obtained in human Ss when the US contained electric shock but not when the US consisted of a decrease in intensity of light. The first part of the study reported here was initiated to test the applicability of this finding to the cat, an animal often used in studies of the autonomic nervous system. The PDR of cats has been successfully conditioned in experiments by Girden (1942a, 1942b), Harlow and Toltzien (1940), and Harlow and Stagner (1933). In all these experiments the US was an electric shock, and no studies have been reported in which the US was a change in light intensity.

The second part of the present study was concerned with the possibility of conditioning the PDR of cats that have had their skeletal muscles paralyzed by Flaxedil, a curariform drug. This was attempted primarily for methodological reasons since curarization offers one of the best means of immobilizing the cat, which is an extremely difficult animal to keep restrained. In addition, the results should have some bearing on one hypothesis concerned with conditioning of autonomic responses suggested by Kendon Smith (1954). According to this hypothesis, no conditioning of the pupillary or any other smooth-muscle response would be anticipated if the skeletal musculature were completely paralyzed. The findings of Harlow and Stagner (1933), Girden and Culler (1937), and Girden (1942a, 1942b), who report conditioning of the PDR in animals paralyzed by curare and B-erythroidine, were not taken as negative evidence against the artifact hypothesis by Smith since some striate-muscle activity was detectable in the Ss used in these studies. In the present experiment, cats were subdued by doses of Flaxedil more than sufficient to paralyze them completely. If no conditioning could be obtained after this degree of curarization, then Smith's view would be supported.

Lastly, an attempt was made to determine whether PDRs conditioned when the Ss were paralyzed by Flaxedil could be evoked when they were normal and vice versa. Previous experiments by Girden and Culler (1937)

From *Journal of Comparative and Physiological Psychology*, 1962, **55**, 486–491. Copyright 1962 by the American Psychological Association, Washington, D.C.

[1] This research was supported by the National Science Foundation under Grant NSF-61791 and completed at the University of Rochester.

and Girden (1942a, 1942b) indicated that the transfer of CRs from either curarized to normal or normal to curarized states did not occur in cats or dogs. Raw curare and B-erythroidine were used to curarize the *S*s, and it is possible that newer curariform compounds such as Flaxedil may not possess the property of these older drugs to produce dissociation of CRs.

EXPERIMENT 1

METHOD.   *Subjects.*   The *S*s were six cats, three females, two males, and one castrate, between 1.5 and 3.0 yr. old. All were in the laboratory at least 6 mo. prior to experimentation.

Apparatus.   The photographic and timing equipment used has been described in detail elsewhere (Gerall *et al.*, 1957). In brief, infrared motion-picture photography with a film speed of 16 frames/sec was used to record changes in pupillary diameter. Both eyes were illuminated by the infrared and US light sources, but only the right eye was photographed. The US lights were placed above and below the *S*'s head. The intensity of the upper light was greater than the lower one, and together they provided about 100 ft. of illumination.

The cat holder constructed to restrain the *S*s is shown in Fig. 1. It consisted of a galvanized-iron stovepipe hinged along one side. A cat was placed in the holder with its shoulders behind the first yoke, its head in front of the second yoke, and its feet under its body. After the foam-rubber-lined top of the holder was closed snugly around the cat, it was secured tightly by straps on two curved blocks mounted on a platform

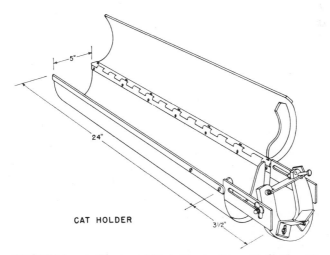

FIGURE 1.   A diagram of the holder used to restrain the cats.

constructed so that the cat holder could be placed close to the part of the box containing the light sources and camera lens. Adjustments of the platform in vertical and horizontal position were possible, and the right eye of the cat could be located directly in front of the camera lens. As shown in Fig. 1, the second yoke was movable so that the cat's neck could be stretched and the head tilted at an angle. Also, the pivoted metal bar on the top of the second yoke could be lowered and secured behind the cat's head. Cats of several sizes could be firmly held in the second yoke by this bar. In general, the cats did not submit to the restraint for more than 15 min. This duration, however, was sufficient for the study.

The CS was a 1000 cps tone approximately 55 db. above human threshold generated by a commercial oscillator. It was 3.5 sec. long and was delivered through two earphones, one phone positioned 3.5 in. directly in front of each pinna.

The US was either light offset or a combination of light offset and electric shock. When the shock was to be part of the US pattern, it was applied to the cat's tail. Two concentric areas separated by 3.0 in. were cut free of hair, and copper electrodes coated with EKG paste were fastened to these areas. The average intensity of the 60 cps shock was 4.0 v., and it lasted for 2.0 sec.

Procedure.   A delayed-conditioning presentation was used with the CS preceding the US by 1.5 sec. and terminating with the offset of the US. The intertrial interval was selected from a preselected random list of five durations averaging 1.0 min. During some intertrial periods, a cat would struggle and the intertrial would be longer than scheduled. Each of the six cats was given the same preliminary and experimental training. About a week before the formal experiment was to begin, each cat was brought up to the experimental room and set free to wander about. Before it was returned to its cage, it was placed in the holder for a short period of time.

On the first experimental day, only adaptation trials were presented. On each of the 7 days, each cat was given 10 trials. Two or three trials would be test trials and the remainder would be conditioning trials in which the CS was followed by the US. The extinction series was started on the eighth day. The order of trials was given according to a prearranged schedule and was the same for all *S*s.

Two *E*s were always present during an experimental period. One *E* operated the switches controlling the equipment, and the other held the cat's lids open. The *E* who held the eyelids open separated them many times during the intertrial interval as well as before the CS was presented. This, of course, was done so that the cat would not become conditioned to *E*'s hand. Before the start of the first trial of each day, a millimeter ruler was aligned with the iris of the cat and photographed. If the cat moved between trials, the precedure was repeated.

Two groups of three *S*s each were given different US. Group I had shock and light offset paired, and Group II had light offset alone as the

US. After the extinction phase was completed, two Ss of Group II were given conditioning trials again but with the US provided Group I.

RESULTS.   To obtain a quantitive estimate of pupil change, the diameter across the major axis of the pupil was measured on every other frame for all adaptation, test, and extinction trials. Skipping alternate frames was done to lessen the task of reading the films and effectively treats the records as though the camera speed were 8 frames/sec. (The films were also projected as motion pictures to permit additional inspection of the activity of the iris. It was for this purpose that the camera speed was set at 16 frames/sec.) An index of anticipatory pupillary change was obtained by subtracting the mean of the first two measured diameters from the mean of the largest measured consecutive diameters during the 1.5-sec. CS-US interval. Maximum pupillary change was computed in the same manner as above except the two largest diameters were chosen from the frames photographed during the 3.5-sec. CS period on test trials. Both measures yielded essentially the same results. For this presentation, anticipatory responses recorded on trials without a US were selected as the primary index of pupillary change.

The anticipatory PDRs obtained during the last six adaptation trials and all acquisition trials are shown in Fig. 2. During the adaptation period, both Group I (shock US) and Group II (nonshock US) showed essentially the same average responsiveness to the CS.

After 52 trials with the paired CS-US, only Group I, the US shock animals, appeared to be modified. All three Ss of this group manifested increasing pupillary dilation to the CS alone with successive training trials

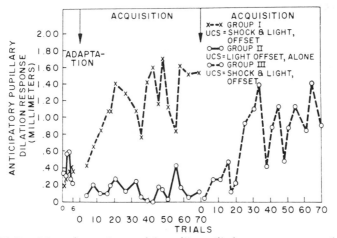

FIGURE 2.   Adaptation and test-trial pupillary dilation responses recorded in two groups that had different US. (After 70 trials, shock was added to the US given to Group II.)

until a level of responsiveness was reached which far exceeded that elicited by the CS during the adaptation trials. Group II Ss, on the other hand, did not exhibit any consistent dilation tendency to the CS as a result of presenting it for 52 trials paired with the US of light offset. The level of responsiveness of the iris of these Ss was slightly below that recorded during the adaptation series. After this first acquisition series, two Ss from Group II were given the same number of conditioning trials as previously but shock was incorporated as a part of the US. As indicated by the last curve in Fig. 2, these animals exhibited increased pupillary dilation to the CS with training and soon exceeded the level evoked during either the adaptation period or the previous conditioning trials when the US consisted of light offset alone. The same results, but to a more obvious degree, were obtained when the maximum pupillary diameters were measured. There was modification when the US contained shock but none when it was omitted. An extinction series of 14 trials was given both groups after the first conditioning series. Group II Ss, as would be expected, responded the same as they had during acquisition. In Group I, the CS was followed by a large dilation of the pupil on all 14 trials. Thus, no extinction tendency was obtained as a result of 14 consecutive omissions of the US.

A comment might be made on the irregularities in the performance curves in Fig. 2 since they reflect one of the difficulties of the index of conditioning used in this study. The extent of dilation that occurs is dependent not only on the effects of the training procedure, but also upon the resting diameter of the pupil present immediately before the onset of the CS. If, at this time, the diameter of the pupil is large, then the dilation change that can be evoked by the CS is limited. In this study, the time of presentation of the CS followed a prearranged schedule. It might have been better to wait until the pupil was relatively constricted before presenting the CS. This procedure was not followed because it might have led to biased results. Some type of transformation of the pupillary dilation score which would compensate for the relationship between basal level and possible dilation needs to be devised. If such a transformation were available and used with the present data, several irregularities in the obtained functions might have been eliminated.

EXPERIMENT 2

METHOD. *Subjects.*   Three female cats approximately 2 yr. old were used. They had lived in the laboratory less than 3 mo. These Ss were not as accustomed to the Es as those in the first study.

Apparatus.   The apparatus was the same as that described above except it was not necessary to secure the S in the restraining tube when it was paralyzed. A Harvard respirator operating at 22 strokes/min provided artificial respiration for the cats. Oxygen was given occasionally to the Ss to overcome initial anoxia.

Procedure. Flaxedil was selected as the curariform drug since it has been reported to have few undesirable side effects (Riker and Wescoe, 1951). Its primary known untoward action is a vagolytic action upon the heart. About 10 min. before Flaxedil was to be injected, cyclaine hydrochloride was sprayed on the tongue and in the pharynx region. This drug immobilized the tongue and desensitized the general area. Shortly after spraying, less than 10 cc of procaine was injected into the subcutaneous areas of the left forelimb of the cat. The cephalic vein was occluded above the elbow and two-thirds the normal paralytic dosage of Flaxedil injected into it. Within 20 sec. the cat usually became limp and would start gasping for air. The mouth was quickly opened, the tongue withdrawn, and the tip of the blade of a baby laryngoscope placed at the point of attachment of the epiglottis. The blade was depressed slighty so that the epiglottis no longer covered the larynx, enabling a catheter to be inserted into the trachea. Artificial respiration was commenced immediately after the catheter was in place.

Once artificial respiration was available to the cat, an additional 2.0 mg/kg of Flaxedil was given to the animal. If there were any evocable responses or detectable twitches, another 1.0 mg/kg of Flaxedil was injected. Before S was placed in the holder, air was blown into the pinna and eye, electric shock delivered to the tail, the surface of the skin pinched, and the legs were stretched. If there were no reactions to these stimuli, the cat was prepared for photography. Throughout the training procedure, the cats were carefully observed for any type of movements. In one cat, the vibrissae were seen to twitch slightly during the conditioning series and an additional 1.0 mg/kg was administered to it before continuing with the presentation of the stimuli.

The training procedure was identical for two Ss. On the first day, adaptation trials were given to the Ss while they were Flaxedilized. The second day they were not drugged and another adaptation series was presented. On Days 3 and 4 the Ss were drugged and conditioning was started. The experimental stimuli and intervals were identical to those in Experiment 1. The US consisted of a light offset paired with an electric shock adjusted to evoke a pupillary dilation response. The extinction phase was given on Day 5, when the Ss were not paralyzed. Both Ss had 18 adaptation, 21 conditioning, 8 test, and 20 extinction trials. The nondrug adaptation series was omitted for the third S. It also had a longer conditioning series than the other two Ss.

RESULTS.   The anticipatory dilation responses recorded from the two Ss that had the same experimental treatment and the third S that did not have a nondrug adaptation series, are shown in Figs. 3 and 4, respectively.

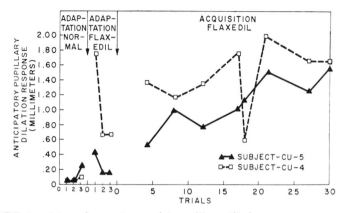

FIGURE 3.   Adaptation and test-trial pupillary dilation responses recorded from two Ss while they were paralyzed by Flaxedil.

It can be seen from an inspection of Fig. 3 that the responsiveness of the iris during adaptation series was greater under the drugged than nondrug condition. But it appears that there was a rapid diminution in the amplitude of the response to the CS during the adaptation series. With successive pairing of the CS with the US during the conditioning series, it appeared to evoke a progressively greater amplitude of the PDR. In general, the performance curves of these two drugged Ss are similar to those found for nondrugged Ss.

The third S was given 70 conditioning trials and according to its performance curve, shown in Fig. 4, the magnitude of the evoked anticipatory PDRs still varied considerably at the end of this prolonged series. How-

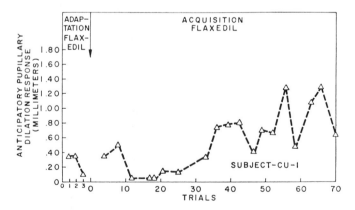

FIGURE 4.   Adaptation and test-trial pupillary dilation responses recorded from one S paralyzed by Flaxedil.

ever, even in this *S* the probability that the CS would evoke a PDR greater than that recorded during the adaptation trials increased during the conditioning series.

EXPERIMENT 3

METHOD. *Subjects and procedure.* Four of the six *S*s used in the first experiment were given a series of 30 reconditioning trials. The day following the reconditioning series, they were paralyzed by Flaxedil and given 20 extinction trials. The three *S*s that were conditioned under Flaxedil were returned to the experimental situation the following day and given 20 extinction trials when they were in their normal, nondrugged condition. In both groups, only 12 of the 20 extinction trials were photographed.

RESULTS.   The magnitude of the extinction responses recorded in both the paralyzed and normal *S*s is shown in Fig. 5 along with the mean of the last three PDRs measured during the previous adaptation and conditioning series. The mean diameter of the PDR evoked by the CS during the adaptation and reconditioning series of the four normal *S*s is shown by the open circles. During extinction, when these animals were drugged, the mean PDR evoked by the CS was considerably larger, as indicated by the solid circles, than that recorded during the reconditioning trials. The initial magnitude of these extinction responses approximately corre-

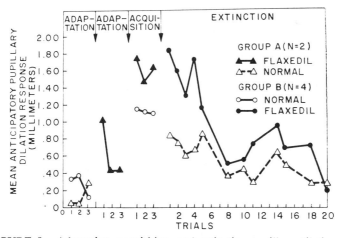

FIGURE 5.   Adaptation, acquisition, and extinction pupillary dilation responses recorded from *S*s either given conditioning trials while normal and extinction trials while paralyzed by Flaxedil or conditioning trials while paralyzed and extinction trials while normal.

sponds to that exhibited by the two drugged *S*s during their last conditioning trials. With successive presentations of the CS alone, there was a progressive decrease in the diameter of the evoked PDR, indicating that extinction was occurring. These data suggest that the PDR conditioned in normal *S*s could be evoked when they are paralyzed by Flaxedil. The rate of extinction of this response, however, is considerably greater than that found when both acquisition and extinction occurs in the nondrugged condition.

The *S*s conditioned while paralyzed by Flaxedil exhibited considerably smaller PDRs to the CS, as shown in Fig. 5, when it was presented to them in their normal state. These responses, however, were initially greater than those recorded during the last adaptation while these *S*s were either normal or paralyzed. Hence, capacity of the CS to evoke the PDR acquired while the *S*s were paralyzed by Flaxedil appears to be maintained to some extent when the *S*s recovered from the paralytic action of the drug.

DISCUSSION

Although either a painful stimulus such as an electric shock or a decrease in illumination could serve as a US for evoking the PDR, results from an experiment using human *S*s (Gerall *et al.*, 1957) indicated that the PDR could be conditioned only to the CS paired with the US containing shock. In the present investigation, cats were used as *S*s, and again no consistent dilation tendency to the CS was found when the US was a decrease in illumination. When the US contained shock, the CS paired with it readily gained the capacity to evoke the PDR. It is concluded, therefore, that the stimulus conditions sufficient for establishing conditioned pupillary dilation responses are similar in human *S*s and the cat.

In the second part of the present study an attempt was made to condition cats paralyzed by Flaxedil. In general, the CS after pairing with a US evoked dilation responses in the *S*s that were greater than the responses elicited before training. Also, the magnitude of the dilation response elicited by the CS increased as the conditioning series progressed. Because no pseudoconditioning control groups were used, it is not possible to state that all the recorded dilation responses were CRs. But if it is accepted that some of the dilation responses were evoked by the CS because of the pairing of the CS and US, then the results have some relevance to the status of the artifact hypothesis (Smith, 1954). Although striate-muscle groups including the extrinsic muscles of the eyes, which to our knowledge could influence the pupillary response, were paralyzed, the efficacy of the CS to evoke dilation increased with training. The results are interpreted, therefore, as not supporting the hypothesis that responses innervated by the autonomic nervous system cannot be directly modified by the classical conditioning method.

In the third part of the present study, Ss conditioned under Flaxedil were extinguished without the drug and Ss conditioned in their normal state were extinguished with Flaxedil. Investigations of the effect of curariform drugs such as B-erythroidine and raw curare showed that the CR could only be evoked by the CS when the Ss were in the state, drugged or nondrugged, under which they had been conditioned (Culler and Girden, 1937; Girden, 1942a, 1942b). In the present study, the pupillary response could be evoked by the CS in paralyzed and nondrugged Ss regardless of their state when they were conditioned. Recent conditioning experiments using another curariform agent, d-tubocurarine chloride, by Lauer (1951) and Black (1958) also have not reported dissociation of CRs. Additional investigation will be required to determine what properties of the earlier curariform drugs produced the dissociation of CRs. The data presently available can be interpreted to indicate that the dissociation effect was not due to the curariform properties of curare or of B-erythroidine but to their other actions on the central nervous system.

Additional research is also required to delineate the characteristics of the pupillary response of the Flaxedilized cats. In the present study, the iris showed greater than normal reactivity when the cats were paralyzed. In general, the resting level of the pupil was narrower and fluctuated less in the paralyzed animals. It is our judgment, with due regard to the limitation placed on the observations by the small number of Ss and few variations in the experimental conditions employed, that Flaxedil provides a useful agent for restricting movement and thereby facilitating certain types of studies of autonomic responses.

SUMMARY

The purpose of this study was to examine several variables that might influence the conditioning of the PDR of cats. First, the relative efficacy of two types of US was investigated. The results indicated that a CS acquired the capacity to evoked the PDR when it was paired with a US containing electric shock but not with one consisting only of a decrease in illumination. Since conditioning of the PDR was also found in human Ss with a US containing shock, it appears that the stimulus conditions sufficient for establishing conditioned PDRs are similar in both human and cat Ss. Secondly, an attempt was made to condition the PDR of three cats that had their skeletal muscles paralyzed by Flaxedil, a curariform drug. All Ss exhibited a systematic change of the pupil to the CS as the training proceeded. These results were interpreted as indicating that conditioning of the PDR, which is an autonomically innervated response, can occur without skeletal-muscle participation. Lastly, extinction of the conditioned PDR was observed in four Flaxedilized cats conditioned originally while uninfluenced by this drug and in three nondrugged cats conditioned previously while paralyzed. The PDR was evoked by the CS during extinction whether or not the *S*s were paralyzed during the conditioning series. Thus, Flaxedil was not found to possess a dissociation effect upon the PDR reported for some types of curariform drugs.

REFERENCES

Black, A. H. The extinction of avoidance responses under curare. *J. comp. physiol. Psychol.*, 1958, **51**, 519–524.

Gerall, A. A., Sampson, P. B., and Boslov, G. L. Classical conditioning of human pupillary dilation. *J. exp. Psychol.*, 1957, **54**, 467–474.

Girden, E. The dissociation of pupillary conditioned reflexes under erythroidine and curare. *J. exp. Psychol.*, 1942, **31**, 322–332. (a)

Girden, E. Generalized conditioned responses under curare and erythroidine. *J. exp. Psychol.*, 1942, **31**, 105–119. (b)

Girden, E., and Culler, E. Conditioned responses in curarized striate muscle in dogs. *J. comp. Psychol.*, 1937, **23**, 261–274.

Harlow, H. F., and Toltzien, F. Formation of pseudo-conditioned response in the learning process. *J. exp. Psychol.*, 1933, **16**, 283–294.

Harlow, H. F., and Toltzien, F. Foramation of pseudo-conditioned response in the cat. *J. gen. Psychol.*, 1940, **23**, 367–375.

Lauer, D. W. The role of the motor responses in learning. Unpublished doctoral dissertation, University of Michigan, 1951.

Riker, W. F., and Wescoe, W. C. The pharmacology of Flaxedil with observations on certain analogs. *Ann. N.Y. Acad. Sci.*, 1951, **54**, 373–394.

Smith, K. Conditioning as an artifact. *Psychol. Rev.*, 1954, **61**, 226–234.

Part II OPERANT CONDITIONING

Operant behavior is controlled by an array of antecedent variables, current circumstances, characteristics of the response, and response-consequence variables. A drug, therefore, can effect a change in operant behavior by interacting with any of these factors. Such an interaction can be viewed as a behavioral mechanism of drug action. Of the following sections, Section A is introductory and Sections B–F deal with each of the classes of factors.

INTRODUCTION

Behavioral pharmacology was born out of necessity during the early 1950's when numerous drug manufactures sought behavioral preparations for predicting clinical efficacy of drugs. The period 1950–1955 was marked by a growing number of publications reporting that a given drug "affected behavior." A small number of investigators recognized that it was not enough to show that drugs could change behavior. More serious efforts to relate behavioral effects of drugs to general principles of behavioral control were required. Among the first systematic explorations of the role of behavioral variables in drug action was a series of experiments initiated by Dews in 1955. These and related studies by Sidman in 1955 and Brady in 1956 led to the publication of several papers representing the methodological foundation of behavioral pharmacology. Numbered among the most significant of these papers are Dews' "Analysis of Effects of Psychopharmacological Agents in Behavioral Terms" (Article 8) and Sidman's "Behavioral Pharmacology" (Article 9). These papers, reproduced in this volume, provide a fitting introduction to the papers that follow.

8

Analysis of effects of psychopharmacological agents in behavioral terms [1]

PETER B. DEWS

Neuropharmacology is concerned with effects of drugs on nervous tissue; psychopharmacology is concerned with the effects of drugs on the behavior of a more or less intact animal. There is an area where the two sciences meet and correlations are sought and it is, of course, no accident that neuropharmacologists and psychopharmacologists tend to be interested in the same sorts of drugs. Nevertheless, the distinction between neuro- and psychopharmacology will probably continue to be useful in the foreseeable future. The aim of this contribution is to show by example how psychopharmacology qualifies as a basic medical science.

The great increase of interest in psychopharmacology during the last few years has not been due to the formulations of new theories or the impact of cogent arguments. It has been due mainly to the remarkable success which experimental pharmacologists and observant clinicians have had in discovering new drugs with hitherto unsuspected kinds of effects on behavior. This success has made it extremely important that a basic science of psychopharmacology should develop as fast as possible. Only by fundamental studies can we hope to achieve a coherent understanding of these drugs and, incidentally, to learn how to use them to best advantage. Much information is already available, but it is mostly unsystematic and fragmentary (1).

The first difficulty facing experimental psychopharmacology is the complexity of behavior. Physiology is complicated too, yet it has been found that an understanding of the effects of a drug on the physiology of an animal can be attained if the effects are studied system by system, even cell by cell. It would seem reasonable to study the effects of drugs on behavior in a similarly analytical way. One method of doing so is to follow Skinner (2) and to study the frequency of occurrence of a "given" response. Many of the things an animal or man can do may be chosen and designated as the "response." (The word "response" is used in the sense prevalent among psychologists; it means simply "a bit of behavior" and does not imply an identifiable eliciting stimulus. A "response" need not be

From *Federation Proceedings,* 1958, **17,** 1024–1030. Copyright 1958 by the Federation of American Societies for Experimental Biology, Bethesda, Md.

[1] Some of the work described in this paper was supported by grants from the Public Health Service (M-1226 and M-2094) and from Burroughs Wellcome & Co., Inc.

a response "to" something; it may be emitted "spontaneously.") For convenience a response is chosen whose occurrences can be recorded objectively; and also for convenience, one that the animal can make repeatedly —can make a large number of times during a reasonable period of time. Then, the factors which determine the distribution of occurrences of the response in time can be studied. Examples of actual responses which fulfill these criteria, and have been studied, are: rats pressing a lever or nuzzling a plastic key or licking water from a bottle; dogs pressing a panel; primates —monkeys, chimpanzees, man—pressing push buttons of various kinds.

In the great majority of studies, the only dependent variable has been the distribution of occurrences of the selected response in time; no attempt has been made to measure all behavior simultaneously; even the response as such is taken for granted, and only its occurrences noted. It is suggested that this type of deliberate restrictiveness is desirable if not essential in basic psychopharmacology at this stage of its development. Why is it, that when somebody learns how to study a single nerve cell or a single renal tubule or to isolate a single enzyme everyone (rightly) says "Bravo"; but when attempts are made to isolate functional units of behavior for study many people say "Ah, but you are neglecting all other concurrent behavior and therefore your results are meaningless"? Surely, in both situations a sufficient justification for the line of study is the help it gives in understanding the total organism.

Already many drugs have been shown to influence the rates with which animals, including man, makes responses of the kinds described. The effects of a given dose of a drug depend on 4 classes of factors: (1) What the animal is; the species chosen and the particular individual chosen. All genetic factors fall into this category. (2) What the animal is doing; (a) the nature of the response chosen for study and (b) the frequency with which it is occurring under control conditions. (3) What the environment is doing to the animal; the eliciting, reinforcing, and discriminative stimuli playing on the animal. It is convenient to include in this class "self-engendered" stimuli. (4) What has happened to the animal in the past; the nature of training to which the animal has been exposed, and also previous administrations of drugs leading to the possibilities of adaptation, tolerance or cumulation.

An example of a drug effect on behavior is the effect of methamphetamine in the following experiments. A pigeon is maintained on a regime of partial food deprivation. After appropriate training, it is given access to a piece of translucent plastic, the key, for several hours a day (3, 4). Periodically, a light comes on behind the key. When it has been on for some fixed period, such as 15 minutes, the bird can get access to food for 4 seconds by giving a single peck to the key; that is, by responding once. The key light goes out when food is presented; it comes on again sometime later and the whole cycle can be repeated indefinitely. A characteristic performance engendered by this schedule is shown in Fig. 1. When the light is not on the pigeon never pecks. When the light comes on, the pigeon still does not peck for a time; there is then a period of progressively increasing rate of pecking to a rate which is maintained until a peck produces the food at the end of 15 minutes. This performance is probably not what would have been expected intuitively, which is one of the reasons it was chosen as an illustration. These curves should be taken at their face value; do not sit in judgment of the intelligence of the pigeon. They should be treated, for example, with the same detached objectivity as an infrared absorption spectrum; one would not try to put oneself in the place of a molecule being irradiated to decide which wave lengths one would expect to be absorbed!

The effects of a rather large dose of methamphetamine on this performance are shown in the lower part of Fig. 1. The difference between the

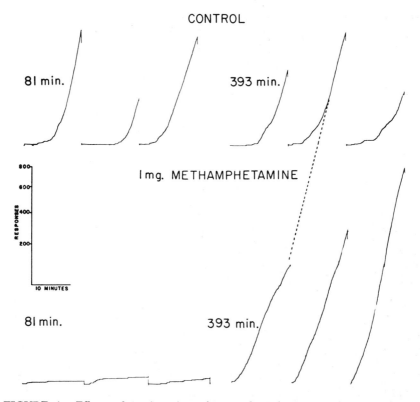

FIGURE 1. Effects of methamphetamine on fixed interval performance in the pigeon. *Ordinate:* cumulative number of responses. *Abscissa:* time with key light on. The pen resets to the base line at each reinforcement. The figure shows samples of the performance at two periods during the daily session. Note the initial "depressive" effect of the large dose of methamphetamine. The dotted line was added to show that the maximum rate following methamphetamine did not exceed the maximum control rate.

effects at 81 minutes and at 393 minutes is due to a change in the effective concentration of the drug; it is the later effect which is of main interest. The biphasic effect is shown here to emphasize the necessity of exploring along the dose effect curve before any reliable statement about a drug effect can be made.

The characteristic effect of methamphetamine is to lead to an increase in the number of responses made per interval. But the maximum rate of responding is not increased (Fig. 1); what happens is that the animal responds steadily at the beginning of the interval at a time when, under control conditions, there is little or no responding.

There is, of course, no more *a priori* reason why studies on pigeons pecking should help us understand human behavior than there is that studies on squid axons or crayfish stretch receptors or even cats' cortices should help us understand human nerves or receptors or synapses. In all cases, direct evidence of generality is needed. Fixed interval performance does, in fact, seem to be a phenomenon of some generality (Fig. 2). The general pattern of the performance (no responding, then acceleration, then maintained steady rate) remains recognizably similar as the parameter of the schedule varies over a considerable range. Similar performances are found in other species—rat and chimpanzee—and for different specific responses—pressing a level with paw or fingers or nuzzling a key—and for different kinds of deprivation and reinforcement—viz, water instead of food. Finally, Holland (5) has shown that a similar performance emerges when a man presses a push button under fixed interval contingencies. While these performances are not necessarily identical, the differences between them are much less than the change which can be caused by administration of a drug in any one of the situations.

The effects of the amphetamines have now been studied in a variety of species on a variety of responses under a variety of conditions. The following generalization seems warranted. If responses are occurring infrequently or intermittently, appropriate doses of the amphetamines lead to an increase in rate of occurrence. If a response is occurring steadily, then the amphetamines do not cause an increase in rate (even though the animal is physically capable of a several-fold increase in rate). This statement is based on the following evidence:

1. Dose effect curves for methamphetamine have been obtained in pigeons working under 4 different schedules of reinforcement (6). Two of these schedules gave rise to steady responding; methamphetamine had no appreciable effect on these performances until large doses were given (when the effect was to decrease responding). The other two schedules engendered intermittent responding; in these, methamphetamine caused a considerable increase in over-all rate.

2. Very low rates of responding in pigeons can be brought about by delay of reinforcement following a response. Methamphetamine caused increase in rate in this situation (7).

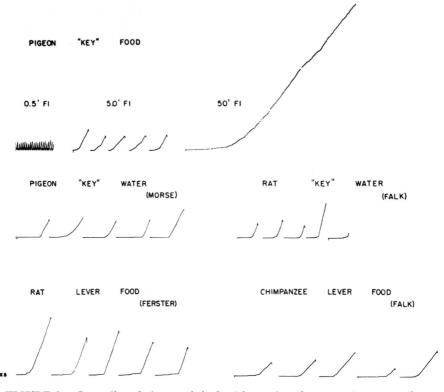

FIGURE 2. Generality of characteristic fixed interval performance (no responding then acceleration then maintained steady rate). A fixed interval schedule of positive reinforcement was in operation in all examples shown in this figure. *Upper row:* pigeon pecking plastic disk (key) for food. Three different lengths of fixed interval are shown, illustrating that the general pattern persists despite the 100-fold change in the schedule parameter. *Middle row:* pigeon pecking key and rat operating similar key with snout; both for water reinforcement. *Bottom row:* rat pressing lever with front paw or paws and chimpanzee pressing lever with fingers; both for food. Note generality of characteristic form of fixed interval performance. (I am grateful to Drs. Morse, Falk and Ferster for providing me with the examples indicated.)

3. Sidman (8) has studied rats pressing a lever to postpone an electric shock and Teitelbaum (9) has studied rats licking water from a bottle, also to postpone an electric shock. In both these situations, after a response or group of responses, there is a period during which the rat rarely responds. In both these situations amphetamine caused a considerable increase in rate. Under control conditions, in Teitelbaum's situation, the animal responds (licks) so infrequently that he receives many shocks. Following amphetamine, for a considerable period the animal got very few shocks, so in this case the amphetamine made the behavior *more* "appropriate."

4. The effects of amphetamines have been studied on a variety of schedules in which periods without a response were a condition for reinforcement (so-called "DRL" schedules). On these schedules, some specified interval (usually of the order of several seconds) must elapse between responses if a response is to lead to food, water, etc. Responding occurs relatively infrequently on these schedules under control conditions, although under many circumstances, usually too frequently for more than a small proportion of the potential number of reinforcements to occur. In pigeons, following the amphetamines, the frequency of responses increased while the frequency of reinforcements decreased. In this case the behavior became less "appropriate." Although the form of the distribution of inter-response times differs in the pigeon and man, the effects of the amphetamines are similar (Fig. 3) (10). Sidman (11) has demonstrated a similar effect in rats.

In conclusion, the effects of amphetamines seem to be determined largely (but, of course, not exclusively) by the frequency of occurrence of the response (class 2*b* determinant in the scheme presented above); the effects are generally similar irrespective of species, nature of response,

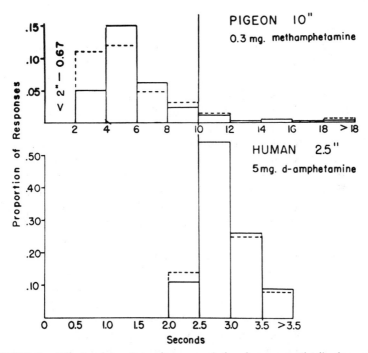

FIGURE 3. Effects of amphetamines on relative frequency distributions of inter-response times. In the pigeons, the 10th response following a previous response by not less than 10 seconds was reinforced. In the humans, the 100th response following a previous response by not less than 2.5 seconds was reinforced. The solid line shows the control performance and the dotted line the performance after the designated dose of drug. Note the much greater tendency of the birds than the men to respond "too soon" under the conditions of these experiments, but the similarity of the effects of the amphetamines in the two situations (movement of the distribution to the left).

motivation, appropriateness of the performance, etc. This general statement agrees well with clinical descriptions of the effects of these drugs.

In contrast, many of the effects of chlorpromazine seem to be determined by class 3 effects. Chlorpromazine seems to weaken the control which some stimuli have over behavior. An example of this is the effect of chlorpromazine on a multiple schedule controlled performance in the pigeon (3, 12). Pigeons receive food for every 50th peck made when a red light is behind the key, but for a response only when 15 minutes has elapsed (fixed interval) when a blue light is behind the key. When the red light is on, the pigeon pecks continually at a high rate; when the blue is on, a more or less characteristic fixed interval performance is seen (Fig. 4). When a dose of chlorpromazine was given, the difference between the performances in the presence of the two stimuli became less (Fig. 4); it was as though the stimuli had become less different.

The effects of chlorpromazine in this regard could be mimicked by making the stimuli more alike—in fact, indistinguishable—by simply having both red and blue lights on all the time during a whole single session. There is a clear resemblance of the performance on this day to the performance after chlorpromazine.

Perhaps one of the best known effects of chlorpromazine on experimental animals, the so-called effects on conditioned versus unconditioned reflexes, is really an example of an effect on stimulus control (13). In these experiments a rat is trained to climb a pole when a buzzer sounds to avoid receiving an electric shock through the grid floor. Chlorpromazine leads to the rat failing to climb the pole when the buzzer sounds, though it still does so when the shock comes. Climbing the pole to the shock is regarded as an unconditioned response; but after a few trials, surely the response to the shock in the form in which it is executed must be largely conditioned. The first time an animal is exposed to the shock it usually shows a very obvious motor response, but this consists of more or less "random" movements. Only after a number of exposures does the animal come to escape from the shock by an immediate jump to the pole; thus this is, by definition, a conditioned response. That the shock can elicit unconditioned responses is no reason for supposing that all responses to the shock must be unconditioned. The differential effect of chlorpromazine must thus be based on the functions of the buzzer and shock as discriminant stimuli; even when attenuated by chlorpromazine, the shock is such an overwhelming stimulus that it still increases the tendency of the rat to climb sufficiently so that it climbs in a large proportion of the trials.

Most of the clinically described effects of chlorpromazine—loss of initiative and reactivity, reduction of tension and compulsiveness, etc.—can be translated into terms of stimulus control. But mere change of terminology does not necessarily contribute much to an understanding of the drug. If it is accepted that a main action of chlorpromazine is on stimu-

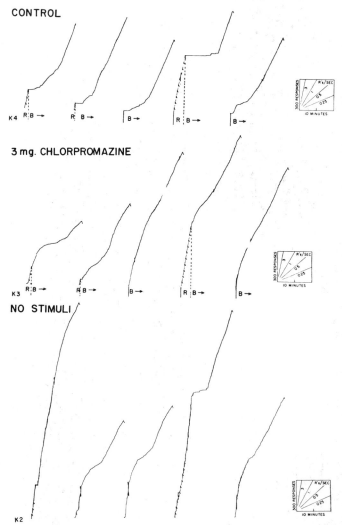

FIGURE 4.   Studies on multiple schedule performance. Each row shows the record of a single complete day's session of the same bird. The record on each row is continuous and has been arranged as shown only for convenience. In the *upper* and *middle rows* the letters R and B indicate the times when red and blue lights respectively were behind the key. When the red light was on, each 50th response was reinforced (shown by small diagonal hatch mark); whein the blue light was on the first response after 15 minutes was reinforced. In the *bottom row* for the first time, both red and blue lights were on throughout the session, although the sequence of reinforcement contingencies was as in previous days.

lus control, this is only the beginning of the full description of the behavioral effects of the drug. The next question is—is the control of all kinds of stimuli equally weakened by chlorpromazine? The fact that the pigeon continued to respond at much the same over-all rate following chlorpromazine in the experiments described earlier suggests that the control of stimuli occasioning responding was not affected by chlorpromazine. In other experiments, on a modified fixed interval type performance, chlorpromazine had but a slight effect on total numbers of responses made over the complete dosage range studied (a hundred-fold range of doses) (14). Clearly the control over behavior of certain types of environmental stimuli (such as, perhaps, reinforcing stimuli) is not readily modified by chlorpromazine. Many experiments are currently in progress to characterize more specifically the behavioral effects of chlorpromazine. A case in point is the recent series of experiments by Blough (15) in which he has shown that chlorpromazine "helps" a pigeon stand still. Perhaps chlorpromazine reduces the tendency of environmental stimuli generally to lead to behavior incompatible with standing still; but many other possibilities remain to be explored.

It is hoped that the following conclusions will be drawn from the preceding discussion: (1) A great deal can be said about the psychological effects of drugs in an entirely objective framework. (2) Even taking a fairly simple situation—one in which the only observed variable is the occurrence of a "given" response—a start can be made towards a systematic description of drug effects. In proceeding thus, it is not necessary to make assumptions about what animals are thinking or feeling. By and large, intuition is proving a misleading guide in sorting out the complexities in this area, and probably the fastest progress will be made if empathy with either experimental animals or even human subjects is avoided.

Although the preceding discussion has been limited to psychopharmacology, this does not bespeak a lack of interest in neuropharmacology. On the contrary, I would like to suggest that proper use of the common element of pharmacology in psychopharmacology and neuropharmacology may give extremely useful information, not only on drugs, but also on the relations between psychology and neurophysiology. It may well be that many "obvious" features of behavior for which neurophysiological explanations are currently being sought will turn out to be chimera; for example, some of the "emotions" may prove to be as useless as scientific concepts as the humors of the ancients are to the biochemists of today. The neurophysiologist may be misled by what he supposes to be incontrovertible psychology. On the other hand, neuropharmacologists and psychopharmacologists can pursue their rigorous studies independently; though, being good friends, they watch one another's progress with interest. The mere fact that they study the same drugs inevitably provides points of correspondence between the two systems; and one may confidently expect that clear and unforced correlations will emerge of an altogether higher order of generality than the ad hoc fragmentary hypotheses of today.

REFERENCES

1. Wikler, A. *The relation of psychiatry to pharmacology*. Baltimore: Williams & Wilkins, 1957.
2. Skinner, B. F. *The behavior of organisms*. New York: Appleton-Century-Crofts, 1938.
3. Ferster, C. B., and Skinner, B. F. *Schedules of reinforcement*. New York: Appleton-Century-Crofts, 1957.
4. Dews, P. B. *J. Pharmacol. & Exper. Therap.* 113:393, 1955.
5. Holland, J. G. *Science* 125:348, 1957.
6. Dews, P. B. *J. Pharmacol. & Exper. Therap.* 122:137, 1958.
7. Dews, P. B. *J. Pharmacol. & Exper. Therap.* 119:141, 1957.
8. Sidman, M. *New York Acad. Sci.* 65:282, 1956.
9. Teitelbaum, P. *J. Comp. Physiol. Psychol.* 51:801, 1958.
10. Dews, P. B. *J. Pharmacol. & Exper. Therap.* 122:18A, 1958.
11. Sidman, M. *Science* 122:925, 1955.
12. Dews, P. B. *New York Acad. Sci.* 65:268, 1956.
13. Cook, L., and Weidley, E. *New York Acad. Sci.* 66:740, 1957.
14. Dews, P. B. *J. exp. anal. Behav.* 1:73, 1958.
15. Blough, D. S. *Science* 127:586, 1958.

9

Behavioral pharmacology

MURRAY SIDMAN

Pharmacologic agents that exercise effects upon behavior have been known since antiquity. But intensive and systematic efforts to investigate the relations between drugs and behavior have only recently begun. A major factor contributing to the slowness of development of a science of Behavioral Pharmacology was the late recognition that behavior is a phenomenon amenable to study by the methods of Natural Science. The overt behavioral effects of drugs were disguised, in conformity with general psychological practice, by such terms as "alertness," "stimulation," "euphoria," "sedation," and, more recently, "tranquilizing." These and other supposedly descriptive terms provided a catchall classificatory scheme in which to deposit a bewildering variety of behavioral observations. They served to impose a beguiling but false veneer of simplicity upon the behavioral changes associated with the administration of chemical agents. Behavior disorders are difficult enough to describe at the human level, and in animals, with which we share neither a common verbal intercourse nor a common behavioral topography, a description in terms of the traditional classfications is virtually impossible. It is apparent that the less precise our behavioral specification, the less precise will be our knowledge of the relations between drugs and behavior. Furthermore, decreased descriptive precision will inevitably be accompanied by increased claims for the effectiveness of a given drug in influencing behavior.

The advent of tranquilizing drugs, accompanied by assertions that they serve to ameliorate behavior disorders, has focussed attention upon the need for more precise specification of behavior and behavioral processes. This is particularly true at the preclinical level, where, fortunately, experimental psychology has produced some of its most striking developments in the past few decades. Behavioral Pharmacology, profiting from recent advances in both Psychology and Pharmacology, has now extended to the study of other types of drugs than tranquilizers, and employs an ever-widening range of behavioral techniques. An excellent historical summary of preclinical research on drug-behavior relationships has been provided by Brady (1956c) and this review will, therefore, be confined to recent developments.

From *Psychopharmacologia* (Berl.), 1959, 1, 1–19. Copyright 1959 by Springer-Verlag, Heidelberg, Germany.

OPERANT CONDITIONING TECHNIQUES. A basic requirement in the assessment of drug-behavior relationships is an experimental repertoire of reproducible behavioral baselines from which to measure drug-correlated changes. Furthermore, reproducibility in terms of averaged data from a group of experimental subjects is not sufficient. Because of the great quantitative variability in dose-response effects from one subject to another, averaged data are likely to obscure, or even falsify, the effects of a drug in the individual organism. Also, the use of statistical control in testing the effects of drugs implies a lack of experimental control over behavior that bodies ill for a program of research on such a complex subject-matter as drug-behavior relationships.

The most precise, sensitive, and reproducible techniques for controlling the behavior of the individual subject are those that have been developed over the past 25 years by B. F. Skinner, his co-workers, and others who have extended the techniques in various directions (Skinner, 1938; Ferster and Skinner, 1958; Brady and Hunt, 1955; Keller, 1941; Blough, 1955; Sidman, 1953; Guttman and Kalish, 1956; Ferster, 1953). The methods are based upon a simple principle; namely, that the characteristics of behavior are, to a large extent, determined by the environmental events that have been consequent upon past occurrences of the behavior. Behavior that operates upon the environment has been termed "operant behavior," and the process of manipulating such behavior by means of its environmental consequences has been termed, "operant conditioning" (Skinner, 1938). Reproducibility among subjects within a given species, and between species, has been enhanced by selecting, for measurement and manipulation, a response whose topography is congenial to the organism, and one that the organism can perform and immediately be in a position to repeat; by selecting an environmental consequence, or "reinforcement," that is appropriate to the particular individual; by limiting the experimental environment; and by utilizing motivational levels that are strong enough to override many experimentally irrelevant variables. For example: the subject may be a hungry pigeon, pecking at a lighted spot on the wall, and reinforced by a small amount of grain; or a thirsty rat may press a level, thereby obtaining a small drop of water; or a monkey may press a pedal, the consequence of which is postponement of shock. The object is not the study of eating or drinking behavior *per se,* or of pain. The purpose of these techniques is to place an arbitrary sample of behavior under experimental control so that *behavioral processes* may be investigated as a function of various operations.

Many types of behavioral baselines have been developed against which to measure the effects of pharmacologic agents. But before describing investigations that have been directed at the evaluation of specific drug-behavior relationships, it will be useful to examine some more general problems that arise whenever overt behavior is employed in an assay technique. These are the problems of general excitatory or depressant effects, motor debilitation, sensory deficit, and motivational effects. For example, if a given drug abolishes behavior whose function it has been to avoid an electric shock, can we draw the conclusion that the drug is specific to this type of behavior? Is it safe to classify the drug as an anxiety reducer? The possibility exists that the drug would have produced a depressant effect upon any type of behavior that had been used as a baseline. Or perhaps the subjects were so debilitated that all motor behavior was virtually impossible, thus invalidating any inference in terms of a particular type of behavior.

One method of meeting such problems has been to provide the experimental animal with a behavioral repertoire, any component of which can be elicited at any time. Then a given drug may be tested over a spectrum of behavior in the same animal at different times. An excellent example has been provided by Dews (1956), working with pigeons. In the procedure employed by Dews, two types of behavior were placed under stimulus control by means of a variant of Ferster and Skinner's "multiple schedule" technique. The birds were rewarded with grain for pecking at a lighted key. When the key was red, 60 pecks were required to produce the grain, and when the key was blue the bird was rewarded for the first peck made after 15 minutes had elapsed since the preceding reward. Thus there were two reward schedules employed. A *fixed ratio* of 60 pecks per reward was required in the presence of the red key. In the presence of the blue key, reward was based upon responses emitted after the passage of a *fixed interval* of time. Under appropriate deprivation conditions, the fixed ratio and fixed interval reward schedules typically generate markedly different rates and temporal patterns of responding, as is illustrated in section D of Fig. 1. On the fixed interval schedule there is no response at all at the beginning of the interval, and then there is accelerated responding up to receipt of the reward. The fixed ratio performance is characterized by high, sustained rates.

Figure 1 shows the time course of action of phenobarbital sodium, as reflected in the fixed ratio and fixed interval behavior. Three hours after injection (section A) there was almost no pecking behavior on the fixed interval schedule. While the fixed ratio behavior was severely disturbed, there was still a substantial output. It was thus economically demonstrated that the drug did not exercise a general depressive effect upon all behavior. Herrnstein and Morse (1956) have confirmed this finding with pentobarbital by means of an experimental arrangement in which the ratio and interval behavior were blended into a single, smooth performance. Sodium pentobarbital acted to fractionate this performance, selectively eliminating the fixed-interval behavior and leaving the rapid fixed-ratio component of the response rate untouched.

Sections B and C of Fig. 1 demonstrate a second method of determining

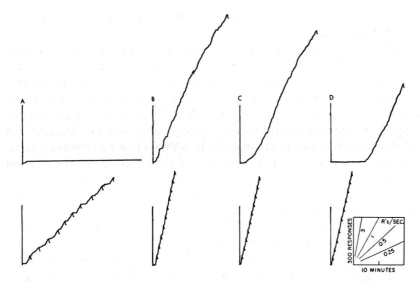

FIGURE 1.   The effects of phenobarbital on performance at various time intervals after injection. Responses are recorded cumulatively as a function of time. A = 18 hours after injection, B = 24 hours, C = 36 hours, and D = 48 hours. The upper series shows the interval behavior, and the lower series shows the corresponding ratio behavior. The performance in Section D is essentially normal. (From Dews, 1956)

the specificity of drug effects upon behavior. Section B, 24 hours after injection, shows a high rate of pecking on the fixed interval performance, but the temporal pattern of responding is markedly different from normal. The bird pecks irregularly throughout the whole interval, with no sign of the initial pause. The ratio behavior is essentially normal at this stage. Boren has reported a similar effect with benactyzine. On the fixed interval schedule, benactyzine allowed responding throughout the interval and, as a result, caused an over-all increased rate. Chlorpromazine decreased the over-all rate and somewhat lengthened the pause after reinforcement, while adiphenine produced no noticeable change. Herrnstein and Morse (1957) have reported a quantitative technique for measuring the curvature in the cumulative record of fixed-interval performance, and have shown that their "quarter-life" measure is sensitive to the effects of pharmacologic agents. These data demonstrate that a drug effect need not appear in the form of a simple depressant or excitatory action upon behavior. The consequence of drug administration may be a shift in the *pattern* of behavior, with over-all changes in response frequency only indirectly reflecting the new temporal pattern. When the consequence of drug administration is a change in the pattern of behavior, rather than an all-or-none depression or excitation, the problem of general debilitating effects is largely circumvented.

There are other dangers inherent in an approach to drug-behavior relationships that would take as its datum an all-or-none change in frequency or probability of occurrence of a response. Dews (1955a) has shown, for example, that pentobarbital may completely depress behavior on both fixed interval and fixed ratio reward schedules. But the dose-response curves are markedly different for the two types of behavior. Fixed-ratio performance is considerably more resistant to pentobarbital than is fixed-interval performance. A relatively low dose of pentobarbital that almost completely depresses fixed-interval behavior may actually increase the response rate on a fixed-ratio schedule. In addition to dose-response effects, there may be differences in the way various types of behavior are affected by a drug as a function of time. Figure 1 demonstrates that the apparent time course of action of phenobarbital is strongly modified by the reward schedule employed to maintain the baseline behavior. In evaluating the specificity of a drug effect, therefore, a family of dose-response curves, determined over a wide range of time intervals following drug administration, is the only sure method of preventing overgeneralization. There have, as yet, been few published studies that possess such a high degree of inclusiveness. Dews (1956), however, has suggested, on the basis of data that deal with the effects of phenobarbital and meth-amphetamine on behavior generated by multiple fixed interval-fixed ratio reward schedules, that the sequential changes at various time intervals following a single large dose of a drug are equivalent to those caused by graded doses at a constant-time interval. If further research proves this finding to be generalizable to other drugs and other types of behavior, the difficulties in studying drug-behavior relationships will be greatly reduced.

The possibility of sensory deficit, i.e., drug effects upon the discriminative capacity of the organism, is not only worthy of study for its pharmacologic implications, but also poses a technical problem when multiple procedures under stimulus control are employed to generate behavioral baselines. For example, Sidman (1956) reports an experiment in which a rat was trained to press a level for a water reward according to three reinforcement contingencies, each under stimulus control. When a clicking noise was presented, 10 lever presses were required to produce the reward. The typical high rate of responding was observed under this *fixed-ratio* schedule. If a tone was present, lever pressing responses were reinforced only when 30 seconds or more had elapsed since the preceding response. When *spaced responses* were thus required, the customary low rate of lever pressing (Wilson and Keller) was observed. When neither the tone nor the clicker was present, a *variable-interval* schedule was in effect, in which responses were rewarded at irregular time intervals. This schedule generated a rate of response intermediate between the fixed ratio and spaced responding performances. Administration of reserpine abolished the differential performance on the three schedules and brought the variable-interval and fixed-ratio rates down to the level normally maintained under the requirement of spaced responding. The problem now arises as to whether the drug affected only the ratio and interval behavior while leaving the spaced responding untouched, or whether the animal, under the influence of the drug, simply could no longer discriminate among the three stimulus conditions. One method of determining the answer to such a question is to obtain dose-response and time-course data. If the several types of behavior display different dose-response curves, or if the time course of action of the drug is different for each behavior, as was the case in Sidman's (1956) experiment, then the behavioral changes are less easily attributable to a loss of discriminative capacity.

A more direct procedure is to make an explicit study of the effects of drugs upon discriminative capacity. Dews (1955b) initiated a study to determine whether a number of drugs alter the pigeon's capacity to discriminate between the two key lights. He found that the behavioral control exercised by a simple pair of stimuli was not appreciably affected by the drugs, but that when more complex conditional discriminations were required, clear discriminative deficits appeared. Similar studies have been carried out by Blough (1957). In Blough's technique, the pigeon was presented with two response keys, separated by a vertical bar. The keys and the bar could be independently illuminated. Hungry birds were rewarded with food, on a variable-interval schedule, only when they pecked the correct key. The correct key was cued as follows: If the vertical bar was lighted, pecking on the darker of the two keys caused food to be presented to the bird. If the bar was dark, pecks on the brighter key brought food. Thus, the pigeons had to discriminate not only between bright and dark keys, but their choice was conditional upon the illumination of the center bar.

Blough presented two measures of the drug effects. One of these was the total number of responses emitted by the birds, and the other was the percentage of the responses that were correct. Figure 2 illustrates the effects of LSD-25 upon these measures, expressed as deviations from control performance. It may be seen that LSD-25, soon after administration, produces a *decline in total responses* but an *increase in accuracy.* There is a clear effect of this drug upon complex discriminative behavior, an effect that was not apparent from the measures of total output. Blough found, in addition, that chlorpromazine *decreased both accuracy and output;* that pentobarbital *decreased accuracy* and *increased output;* that meperidine, like chlorpromazine, *reduced both accuracy and output;* and that caffeine had little effect upon either measure. In another study, Blough (1956) also demonstrated that both alcohol and sodium pentobarbital *increase* the total response output while decreasing the accuracy of the discrimination. Differences in the time course of action also appeared

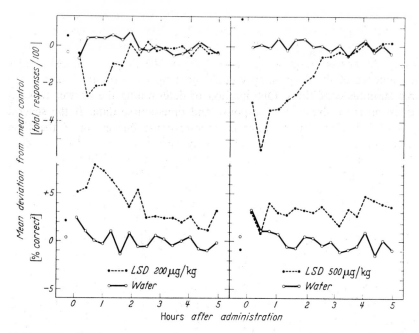

FIGURE 2   Total responses and percent correct responses in a conditional discrimination. Performance is plotted as a function of time following oral administration of LSD-25. (From Blough, 1957)

not only among the drugs, but, in some cases, between the two measures
for a given drug.

It should be emphasized that a drug effect can be attributed to a loss
of discriminative capacity by the organism only if the two or more types
of behavior in a multiple schedule procedure fail to display a differential
response to the drug. When each of the behavioral members of a multiple
baseline reacts similarly to the drug, then it becomes necessary to employ
techniques, such as those of Dews (1955b) or Blough (1956), for a direct
test of stimulus discrimination.

BEHAVIORAL TOXICITY.   A problem closely related to non-specific behavioral effects is that of behavioral toxicity. While physiological toxicity has
long been recognized as a major problem in the evaluation of any drug,
the corresponding behavioral problem has only recently been explicitly
stated. No drug that affects behavior has yet been found to confine its
action to a single type of behavior. The problem of behavioral toxicity is
raised by the question, "Are any of the behavioral 'side effects' of such a
nature as to prevent the organism from functioning adequately in its behavioral adaptations to the normal environment?" Hunt (1956a, 1956b)

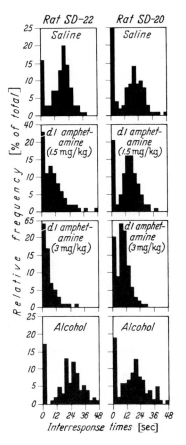

FIGURE 3. Relative frequency distributions of the time intervals between successive lever presses. Each distribution represents one animal's performance in a single two-hour session. (From Sidman, 1955)

has pointed out, for example, that the ideal tranquilizing drug is not necessarily one that weakens avoidance or fear-type behavior. Such a drug might lead to a sort of psychopathic irresponsibility, or to a loss of the anticipatory behavior that serves to protect organisms from impending harmful events.

The first experimental investigation explicitly directed at the problem of behavioral toxicity was that of Sidman (1955), who utilized the technique of Wilson and Keller to determine whether amphetamine had any effect upon temporal orientation. White rats were rewarded for lever pressing only when they spaced their lever pressing responses at least 20 seconds apart. The temporal pattern of responding that develops with this procedure may be seen in the "saline" records of Fig. 3. The relative frequency distribution of time intervals between successive lever pressing responses rises sharply to a peak at 16–20 seconds, indicating relatively well-developed timing behavior. Amphetamine, in increasing doses, shifted the peak of the distribution toward the shorter values, indicating that the animals were responding too early. The orderly shift in the temporal patterning of responses indicates that the effect of the drug was not a simple excitatory one, even though rate increases were also observed. The effects of alcohol, sodium pentobarbital, and reserpine were also tested against a baseline of spaced responding, and markedly different effects were observed in each case [Sidman (1956)]. Sodium pentobarbital, unlike amphetamine, completely destroyed all evidence of timing. While responding was eventually completely suppressed by reserpine, the timing remained as long as there was enough behavior to provide an adequate measure.

There are many different techniques for generating timing behavior in experimental animals, and it is likely that the effect of a given drug will depend upon the technique and the measures employed. The same may be expected in other areas in which behavioral toxicity will be of concern. Herrnstein and Morse (1957), utilizing the characteristic performance on a fixed-interval reinforcement schedule as a measure of timing behavior, have demonstrated the disrupting effect of pentobarbital. Weiss, using a similar technique, has demonstrated a breakdown of timing under the influence of nalorphine. It is likely that toxic effects of a more subtle nature will be detectable either by means of more complex behavioral procedures, or by more complex analysis of simpler situations. Morse and Herrnstein (1956a) have shown that complex behavior, when measured and analyzed appropriately, will display changes in response to drug administration that are not evident upon gross inspection of the behavior. Stone, Calhoun, and Hemmer have demonstrated that even relatively simple behavior may, upon finer analysis, be found to consist of several components that are differentially susceptible to drugs. It will remain for future clinical observation to correlate such laboratory findings with possible adaptive malfunctioning.

EMOTIONAL BEHAVIOR.   The possibility of drug effects upon emotional behavior is receiving considerable attention, largely as a result of the current interest in tranquilizing drugs. The problem is a difficult one, because of the poor specification of what is meant by the term, "emotional behavior." The usual course, in investigating drug-behavior relations in this area, is to employ experimental operations that contain elements analogous to those commonly supposed to be present in certain types of "emotional" situations. Such operations have typically involved the use of noxious stimuli, such as electric shocks, to generate behavior that is often labelled "anxiety"- or "fear"-type behavior.

A commonly employed technique is that of avoidance conditioning. The animals are permitted to prevent the occurrence of an electric shock by making some arbitrary response. When the avoidance response fails to occur, the animal receives a shock, which may or may not have been preceded by a warning stimulus. As Brady (1957) has pointed out, "few of these studies have adequately controlled for generalized motor effects, sensory decrements, and general malaise, any or all of which could produce depression of avoidance behavior independently of any specific emotional change." In illustration, Weiskrantz and Wilson have shown that a dose of reserpine that depressed avoidance behavior in the monkey also completely depressed behavior that was maintained by food reinforcement. Verhave, on the other hand, has shown that doses of *d*-desoxyephedrine that *depress* food-reinforced behavior produce an *increase* in avoidance responding.

The problem of "emotional specificity" of a drug was partially resolved by Verhave, Owen and Slater, who required their animals not only to avoid the shock but also to terminate, or escape, the shock whenever it was permitted to occur. They were then able to use this escape response as a control for nonspecific effects of the drugs. That is to say, if a drug eliminates avoidance responding but has no effect upon the escape behavior, a more satisfactory case can be made for a specific effect of the drug upon avoidance behavior. Using this technique, Verhave, Owen, and Slater demonstrated that increasing doses of chlorpromazine were directly related to the magnitude of depression of shock-avoidance behavior. A lesser effect upon shock-escape behavior was observed, with doses that completely abolished all avoidance responses producing only minor decrements in the escape behavior. A similar effect was noted for morphine.

Sidman (1956) has demonstrated that avoidance behavior is sensitive to reserpine, with the magnitude of the effect depending not only upon the drug but also upon the behavioral variables involved in the avoidance situation. When the rats received a shock every time they permitted 20 seconds to elapse without depressing a lever, a given dose of reserpine produced no decrement in lever pressing. But when the animals received a shock only on 20 percent of the occasions when it became due because of a failure to press the lever, the same dose of reserpine produced a marked depression in the rate of avoidance responding. A finding such as this points up the necessity of investigating not only a wide range of drug doses over the total acting time of the drug, but also a wide range of the behavioral parameters that are involved in the test situation. Drug effects are dependent not only upon the nature of the chemical agent, the physiological state of the organism, and the qualitative nature of the reinforcement schedule, but also upon the quantitative properties of the contingencies maintaining the behavior in question. Further evidence of this factor has been demonstrated in the case of behavior generated by fixed-ratio reward schedules, Dews (1956) found that methamphetamine did not appreciably alter fixed ratio behavior when 30 to 60 responses were required to produce the reinforcement. But when a ratio of 160 responses per reinforcement was used to maintain behavior, Morse and Herrnstein (1956a) observed marked alteration in both the normal baseline performance and in the behavior following administration of methamphetamine.

A different type of "emotional" situation than avoidance has also been successfully employed to evaluate tranquilizing and other types of drugs. Estes and Skinner pointed out that one defining aspect of emotional situations is the widespread and simultaneous alteration of large classes of behavior. Based upon this observation they introduced a method of measuring "anxiety" in terms of changes in base-line responding as a function of a stimulus that was not contingent upon the ongoing behavior. A stable level of baseline behavior was first generated by reinforcing lever pressing responses with food on a variable-interval schedule. Then while the animal was lever-pressing, a stimulus of several minutes duration was presented and terminated contiguously with the delivery of an electric shock. After several such pairings of stimulus and shock, the stimulus came to produce a complete disruption of the animal's ongoing behavior. Lever-pressing ceased during the stimulus and was resumed only after receipt of the unavoidable shock. While this conditioned suppression of ongoing behavior may or may not correspond with one's favorite definition of "anxiety," the situation in which some event signals the occurrence of a noxious, unavoidable stimulus is a common one, perhaps basic to many behavioral processes generated by aversive control (Schoenfeld).

Employing the conditioned suppression technique, Brady (1956a) has demonstrated some striking behavioral changes as a consequence of amphetamine and reserpine administration. The normal disruption of ongoing behavior in the presence of a stimulus that has been paired with unavoidable shocks may be "cured" by continued reserpine treatment (Fig. 4). Amphetamine may exercise an opposite effect, intensifying the degree of behavioral suppression. Examination of Fig. 4 demonstrates that the conditioned suppression technique has a built-in control for nonspecific side effects. This control is provided by the rate of responding on the variable-interval reinforcement schedule during the periods between stimulus presentations. It may be seen that amphetamine, which produced a greater suppression of responding during the warning stimulus, actually increased the response output in the absence of the stimulus. Reserpine, while it increased the response rate during the warning stimulus, produced a lowered output between stimuli. When a drug can be shown to produce such diametrically opposite effects nearly simultaneously in a single organism, general behavioral and motor disturbances can virtually be eliminated as explanations of the changes in emotional behavior. It may be possible to invoke sensory impairment as a factor in the reserpine effect, but other data have failed to demonstrate a breakdown of discrimination as a consequence of reserpine administration (Sidman, 1956).

While the effect of reserpine on the emotional response (suppression of ongoing behavior) is not easily attributable to some sort of generalized behavioral malfunction, the side effect demonstrated in Fig. 4 should not

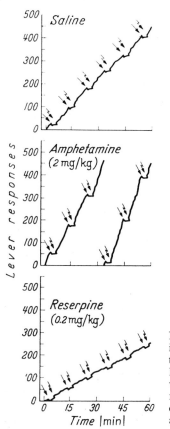

FIGURE 4.   Cumulative response curves showing the effect of amphetamine and reserpine on the conditioned emotional suppression. The oblique solid arrows indicate the onset of the warning stimulus, and the oblique broken arrows indicate the termination of the stimulus contiguously with the brief electric shock to the animal's feet. (From Brady, 1956a)

be ignored. The lowered baseline rate of response during the absence of the warning stimulus suggests that reserpine may have a "toxic" effect upon adaptive behavior as well as a palliative effect upon anxiety behavior.

Hunt (1957) failed to observe any clear attenuation of the conditioned suppression as a consequence of meprobamate administration, although there was a suggestion that meprobamate may slightly retard the acquisition, or learning, of the suppression. Hunt (1956) also found that chlorpromazine, in heavy doses, does not block conditioning of the emotional suppression. Similar results were obtained in a well-controlled experiment by Stein, working with reserpine. Even a dose of the drug that completely abolished all lever-pressing behavior failed to interfere with the acquisition of the conditioned suppression, tested after the drug had worn off.

Hill, Belleville and Wikler (1954a) have found striking effects of morphine upon the conditioned suppression in rats. They report an increasing attenuation of the emotional suppression with increasing doses of morphine sulfate (Hill et al., 1954b). These writers interpret their data as an indication that "one of the major actions of a potent analgesic is the reduction of behavior-disrupting anticipatory response to noxious stimuli" (Hill *et al.,* 1954b). It is possible, however, that the alleviation of the conditioned suppression is only incidental to the analgesic effect. If the shock is made less painful, it is likely that the anticipatory disruption of behavior will disappear through the normal extinction process Brady (1955). More conclusive support for the attractive hypothesis that analgesic agents exercise at least part of their effect through anxiety reduction may be obtained by employing a non-painful aversive stimulus instead of electric shock, e.g., Lindsley and Jetter, Morse and Herrnstein (1956b). This would permit a test of the effect of morphine upon the anticipatory disruption of behavior, while at the same time ruling out the analgesic effect.

DRUG-BEHAVIOR INTERACTIONS. Recent research has made it abundantly clear that drugs and behavior are, in a wide sense, interactive. The behavioral effect of a drug depends qualitatively and quantitatively upon the variables that are maintaining the behavior at the time. Sidman (1956) has suggested that such dependence may be responsible for the notorious variability that almost inevitably hampers the clinical evaluation of a CNS-acting drug. Miller has also demonstrated that even under a constant set of behavioral variables, various aspects of a given type of behavior may react differently to a drug.

But drug-behavior interactions may be considered in a more restricted sense. If a drug alters the frequency or temporal pattern of some form of behavior, it is possible that the new pattern may, itself, be perpetuated after the drug has been withdrawn. This might occur especially if the drug-induced change in behavior were more advantageous to the organism than the previous mode of behavior. While the original conditions maintaining the behavior may have been such as to hamper an adaptive adjustment, the drug, by reducing the degree of control of these factors, may permit the organism to learn a more adaptive response. An effect such as this is probably the one most to be sought in testing drugs for efficacy in the treatment of behavior disorders.

Unfortunately, there has been almost a complete lack of experimental attention to this type of drug-behavior interaction. Relevant observations have, for the most part, been secondary ones in experiments directed at other problems. In one of the few direct attacks upon the problem, Hunt (1956) checked the effect of chlorpromazine upon the extinction of a conditioned emotional response. Suppression of ongoing behavior was first established by pairing a stimulus with shock until the ongoing behavior was completely disrupted during the anticipatory signal. Extinction was then carried out, with and without the drug, by presenting the warning signal but omitting the shock. Hunt found that animals which were drugged during the extinction procedure still displayed the anticipatory behavioral disruption after the drug was discontinued. In animals which were not drugged, the extinction procedure had its usual effect of eliminating the emotional response. Thus chlorpromazine, far from permitting the animals to unlearn their fear, actually prevented the normal extinction process from occurring.

Sidman (1956) has investigated the permanence of a reserpine effect upon avoidance behavior. Boren and Sidman had demonstrated that even when 80 percent of the shocks normally received by the animal for failure to make the avoidance response were withheld, the rate of avoidance behavior did not diminish. Under the influence of reserpine, however, the rate of avoidance responding fell to a more appropriate level on this intermittent shock procedure (Sidman, 1956). But when the drug was discontinued, avoidance responding returned to the unnecessarily high level that had prevailed prior to "treatment." Again, then, we observe the failure of an adaptive behavioral effect to perpetuate itself after the drug was withdrawn.

Morse and Herrnstein (1956a) demonstrated an effect that may be classified as at least partially successful in revealing a continued behavioral change following administration of a drug. Using a fixed-ratio reinforcement procedure, they required 160 responses before a food reinforcement could be procured. With such a large ratio of responses to reinforcements, the behavior typically was characterized by high rates alternating with long pauses during which no responses were emitted. The pauses were almost completely eliminated by a large dose of methamphetamine, so that a great many more food reinforcements were obtained under the drug. On the following day, 23 hours after the drug had been administered, there was a clear residual effect of the drug, with higher response rates, few pauses, and more frequent reinforcements. Eventually, however, the behavior returned to its normal "strained" state, indicating that the residual effect of the drug was not permanent.

DRUGS, BEHAVIOR, AND THE NERVOUS SYSTEM. With the advent of more precise methods for generating and measuring behavior, there has developed an increasing experimental interest in the relations between behavior and other biological processes. By means of central nervous system lesions, electrical stimulation and recording, and biochemical assay techniques, knowledge of the relations between behavior and the internal functioning of living organisms is steadily increasing in scope. Drugs, too, promise to add to the understanding of both behavior and the nervous system. A relatively sophisticated area of research, barely initiated as yet, is the investigation not simply of the effects of drugs upon behavior, or upon the nervous system, but of the effects of drug activity upon known *relations between* behavior and the nervous system.

An experiment that is likely to become a classic prototype in this area is that of Mason and Brady. It had first been determined that the conditioned emotional suppression was accompanied by significant elevations of plasma 17-hydroxycorticosteroid levels (Mason *et al.*). Other experiments demonstrated that reserpine markedly attentuates the conditioned emotional suppression of ongoing behavior (Brady, 1956b). The next step was to examine the relation between reserpine activity and the adrenal-cortical response to emotional conditioning. Mason and Brady found that when the behavioral suppression had been abolished by reserpine, the corticosteroid elevation also failed to appear during the "anxiety" stimulus. When the drug treatments were discontinued, the behavioral suppression reappeared and corticosteroid elevations were again recorded. Although the behavioral and endocrine responses thus appeared to be intimately related, as was suggested by their correlated changes, the recovery of the behavioral suppression and the corticosteroid response did not follow precisely the same time course after the drug had been withdrawn. The steroid response returned to normal well after the conditioned suppression had reappeared. The writers suggest that this difference in recovery time may indicate at least partially independent neural mechanisms underlying the two responses.

Research such as this, in which information concerning drug action is obtained and, *in addition,* the drug effect is utilized to clarify relations between behavior and physiology, has been rare. In most of the experiment of this sort that are reported, the physiological variables involved have been those that *produce,* rather than *accompany,* behavioral effects. A major problem in these experiments is the lack of precise information, behavioral or otherwise, concerning the effects of the physiological operations involved. One such operation consists of experimental lesions of the central nervous system. Weiskrantz and Wilson, testing the action of reserpine upon normal and amygdaloidectomized monkeys in an avoidance situation, found that the lesions did not interfere with the depressant effect of a large dose of the drug. Hunt and Beckwith utilized phenurone, dilantin, and amphetamine to investigate the effects of electro-convulsive shock (ECS) upon the conditioned emotional suppression. It had previously been shown that electro-convulsive therapy attenuated the emotional suppression (Brady and Hunt). Hunt and Beckwith found that when the drugs were given intercurrently with ECS, phenurone blocked the attenuating effect of ECS while dilantin or amphetamine increased the attenuating effect. Olds, Killam and Bach-y-Rita have presented data in yet another area, investigating the effects of drugs upon behavior that is involved in electrical self-stimulation of the brain. Their technique made use of the finding, by Olds and Milner, that when rats are permitted to press a lever and thereby electrically stimulate specific brain structures, such stimulation acts as a reinforcement. That is, the animals press the lever at a high rate. Olds, Killam and Bach-y-Rita designed their experiment to determine whether different drugs would affect self-stimulation rates for some electrode loci more than for others. They found that reserpine depressed the response rate markedly in animals that were stimulated in the hypothalamus or in the amygdala, but produced only a minor depression when the electrodes were located in the septal region. Chlorpromazine produced similar effects, while pentobarbital did not show selective effects among the stimulated areas. Although the close temporal spacing of drug administrations somewhat clouds the data of these experiments, particularly in the case of reserpine, whose long-term effects are well-known, the technique will undoubtedly yield basic information concerning both drug action and behavior-nervous system interrelations. There have been, finally, a few experiments in which the chief interest has been in the influence of chemical agents upon the efficacy of specific motivating operations, e.g., deprivation of food, oxygen, or heat. Miller found that amphetamine decreased the amount of food consumption by hungry rats, and lowered the concentration of quinine, mixed with milk, that the animals would accept. The rate of lever-pressing, reinforced on a variable-interval schedule, declined with higher doses of amphetamine and increased with lower doses. The rate increase was consistent with earlier reports by Skinner and Heron and Wentink. Weiss and Danford utilized an ingenious technique whereby rats subjected to cold temperatures were reinforced for lever-pressing by the activation of an infrared heat lamp. They found that animals which were severely deprived of both food and pantothenic acid markedly increased the rate of lever pressing for the heat reward. Berryman, Mechner, Keller and Metlay employed behavioral techniques to assess possible interactions between anoxia and tocopherol. They found that anoxia produced an early and abrupt interruption of behavior maintained by food reinforcement, and a slow, gradual depression of avoidance behavior. Tocopherol appeared to have some tendency to postpone the behavioral effects of anoxia, the drug effect being most pronounced on avoidance behavior.

HUMAN BEHAVIOR. This has been a review of experimental data on drug-behavior relationships obtained largely by means of operant conditioning techniques with animal subjects. It will be noted that the vast majority of the references were published after 1950. The validity of extrapolations to the human sphere remains an empirical problem which will require a considerably longer period of time to evaluate. There are, however, encouraging signs. Operant methods have been successfully employed with mice, rats, guinea pigs, pigeons, cats, dogs, monkeys, chimpanzees, and both normal and psychotic human children and adults. The behavioral principles based on this work appear to possess great species generality, and even in those cases where the behavior differs from one species to the next, the control techniques themselves remain generally applicable. To the extent that the behavioral principles are applicable to humans, we may have confidence in the applicability of data on drug-behavior relationships also. A major obstacle in the way of determining the validity of extrapolations from the animal laboratory to the clinic is the lack of precise and reliable methods for evaluating human behavior problems. Brady (1956) has provided a succinct statement of the problem. "It seems reasonable, for the present, to define differential behavioral properties of various pharmacologic agents at any level where experimental controls permit operational analysis, allowing empirical relationships to take form as refinements in clinical methods provided reliable comparative information."

A promising beginning has been made in the direction of refining clinical observations through the use of operant conditioning techniques with psychotic patients. An outline of the methodology has been presented by Skinner, Solomon and Lindsley (1954). Although some data have been reported on the effects of chlorpromazine and lysergic acid, adequate control data are not yet available (Skinner *et al.,* 1956). While other laboratories have also begun to extend the techniques to human subjects, there have as yet been no published reports on the effects of pharmacologic agents.

REFERENCES

Berryman, R., Mechner, F., Keller, F. S., and Metlay, M.: Effects of vitamin E on behavior in anoxia. School of Aviation Medicine, USAF, Randolph AFB, Texas.

Blough, D. S.: Method of tracing dark-adaptation in the pigeon. *Science* 121, 703–704 (1955).—Technique for studying the effects of drugs on discrimination in the pigeon. *Ann. N.Y. Acad. Sci.* 65, 334–344 (1956).—Some effects of drugs on visual discrimination in the pigeon. *Ann. N.Y. Acad. Sci.* 66, 733–739 (1957).

Boren, J. J.: Some effects of benactyzine upon operant behavior. *J. Pharmacol. exp. Ther.* In press at time of publication.

Boren, J. J., and Sidman, M.: Maintenance of avoidance behavior as a function of intermittent shocks. *Canad. J. Psychol.* 11, 185 (1957).

Brady, J. V.: Extinction of a conditioned "fear" response as a function of reinforcement schedules for competing behavior. *J. Psychol.* 40, 25–34 (1955).—Assessment of drug effects on emotional behavior. *Science* 123, 1033–1034 (1956a). —A comparative approach to the evaluation of drug effects upon affect behavior. *Ann. N.Y. Acad. Sci.* 64, 632–643 (1956b).—A comparative approach to the evaluation of drug effects upon behavior. *Brain mechanisms and drug action,* W. S. Fields (ed.). Springfield, Ill.: Ch. C. Thomas 1957.—Comparative Psychopharmacology: Animal experimental studies on the effects of drugs on behavior. Conference on Drugs in Psychiatry, National Research Council 1956c.

Brady, J. V., and Hunt, H. F.: An experimental approach to the analysis of emotional behavior. *J. Psychol.* 40, 313–324 (1955).

Dews, P. B.: Studies on behavior. I. Differential sensitivity to pentobarbital of pecking performance in pigeons depending on the schedule of reward. *J. Pharmacol.*

exp. Ther. 113, 393–401 (1955a).—Studies on behavior. II. The effects of pentobarbital, methamphetamine, and scopolamine on performance in pigeons involving discriminations. *J. Pharmacol. exp. Ther.* 115, 380–389 (1955b).— Modification by drugs of performance on simple schedules of positive reinforcement. *Ann. N.Y. Acad. Sci.* 65, 268–281 (1956).

Estes, W. K., and Skinner, B. F.: Some quantitative properties of anxiety. *J. exp. Psychol.* 29, 390–400 (1941).

Ferster, C. B.: The use of the free operant in the analysis of behavior. *Psychol. Bull.* 50, 263–274 (1953).

Ferster, C. B., and Skinner, B. F.: *Schedules of reinforcement.* New York: Appleton-Century-Crofts 1958.

Guttman, N., and Kalish, H. I.: Discriminability and stimulus generalization. *J. exp. Psychol.* 51, 79–88 (1956).

Herrnstein, R. J., and Morse, W. H.: Selective action of pentobarbital on component behaviors of a reinforcement schedule. *Science* 124, 367–268 (1956).—Effects of pentobarbital on intermittently reinforced behavior. *Science* 125, 929–931 (1957)

Hill, H. E., Belleville, R. E., and Wikler, A.: Anxiety reduction as a measure of the analgesic effectiveness of drugs. *Science* 120, 153 (1954a).—Reduction of pain-controlled anxiety by analgesic doses of morphine in rats. *Proc. Soc. exp. Biol. Med.* 86, 881–884 (1954).

Hunt, H. F.: Some effects of drugs on classical (Type S) conditioning. *Ann. N.Y. Acad. Sci.* 65, 258–267 (1956a).—Effects of drugs on emotional responses and abnormal behavior in animals. Conference on Drugs in Psychiatry, National Research Council 1956b.—Some effects of meprobamate on conditioned fear and emotional behavior. *Ann. N.Y. Acad. Sci.* 67, 712 (1957).

Hunt, H. F., and Beckwith, W. C.: The effect of electroconvulsive shock under phenurone, dilantin, or amphetamine medication on a conditioned emotional response. *Amer. Psychologist* 11, 442 (1956).

Keller, F. S.: Light aversion in the white rat. *Psychol. Rec.* 4, 235–250 (1941).

Lindsley, O. R., and Jetter, W. W.: The temporary elimination of discrimination and fear by sodium pentobarbital injections. *Amer. Psychologist* 8, 390 (1953).

Mason. J. W., and Brady, J. V.: Plasma 17-hydroxycorticosteroid changes related to reserpine effects on emotional behavior. *Science* 124, 983–984 (1956).

Mason, J. W., Brady, J. V., and Sidman, M.: Plasma 17-hydroxycorticosteroid levels and conditioned behavior in the rhesus monkey. *Endocrinology* 60, 741 (1957).

Miller, N. E.: Effects of drugs on motivation: the value of using a variety of measures. *Ann. N.Y. Acad. Sci.* 65, 318–333 (1956).

Morse, W. H., and Herrnstein, R. J.: Effects of drugs on characteristics of behavior maintained by complex schedules of intermittent positive reinforcement. *Ann. N.Y. Acad. Sci.* 65, 303–317 (1956a).—The maintenance of avoidance behavior using the removal of a conditioned positive reinforcer as the aversive stimulus. *Amer. Psychologist* 11, 430 (1956b).

Olds, J., Killam, K. F., and Bach-y-Rita, P.: Self-stimulation of the brain used as a screening method for tranquilizing drugs. *Science* 124, 265–266 (1956).

Olds, J., and Milner, P.: Positive reinforcement produced by electrical stimulation of septal area and other regions of rat brain. *J. comp. physiol. Psychol.* 47, 419–427 (1954).

Schoenfeld, W. N.: An experimental approach to anxiety, escape, and avoidance behavior. *Anxiety,* P. H. Hoch and J. Zubin (eds.). New York: Grune & Stratton 1950.

Sidman, M.: Avoidance conditioning with brief shock and no exteroceptive warning signal. *Science* 118, 157–158 (1953).—Technique for assessing the effects of drugs on timing behavior. *Science* **122**, 925 (1955).—Drug-behavior interaction. *Ann. N.Y. Acad. Sci.* **65**, 282–302 (1956).

Skinner, B. F.: *The behavior of organisms: An experimental analysis.* New York: Appleton-Century-Crofts 1938.

Skinner, B. F., and Heron, W. T.: Effects of caffeine and benzedrine upon conditioning and extinction. *Psychol. Rec.* **1**, 340–346 (1937).

Skinner, B. F., Solomon, H. C., and Lindsley, O. R.: A new method for the experimental analysis of the behavior of psychotic patients. *J. nerv. ment. Dis.* **120**, 403–406 (1954).—New techniques of analysis of psychotic behavior. Annual Technical Report No. 3. Metropolitan State Hospital, Waltham, Mass., 1956.

Stein, L.: Reserpine and the learning of fear. *Science* **124**, 1082–1083 (1956).

Stone, G. C., Calhoun, D. W., and Hemmer, M. L.: The interresponse interval as a measure of bar-pressing behavior in normal and drugged rats. *Amer. Psychologist* **11**, 447 (1956).

Verhave, T.: Differential effects of *d*-desoxyephedrine, caffeine, and picrotoxin on operant behavior. *J. Pharmacol. exp. Ther.* **119**, 120 (1957).

Verhave, T., Owen, J. E., and Slater, I. H.: Effects of various drugs on escape and avoidance behavior. *Progr. Neurolbol. Psychiat.* **3**, 267–280 (1958).

Weiskrantz, L., and Wilson, W. A., Jr.: The effects of reserpine on emotional behavior of normal and brain-operated monkeys. *Ann. N.Y. Acad. Sci.* **61**, 36–55 (1955).

Weiss, B.: The effects of various morphine-*N*-Allyl-Normorphine ratios on behavior. *Arch. int. Pharmacodyn.* **105**, 381–388 (1956).

Weiss, B., and Danford, M. B.: Reward value of heat at low temperatures during inanition and pantothenic acid deprivation. School of Aviation Medicine, USAF, Randolph AFB, Texas. Report No. 56–72, 1956.

Wentink, E.: The effects of certain drugs and hormones upon conditioning. *J. exp. Psychol.* **22**, 150–163 (1938).

Wilson, M. P., and Keller, F. S.: On the selective reinforcement of spaced responses. *J. comp. physiol. Psychol.* **46**, 190–193 (1953).

Section **B**   ANTECEDENT VARIABLES

Phenotypically similar behavior can be generated by quite different conditioning procedures. As a result, the same manipulation of the current reinforcement contingencies might reasonably be expected to produce different changes in the two apparently similar operants. Similarly, drug administration might be expected to alter behaviors established in different ways. A demonstration of such drug-conditioning history interaction is given in Article 10, where the effects of chlorpromazine and imipramine are determined on discriminated operants established with and without a history of unreinforced responding. This work, which provided the first sound evidence supporting the generalization that reinforcement history can alter drug action, opened up an entirely new field in behavioral pharmacology.

Deprivation conditions are widely known to affect the strength of operant behaviors. Overall response rate, detailed features of performance, and response latencies can all vary as a function of the level of deprivation. Drugs can have effects that resemble changes in deprivation level, and they can interact with the effects of level of deprivation. Article 11 explores the interactions between water deprivation level and the effects of methylphenidate and chlorpromazine on a water-reinforced response. Article 12 extends this line of investigation to include the role of reinforcement history as well as deprivation level. These papers clearly indicate that the behavioral actions of drugs depends, at least in part, on the organism's past reinforcement history and the current deprivation state.

111

10

Errorless discrimination learning in the pigeon: Effects of chlorpromazine and imipramine

HERBERT S. TERRACE

Recent experiments (1) have shown that a pigeon is able to acquire a discrimination of color and the orientation of a line without any "errors." An "error" is the failure to respond to the stimulus correlated with reinforcement (S+) or a response to the stimulus correlated with nonreinforcement (S−). Errorless learning is accomplished by starting discrimination training immediately after the response to S+ has been conditioned, and by progressively reducing the difference between S+ and S− from an initially large value to the relatively smaller final value.

When a discrimination is learned without errors, certain characteristics of performance, normally observed in discrimination performance after learning with errors, are lacking (1). These are (i) an increase in the rate (or decrease in the latency) of the response to S+, (ii) sporadic bursts of responses to S−, separated by long intervals of no responses to S−, and (iii) "emotional" responses to S−. The present study investigates another frequently observed characteristic of discrimination performance, the disruption of performance that follows the administration of certain drugs (2). Specifically, the effects of chlorpromazine and imipramine were studied after discrimination learning by the pigeon with, and without, errors. These drugs disrupt discrimination performance in the pigeon (3).

Discrimination training was carried out in a standard operant conditioning appartus (1). The discriminative stimuli were projected on the response key during discrete, automatically programmed trials. Each trial was terminated by a single response or by the failure to respond within 5 seconds of the onset of the trial. A response that occurred during an S+ trial was immediately reinforced. Between trials, the "house light" remained on but the key was dark for intervals (mean length 30 seconds). S+ and S− trials alternated in random succession, unless an error was made, in which case the trial was repeated.

The subjects were four White Carneau male pigeons with no prior experimental history. Two pigeons (Nos. 75 and 100) were trained to discriminate between a vertical S+ and a horizontal S− line without errors. The details of the training procedure, which are described elsewhere (1), may be summarized as follows. Initially a red S+-green S− discrimination,

From *Science*, 1963, **140**, 318–319. Copyright 1963 by the American Association for the Advancement of Science, Washington, D.C.

which is easier to learn than the vertical-horizontal discrimination, was used to train the pigeons. At the start of discrimination training, S+ was a red key which was presented for 5 seconds. S— was a green key presented for 1 second. As training progressed the duration and intensity of S— was progressively increased until it equaled the duration and intensity of S+. In this manner the pigeons were trained to discriminate between red and green without any errors. After ten sessions of red-green training the discriminative stimuli were modified so that, on S+ trials, a white-vertical line was superimposed on the red key, and on S— trials, a white-horizontal line was superimposed on the green key. These compound stimuli presented during sessions 11 to 14 and during the first five trials of session 15. During trials 5 to 30 of the 15th session, the red and the green backgrounds of the compound stimuli were progressively faded out until only the vertical and the horizontal lines appeared as the discriminative stimuli. In this way, the pigeons were trained to discriminate between vertical and horizontal lines without any errors. Birds Nos. 75 and 100 each received 15 sessions of vertical-horizontal training, for a total of 30 discrimination sessions. During these sessions neither subject made an error.

The other two pigeons (Nos. 334 and 217) were trained to discriminate between the vertical and the horizontal lines without any progressive training. The vertical and the horizontal lines were the only stimuli to appear throughout their training. They made 860 and 1372 responses to S—, respectively, in 30 discrimination sessions. For both birds the probability of a response to S+ after the first conditioning session was always 1.0

After 30 discrimination sessions had been completed for each of the four birds, each was given a series of discrimination trials after administration of a drug. Either chlorpromazine, imipramine, or physiological saline was injected intramuscularly every third day. On the two days between the administration of the drugs each bird was given further vertical-horizontal training. Four dose levels of each drug were used: 1, 3, 10, and 17 mg. The drug and the dosage to be used during each session were selected at random with the provision that a given dosage of each drug was to be used only twice. Each session began 30 minutes after the administration of the drug.

Table 1 shows the number of responses to S— emitted by each bird with repetition of a given dose or with increase in dose level of either chlorpromazine or imipramine. The duplicate values for dosage which appear consecutively in Table 1 represent responses at the first and second session, respectively, at that dosage. Table 1 shows very clearly that neither chlorpromazine nor imipramine had any effect on the performance of the two birds (Nos. 75 and 100) that had learned the vertical-horizontal discrimination without errors. The results also show that the performance of the other two birds was greatly impaired by both drugs at all dose levels. Neither of these two birds (Nos. 334 and 217) made more than eight

TABLE 1. Number of responses in pigeons to the S— stimulus during horizontal
(S+)-vertical (S—) discrimination after being given injections of chlorpromazine or
imipramine.

Dose (mg)	Responses (No.)			
	Bird No. 75	Bird No. 100	Bird No. 334	Bird No. 217
Chlorpromazine				
1	0	0	5	76
	0	0	18	86
3	0	0	409	149
	0	0	421	235
10	0	0	496	272
	0	0	521	315
17	0	0	1325	862
	0	0	1514	1655
Imipramine				
1	0	0	137	324
	0	0	161	207
3	0	0	544	522
	0	0	415	254
10	0	0	987	904
	0	0	2084	1186
17	0	0	3655	2651
	0	0	1872	2764

responses to S— in ten sessions prior to, or on the days between the
sessions in which the drug was administered. Injection of physiological
saline had no effect on the performance of any of the birds.

Neither drug had any effect on the frequency of responses to S+. For
all four birds the probability of responding to S+ remained at 1.0 during
each session after drug administration. However, the latency of the response to S+ was, in each instance, lengthened as the dosages of the
two drugs were increased. No systematic relation was observed between
the effect of either drug on the latency of responding to S+ and the manner in which the vertical-horizontal discrimination was acquired.

The use of the correction procedure, repeating each trial during which
an error occurred, makes it difficult to derive a dose-response curve from
the data in Table 1. The correlation suggested by these data, between the
dosage of a drug and its effect, may be attributed to an interaction between
the length of a session and the duration of the effect of different dosages
of a drug. Thus, it is possible that each dose has a similar effect on discrimination performance and that the larger effect of the larger dosages
was the result of longer sessions stemming from the correction procedure.
This possible artifact is currently being studied without employing the
correction procedure.

The lack of any effect of both drugs on discrimination performance after learning without errors, argues strongly against explaining the disruption of performance, after learning with errors, in terms of a sensory deficit. An alternative explanation may stem from the aversive properties of extinction (4) that may be temporarily reduced by chlorpromazine or imipramine. When an extinction curve is obtained during the training of a discrimination, it is possible that S— acquires aversive properties. This is, presumably, not the case when a discrimination is learned without errors. The hypothesis that emerges from these assumptions is that chlorpromazine or imipramine, in the case of a discrimination learned with errors, reduces the aversiveness of S— and thus facilitated the pigeon's S— responses (5).

SUMMARY.   Chlorpromazine or imipramine disrupts a pigeon's performance on a discrimination between a vertical and horizontal line only if the discrimination was learned with errors. Errorless learning is obtained if training starts with an easy-to-learn discrimination of color and shifts progressively to the more difficult horizontal-vertical discrimination.

REFERENCES AND NOTES

1. H. S. Terrace, *J. Exptl. Analysis Behavior* 6, 86 (1963); *ibid.,* in press at time of publication.
2. P. B. Dews, *J. Pharmacol, Exptl. Therap.* 115, 380 (1955); P. B. Dews and B. F. Skinner, Eds., *Ann. N.Y. Acad. Sci.* 65, 247 (1956).
3. D. Blough, *ibid.* 66, 733 (1957); L. Cook and R. T. Kelleher, *ibid.* 96, 315 (1962).
4. A. Amsel, *Psychol. Bull.* 55, 102 (1958).
5. The author thanks W. Morse for his generous and valuable advice. This research was supported by a grant from the National Science Foundation, G-8621, and it was conducted while the author held a U.S. Public Health Service predoctoral fellowship at Harvard University.

11

Combination of drive and drug effects

JOSEPH MENDELSON and DALBIR BINDRA

Does the effect of a drug on a trained response depend upon the current drive level of S? In other words, is the performance of a given response more vulnerable to the effects of a drug when the response is tested at a high drive level than when it is tested at a low drive level? An answer to this simple empirical question is likely to contribute to an understanding of the way in which drive (D) combines with other variables in determining response output, and might clarify the results of the studies (see Hulicka, 1960, for review) of the interaction of D with habit strength (H) and reward (K).

In the present investigation, the combinations of each of several levels of drive (thirst) with two drugs were studied. Variations in thirst drive were obtained by "prefeeding" Ss different amounts of water before testing. The drugs employed were chlorpromazine, a mild depressant ("tranquilizer"), and methylphenidate, an amphetamine-like stimulant. Though, like other drugs described as stimulants, methylphenidate, in medium doses of from 2 to 10 mg/kg, increases general activity (Bindra and Baran, 1959), we have repeatedly observed that it decreases the rate of a water-, food- or saccharin-rewarded lever pressing response; in this respect methylphenidate resembles amphetamine, which is also known to decrease such responding under certain conditions (e.g., Hearst, 1961; Miller, 1956; Owen, 1960). By using doses of chlorpromazine and methylphenidate that would have roughly equal decremental effects, we hoped to study the interactions of drive with these drugs at comparable levels of response output.

METHOD. *Subjects.* Twenty-eight naive male hooded rats, about 90 days old (weighing between 170 and 205 gm.) at the beginning of the experiment, were used as Ss. They were housed in small metal cages, 2 to a cage. Food was available to them at all times except during the experimental sessions. The Ss were placed on a 23-hr. schedule of water deprivation the day after their arrival at the laboratory, and they remained on this schedule for the duration of the experiment. They were allowed access to water in their home cages for 40 min. daily, at the conclusion of the experimental session.

From *Journal of Experimental Psychology*, 1962, **63**, 505–509. Copyright 1962 by the American Psychological Association, Washington, D.C.

Apparatus.   The apparatus consisted of four identical lever boxes, made of plywood and measuring 7 in. wide, 8½ in. deep, and 11½ in. high. All the boxes were painted gray on the inside and were covered by a wire mesh roof. Each was equipped with a water-delivery mechanism and an automatic counter. A lever, measuring 4 × ¾ in., was mounted 3 in. above the floor on one of the smaller walls of each box. A tray for receiving water was located on the same wall, 2½ in. from the center of the lever and 2 in. above the floor. Each lever press delivered .02–.04 cc of water into the tray. The minimum weight required to depress the lever was 44 gm.

Procedure.   After 1 day of water deprivation, each *S* was placed in a lever box for 10 min. The trays were filled with water; by the end of the period most *S*s had begun to drink the water. A 13-day training period was initiated on Day 2. On Days 2–9 each *S* was placed in a lever box for 15 min.; on Days 10–14, for 10 min. A given *S* was always placed in the same one of the four lever boxes. At the end of the training period the 4 *S*s with the lowest lever pressing rates were discarded, leaving 24 for the tests.

Variations in thirst drive were produced by allowing each *S* to drink a predetermined amount of water during a 10-min. period beginning about 40 min. before the daily test session. Each *S* was placed with its allotted quantity of water in a box measuring 7 × 8 in. Except when the highest amount (10 cc) of water was given, all *S*s drank all their allotted water in the given 10-min. period. When *S* did not finish the allotted water, it was placed in its home cage and given an additional 10-min. period to finish the water; at the conclusion of this period there was never more than 1 cc of water left over.

Immediately after water consumption, that is, about 30 min. before testing, each *S* was weighed and injected intraperitoneally with an appropriate amount of distilled water (control), chlorpromazine, or methylphenodate. The test sessions were conducted in three stages, each consisting of six sessions, one per day, with one practice session in between the stages. During each stage, each *S* was tested twice under each of the three drive levels. The two test sessions at each drive level were conducted on consecutive days; one of the tests followed a drug injection, while the other followed a control injection. The order of the three drive levels and the two types of injection (drug vs. control) was varied so that 2 *S*s were tested in each of the 12 possible permutations of drive level and type of injection. Thus, each of the 24 *S*s was tested under the six conditions (3 drive levels × 2 drug conditions) in each of the three stages of the experiment. The exact conditions of drive and drug employed in each stage are summarized in Table 1. It may be seen that, in Stages 1 and 2, *S*s were tested under the influence of 1.5 mg/kg chlorpromazine at five different drive levels; in Stage 3, effects of methylphenidate at three drive levels were determined.

TABLE 1.   Summary of experimental procedure.

Stage	"Predrinking" in cc			Drug Condition	
	High Drive	Medium Drive	Low Drive	Drug Injection	Water Injection
1	0.0	2.5	5.0	1.5 mg/kg Chlorpromazine	0.3cc
2	2.5	7.5	10.0	1.5 mg/kg Chlorpromazine	0.3cc
3	0.5	4.0	8.0	4.0 mg/kg methylphenidate	0.75cc

RESULTS.   The mean numbers of responses made in the 10-min. test sessions under the different conditions of drive and drug are shown in Fig. 1 and 2. The higher scores obtained in Stages 2 and 3 can be accounted

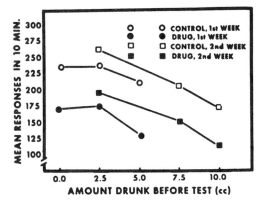

FIGURE 1.   Number of lever presses as a function of five drive levels (high to low) following control (water) and drug (chlorpromazine, 1.5 mg/kg) injections.

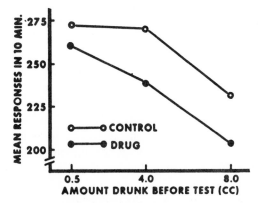

FIGURE 2.   Number of lever presses as a function of three drive levels (high to low) following control (water) and drug (methylphenidate, 4 mg/kg) injections.

TABLE 2.   Values of t for differences between means at different drive levels.

Stage	Control Scores			Drug Scores		
	D_L-D_M	D_M-D_H	D_L-D_H	D_L-D_M	D_M-D_H	D_L-D_H
1	2.72*	0.04	2.39*	3.35**	0.46	2.34*
2	3.93**	4.03**	9.29**	2.61*	2.50*	5.20**
3	3.54**	0.31	3.85**	2.71*	1.48	4.30**

* $P < .05$.
** $P < .01$.

for by the fact that Ss had not been trained to an asymptote before the initiation of the test sessions, so that their performance was still improving during the test sessions. Three features of the curves in these figures should be noted. First, in the control, water-injection, conditions, the higher the drive level (i.e., the less the amount of "predrinking") the greater were Ss' response rates. Two tailed t tests for differences between correlated means indicated that most of the differences between the means at different drive levels were significant (see Table 2); the only nonsignificant differences were those between medium and high drive levels in Stages 1 and 3. Second, the level of performance in the drug conditions was also different at the different drive levels; the relation between drive level and response rate was the same as that exhibited under control conditions—the higher the drive level, the greater the rate of response. Again most of the differences were significant (see Table 2); as in the case of control scores, the differences between the scores at the medium and high drive levels in Stages 1 and 3 were not significant. Third, both drugs led to a decrease in the number of lever presses; the differences between the mean drug and mean control performances were significant at each drive level ($P < .05$), except under the high drive methylphenidate condition.

To determine whether the effects of the drugs on response rate varied with drive level, two measures of response decrement were calculated for each S: (a) the absolute difference between drug and control scores, and (b) the ratio of drug score to control score (D/C). The latter measure was used to minimize the effects of the absolute level of performance on response decrement. Using the absolute measure, the t test for correlated means indicated no significant differences between the means of absolute decrement in response scores at the different drive levels; this was true for both drugs. Using the ratio measure (Table 3) it was also found that the mean ratio of drug to control performance was independent of the drive level at the time of test. In the case of chlorpromazine, the ratios at the lowest drive level were somewhat smaller than those at the two higher drive levels, but this apparent trend is not reliable.

TABLE 3. Means and *SD*s of ratios of drug to control performance at different drive levels.

Stage	Drive Level					
	Low		Medium		High	
	Mean	SD	Mean	SD	Mean	SD
1	.58	.31	.73	.28	.75	.22
2	.60	.36	.79	.30	.76	.28
3	.94	28	.89	.29	.97	.19

DISCUSSION. Under the conditions of the present experiment, mild doses of chlorpromazine and methylphenidate decreased the rate of lever pressing for water. The decremental effect of methylphenidate requires a word of comment. Even a cursory glance at the results of studies of the effects of stimulants on a lever pressing response (e.g., Hearst, 1961; Miller, 1956; Owen, 1960; Skinner and Heron, 1937; Teitelbaum and Derks, 1958) shows these effects to be quite variable; incremental effects are found together with decremental effects, sometimes in the same experiment. We believe that these discrepancies have arisen mainly from three types of differences in procedure: (*a*) Dose level: in general, the higher the dose the more likely it is that the stimulant will produce a decremental effect. (*b*) Schedule of reinforcement: continuous reinforcement schedules are more likely to yield decremental effects; schedules, such as partial and extinction, under which the animal makes many multiple responses (lever presses without entering the goal area) are likely to yield incremental effects. (*c*) Distance between the lever and the reward area: in general, the greater this distance, the more likely it is that the stimulant will decrease response rate. (It may be that the crucial factor here is the size of the lever box rather than the distance between the lever and the reward area.) Using the specifications of the procedure employed in the present experiment, we have consistently obtained decremental effects with from 2 to 10 mg/kg of methylphenidate. As methylphenidate, like amphetamine, has an anorexic effect (Karczmar and Howard, 1959), it cannot be said whether the obtained decrease in lever pressing rate arises from anorexia or from interference caused by increased general activity; however, we are inclined to attribute greater importance to the latter factor (Bindra, 1961).

The decremental effects of both chlorpromazine and methylphenidate, as measured by the absolute and proportionate decrement in response scores in the present study, were fairly constant over a wide range of drive levels. For chlorpromazine, the effects were constant over the entire range of drive levels used (see Fig. 1 and Table 3). For methylphenidate, although the effects at different drive levels were not significantly different from each other, the absolute decrement in response rate was significantly different from zero at the two lowest drive levels, but not at the highest drive level (see Fig. 2 and Table 3). Our casual observations suggested one possible basis for the difference between chlorpromazine-drive and methylphenidate-drive interactions. It seemed to us that while the decrement in the response rate under the influence of chlorpromazine resulted from over-all slowing of S's movements, the methylphenidate-induced decrement was associated with an increase in general activity, mainly repeated sniffing of different parts of the apparatus. Whether this difference is in any way related to the observed differences in interaction effects is a question that we are now investigating.

Payne (1958), in extending Hullian theory to account for response decrements resulting from drugs, concluded that "manipulations resulting in higher reaction potential will, under constant dosage, attenuate the degrating effect of a drug" (p. 342). According to Payne's analysis, one would expect the depressing effects of drugs to be less when the response is tested at high drive than when it is tested at a low drive level. The present results show this to be true only in the case of methylphenidate. Apparently, the simple relation suggested by Payne has limited applicability. The factors that determine the exact manner in which various drive and drug effects combine remain to be determined.

SUMMARY.   Is the effect of the injection of a given drug on a response dependent upon the drive level at which the response is tested? The effects of injections of chlorpromazine (1.5 mg/kg) and methylphenidate (4 mg/kg) on a water rewarded lever pressing response were studied at several levels of thirst. Within three phases of the experiment all Ss were tested, in a balanced order, under each of the six conditions (3 drive levels × 2 drug conditions).

The following results were found: (a) The higher the drive level, the greater the response rate in both the control and the drug conditions. (b) Both chlorpromazine and methylphenidate decreased response rate, though the former drug is a mild depressant ("tranquilizer") and the latter a stimulant. (c) There were no significant differences between the mean absolute, or relative, decrements in response score produced by either of the drugs at the different drive levels. (d) Methylphenidate failed to produce any marked decrement at the highest drive level; thus the response was less vulnerable to the effects of this drug at a high drive level than at low drive levels.

The decremental effects on the response of stimulants such as methylphenidate and amphetamine are discussed. Some suggestions are presented regarding the basis of the difference in methylphenidate-drive and chlorpromazine-drive combinations.

REFERENCES

Bindra, D. Components of general activity and the analysis of behavior. *Psychol. Rev.*, 1961, 68, 205–215.

Bindra, D., and Baran, D. Effects of methylphenidylacetate and chlorpromazine on certain components of general activity. *J. exp. Anal. Behav.*, 1959, 2, 343–350.

Hearst, E. Effects of *d*-amphetamine on behavior reinforced by food and water. *Psychol. Rep.*, 1961, 8, 301–309.

Hulicka, I. M. Combination of drive and incentive. *Quart. J. exp. Psychol.*, 1960, 12, 185–189.

Karczmar, A. G., and Howard, J. H. Anorexigenic action and methylphenidate (Ritalin) and Pipradrol (Meratran). *Proc. Soc. Exp. Biol. Med.*, 1959, 102, 163–167.

Miller, N. E. Effects of drugs on motivation: The value of using a variety of measures. *Ann. N.Y. Acad. Sci.*, 1956, 65, 318–333.

Owen, J. E., Jr. The influence of *dl-, d-,* and *l*-amphetamine and *d*-methamphetamine on a fixed-ratio schedule. *J. exp. Anal. Behav.*, 1960, 3, 293–310.

Payne, R. B. An extension of Hullian theory to response decrements resulting from drugs. *J. exp. Psychol.*, 1958, 55, 342–346.

Skinner, B. F., and Heron, W. T. Effects of caffeine and benzedrine upon conditioning and extinction. *Psychol. Rec.*, 1937, 1, 340–346.

Teitelbaum, P., and Derks, P. The effect of amphetamine on forced drinking in the rat. *J. comp. physiol. Psychol.*, 1958, 51, 801–810.

12

The interaction of drug effects with drive level and habit strength

SHEO D. SINGH and SATINDER N. MANOCHA

In contrast to the reports of Bindra and Mendelson (1962, 1963), we have previously published data (Singh, 1964; Singh, Sharma and Manocha, 1965) which indicate that more highly learned responses become less susceptible to drug effects than less highly learned responses. The stronger the habit strength of a lever-pressing response in the rat, the weaker was the deleterious effect of a "tranquilizing" drug, chlorpromazine, upon it. According to Singh (1964), it was Bindra and Mendelson's use of an ambiguous measure, the performance level, as an index of habit strength which was mostly responsible for the contrasting nature of their results. In another similar study (Singh, Sharma and Manocha, 1965), we have observed that the effects of the same drug on the lever-pressing behaviour also decreased with an increase in drive level, but less reliably. In view of the important theoretical and practical implications of the knowledge concerning the way in which drug effects combine with those of such behavioural parameters as drive and habit (Mendelson and Bindra, 1962; Payne, 1958; Russel, 1964) the present study was undertaken (a) to verify our previous findings, and also (b) to examine what manner habit and drive variables combine with each other to influencing the deleterious effects of drugs on learned behaviours.

Specifically, combinations of various levels of drive and habit variables with a small dose of chlorpromazine were studied in the present experiment. Variations in this drive were introduced by "prefeeding" different amounts of water before testing; variations in habit were attained by the provision of varying number of training sessions.

METHOD. *Subjects.* The subjects were 27 naive white male albino rats, approximately 75 days old and weighing 50–75 g at the beginning of the training trials. They were housed in 25 by 25 by 25 cm cages, four to a cage, with food available at all times. They were gradually initiated to a 23-hr. water deprivation schedule, on which they remained throughout the experiment.

Apparatus. The apparatus consisted of a Skinner box as described elsewhere (Singh, 1964). In brief, it contained a lever measuring 2.5 by

From *Psychopharmacologia* (Berl.), 1966, 9, 205–209. Copyright 1966 by Springer-Verlag, Heidelberg, Germany.

1.9 cm and mounted 5 cm above the floor on one wall of the box. The lever required a pressure of 12 g to be depressed. Each lever-press delivered approximately .06 ml water into a water tray, which was located 6 cm to the left of the lever. The inside of the box was painted gray, and illuminated by a 2.5 w. bulb.

Procedure. Training in the lever-pressing behaviour was managed as follows. Each subject was placed individually in the box for 5 min. a day, and the number of times it pressed the lever was recorded. This procedure continued till the animal showed a stable lever-pressing performance as defined by two or more equal scores on three successive training sessions. The subjects reaching this level earlier than others were suspended from training until the others also reached the criterion of stable performance. Then they were randomly assigned in groups of nine to three habit groups designated H1, H2, and H3. The H1 group was put to the testing schedule immediately after attaining the defined criterion, and the H2 and H3 groups after seven and fifteen days of overtraining respectively. The subjects in each group were further subdivided equally into three drive groups designated by D_1, D_2, and D_3 according to the variations in the D level. The animals in the D_1, D_2, and D_3 groups were allowed to drink 0.2, 3 and 7 ml water respectively approximately 55 min. before the testing session. For this purpose the animal was placed with its allotted amount of water in a cage measuring 25 by 25 by 25 cm.

The same testing schedule was employed for all the subjects. Each subject was tested for two days under both the drug and placebo conditions in a random order. The drug treatment consisted of giving an i. p. injection of 2 mg/kg dose of chlorpromazine, and the placebo treatment was an i. p. injection of 0.25 ml distilled water. Forty-five minutes after the treatment the subject's performance in the Skinner box was observed for a 5-minute period. Almost 24 hours elapsed between the test sessions.

RESULTS. At the time of allocation of the subjects to the experimental groups their stable lever-pressing scores ranged from 33 to 90, with a mean = 52.26 and SD = 11.10. The groups and sub-groups were comparable in respect of these performance scores, as the analysis of variance results disclosed no significant differences among them.

Table 1 summarizes the performance scores of the sub-groups under both the drug and placebo conditions. In respect of placebo scores, as is apparent from Table 1, the groups varied largely. Analysis of variance showed that such differences among them resulted mainly from variations in drive (F = 39.61; d. f. = 2/18; $p < .001$) rather than in habit; as expected, the higher the level of drive (i.e., the less the amount of "predrinking") the greater were subjects' response rates under the placebo condition. Therefore, mainly in view of the large variations in the placebo scores of the subjects in different drive groups, reduction in a subject's performance

TABLE 1. Means and standard deviations of the placebo and drug scores of the experimental groups.

Drive levels	Habit levels											
	H_1				H_2				H_3			
	Placebo		Drug		Placebo		Drug		Placebo		Drug	
	M	SD	M	SD	M	SD	M	SD	M	SD	M	SD
D_1	48.00	5.61	29.35	5.32	46.65	9.06	31.80	4.71	52.51	10.72	45.50	12.25
D_2	36.16	8.41	14.50	1.80	38.65	8.91	24.51	9.80	41.15	0.23	32.85	5.03
D_3	19.67	5.21	3.00	1.08	17.82	6.71	10.15	5.89	22.35	6.86	16.67	5.57

under drug conditions was evaluated against its placebo performance by way of transforming the test scores into an inflection ratio using the formula: Inflection ratio = $(B - A)/A$ (A = mean of the two placebo scores, and B = mean of the drug scores of a subject). Negative and positive values of the ratios indicate decreases and increases respectively in a subject's rate of lever-pressing response on the drug trials. An analysis of variance was performed on these ratios, the results of which are presented in Table 2.

As shown in the table each of the two behavioural parameters, drive and habit, was found to affect significantly the drug's deleterious action on performance efficiency; an insignificant interaction between them simply indicates that their combination with each other was no more than additive in its influence on the degrading effects of the drug. Figure 1 clearly illustrates the nature of the relationship between these parameters and the drug effects on the learned response. As shown in the figure, the deleterious effects of the drug on the performance decreased with an increase in drive and habit levels; the drug effects were minimal and maximal at the highest and lowest levels of both of these parameters respectively. The two tailed t test, using the error term of the analysis of variance, indicated significant differences among the habit groups, the levels of significance being not less than .05 in any case; the differences among the drive groups, on the other hand, were not very marked, as only the D1 and D3 groups differed significantly ($P < .02$).

TABLE 2. Results of analysis of variance.

Source	df	Ms	F
Habit (H)	2	0.376	10.08*
Drive (D)	2	0.132	3.54**
H × D	4	0.026	0.69
Error	18	0.037	
Total	26		

* Significant at .001 level.
** Significant at .05 level.

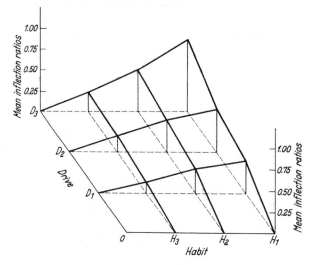

FIGURE 1. A three-dimensional graph of the results showing the relationship of the drug effects on learned behavior with those of drive level and habit strength.

DISCUSSION. It is clear from the results of the experiment that over-learning and high drive level attenuate the effects of chlorpromazine on learned behaviours. Further, these behavioural parameters seem to combine with each other in an additive fashion to influence the effects.

Extending the Hullian model (1943) to account for the effects of depressant drugs upon learned behaviour, Payne (1958) proposed that "manipulation resulting in higher reaction potential will, under constant dose, attenuate the degrading effect of a drug." In other words, according to Payne's analysis, more highly learned or more highly motivated responses will be less susceptible to the deleterious effects of drugs than the less highly learned or less highly motivated responses. The present results, along with the results of our previous studies (Singh, 1964; Singh, Sharma and Manocha, 1965), lend strong support to Payne's hypotheses in regard to the nature of combinations of the effects of depressant drugs with those of drive level and habit strength mediating a learned form of behaviour.

SUMMARY. Combinations of effects of chlorpromazine with those of various levels of drive and habit on the lever-pressing response in the rat were studied in a factorially designed experiment. Twenty-seven white male albino rats served as subjects. Variations in drive level were obtained by "prefeeding" subjects different amount of water before testing, and in habit level by giving them varying number of training sessions. The results indicate that over-learning and high drive level attenuate the effects of chlorpromazine, and that, drive and habit seem to combine with each other in an additive fashion in influencing the drug effects. These results were interpreted to support Payne's hypothesis with regard to the combinations of the effects of drive and training level with the effects of depressant drugs on learned behaviour.

REFERENCES

Bindra, D., and Mendelson, J.: Interaction of habit strength and drug effects. *J. comp. physiol. Psychol.* **55**, 217–219 (1962).

Bindra, D., and Mendelson, J.: Training, drive level, and drug effects: A temporal analysis of their combined influence on behavior. *J. comp. physiol. Psychol.* **56**, 183–189 (1963).

Hull, C. L.: *Principles of behavior.* New York: Appleton-Century-Crofts 1943.

Mendelson, J., and Bindra, D.: Combinations of drive and drug effects. *J. exp. Psychol.* **63**, 505–509 (1962).

Payne, R. B.: An extension of Hullian theory to response decrements resulting from drugs. *J. exp. Psychol.* **55**, 342–346 (1958).

Russell, R. W.: Psychopharmacology. *Ann. Rev. Psychol.* **15**, 87–114 (1964).

Singh, S. D.: Habit strength and drug effects. *J. comp. physiol. Psychol.* **58**, 468–469 (1964).

Singh, S. D, Sharma, S., and Manocha, S. N.: Habit, drive and drug effects. *Psychol. Stud.* **10**, 38–44 (1965).

Section **C**   STIMULUS VARIABLES

Stimulus control refers to the degree to which an antecedent stimulus determines the probability of a given response. The effect of drugs on stimulus control has been the focus of a good deal of research, but distinguishing alterations of stimulus control from other behavioral actions has been difficult. Adding to the complexities of the task is the problem that drug effects themselves may have stimulus properties. Behavior acquired under one set of stimulus conditions and tested for strength under other conditions poses a general problem in drug research. Any drug has the potential for changing stimulus conditions, thereby weakening the strength of the conditioned response. The limits of drug-produced stimulus control have been the subject of increasing research. Methodologically, some of the more important advances have been the use of intravenous route of administration, which provided greater experimental specificity and control, and the use of naturally occurring neurohumors (Articles 13 and 14).

Traditional psychophysical problems of measuring absolute sensory thresholds are further confounded when drug variables are introduced. Operant technology has provided increasingly refined behavioral preparations for studying sensory thresholds, and one of these is discussed in Article 15, with LSD-25 as the investigational drug.

One interpretation of the ability of drugs to alter the

129

strength of behavior is that chemical changes may shift the gradient of stimulus generalization. Obtaining stable gradients of stimulus generalization is difficult, but the method used by Hanson and Guttman (Article 16) provides a basis for exploring the role of drugs in modification of generalization. A related method, used by Hearst (Article 17), yields similar results.

Interactions between kinds or parameters of discriminative stimuli and drugs are a major consideration in evaluating behavioral actions of drugs. Behavior controlled by introceptive stimuli may be more susceptible to alteration by drugs than exteroceptively controlled behavior (Article 19). Behavior controlled by complex discriminative stimuli may be more readily disrupted than that controlled by simpler stimuli (Article 18). Thus, it is of questionable value to say that a drug diminishes stimulus control, unless several modalities have been studied, across a range of intensities and under a variety of conditions of complexity.

13

Epinephrine, norepinephrine, and acetylcholine as conditioned stimuli for avoidance behavior

Leonard Cook, Arnold Davidson, Dixon J. Davis,
and Roger T. Kelleher

Many investigators have suggested the importance of physiological correlates of behavior (1). However, few workers have considered the possible role of physiological changes as stimuli (2). The studies reported here were conducted to determine whether physiological changes produced by *l*-epinephrine, *l*-norepinephrine, acetylcholine, or stimulation of a Thiry-Vella jejunal loop can become conditioned stimuli in avoidance conditioning.

Beagles, surgically prepared with Thiry-Vella jejunal loops, were restrained in a harness in a soundproof chamber. A balloon inserted into the Thiry-Vella loop could be inflated remotely with 10 cm-Hg pressure. The conditioned stimulus was a balloon inflation lasting 2 seconds, terminated by the unconditioned stimulus, a brief electric shock (of intensity sufficient to cause leg flexion) delivered to the left hind leg. After an appropriate number of trials, balloon pressure *alone* consistently produced leg flexion, the conditioned avoidance response.

Other experiments were conducted to determine whether physiological changes produced by pharmacological agents could also act as conditioned stimuli in avoidance conditioning. A polygraph simultaneously recorded respiration, electrocardiogram, and intestinal activity of Thiry-Vella jejunal loops. The electrocardiographic recordings were made with surface electrodes fixed over the heart apex and the right paravertebral line (modified CR_{6L} lead) in order to minimize artifacts from gross body movements (3). Two fine polyethylene catheters were inserted into the external saphenous vein of the right hind leg and attached to syringes outside the soundproof chamber. These catheters permitted the injection of *l*-epinephrine, *l*-norepinephrine, or acetylcholine under remote control.

In each conditioning trial, electric shock was delivered to the left hind limb 30 seconds after the start of the injection. Injections were spaced 5 to 10 minutes apart, to allow time for physiological responses to return to normal levels. No stimuli, other than the physiological effects produced by the injected agents, preceded the shock. Preliminary experiments demonstrated that the monitored physiological responses were generally maximal

From *Science,* 1960, 131, 990–991. Copyright 1960 by the American Association for the Advancement of Science, Washington, D.C.

30 seconds after injection. Leg flexions occurring within the 30-second interval automatically prevented the shock. Prior to conditioning, none of the agents studied produced leg flexion. The effects of *l*-epinephrine (10 μg/kg), *l*-norepinephrine (10 μg/kg), or acetylcholine (20 μg/kg) came to serve as conditioned stimuli for the avoidance response after an appropriate number of training trials.

Figure 1 shows representative curves for the development of avoidance behavior with the various types of conditioned stimuli. For comparative purposes, other dogs were conditioned to an auditory stimulus (tone) as the conditioned stimulus. Differences in rates of acquisition are apparent; however, direct comparison of these rates is limited because the patterns of stimuli vary, due to differences in dose and in the intensity of effects. Figure 2 is a polygraphic recording of a representative trial, showing physiological effects and conditioned leg-flexion avoidance response. Jejunal activity, respiration, and electrocardiograph were monitored for indications of the occurrence of physiological changes and the temporal relationships of these changes to conditioned leg flexion. It was observed that physiological changes consistently preceded the occurrence of the avoidance response.

After dogs had been conditioned to the effects of 10 μg of *l*-epinephrine per kilogram, doses of 1 or 2.5 μg of *l*-epinephrine per kilogram could produce avoidance responses. In a similar manner, dogs conditioned to 20 μg of acetylcholine per kilogram manifested avoidance responses after the injection of 10 μg of acetylcholine per kilogram. Saline, in comparable

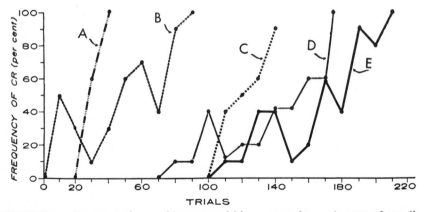

FIGURE 1. Representative avoidance acquisition curves for each type of conditioned stimulus; each curve represents the results obtained with a single animal. Conditioned stimuli: *A,* tone; *B,* acetylcholine; *C, l*-norepinephrine; *D,* jejunal pressure; *E, l*-epinephrine. Different dogs were used in each experiment. Each point represents the percentage of conditioned leg flexions occurring in blocks of ten successive trials.

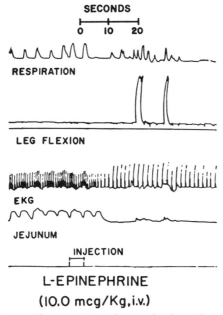

L-EPINEPHRINE

(10.0 mcg/Kg, i.v.)

FIGURE 2.   Polygraphic record showing a trial in which the dog avoided shock. The leg flexion (avoidance response) followed the compensatory bradycardia and decreased intestinal motility produced by the injection of epinephrine.

volumes, was injected on a random basis with all drug injections through the second catheter; saline injections never produced an avoidance response. These control injections eliminate the possibility that local sensation at the site of injection or volume changes acted as the conditioned stimulus. Injections of glucose (5 or 10 mg/kg) also failed to produce conditioned avoidance responses in dogs conditioned with *l*-epinephrine.

This type of conditioning can be due to peripheral physiological effects having an afferent influence centrally, or to direct drug effects on the central nervous system, or to aspects of both (4). The experiments involving pressure in jejunal Thiry-Vella loops suggest that peripheral stimulation alone can act as a conditioned stimulus. Physiological effects produced by *l*-epinephrine, *l*-norepinephrine, or acetylcholine can play a role in the development, as well as the maintenance, of a conditioned avoidance response in dogs.

SUMMARY.   Conditioned leg-flexion responses in dogs were developed with electric shock as an unconditioned stimulus and with intestinal stimulation or the effects of injections of various drugs as conditioned stimuli. It is concluded that physiological effects can play a role in the development and maintenance of conditioned avoidance behavior.

REFERENCES

1. W. B. Cannon, *Bodily changes in pain, hunger, fear and rage* (Branford, Boston, Mass., ed. 2, 1953); F. Dunbar, *Emotions and bodily changes* (Columbia Univ. Press, New York, ed. 4, 1954).
2. K. M. Bykov, *The cerebral cortex and the internal organs,* W. H. Gantt, trans. (Chemical Publishing Co., New York, 1957); G. Razran, *Science* **128**, 1187 (1958).
3. N. Lannek, *A clinical and experimental study on the electrocardiogram in dogs* (Hoeggströms, Stockholm, 1949).
4. A. B. Rothballer, *Pharmacol. Revs.* **11**, 494 (1959); H. Weil-Malherbe, J. Axelrod, R. Tomchick, *Science* **129**, 1226 (1959).

14

The discriminative control of a food-reinforced operant by interoceptive stimulation [1]

CHARLES R. SCHUSTER and JOSEPH V. BRADY

In 1928 Bykov and Ivonova provided the first demonstration that interoceptive stimulation could become a conditioned stimulus in a classical conditioning paradigm (1). Utilizing the classical conditioning technique, Bykov and his co-workers have subsequently demonstrated the existence of interoceptors in a wide variety of organs and tissues in the body. The extent of general scientific interest in this area is indicated by the fact that Bykov's major report of his thirty-year program on interoception has been translated into more foreign languages than any other Russian book in the field of medicine or biology (2).

The role of interoceptors in the control of operant behavior has unfortunately received only limited experimental attention. That operants may be brought under the stimulus control of interoceptors has been strongly suggested by the numerous studies requiring subjects to respond differentially on the basis of inferred physiological changes induced by such manipulations as drug administration or by deprivation of food or water (3, 4, 5, 6, 7, 8). More recently, Cook *et al.,* have demonstrated that avoidance responses can be brought under the stimulus control of physiological changes associated with the intravenous administration of epinephrine, nor-epinephrine, and acetylcholine (9).

The present investigation was concerned with demonstrating whether a food-reinforced operant could be brought under the discriminative control of interoceptive stimulation induced by: (*a*) the intravenous infusion of epinephrine and (*b*) the intravenous infusion of a saline-dextrose mixture into the superior vena-cava. Manipulations were carried out not only to determine the existence of receptors in the superior vena-cava, but also to define their characteristics and sensitivity.

METHOD

Subjects. The subjects in this investigation were 4 adult male rhesus monkeys selected from a stock colony on the basis of health and size.

From *Pavlov Journal of Higher Nervous Activity,* 1964, 14, 448–458. Copyright 1964 by Elsevier Publishing Company, Amsterdam, The Netherlands.

[1] This research was supported by Research Grant MY-1604 from the National Institute of Mental Health.

All subjects weighed between 4.0 and 6.0 kg. Prior to this investigation the subjects were experimentally naive. The principles of laboratory animal care as promulgated by the National Society for Medical Research were observed.

Surgical procedure for the implantation of a chronic indwelling jugular catheter. Each subject was surgically prepared with a chronic polyethylene tubing catheter introduced into the internal jugular and terminating in the superior vena-cava. The tubing was run subcutaneously to a midpoint on the animal's skull, where it was fixed in a skull-mounted bolt. Details of the surgical procedure are described elsewhere (10).

Apparatus. Each subject was restrained in a standard Foringer Primate Chair to which was attached a lever manipulandum, a food-pellet magazine, and a visual stimulus display panel. To prevent the subject from dislocating the catheter, the hand-hole covers on the restraining chair were kept closed. This necessitated utilization of a special mouth feeder in order to dispense pellets of food to the subject automatically. A cable, led through the wall, connected this equipment to a relay rack situated in an adjacent room. Stimulus presentations, food reinforcements, and recording of the subject's lever responses were accomplished automatically by means of electrical timers, counters, running time meters, stepping switches, and associated relay circuitry. In Experiment 2 cumulative records were obtained by use of a Gerbrands Model C Cumulative Recorder.

Each subject was housed individually in an $8 \times 8 \times 10$-foot room, with the back of the primate chair situated approximately 6 inches from the side wall. A 6-foot length of sterile polyethylene tubing (PE 100) was fixed with a needle juncture to the implanted catheter. This tubing was next run through a rubber stopper in the wall behind the chair. The tubing was fixed in the rubber stopper with epoxy resin glue.

White noise was on continuously in the experimental room to mask noises made by the experimenter and associated mechanical and electrical apparatus.

In Experiment 1, epinephrine and saline solutions were infused manually from 1 cc tuberculin syringes. The rate of infusion was held constant by careful attention to a wall clock with a sweep second hand.

In Experiment 2, infusions were made automatically by a Harvard Infusion Apparatus (Model 410). This apparatus had been modified so that periods of infusion could be programmed intermittently.

General behavioral procedures. The general procedure followed in this series of experiments was to bring a food-reinforced lever-pressing operant under the discriminative control of an interoceptive stimulus. A precise description of the nature of the interoceptive stimulation will be given in connection with each experiment. Certain features of the training regimen common to both experiments are given here

Deprivation conditions. At the start of each experimental session the subjects had been deprived of food for approximately 18 hours. Whenever possible, the subjects received their total daily food ration in the experimental session. In instances where this was not possible, the animals received the remainder of their daily food ration at the end of the experimental session. Water was available continuously.

Session 1: Magazine training. In this and in all subsequent sessions a white light in the visual display panel was illuminated during the experimental session. On a variable time schedule, with an average of 4 minutes, food pellets were automatically presented in the mouth feeder. The animals' ability to obtain these pellets was monitored by the experimenter. All the subjects were observed to obtain and eat the food pellets in the first 4-hour session. The sound of the electric motor in the food magazine accompanied the presentation of the food pellets. A total of 60 food pellets were given to each subject in this session.

Session 2: Lever training. The subjects were given access to the lever manipulandum for the first time during the second experimental session. In the presence of the white house light each lever response was reinforced with the presentation of a single pellet of food. All subjects were conditioned to emit this response and received a total of 75 reinforcements within a 2-hour experimental session.

In both experiments, discrimination training was initiated in Session 3. The details of the exact procedure will be described in conjunction with each of the experiments.

EXPERIMENT I

Methods. Two subjects, surgically prepared and lever-trained as previously described, were used in this experiment.

Interoceptive stimulation was produced by infusion of an epinephrine solution through the chronic indwelling jugular catheter.

The infusion sequence was as follows:

A. In the presence of the white house light a 60-second infusion period was intermittently presented.

B. In the first 20 seconds of the infusion period the animal was infused with 0.20 cc of the epinephrine solution. In this volume 20 mcg/kg of the drug was dissolved.

C. In the next 10 seconds the experimenter changed syringes to one containing 0.9% saline.

D. In the last 30 seconds of the infusion period 0.40 cc of saline was forced through the catheter in order to wash all the epinephrine solution into the subject.

The above procedure will hereafter be referred to as an epinephrine trial.

E. Control infusion trials were carried out in the same manner as described above, with the exception that in section B 0.9% saline was used rather than the epinephrine solution. This will hereafter be referred to as a saline control trial.

Injections were made manually by the experimenter. Every attempt was made to keep the injection procedure constant for both the epinephrine and saline control trials. In each daily session a total of 25 epinephrine trials were randomly alternated with 25 saline control trials. All trials were presented on a variable time schedule with a minimum of 120 and a maximum of 480 seconds. A response occurring within 60 seconds after the termination of the epinephrine trial was reinforced with three pellets of food. Responses in the 60-second interval following the saline control infusion sequence were never reinforced with food.

Table 1 gives the procedure followed in the discrimination training.

Beginning with Session 11 the number of responses required for delivery of the food reinforcement was increased to five (FR 5).

Following Sessions 18 and 27 the dosage of epinephrine was decreased. This was done because of certain toxic effects produced by the drug. At the higher dosages employed, the subjects showed frequent vomiting in close temporal contiguity with the drug administration. Further, both subjects suffered chronic diarrhea.

The number of responses made in the 60-second interval following epinephrine and saline infusions were recorded for each presentation. This was coverted to a percentage of times that the subject met the ratio requirement in saline and epinephrine trials in each daily session.

RESULTS.   Figure 1 shows the percentage of saline control and epinephrine trials in which the subjects met the fixed-ratio requirements. In Sessions 3 to 10 this percentage shows a gradual increase for both the epinephrine and saline control trials. When the response requirement was increased to FR 5 in Session 11, this percentage shows a slight decline. In subsequent sessions, however, the percentage continues to increase. By Session 18 the subjects met the fixed-ratio requirement more than 75%

TABLE 1.   Discrimination training procedure.

Session	Epinephrine dosage mcg/kg	No. of epinephrine trials	No. of saline-control trials	No. of responses required for reinforcement
3–4	20	25	25	1
5–10	20	25	25	1
11–17	20	25	25	5
18–27*	15	25	25	5
28–57	10	25	25	5

* Subject E-1 only following Session 27.

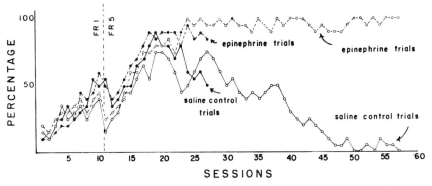

FIGURE 1. Percentage of epinephrine and saline control trials in which the subject met the response requirements for reinforcement.

of the time. There was, however, no difference between the non-reinforced saline control trials and the reinforced epinephrine trials. Evidence of differential stimulus control by the epinephrine infusion is not observed until Session 23. Beginning with Session 23 the subjects showed a gradual decrement in emitting the fixed ratio of five responses in the saline control trials.

Subject E-2 died following Session 27. The remaining results were obtained from subject E-1 only.

In subject E-1 the epinephrine infusion has clearly gained discriminative control over the lever-pressing operant by Session 47. In Sessions 47 to 57 the subject rarely responded following the saline control infusion, whereas the subject met the ratio requirement almost 100% of the time following the epinephrine administration. Following Session 57 subject E-1 died.

DISCUSSION.   The demonstration that a food-reinforced operant can be brought under the discriminative control of interoceptive changes produced by the administration of epinephrine is a logical extension of prior reports (9). As previously mentioned, Cook *et al.* have demonstrated that avoidance responding in dogs can be brought under the stimulus control of intravenous administration of epinephrine. The present findings confirm this earlier investigation in showing that drug-induced interoceptive changes can act as a discriminative stimulus.

The most striking result obtained in the present investigation is that the lever-pressing operant readily came under the discriminative control of the infusion of both epinephrine and saline. This is indicated by the increased frequency of responding for both types of trials in the first 15 to 20 sessions. Presumably the subjects are showing generalization from the reinforced epinephrine infusions to the non-reinforced saline infusions. The results suggest that the infusion of saline through the jugular catheter into the superior vena-cava was discriminable to the subjects. Because of this unexpected finding a second experiment was undertaken to specify the conditions under which a monkey's operant behavior could be brought under the discriminative control of this infusion procedure.

EXPERIMENT II

METHODS. *A. Discrimination training sessions.* Two subjects (DM 2 and DM 3), surgically prepared and lever-trained as previously described, were used in the experiment.

Interoceptive stimulation was produced by infusing a 5% dextrose saline solution into the superior vena-cava at a rate of 2.00 cc/minute. These S^D infusion periods were controlled by a Harvard Infusion Apparatus (Model No. 410) modified so that infusion periods could be intermittently programmed. Control infusion periods consisted of the infusion of the saline-dextrose mixture at a rate of 0.04 cc/minute. The rate of infusion for the control and S^D infusion periods was manually preset by the experimenter through the dial adjustment on the Harvard Infusion Apparatus.

The S^D and control infusion periods continued at each presentation until the subject emitted a lever-pressing response or for a period of 30 seconds. A response during the S^D infusion period had two consequences: (*a*) the infusion was terminated and (*b*) a reinforcement of two food pellets was delivered to the subject. Responses during the control infusion periods also had two consequences: (*a*) the termination of the infusion and (*b*) the occurrence of a 2-minute "time-out" period during which all experimental stimuli and the timer controlling infusion-period presentations were turned off. The number of responses required for the above-mentioned consequences was increased in Sessions 4 to 8 from 1 to 10. This will be referred to as a fixed ratio of ten responses or FR 10.

Each daily experimental session lasted for approximately 5 hours. A white light in the visual display was illuminated during the experimental sessions except during "time-out" periods. In the course of the 5-hour session, 50 S^D infusion and 50 control infusion periods were randomly presented on a variable time schedule. A minimum of 60 and a maximum of 300 seconds separated each infusion presentation.

Latency measures, from the onset of the infusion period to the emission of the tenth response, were separately recorded in 0.01 of a minute for S^D and control infusion periods. In addition the frequency of S^D and control infusion periods in which the fixed ratio of ten responses occurred was recorded and converted into percentages for each experimental session. Cumulative records of each daily session were obtained.

B. Parametric investigation of discriminative control as a function of infusion rate. Following stabilization of the subject's behavior, the rate of infusion was varied systematically over five values: 0.125, 0.25, 0.50, 1.00, and 2.00 cc/minute. Emission of ten responses during the 30-second infusion period at all values was reinforced with a single food pellet. In Sessions 46 to 55 each subject was given 100 S^D infusion presentations at each of these values to allow stabilization of its performance. During the next ten sessions (56 to 65) the five infusion rates were presented systematically. In each daily session ten S^D infusion periods were given at each rate. Ten control infusion periods were also presented daily. The sequence of presentation was randomized immediately prior to each daily session.

Latency measures, from the onset of the infusion period to the time taken for the subjects to emit ten responses, were separately recorded in units of 0.01 of a minute for all the infusion rates. The frequency of meeting the FR 10 requirement was also separately recorded for all infusion rates.

RESULTS.   *A. Discrimination training sessions.*   After approximately 35 sessions, the lever-pressing operant of both subjects was seen to be under the discriminative control of the S^D infusion periods. Figure 2 shows a one-hour sample cumulative record taken from Session 39 for both subjects. This record shows that the subjects consistently emitted the FR 10 in the S^D infusion periods. By contrast, the animals rarely responded as frequently as ten times in the 30-second control infusion period. Table 2 shows these percentages for both subjects in Sessions 41 to 45. The subjects met the FR 10 requirement over 90% of the time in the S^D infusion periods while the percentage of control trials in which the subjects emitted ten responses was consistently below 35%.

Table 3 shows the average latencies from the same sessions in 0.01 of a

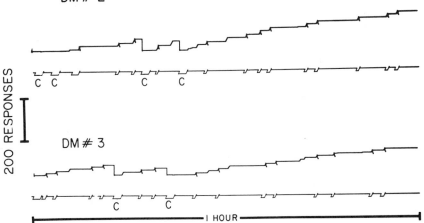

FIGURE 2.   Representative cumulative records under baseline performance conditions. C = Control infusion periods.

TABLE 2.   Percentage of S^D and control infusion periods in which subjects emitted ten responses.

	Subject DM 2		Subject DM 3	
Session no.	% S^D infusion	% Control infusion	% S^D infusion	% Control infusion
41	96	20	100	32
42	100	32	92	24
43	92	32	96	20
44	100	24	100	32
45	100	28	96	32

minute from the onset of the S^D and control infusion periods to the occurrence of the tenth response. The consistent and marked difference in the latencies between the control and S^D infusion periods reflects the degree of stimulus control exercised by the S^D infusion procedure.

Since the latency measure and the percentage of trials in which the subjects met the FR 10 requirement was found to be stable over Sessions 41 to 45, the second phase of this experiment was started in Session 46.

B. Parametric investigation of discriminative control as a function of infusion rate.   Figure 3 shows the percentage of trials in which the subjects met FR 10 requirement as a function of the five S^D infusion rates and control infusions. At the highest infusion rate of 2.00 cc/minute both subjects met the FR 10 requirement over 90% of the time.

The percentage of trials in which the subjects met the FR 10 requirement varies directly as a function of infusion rate. At the lower infusion rates of 0.25 and 0.125 cc/minute the percentage approximates that obtained in the non-reinforced control infusion periods.

Figure 4 illustrates changes in latencies to the tenth response as a function of the rate of infusion. As the rate of infusion decreased, latencies to the tenth response show a consistent increment. At the lowest infusion rates of 0.25

TABLE 3.   Average latencies in 0.01 of a minute from S^D or control infusion onset to emission of the tenth response.

	Subject DM 2		Subject DM 3	
Session no.	S^D infusion latencies	Control infusion latencies	S^D infusion latencies	Control infusion latencies
41	0.13	0.46	0.11	0.42
42	0.10	0.42	0.10	0.40
43	0.11	0.44	0.13	0.41
44	0.09	0.39	0.12	0.45
45	0.13	0.42	0.11	0.40

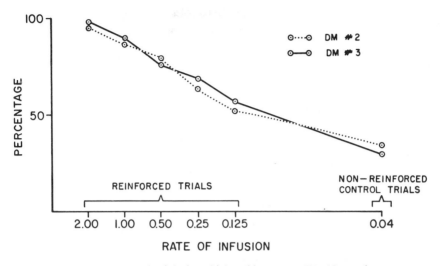

FIGURE 3.   Percentage of trials in which subjects met FR 10 requirement as a function of rate of infusion. Each point represents 100 trials.

and 0.125 cc/minute the latencies for both subjects approximate those obtained for the non-reinforced control infusion periods.

DISCUSSION.   The results of this experiment demonstrate that an operant can be brought under the control of the infusion of a saline-dextrose mixture into the superior vena-cava. From the parametric study of infusion rates it can be stated that rates at least as low as 0.50 cc/minute can require significant discriminative control over the lever-pressing operant. These con-

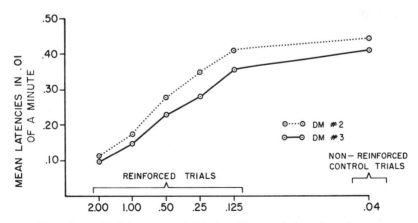

FIGURE 4.   Latencies from onset of infusion S^D to emission of tenth response as a function of rate of infusion. Each point represents mean of 100 trials.

clusions are based on the observed differences in the subjects' performance in the S^D infusion periods and the control infusion periods. Before concluding that the discrimination is based upon differential interoceptive stimulation, however, it is necessary to rule out any possible differential exteroceptive cues associated with the different infusion rates. The two most likely sources of exteroceptive stimulation were those associated with temperature of the infused solution and with vibrations of the catheter induced by the Harvard Infusion Apparatus. Control studies were therefore performed to assess the role of such factors in determining the results of this experiment.

CONTROL STUDIES FOR EXPERIMENT II

METHODS.   Following Experiment 2, subjects DM 2 and DM 3 were returned to the baseline condition in which the S^D infusion rate was fixed at 2.00 cc/minute. For five consecutive sessions 50 S^D and 50 control infusion periods were given daily. Latencies, from the onset of the infusion periods to the completion of the tenth response, were recorded separately. The frequency of meeting the FR 10 requirement under the different conditions was also recorded separately. These contingencies prevailed during the following three experimental manipulations.

A. Vibration control study.   In Session 71 the polyethylene catheter was firmly taped to a 3-inch, 8-ohm Varsity speaker at a distance of 15 inches above the insertion point of the tubing into the subject. The speaker was driven continuously during this session by a Foringer White Noise Generator.

B. Thermal control study.   In Session 74 the saline-dextrose mixture was heated to a temperature of 100°F. at the point of entry of the catheter into the subject.

C. Chemical constituents study.   In Sessions 76, 77, and 78 the infused solution was systematically varied from 0.9% saline–5% dextrose mixture to either 5% dextrose in sterile water or 0.9% saline. Blocks of six S^D infusions using each of the three solutions were randomly presented over the course of these three sessions. The subjects were reinforced for emitting the FR 10 in all of the S^D infusion periods regardless of the constituents of the solution. Since it was impossible to drain the catheter connection to the subject, the data from the first S^D infusion period following a change in solutions were discounted. This trial served essentially to refill the catheter with the new solution being tested. This gave a total of 50 S^D infusion periods with each of the three solutions from which the subjects' performance was recorded.

RESULTS.   *A. Vibration control study.*   Figure 5 shows the percentage of times that the subjects met the FR 10 requirement in the S^D infusion pe-

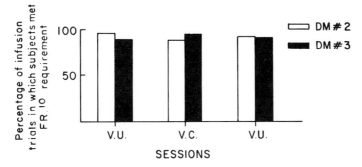

FIGURE 5. Percentage of trials (N = 50) in which subjects met FR 10 requirement in sessions with (V.C.) and without (V.U.) vibration of catheter.

riods 70, 71, and 72. In Sessions 70 and 72 the baseline procedure was followed. In Session 71 the catheter was vibrated by being taped over the 3-inch Varsity speaker. The percentage of trials in which the subjects met the FR 10 requirement was not significantly affected by the addition of the vibration to the catheter. The ineffectiveness of this vibratory procedure to mask the infusion S^D is further shown by the latency data in Figure 6. The latencies in Sessions 70 and 72 were not significantly from those obtained in Session 71.

Figure 7 reveals an especially pertinent fact. In Session 71, where the catheter was purposely vibrated, the percentage of control trials in which the subjects emitted ten responses is consistently below that seen in Sessions 70 and 72.

B. Temperature control study. Figure 8 shows the percentage of time that the subjects met the FR 10 requirement in the S^D infusion periods in Sessions 73, 74, and 75. In Sessions 73 and 75 the temperature of the infused solution was uncontrolled to the extent that room temperature fluctuations occurred. In Session 74 the solution reached the subject at a

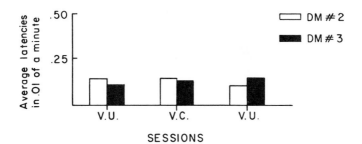

FIGURE 6. Percentage of control trials (N = 50) in which subjects emitted ten responses in sessions with (V.C.) and without (V.U.) vibration of catheter.

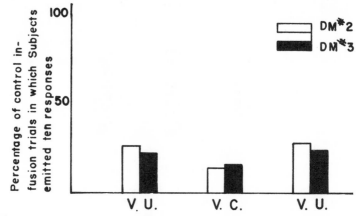

FIGURE 7.   Latencies to the tenth response in infusion S^D in sessions with (V.C.) and without (V.U.) vibration of catheter.

temperature of approximately 100–102°F. The manipulation produced no change in the frequency with which the subjects met the FR 10 requirement in the S^D infusion periods. The failure of this manipulation to alter the subjects' discrimination is also reflected by the latency data given in Fig. 9. The latencies shown here for sessions without the temperature control are not significantly different from the session where the solution was heated to approximately 100°F.

C. Chemical constituents study.   Figure 10 shows the percentage of trials in which the subjects met the FR 10 requirement in S^D infusion periods as a function of the three types of solution: 0.9% saline–5% dextrose, 0.9% saline, and 5% dextrose in sterile water. The results in Fig. 10 fail to reflect any differences in the stimulus control of the infusion S^D as a function of the different constituents in the solution. The latency measures, shown in Fig. 11, also fail to reflect any change in the discriminative con-

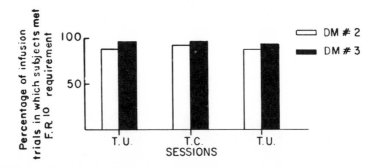

FIGURE 8.   Percentage of trials (N = 50) in which subjects met FR 10 requirement when infusion temperature was uncontrolled (Sessions T.U.) and when heated to 100°F. (Session T.C.).

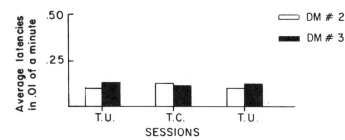

FIGURE 9.   Latencies to the tenth response in infusion S^D when infusion temperature was uncontrolled (T.U.) and when heated to 100°F. (Session T.C.).

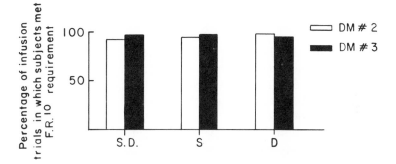

FIGURE 10.   Percentage of trials (N = 50) in which subjects met FR 10 requirement as a function of the chemical constituents of the infusion S^D.

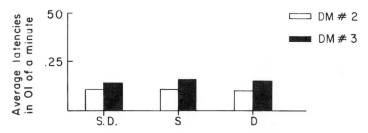

FIGURE 11.   Latencies to the tenth response in infusion S^D as a function of the chemical constituents of the infusion.

trol of the infusion procedures as a function of the different chemical constituents.

GENERAL DISCUSSION

The control studies in the previous section fail to give any evidence that the discriminative control exerted by the S^D infusion procedure was based upon thermal or vibratory stimulation. It seems likely, however, that vibratory stimulation common to both S^D and control infusion periods may account for the subjects' responding periodically in the control infusion periods. The decrement seen in the frequency of responding in the control infusion periods when the catheter was continuously vibrated may have been caused by the "masking" of the vibratory cues induced by energizing the Harvard Infusion Apparatus. The fact that the stimulus control exerted by the infusion S^D was not disrupted by the continuous vibration of the catheter indicated, however, that the vibratory stimulation caused by the Harvard Infusion Apparatus was not a necessary condition for the discrimination. The procedure of continuously vibrating the catheter may be found useful in future research for "masking" potential sources of vibratory stimulation.

On the basis of the evidence obtained in the control studies, it may be concluded that the discriminative control exerted by the infusion of the saline-dextrose solution into the superior vena-cava is based upon the stimulation of interoceptors. The exact nature and location of these interoceptors cannot as yet be specified, since the data in this report suggest only certain logical possibilities.

The fact that the discriminative control exerted by the S^D infusion procedure was comparably effective when the infused solution was changed from saline-dextrose to 0.9% saline indicates that neither systemic nor local effects of the dextrose were necessary conditions for this discrimination. The comparable stimulus control exerted by the infusion of the 5% dextrose in sterile water also rules out systemic or local effects of the NaCl as the basis of this discrimination.

The existence of baroreceptors in the circulatory system has been demonstrated (1) and suggests the possibility that such receptors located in the superior vena-cava could be involved in the present discrimination. This possibility seems unlikely, however, since rates of infusion as low as 0.50 cc/minute were found to exert significant discriminative control over the subjects' behavior. The average volume of the saline-dextrose mixture which the subjects received in each S^D infusion period at the rate of 0.50 cc/minute was less than 0.40 cc. In the same time period as this infusion, approximately 300–400 cc of venous blood was returned into the superior vena-cava (11). Normal fluctuations in the volume of venous blood returning through the superior vena-cava are far greater than that produced by the infusion procedure, and it would be difficult to conceive how the baroreceptors could serve as the basis for the observed discrimination under these conditions.

The results of the thermal control study, in which the saline-dextrose solution was heated to approximately the subjects' body temperature, would seem to rule out thermal receptors in any location as the basis of this discrimination. Further, the warming of the saline-dextrose mixture by the blood in the superior vena-cava would be extremely rapid because of the volume differences involved.

Several experimental manipulations remain to be explored in future investigations in an effort to specify the exact nature of the stimulus and interoceptors involved in this discrimination. A technique is currently being developed which will allow the use of the subject's own venous blood as the infused solution. The physical and chemical properties of the withdrawn blood will be maintained unchanged. If the infusion of blood can be shown to gain discriminative control over the lever-pressing operant, then chemoreceptors can be excluded as the possible neural basis of this discrimination.

SOME GENERAL COMMENTS.   Both Experiments 1 and 2 demonstrate that a food-reinforced operant can be brought under the discriminative control of interoceptive stimulation. This fact has both methodological and theoretical implications.

First, the use of the operant paradigm for establishing discrimination has been shown applicable to investigating the existence and sensitivity of at least certain types of interoceptors. Neurophysiologists, psychopharmacologists, as well as psychologists may find this a valuable procedure for establishing a behavioral baseline for studying changes in the sensitivity of interoceptors as a function of experimental manipulations appropriate to these disciplines. Future research will determine the relative efficacy of this procedure, as compared to the classical conditioning paradigm, as a means of studying interoceptors. Hopefully. both methods can be used to confirm and extend important new facts relevant to the experimental analysis of behavior.

REFERENCES

1. Bykov, K. M. trans. and ed. by W. H. Gantt. *The cerebral cortex and the internal organs.* Chemical Publishing Co., Inc., New York, N.Y., 1957.
2. Razran, G. The observable unconscious and the inferable conscious in current Soviet psychophysiology: Interoceptive conditioning, semantic conditioning, orienting reflex. *Psychol. Rev.,* 1961, **68**, 81–147.
3. Hull, C. L. Differential habituation to internal stimuli in the albino rat. *J. comp. Psychol.,* 1933, **16**, 255–273.
4. Leeper, R. The role of motivation in learning: A study of the phenomenon of differential motivational control of the utilization of habits. *J. genet. Psychol.,* 1935, **46**, 3–40.
5. Kendler, H. H. The influence of simultaneous hunger and thirst drives upon the learning of two opposed spatial responses of the white rat. *J. exp. Psychol.,* 1946, 36, 212–220.
6. Amsel, A. Selective association and the anticipatory goal response mechanism as explanatory concepts in learning theory. *J. exp. Psychol.,* 1949, **59**, 785–799.

7. Conger, J. J. The effects of alcohol on conflict behavior in the albino rat. *Quart. J. Stud. Alc.*, 1951, 12, 1–29.

8. Heistad, G. T. A biopsychological approach to somatic treatments in psychiatry. *Amer. J. Psychiat.*, 1957, 114, 540.

9. Cook, L., Davidson, A., Davis, D. J., and Kelleher, R. T. Epinephrine, norepinephrine, and actylcholine as conditioned stimuli for avoidance behavior. *Science*, 1960, 131, 990–991.

10. Nieman, W. I., Schuster, R. C., and Thompson, T. A surgical preparation for chronic intravenous infusion in rhesus monkeys. Technical Report #6230, Laboratory of Psychopharmacology, The University of Maryland, 1962.

11. Spector, W. S. (Ed.) *Handbook of biological data.* Philadelphia, Pa., W. B. Saunders Co., 1956.

15

Effect of lysergic acid diethylamide on absolute visual threshold of the pigeon

Donald S. Blough

There have been many recent reports that human subjects receiving small doses of lysergic acid diethylamide (LSD) tend to behave in some ways like psychotic patients. These reports have stimulated efforts at careful specification of the psychological and physiological effects of LSD. Prominent among the effects found thus far have been disturbances of visual functions, including apparent changes in visual sensitivity. E. V. Evarts (1) recently reported that monkeys recovering from large doses of LSD were active but behaved as though they were blind. Carlson (2) has noted a slight rise in the absolute visual threshold of human subjects following intravenous administration of 100 μg of LSD. In a related neurophysiological study (3), LSD markedly reduced the postsynaptic response in the lateral geniculate nucleus to stimulation of the optic nerve of the cat.

Such findings suggest that elevation of the absolute visual threshold is characteristic of the action of LSD. The present study (4) uses a recently devised technique (5) to measure this effect in the pigeon. The method is rather complex and its restatement here will be brief. The pigeon stands in a light-tight box and views a stimulus patch fixed in the wall. It pecks one response key when the stimulus patch is visible and another key when the patch appears dark. These pecks, operating through automatic control circuits, cause the intensity of the stimulus to vary up and down across the pigeon's absolute threshold. A recorder charts the stimulus intensity, indicating the bird's threshold through time. The automatic controls provided the pigeon with periodic rewards of food for correct responses.

The subjects were three male domestic pigeons (White Carneaux). The bird to be tested first was dark-adapted for at least 1 hour in the experimental box. The stimulus patch was then illuminated by a light beam of 500-mμ wavelength from a Bausch and Lomb grating monochromator. The bird responded to this stimulus for at least 30 minutes, or until its threshold appeared to be stable. Then the experimental box was opened in darkness, and a dose of water or LSD solution (100 or 300 μg/kg) was administered either orally or by intraperitoneal injection. Following administration, the bird's threshold was recorded for 2 hours. The bird then rested in the dark until a 30-minute test was made during the fifth hour after administration of the dose. In several instances, a final test was made about 22 hours after

From *Science*, 1957, **126**, 304–305.

administration of LSD. The birds were allowed from 3 days to 2 weeks for recovery between doses of LSD.

Some of the original data are reproduce in Fig. 1. The curves represent the brightness of the stimulus patch as a function of time before and after dosage. The base line for each curve extends through the midpoint of the threshold recorded before a dose was given. Three curves from single sessions are superimposed in the case of data obtained after administration of oral doses, while two curves make up each function in the case of data obtained after intraperitoneal administration. The uppermost function in Fig. 1 illustrates typical control data. Gaps appear in the records when the bird failed to respond. This often happened for a time after administration of the larger doses of LSD.

It is apparent that LSD caused a striking rise in absolute threshold. Bird

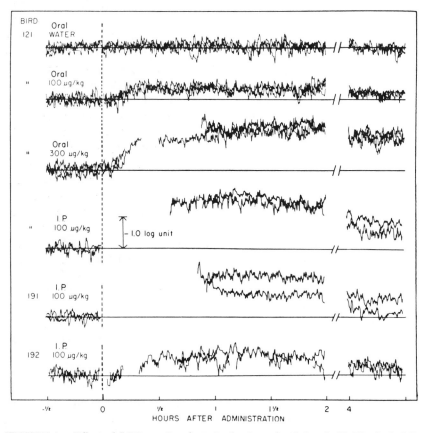

FIGURE 1. Effect of LSD on the pigeon's absolute visual threshold. Vertical shifts in the curves represent changes in the brightness of a "just visible" stimulus patch. A single oral dose amounted to about 4 ml of solution (10 ml/kg). A single intraperitoneal dose amounted to about .04 ml of solution (1 ml/kg).

121 was affected the most. It showed a swift and substantial rise in threshold with both doses and with both routes of administration. Intraperitoneal doses of 100 μg/kg given to this bird produced the largest threshold rise that was observed. The rise amounts to approximately 1.8 log units, a linear increase of roughly 60-fold.

Samples of the data from the other two pigeons are plotted as the lowest two functions in Fig. 1. The threshold changes observed in these birds were similar to those found with pigeon 121, though of somewhat smaller magnitude.

In most cases, the effect of LSD had diminished considerably by the fifth hour after administration. This was especially true in the case of intraperitoneal dosage. In no case was a threshold elevation still evident in the tests made after 22 hours.

It might be argued that the rise in threshold is only apparent and that the findings actually represent a failure by the birds to perform correctly in the discrimination situation. However, in a previous study, LSD at these dose levels improved the pigeon's performance on a visual discrimination task, rather than producing a decrement (6). Furthermore, spurious departures from a stable threshold have been marked in past studies by increased variability, rather than by the stable shift in level evidenced here.

Small doses of LSD thus appear to affect the visual threshold of the pigeon without grossly disturbing motor or discriminative functions. This fact may be a valuable clue in understanding the physiological action of the drug. It also suggests the use of visual threshold measurement as an assay technique in the study of LSD and related substances.

REFERENCES AND NOTES

1. E. V. Evarts, *Arch. Neurol. Psychiat.* **75**, 49 (1956).
2. V. R. Carlson, personal communication.
3. E. V. Evarts *et al., Am. J. Physiol.* **182**, 594 (1955).
4. The author acknowledges the aid of William H. Jones in running the experiments and in preparing the figures.
5. D. S. Blough, *Science* **121**, 703 (1955).
6. D. S. Blough, *Ann. N.Y. Acad. Sci.* **66**, 733 (1957).

16

The use of a behavioral stimulant in the study of
stimulus generalization [1]

HARLEY M. HANSON and NORMAN GUTTMAN

Pipradrol, a CNS stimulant, has been shown to affect the performance of
pigeons trained in the operant situation (Dews, 1956). In the present study,
the drug was used to modify response rates during tests of stimulus generalization in the pigeon.

METHOD. *Subjects.* Fifteen male White Carneaux pigeons (Palmetto
Pigeon Plant) maintained at 70–80% free-feeding body weight by restricted
feeding, were used.

Apparatus. An automatic key-pecking apparatus especially designed
for the study of stimulus generalization was used. A monochromatic light
source illuminated the key with any desired wavelength. Details of the
apparatus have been published elsewhere (Hanson, 1959).

Procedure. All pigeons were magazine-trained and conditioned to key
peck with monochromatic light of 550 millimicrons on the key. After two
daily sessions during which 50 continuous reinforcements were given, all
birds received 165 minutes of VI 1 traning to the same stimulus (550 millimicrons). Daily sessions consisted of sixty 30-second work periods separated by 10-second blackouts. The tenth daily session consisted of 120 such
work periods. After the tenth and final day of training, the pigeons were
divided into two groups: the experimental group N = 10, and the control
group N = 5.

All pigeons received generalization tests consisting of the repeated presentation of 11 monochromatic stimuli ranging from 490 to 640 millimicrons
under extinction conditions. Each stimulus was presented 10 times for 30
seconds according to a predetermined schedule of random permutations of
of the 11 stimuli. Ten-second blackouts separated presentations. A different
randomized schedule was used for each bird. On the day following the first
test, a second identical test was given. No training intervened between tests.

From *Journal of the Experimental Analysis of Behavior,* 1961, 4, 209–212. Copyright
1961 by the Society for the Experimental Analysis of Behavior, Inc., Bloomington,
Ind.

[1] This investigation was carried out during the senior author's tenure of a Public
Health Service Postdoctoral Research Fellowship. Support was derived from Grant
MH-1002, National Institute of Mental Health. Fellowship Supply Grant MF-6653
awarded by the Public Health Service also contributed to the research. Thanks are
due Mr. Arthur G. Itkin of the Merck Institute for statistical analysis of the data.

Approximately 80 minutes preceding generalization testing, the pigeons were injected intramuscularly with either 8 milligrams per kilogram of pipradrol [2] dissolved in saline or with a comparable volume of saline. The injection was given at two sites in the pectoral muscle.

RESULTS AND DISCUSSION.   The course of the rates of responding during generalization testing is shown in Fig. 1. The average number of responses emitted during 5.5-minute periods of the test (the time required, ignoring blackouts, for a single presentation of each of the test stimuli) is plotted against elapsed test time. The control group shows an orderly decrease, typical of extinction, in the number of responses emitted during testing for both Tests 1 and 2. The average number of responses emitted in the first 5.5-minute period of the second test is higher than the number of responses emitted during the last period of the first generalization test. This increase in responding (spontaneous recovery) is significant at better than the .05 level of confidence by the Mann-Whitney U test (Siegel, 1956).

The course of extinction was clearly different for the experimental group. The average rate of responding during the first period of the first test was significantly lower than that of the control group (.05 level by the Mann-Whitney U test). The response rates did not decrease during the course of extinction for either the experimental group or the control group.

[2] Pipradrol (Meratran) was kindly supplied by William S. Merill and Company.

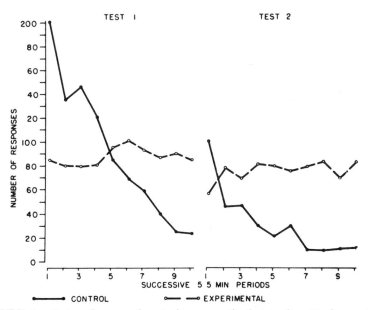

FIGURE 1.   Rates of responding during generalization testing. During each 5.5-minute period, each of the 11 test stimuli was presented once.

No significant differences were found between the average rates of responding for Periods 1 and 10 of the first generalization test. The average rates of responding of the experimental group during the first period of the second test are significantly lower than the average rates in the final period of the first test (P < .05 by the Mann-Whitney U test). During the second generalization test as during the first, the rate of responding of the drugged group did not decrease significantly.

From the data in Fig. 1, it would appear that pipradrol has a pronounced effect upon the behavior recorded during generalization testing. The initial rate of responding is lower for the drugged group, but this response level is sustained, essentially without decrement, during both test sessions. Thus, there is little evidence for experimental extinction within sessions and none for "spontaneous recovery" between sessions. It would seem safe to conclude that the compound injected was behaviorally active during the major part of generalization testing.

The generalization gradients in Fig. 2 were constructed by plotting the average number of responses emitted to each stimulus during testing against the wavelength of that stimulus. The gradients for the first and second tests were plotted separately. The average gradients produced during the first test by the two groups appear to be very similar in shape and height, and no significant differences between them were demonstrable. The gradient produced by the experimental group during the second test is markedly higher than that of the control group; both curves, however,

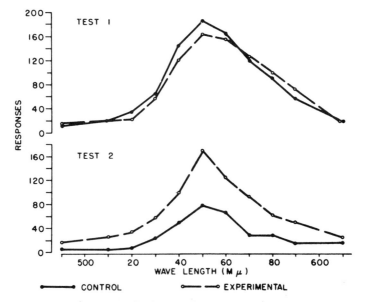

FIGURE 2. Mean generalization gradients for the drug and control groups.

would appear to belong to the same family of multiplicative curves published by Guttman and Kalish (1956). No gross changes or effects other than those attributable to changes in the total number of responses emitted are apparent.

This lack of effect on the gradient is supported by the curves in Fig. 3. To eliminate any difficulties in interpretation due to different response rates (interest being focused on possible effects on the shape of the gradient), only those data were plotted which were collected during the fourth and fifth presentations of the 11 stimuli in the first generalization test and during the first and second presentations of the 11 stimuli in the second test. At these times in the experiment, the response rates were essentially equal for the two groups. (See Fig. 1.) The per cent total average responses to each wavelength were plotted against wavelength. As was true for the original gradients, no significant differences are demonstrable between the two groups.

Figure 4 shows the percentage of the total number of individual stimulus presentations, *i.e.,* 30 seconds' exposure to one of the 11 stimuli, during which one or more responses were emitted during generalization testing, plotted against wavelength. The curves are bowl-shaped and essentially symmetrical around 550 millimicrons. For the first generalization test the curves are very similar, with only a nonsignificant difference in height separating them. These curves indicate that in the region where

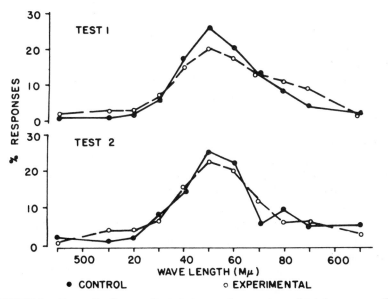

FIGURE 3. Generalization gradients in terms of percentage of total responses. Each point represents the group average for two stimulus presentations, at the stage of testing when the rates of responding of the drug and control groups were equal.

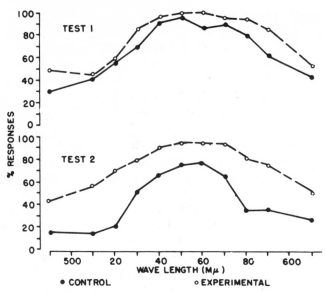

FIGURE 4. The group average percentage of stimulus presentations to which one or more responses were emitted plotted against wavelength of stimulus.

high rates of responding were found (*i.e.,* those stimuli close to the reinforced stimulus), nearly every stimulus presentation elicited one or more responses. In the second test the rates of the control group were lower and the general form of the curve is "contracted," *i.e.,* fewer stimuli elicited responses. In the experimental group, however, the over-all rates were high during the second test, and the per cent response curve is approximately that of the first test.

If the effect of the drug studied had been to lessen the stimulus control exerted by the earlier training, or if the effect of the drug was to increase responding to all stimuli additively, the experimental curves produced would be flatter. That this was not the case is apparent.

The effective control of responding along the wave-length continuum is dependent on both the over-all rate of responding and upon the proximity of a particular stimulus to the original positive stimulus. As the over-all rate of responding drops during generalization testing, the range of the stimuli eliciting responding decreases until, in the last stages of extinction, only the conditioned stimulus and one or two surrounding stimuli are responded to. This relationship is presented graphically in Fig. 5. The average number of responses emitted to any particular series of the 11 stimuli is plotted against the number (group average) of stimuli that elicited one or more responses. No curve has been fitted to the data, but a logarithmic function clearly represents them. When the response rate during generalization testing is low, the number of "active" stimuli is small. When the momentary response rate is high, the number of stimuli responded to is large.

The response rates for the pipradrol-treated animals did not drop appreciably during the generalization tests, as Fig. 1 shows. The points plotted for this group in Fig. 5 do not diverge appreciably from a function representing the control group; this fact may be considered additional evidence that the effect of this dose of pipradrol was to modify the over-all response rate but not the shape of the generalization gradient.

The data in Fig. 5 are strong evidence for the belief that if preliminary training is constant, the factors controlling responding during any single stimulus presentation during generalization testing are essentially *independent* of the serial effects of the testing procedure, and are mainly determined by: (1) the relationship along some dimension of the test stimulus to the conditioned stimulus; and (2) the momentary response rates obtaining during testing. The present experiment would suggest that these factors can be independent of factors controlling over-all response rates.

SUMMARY AND CONCLUSIONS.   Responding during generalization testing was modified by the administration of pipradrol. Although the pattern of responding occurring during testing was changed, no modifications in the gradients collected were detected.

The control of responding during generalization testing appears to be independent of both over-all response rates and the serial effects of the

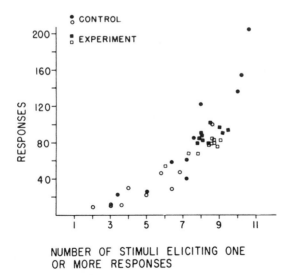

FIGURE 5.   Responses emitted to any individual series of the 11 stimuli, versus number of stimuli in the series eliciting one or more responses. (The filled points represent the data from the first generalization test.)

testing procedure. The essential controls during testing would appear to be the test stimulus-conditioned stimulus relationship on the test dimension and the momentary response rate.

REFERENCES

Dews, P. B. Modification by drugs of performance on simple schedules of positive reinforcement. *Ann. N.Y. Acad. Sci.,* 1956, 65, 268–281.

Guttman, P., and Kalish, H. Discriminability and stimulus generalization. *J. exp. Psychol.,* 1956, 51, 79–88.

Hanson, H. M. Effects of discrimination training on stimulus generalization. *J. exp. Psychol.,* 1959, 58, 321–334.

Siegel, Sidney. *Nonparametric statistics for the behavioral sciences.* New York: 1956.

17

Drug effects on stimulus generalization gradients in the monkey *

ELIOT HEARST

Drugs often affect the power of stimuli to evoke learned responses (Dews and Morse, 1961). Impairment of simple auditory or visual discriminations has been a common finding in the psychopharmacological literature, but there have been only a few studies in which the properties of conditioned stimuli were varied over a wide enough range so that an actual "gradient of stimulus control" could be obtained. Such gradients may serve as a useful tool for analyzing the relative sensitivity of normal and drugged animals to changes in their external environment.

In the present study, monkeys were trained to press a lever to avoid shock whenever one specific light intensity out of eight possible intensities illuminated the experimental chamber. The monkeys did not have to press the lever in the presence of the other seven intensities, since shocks could not occur in these other intensities. Even after prolonged training the monkeys never stopped responding in the seven "safe" intensities; however, they did press the lever much more often during intensities that were very similar to the one dangerous intensity than during intensities that were very different. In other words, responding along the light intensity continuum showed a gradient of stimulus generalization.

Drug tests with d-amphetamine, scopolamine and caffeine were then scheduled and their effects on gradients of stimulus generalization were observed.

METHOD. *Subjects.* The subjects were three mature rhesus monkeys, two males (No. 556 and No. 70) and one female (No. 240). Each monkey was housed in an individual home cage that was provided with an ample supply of water and food (NIH Primate Diet Pellets and an occasional orange or apple). All the monkeys had been subjects in prior studies that involved lever pressing for food reward or shock avoidance in various visual discrimination tasks.

Apparatus. The experimental chamber and accessory equipment

From *Psychopharmacologia* (Berl.), 1964, 6, 57–70. Copyright 1964 by Springer-Verlag, Heidelberg, Germany.

* The expert technical assistance of Peter Edmondo, Roger Poppen, and Joe Whitley is gratefully acknowledged. Some of the early experimental results have been briefly described in Hearst (1963).

have been described in detail in a previous report (Hearst, 1962). The monkeys pressed a lever mounted on one sidewall of the experimental chamber. Shocks of approximately 5 ma. for 0.5 sec. could be administered through the grid floor and walls of the chamber. A 110-vac., 60-watt Sylvania bulb, which was mounted above a milk glass screen in the far ceiling of the chamber, served both as a general illuminant (house light) and as the generalization test stimulus.

A group of potentiometers in series with the house light provided eight different test intensities. From time to time during the experiment, and on the rare occasions when the house light bulb burned out, the test intensities were recalibrated by adjustment of the potentiometer values. A Photovolt Corp. Model 210 Photometer was used in making the intensity measurements and calibrations.

The test chamber was located in a small lightproof cubicle. A white noise generator remained on at all times to mask sounds from outside the chamber. In another room a system of relays, timers, and counters automatically controlled variation of stimulus intensities, programming of the avoidance schedule, tabulation of lever presses, etc. A Gerbrands recorder was used to obtain cumulative response curves.

Procedure. Since the monkeys had previously learned to press the lever to avoid shock, they were immediately placed on the generalization procedure. Eight different light intensities, approximately equally spaced along a logarithmic scale from "very bright" (5.8 ft. ca., measured with the photometer at the grid floor of the chamber) to "very dim" (0.003 ft. ca.) were presented during each experimental session. The absolute intensity of the critical stimulus (henceforth to be abbreviated CS) was different for different subjects: Two monkeys (No. 556 and No. 70) had to press the lever to avoid shock during the brightest intensity, whereas the other monkey (No. 240) had to press the lever during the dimmest intensity.

Whenever CS was on, the subject had to respond at least once every 10 sec. to avoid shock; this is a continuous avoidance schedule of the kind described by Sidman (1953) and Heise and Boff (1962), in which the response-shock and shock-shock intervals are both equal to 10 sec. Each presentation of a specific intensity was 2 min. long. Every one of the eight intensity values occurred about 16 times during a standard test session, which lasted slightly more than 4 hrs. A mixed order of presentation of the 16 exposures of the eight different intensities was used, and the sequence was changed periodically during the months of experimentation in order to prevent possible learning of a particular sequence.

Two monkeys (No. 556 and No. 240) were tested during the normal working day. The other monkey (No. 70) was placed in the chamber in late afternoon and stayed there overnight; the house light went out at the termination of the session and this monkey was left in the darkened chamber until the next morning. With few exceptions, all animals were tested every weekday.

Since the monkeys were presented with all the different test intensities during every experimental session, this procedure was a combination of discrimination training and generalization testing. All subjects showed a peak of response strength at the CS, and decreasing response frequency as the light intensity was varied further and further from the CS.

After more than 20 sessions on this procedure, the behavior of the subjects no longer showed further improvement. The generalization gradients provided by each monkey were very consistent from day to day. Drug effects were then studied.

Drug administration. Three drugs were tested in the following order [1] in all the monkeys: *d*-amphetamine (1.0 and 2.0 mg/kg), scopolamine (0.01, 0.033, and 0.1 mg/kg), and caffeine (10.0, 20.0, and 40.0 mg/kg). The order of testing the different doses of each drug was different for each subject, but all tests with a given drug were completed before tests with a new compound began. Drug sessions occurred no more than once per week, usually on Wednesdays or Thursdays.

The average weights of the monkeys throughout the experiment were as follows: No. 556, 6.4 kg; No. 240, 5.2 kg; No. 70, 4.7 kg.

All injections were given intramuscularly less than a minute before the monkey was placed in the experimental chamber. Placebo injections (Ringer's solution) were administered on at least one occasion during each drug series. The data of these placebo tests, along with the results obtained on the no-injection days immediately preceding drug days, provided control records with which to compare the drug effects.

After the above drug determinations had been made, additional comparisons of *d*-amphetamine and caffeine were arranged. During these new determinations, higher doses of caffeine (60.0 and 80.0 mg/kg) were injected. These were compared with the standard 1.0 and 2.0 mg/kg doses of *d*-amphetamine. The various doses of the two drugs were administered in an irregular order to each subject. Just as before, only one drug test was scheduled weekly. During this new phase of the experiment, gradient readings were recorded every hour for Monkey No. 556 in order to secure information concerning the time course of the drug effects. Hourly readings for the other two monkeys could be recorded only occasionally, and the collected data were too incomplete for description in this report.

---

[1] All subjects were tested with several doses of chlorpromazine for a few months after the *d*-amphetamine data had been gathered and before the scopolamine phase began. The effects of chlorpromazine on stimulus generalization gradients were rather unreliable and differed from animal to animal, probably because of complicated interactions arising from the large number of shocks that often occurred after administration of chlorpromazine. The drug effects were therefore very difficult to interpret without further control experiments, and will not be discussed here.

Besides providing additional comparisons of *d*-amphetamine and caffeine, this final phase of the experiment permitted us to check on the reliability of the *d*-amphetamine effects obtained in the earlier test series, which occurred approximately seven months before. Any possible influences of the intervening tests with all the other compounds could also have been detected by these final *d*-amphetamine trials.

RESULTS.   Generalization gradients are plotted in two ways throughout the presentation of result in Figs 1–6. One of these uses response frequency as an absolute measure of generalization. The other is a relative measure that corrects for differences in overall response output.

The average number of lever presses per 2-min. presentation of each light intensity served as the absolute measure. Relative generalization was derived from the absolute measures by assigning the value of 1.00 to the peak of each gradient, the stimulus intensity at which the monkey pressed the lever most frequently; the other response frequencies were expressed as decimal fractions of this maximum value. The effect of a given drug on the actual frequency of lever pressing at each intensity can be seen only in the gradients of absolute generalization, whereas drug influences on the relative control that was exerted by each stimulus intensity can perhaps be most clearly observed in the other gradients.

The effects of different drugs will be discussed in the same order as the drugs themselves were tested. Figure 1 presents data obtained during the *d*-amphetamine series. Two doses (1.0 and 2.0 mg/kg) were tested twice each in all subjects. Each drug curve of Fig. 1 represents combined results for the two tests. The control (no injection) gradients were obtained on days immediately preceding drug days and therefore are means from a total of four sessions. One placebo injection was given during the series, on a day on which a drug would normally have been given. Gradients during this placebo test are also indicated in Fig. 1.

Although the effect of *d*-amphetamine on number of responses to the CS differed from monkey to monkey, frequency of response to the non-CS intensities was disproportionately facilitated in every monkey and therefore all relative generalization gradients became flatter after drug injection. Monkey No. 556 showed the largest effect; under *d*-amphetamine it pressed the lever very frequently in the presence of all the "safe" stimuli, and showed a facilitation of response during the CS as well. Monkey No. 70 displayed a similar flattening of gradients under *d*-amphetamine, even though it emitted fewer responses to the CS than under no-drug conditions.

Monkey No. 240 showed little or no effect of *d*-amphetamine on number of lever presses during CS. However, this subject did press the lever more often to safe stimuli when given *d*-amphetamine, which resulted in a flattening of relative gradients. The flattening was not as pronounced

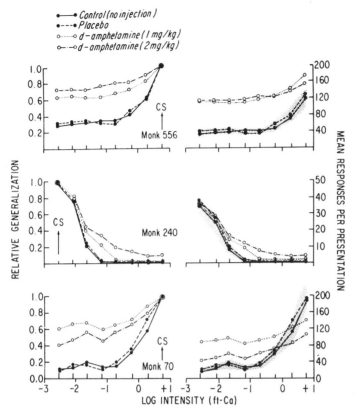

FIGURE 1.   Absolute and relative gradients of generalization during the *d*-amphet-amine series. The shaded areas in the absolute curves indicate the range of scores during the control sessions. All data are for entire (4 hr.) sessions.

as for the other two subjects. This may be related to the fact that No. 240's normal gradient was much sharper than that of the other two subjects, perhaps because the discrimination of CS-"dim" was easier to form than that of CS-"bright."

Absolute and relative generalization gradients obtained after placebo injections fell within the normal, non-drugged range for all monkeys.

One additional fact concerning avoidance performance on drug days ought to be emphasized: *d*-amphetamine did not have a significant effect on the number of shocks received by any of the subjects. During no-injection sessions the monkeys almost never received more than one shock per day (usually none), and this level was exceeded on only one occasion under the drug: Monkey No. 240 obtained 3 shocks during one of its *d*-amphetamine tests at 1.0 mg/kg. It is clear, then, that the flattening of generalization gradients was not associated with an increase in number of shocks on drug days. Past results (Sidman, 1958; Hearst,

1962), which suggest that shocks themselves may broaden stimulus generalization gradients, therefore do not seem to have very much applicability to the present findings.

Figure 2 summarizes the effects of scopolamine on absolute and relative measures of stimulus generalization. Procedures used in the analysis of data were exactly the same as for *d*-amphetamine, except that three different doses of scopolamine were tested twice each in this series. Consequently there were six no-injection sessions which entered into the calculation of the control means.

The effects of scopolamine on gradients of relative generalization were generally quite similar to those of *d*-amphetamine. Even though lower doses of scopolamine tended to facilitate responding to the CS in every subject—which had not been a consistent finding with the *d*-amphetamine doses tested—all gradients became flatter after drug administration. Once again, placebo results fell within the normal range for all subjects.

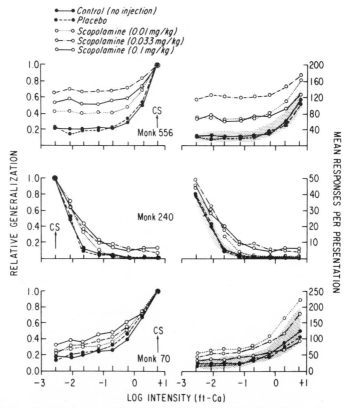

FIGURE 2.   Absolute and relative gradients of generalization during the scopolamine series.

The highest dose of scopolamine (0.1 mg/kg) had a detrimental effect on the efficiency of avoidance behavior in every subject. No monkey received more than one shock per session under the 0.01 and 0.033 mg/kg doses, and on no-injection days subjects rarely obtained even a single shock. On two occasions on which the 0.1 mg/kg dose was injected, however, Monkey No. 556 received 3 and 2 shocks, Monkey No. 240 received 6 and 4 shocks, and Monkey No. 70 received 26 and 3 shocks. Despite this impairment of performance at the highest dose, it seems unlikely that the number of shocks was a critical factor in the flattening of gradients, since the lower scopolamine doses also produced flatter than normal gradients and had no effect on number of shocks received.

Caffeine effects on generalization and response output can be seen in Fig. 3. The two highest doses (20.0 and 40.0 mg/kg) clearly increased the frequency of lever pressing to the CS and the safe stimuli in

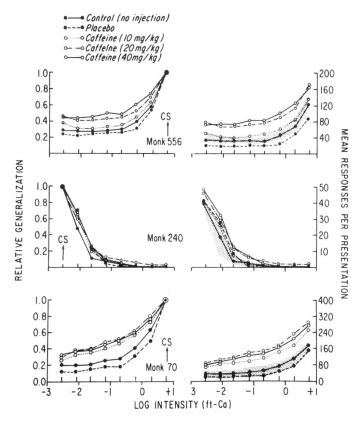

FIGURE 3.   Absolute and relative gradients of generalization during the caffeine series.

all monkeys. However, the influence of caffeine on the slope of the relative gradients was not as large as that of *d*-amphetamine, even though a flattening of gradients is certainly present for at least two of the three monkeys. In the next phase of the experiment (see ahead) still higher doses (80.0 mg/kg) of caffeine were injected and, although response output to the CS and the safe stimuli became even higher than at the lower doses, the flattening effect did not attain levels produced by 1.0 and 2.0 mg/kg doses of *d*-amphetamine—which had less effect than caffeine on absolute response frequency.

The major effect of caffeine in this situation therefore appears to be a facilitation of response output; its effect on gradient slope is less obvious than for *d*-amphetamine and possibly for scopolamine, too. On the other hand, the most obvious effects of *d*-amphetamine are on the slope of the generalization function rather than on frequency of lever-pressing to the CS and adjacent intensities. Absolute response frequency and gradient slope do not appear to be related in any obvious way.

Caffeine, like *d*-amphetamine, did not result in any impairment of avoidance behavior. On control and drug days monkeys rarely received even a single shock.

The final phases of the experiment involved specific comparisons of *d*-amphetamine and caffeine. These comparisons were made primarily to examine in more detail the suggestion of Figs. 1 and 3 that overall response level and relative slope may be independent of one another. By using even higher doses of caffeine, we could presumably increase response output to the various stimuli still further, and then check to see if flatter gradients would be obtained for caffeine than for *d*-amphetamine under these conditions.

Figure 4 presents some of these comparisons. For each monkey the mean performance for two sessions under caffeine (80.0 mg/kg) is compared with (a) mean performance during caffeine-control sessions (days immediately preceding the two caffeine days), (b) mean performance for two *d*-amphetamine tests [2.0 mg/kg for Monkeys No. 556 and No. 240, and 1.0 mg/kg for Monkey No. 70; the 1.0 mg/kg dose was used for No. 70 because this dose had consistently produced a greater effect than the 2.0 mg/kg dose during the earlier drug series (Fig. 1)], and (c) mean performance during the two *d*-amphetamine-control sessions.

Unfortunately, Monkey No. 240 became very ill after one of its tests at the 2.0 mg/kg dose of *d*-amphetamine and died a few days later. Therefore, in the presentation of this monkey's data in Fig. 4 we have had to compare the recent caffeine data with *d*-amphetamine data obtained from this monkey 6–7 months previously (the same data as plotted for the 2.0 mg/kg dose in Fig. 1).

It was noted in the procedure section of this report that 60.0 mg/kg doses of caffeine were also administered to the subjects during this final

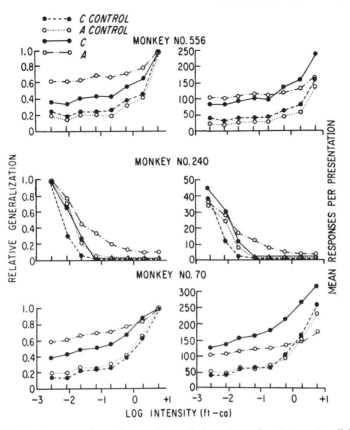

FIGURE 4. A comparison of the effects of d-amphetamine (A) and caffeine (C). The sessions immediately preceding each drug session provided the C-Control and A-Control data.

stage of the experiment. Since the results of tests at this dose merely supplement and confirm the other caffeine data of Fig. 3 and Figs. 4–6, the 60 mg/kg data will not be discussed further here.

In Fig. 4 all monkeys show a qualitatively similar effect: Caffeine had a much greater effect than d-amphetamine on overall response output, but d-amphetamine produced flatter gradients than caffeine. The effects of d-amphetamine on the absolute and relative gradients of Monkeys No. 556 and 70 were very similar to the earlier results of Fig. 1, even though a half-year of additional training and various drug injections had intervened between the determinations. The former monkey displayed, if anything, a tendency toward increased responding to the CS under d-amphetamine, the latter a tendency toward decreased responding.

The C- and A-control gradients are very similar to each other for

Monkeys No. 556 and 70, but are not particularly similar for Monkey 240, especially at intensity values close to the CS. It will be remembered that because of this subject's death the *d*-amphetamine gradients had to be taken from data obtained more than 6 months earlier than the caffeine gradients. Despite these discrepancies between C- and A-controls, Monkey 240 still showed an effect qualitatively similar to that of the other subjects.

Figures 5 and 6 present some data on the time course of the effects of *d*-amphetamine and caffeine for Monkey No. 556 only. Due to Monkey No. 240's death and No. 70's nighttime working hours, the hourly data of these other subjects were too fragmentary for presentation here. Monkey No. 556's records in Figs. 5 and 6 were obtained during the same sessions for which complete 4-hr. results were shown in Fig. 4.

During Hour 1 the effects of caffeine and *d*-amphetamine on both the absolute (Fig. 5) and relative (Fig. 6) measures were very similar; response output to the CS and to the other stimuli was significantly increased over control levels by both drugs, and the slopes of the relative gradients were flattened. During the next three hours, however, the

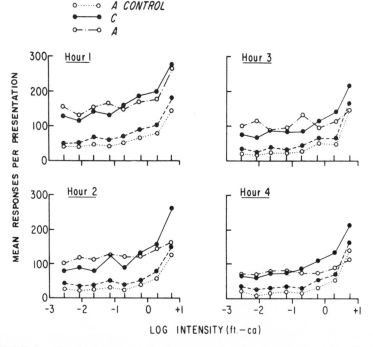

FIGURE 5.   Hourly records of absolute generalization for Monkey No. 556 during tests summarized for the entire session in Fig. 4.

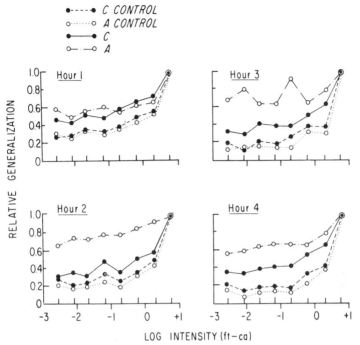

FIGURE 6.   Hourly records of relative generalization from the results of Fig. 5.

flattening of relative gradients was much more obvious with *d*-amphet-amine than with caffeine, even though overall response output (due primarily to high response frequencies at values near the CS) was much greater with caffeine.

Clear effects of *d*-amphetamine, scopolamine, and caffeine on gradi-ents of stimulus generalization were observed in this experiment. All drugs produced a flattening of gradients, that is, responding to the seven safe stimuli showed a proportionately greater increase over control levels than did responding to the CS. The effect was most pronounced with *d*-amphetamine, even though this drug did not have as great a facilitating effect on overall response output as did selected doses of caffeine.

This result indicates that gradient slope and overall response level may be relatively independent of one another, a finding which is some-what similar to that obtained in the psychopharmacological studies of Honig and Worst (1960), Hanson and Guttman (1961), and Key (1961). All of these workers found that increases or decreases in overall response strength after injections of such drugs as chlorpromazine, LSD-25, *d*-amphetamine, sodium pentobarbital, or pipradol were not accompanied by consistent changes in the slope of generalization gradi-ents. As a matter of fact, with the exception of sodium pentobarbital in Honig and Worst's food reward situation, the relative gradients of drugged subjects in these prior studies remained essentially unchanged despite changes in response level. In the present study the gradients did change in slope after drug injections, but these changes were not obviously correlated with changes in overall response level.

Certain specific details of our procedure make direct comparisons with prior studies of drug effects on stimulus generalization very difficult. The other studies involved tests for stimulus generalization during response extinction, and some were carried out with food reward as the incentive during training. In addition, the present procedure was a combination of discrimination training and generalization testing so that earlier methods, which focused on either one of these two aspects of stimulus control, are not especially comparable to ours. In the past, differential drug effects have occasionally been observed between discrimination and generalization procedures. For example, Key (1961) observed large effects of LSD and chlorpromazine on a trained discrimination between two auditory stimuli, but obtained negligible effects of these drugs in a multiple-auditory-stimulus test of gradient slope that involved no explicit discrimination training. Honig and Worst found no effect of d-amphetamine on the relative slope of visual wave length generalization gradients when no prior discrimination training had been given; however, these workers obtained deterimental effects of d-amphetamine in a trained positional discrimination. Honig and Worst commented that the processes of stimulus control in the "discrimination" and "generalization" procedures may well be different and that one way of illustrating this point is through such differential drug effects.

Perhaps somewhat similar to our caffeine results were those of Blough (1957), who found that caffeine had no apparent effect on accuracy of a visual discrimination in pigeons, but did bring about an increase in total response output.

In comparison to most of these prior studies, the present procedure for studying generalization appears to have the advantage that a large number of generalization tests may be given to individual subjects, which can therefore provide their own control data.

The flattening of gradients after administration of scopolamine supports the results and theoretical framework of Carlton (1963) who suggested that there is a cholinergic involvement in the mediation of the effects of nonreward. According to his analysis, anticholinergics like scopolamine ought to reactivate behavior that has been weakened by extinction, as was the case in the non-CS intensities of the present experiment. Whether the flattening effect produced by scopolamine occurs through a different "neurochemical-behavioral" mechanism than the effect produced by d-amphetamine or caffeine, which is an implication of Carlton's analysis, cannot be answered at the present time.

SUMMARY. Monkeys that had been trained to avoid shock in the presence of only one of eight possible light intensities showed maximal responding during the one dangerous intensity and a decreasing response frequency as the light intensity was varied further and further from the dangerous value. The effects of *d*-amphetamine, scopolamine, and caffeine were studied on these maintained gradients of stimulus generalization. The drugs had varying effects on specific measures of response output, but all drugs flattened the slopes of the generalization gradients; monkeys responded much more often than normally to intensities that were very different from the dangerous intensity. Since selected doses of caffeine facilitated overall response output more than *d*-amphetamine did, but had less of a gradient-flattening effect than *d*-amphetamine, variations in gradient slope are apparently more or less independent of effects on response strength.

REFERENCES

Blough, D.: Some effects of drugs on visual discrimination in the pigeon. *Ann. N.Y. Acad. Sci.* **66**, 733–739 (1957).

Carlton, P.: Cholinergic mechanisms in the control of behavior by the brain. *Psychol. Rev.* **70**, 19–39 (1963).

Dews, P. B., and Morse, W.: Behavioral pharmacology. *Ann. Rev. Pharmacol.* **1**, 145–174 (1961).

Hanson, H., and Guttman, N.: The use of a behavioral stimulant in the study of stimulus generalization. *J. exp. Anal. Behav.* **4**, 209–212 (1961).

Hearst, E.: Concurrent generalization gradients for food-controlled and shock-controlled behavior. *J. exp. Anal. Behav.* **5**, 19–31 (1962).

Hearst, E.: Studies in stimulus generalization: Some behavioral, pharmacological, and neuroanatomical factors. In: Proceedings of the Symposium on Feedback Mechanisms in the Central Nervous System. *Bol. Inst. Estud. méd. biol.* (Méx.) **21**, 485–496 (1963).

Heise, G., and Boff, E.: Continuous avoidance as a baseline for measuring behavioral effects of drugs. *Psychopharmacologia* (Berl.) **3**, 264–282 (1962).

Honig, W. K., and Worst, R. W.: Differential effects of drugs on generalization and discrimination in pigeons. Paper presented at the Amer. Psychological Ass. meetings, Chicago 1960.

Key, B. J.: The effect of drugs on discrimination and sensory generalization of auditory stimuli in cats. *Psychopharmacologia* (Berl.) **2**, 352–363 (1961).

Sidman, M.: Avoidance conditioning with brief shock and no exteroceptive warning signal. *Science* **118**, 157–158 (1953).

Sidman, M.: Avoidance conditioning with brief shock and no exteroceptive warning signal. *Science* **118**, 157–158 (1953).

Sidman, M.: Some notes on "bursts" in free-operant avoidance experiments. *J. exp. Anal. Behav.* **1**, 167–172 (1958).

18

The effects of pentobarbital, methamphetamine, and scopolamine on performances in pigeons involving discriminations [1]

PETER B. DEWS

The application of the Skinner box technique to study the behavioral effects of drugs has been described in a previous communication (Dews, 1955). The work was done on pigeons; the birds were intermittently rewarded with food for pecking a transilluminated plastic disc (the key). Two different schedules of reward were used; each gave rise to a characteristic pecking performance. The two different performances showed differential sensitivity to modification by pentobarbital. The schedule of reward was thus shown to be a relevant environmental variable in determining the behavioral effect of pentobarbital.

It is a characteristic feature of this type of behavior ("operant behavior"—Skinner, 1938) that it may be brought under "stimulus control." If a pigeon is rewarded according to an appropriate schedule for pecking the key when certain suitable environmental stimuli [2] are present, but is never rewarded when other stimuli are present, then the pecking performance comes to differ according to which of the stimuli are present. The pigeon "discriminates" between the stimuli, and behaves more or less appropriately to each. Alternatively, it may be said that the stimuli "control" the behavior of the animal. In the present work, the effect of three drugs (pentobarbital, methamphetamine, and scopolamine) on some aspects of such discriminatory behavior has been studied. It has been shown that these drugs, in doses up to those abolishing all pecking behavior under the conditions of study, did not interfere with the differential performance to a simple pair of stimuli. On the other hand, when a more complicated set of stimuli was used, it was found that pentobarbital, and methamphetamine but not scopolamine reduced the usual difference between the performance when the stimuli were appro-

From *Journal of Pharmacology and Experimental Therapeutics*, 1955, **115**, 380–389. Copyright © 1955 by The Williams and Wilkins Co., Baltimore, Md.

[1] This work was supported in part by funds received from the William F. Milton Fund of Harvard University, and in part by funds received from The Roche Anniversary Foundation of Hoffmann-La Roche Inc. The author wishes to thank Mr. Briah Connor for conscientious assistance throughout these experiments.

[2] The term "stimulus" is used here in its usual physiological sense of an environmental influence which causes, or tends to cause, a change in a living system.

DIAGRAMMATIC   REPRESENTATION
OF   SCHEDULES

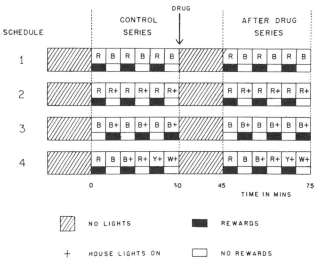

FIGURE 1.   Diagram showing sequence of stimuli in the various schedules used. R, B, Y and W indicate that the red, blue, yellow and white lights respectively were on behind the key.

priate for rewards and the performance when the stimuli were inappropriate for rewards.

MATERIALS AND METHODS. *Apparatus.* The Skinner pigeon box previously described (Dews, 1955) was modified for the present work. Four different colored bulbs (G.E. C 7½) were arranged so that the key could be transilluminated by any one of them, giving four possible "key colors." In addition, a 12 watt source of white light was put in the roof of the pigeon compartment at the opposite end to the key; this light (the "house light"), when on, brightly illuminated the whole pigeon compartment. Hence 8 different combinations of stimuli were possible, viz. 4 different key colors each with or without the house light; of these, 6 combinations were actually used. In the presence of certain of these combinations, the pigeon was intermittently rewarded with access to food for 4–5 seconds for pecking the key; these combinations of stimuli will be referred to as S+. In the presence of other combinations, the pigeon was never rewarded; these combinations of stimuli will be referred to as S—.[3] Responses made in the presence of S+ and S— were counted sepa-

[3] The symbols S+ and S— as here defined correspond to the symbols S^D and S^Δ respectively used in the psychological literature in this field. S+ and S— have been used for typographical convenience and because they suggest their meaning more obviously.

rately on digital counters; in addition a permanent time-cumulative response record was taken in all experiments, as previously described.

Schedules. In the presence of S+ rewards were arranged as follows. For a predetermined period of time following a reward (or the start of the S+ period) no peck was rewarded; when this time had elapsed, the first peck made was rewarded. The minimum interval which necessarily intervened between successive rewards was not constant; in the present work 15 different intervals were used, varying from 0 (two consecutive pecks rewarded) to 2 minutes, with an arithmetic mean of 1 minute. The sequence of the intervals was randomly determined in the first instance but then kept the same through all the experiments. This scheme is an example of a "variable interval" schedule of reward in the terminology of Skinner (1953). In the presence of S−, by definition, the pigeon never received any food.

In definitive experiments, S+ and S− were presented alternatively, each for 5 minutes. The changeover from one to the other was abrupt. Three alternations, giving a total presentation of S+ and S− of 15 minutes each, comprised a "series." Each experiment started with the bird waiting 15 minutes in the completely darkened box, followed by a control series. The pigeon was then removed from the box, injected with the appropriate dose of drug (or saline alone) and immediately replaced in the darkened box. The after drug series started 15 minutes later.

Four schedules, which differed according to the combinations of key color and presence or absence of house light constituting S+ and S−, were programmed. The arrangements are shown diagramatically in Fig. 1. It will be seen that in schedules 1, 2, and 3, S+ and S− differed in a single constant feature, viz., either key color (schedule 1) or presence or absence of the house light (schedules 2 and 3). On the other hand, in schedule 4, not only were there 3 different S+ and 3 different S− but, in the first four periods of a series, the contingency associated with each individual stimulus was conditional; neither the key color alone nor the presence or absence of the house light alone characterized the stimuli as S+ or S−; e.g. the presence of the house light was part of an S+ combination when the key was blue; but was part of an S− combination when the key was red. In contrast, in the last two periods of a schedule 4 series the yellow and white key colors uniquely characterized the stimuli as S+ and S− respectively exactly as did the red and blue key colors of schedule 1.

Procedure. Male white pigeons of between 400 and 500 grams weight were maintained in a standardized state of food deprivation (but with constant free access to water) and were trained to work in the Skinner box, as previously described (Dews, 1955). They were then assigned to the various schedules just described and run once daily, most days, until the completion of the experiments. The programming circuits were arranged so that each peck in the presence of S− could be made to reset the timer which was timing the 5 minute period of presentation of S−. Thus, when this "S− renewing" device was in operation, the S− periods continued until the pigeon had not pecked for 5 minutes. In general, S− renewing was used only during training of the birds; it was never in operation during definitive experiments. Stable performance developed much more slowly on schedule 4 (2–3 weeks) than on schedules 1, 2, 3 (4–5 days). Three pigeons were studied on schedule 1, one each on schedules 2 and 3 and two on schedule 4.

Pentobarbital sodium,[4] methamphetamine hydrochloride [5] and scopolamine hydrobromide [6] were dissolved in 0.9 per cent sodium chloride solution and were injected intramuscularly. Doses are stated in terms of these salts and give the total dose given to the birds. The various doses of each drug were given in random order; each dose was given on two occasions to the same pigeon. In general, where more than one drug was studied in the same pigeon, the observations on one drug were completed before starting observations on another drug.

Measurements of drug effects. Two indices have been used. (1) The *output ratio* (O.R.) was defined as the ratio of the average rate of response in the presence of S+ in the after drug series to the average rate of response in the presence of S+ in the control series in the same experiment. It is thus a measure of the effect of drugs on performance in the presence of S+. (2) The *discriminative ratio* (D.R.) was defined as the complement of the ratio of the average rate of response in the presence of S− to the average rate of response in the presence of S+ in the same series. Hence if the pigeon does not respond in the presence of S− but responds in the presence of S+ in the same series, the D.R. is 1; while if the rates of response are identical in the presence of both S+ and S− the D.R. is zero.

RESULTS. The 1 minute variable interval schedule of reward, in operation during all the S+ periods, gave rise to a relatively constant rate of response throughout the time of presentation of S+ (see Figs. 2 and 3). While the average rate varied amongst the pigeons from less than 60/min. to more than 130/min. (Table 1), it remained relatively constant for any one pigeon (average coefficient of variation 15 per cent).

On the other hand, the rate of response in the presence of S− fell to very low levels (Figs. 2 and 3, Table 1); i.e. the D.R. became close to 1.

Injections of drug or saline were given only when the D.R. of the control series exceeded 0.9. On 6 occasions with schedule 1 and on 9 occa-

---

[4] Generously donated by Abbott Laboratories.
[5] Generously donated by Burroughs, Wellcome & Co.
[6] Generously donated by Merck & Co.

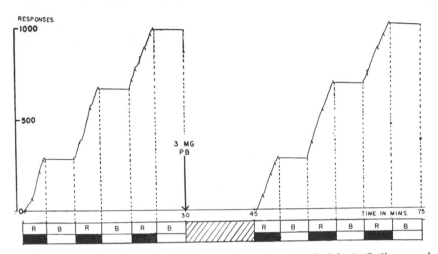

FIGURE 2.   Effect of pentobarbital on performance on schedule 1. Ordinate and abscissa scales have been superimposed on an original record. The short diagonal lines on the original record show the occurrence of rewards. Below the record is a key showing the nature of the stimuli throughout the run. The conventions in the key are the same as those of Fig. 1. Note almost complete absence of responding in S— periods and the lack of effect of 3 mgm. pentobarbital on performance on this schedule.

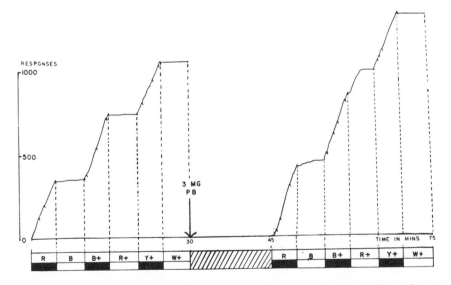

FIGURE 3.   Effect of pentobarbital on performance on schedule 4. Note almost complete absence of responding in S— periods before drug, but large number of responses in the second S— period after drug. Performance in S+ periods not obviously affected by this dose of pentobarbital.

TABLE 1.   Pecking performances of pigeons during control series.

Pigeon No.	Schedule	No. of Experiments	Mean No. of Pecks in 15 Mins of S+	Mean No. of Pecks in 15 Mins of S−	Mean D.R.
1	1	40	858	2.1	> .99
2	1	40	1257	4.6	> .99
3	1	24	1955	8.7	> .99
4	2	11	920	0.3	> .99
5	3	15	905	3.0	> .99
6	4	33	981	23.3	.98
7	4	40	906	19.9	.98

sions with schedule 4, the D.R. of the control series was less than 0.9; these experiments were not continued, and the figures from them are not included in Table 1.

Performance on schedule 1.   The control performances of birds on schedule 1 are summarized in Table 1. In all except 3 (out of 104) experiments, the D.R. was greater than 0.99 (i.e. the average rate in the presence of S+ was more than 100 times greater than in the presence of S−). In 20 control series there were no pecks in the total 15 minute presentation of S−, and in a further 41 there was only a simple peck; more than 5 pecks were made in only 16 experiments.

Following saline, the average D.R. was again 0.99 or higher (Table 2). Bird 1 rather consistently showed a slightly higher average response rate in the presence of S+ after the injection of saline than before (O.R. > 1); the opposite was true for bird 2 (O.R. < 1) (Table 2).

Effect of drugs on performance on schedule 1 (Table 3).   The effects of pentobarbital were studied in birds 2 and 3 (Fig. 2). Following doses of 4.0 mgm. or 5.2 mgm., the average rate of response in the presence of S+ was greatly reduced; but at no dose level did the average D.R. fall below 0.99.

TABLE 2.   Summary of saline control experiments.

Pigeon No.	Schedule No.	No. of Experiments	Mean O.R.	Standard Deviation	Mean D.R. of "After Drug" Series*
1	1	10	1.05	.059	> .99
2	1	14	0.82	.098	> .99
3	1	13	1.01	.108	> .99
4	2	2	0.93	—	> .99
5	3	2	1.02	—	> .99
6	4	8	0.88	.092	.98
7	4	9	1.04	.096	.95

* When saline alone had been given.

TABLE 3.   Effect of pentobarbital, methamphetamine and scopolamine on performance on schedule 1.

Pentobarbital Dosage (mgm.)	Mean[1] O.R.	Mean[1] D.R.	Methamphetamine Dosage (mgm.)	Mean[2] O.R.	Mean[2] D.R.	Scopolamine Dosage (mgm.)	Mean[3] O.R.	Mean[3] D.R.
0[4]	0.90[5]	>.99	0[4]	0.92[6]	>.99	0[4]	1.05[7]	>.99
1.0	0.91	>.99	0.1	0.98	>.99	0.001	1.02	>.99
3.0	1.00	>.99	0.3	0.78	>.99	0.003	0.87	>.99
4.0	0.22	>.99	1.0	0.27	>.99	0.01	0.76	>.99
5.2	0.01	>.99	1.7	0.22	>.99	0.017	0.64	>.99
			3.0	0.01	>.99	0.03	0.14	>.99
						0.052	0.08	>.99
						0.1	0.02	>.99

[1] Mean of birds 2 and 3.   [2] Mean of birds 1 and 2.   [3] Bird 1 only.   [4] Saline alone.
[5] S.E. = .074.   [6] S.E. = .067.   [7] S.E. = .059.

Similar results were obtained with methamphetamine on birds 1 and 2. At no dose level did the birds show any increase in the number of responses in the presence of S−, although doses of 0.3 mgm, or more caused pronounced behavioral effects, shown by the fall in the average rate of response in the presence of S+.

Scopolamine was studied in bird 1 only. Again, even doses sufficient to affect performance grossly in the presence of S+ caused no breakdown of discriminative behavior; the D.R. never fell even to 0.99.

Performance on schedule 4.   The average D.R. in the control series of birds 6 and 7 working on schedule 4 was 0.98 (Table 1, Fig. 3) indicating an approximately 50-fold difference in rates of response in the presence of S+ and S−. Both the O.R. and D.R. were well maintained in experiments in which saline alone was injected (Table 2).

Effect of drugs on performance on schedule 4 (Table 4).   The effects of all three drugs were studied in both pigeon 6 and pigeon 7.

TABLE 4.   Effect of pentobarbital, methamphetamine and scopolamine on performance on schedule 4 of birds 6 and 7.

Pentobarbital			Methamphetamine			Scopolamine		
Dose	Mean O.R.	Mean D.R.	Dose	Mean O.R.	Mean D.R.	Dose	Mean O.R.	Mean D.R.
0	0.95[1]	0.95[2]	0	0.95	0.95	0	0.95	0.95
1	0.97	0.93	0.1	1.00	0.96	0.003	0.86	0.97
3	0.97	0.82	0.3	1.07	0.56	0.01	0.50	0.98
5.2	0.36	0.06	0.52	1.10	0.89	0.03	0.30	>0.99
			1.0	0.71	0.76	0.1	0.02	>0.99

[1] S.E. = .063.   [2] S.E. = .025.

Following 3 mgm. of pentobarbital consistently more responses were made in the presence of S— than following saline alone, although the average rate of response in the presence of S+ was not much affected. This is illustrated in Fig. 3. It will be noted that in this particular experiment, most of the responses in S— occurred in the first part of the second S— period after the drug. The responding in S— often took the form of a period of steady responding, as here. In general, such periods of responding were rare and short in the third S— period (see below), but there was no obvious tendency for them to occur in any particular part of the first or second S— periods. In spite of this variability in the time of occurrence of the pecks during S—, the total number made throughout the presentation of the various S— was reasonably constant. Following 5.2 mgm. of pentobarbital the average rate of response in the presence of S— was almost as high as that in the presence of S+.

Methamphetamine in appropriate doses also caused a fall in D.R. to values below those seen following saline, even when the rate of response in the presence of S+ was well sustained or even increased. The extent of fall of D.R. was variable, and over a considerable range bore no obvious relation to dosage. However, since the D.R. following saline showed great consistency (coefficient of variation 2.5 per cent) there can be no reasonable doubt that the lowering of the D.R. by methamphetamine was a real phenomenon.

Injection of scopolamine led to no fall in the D.R.; on the contrary, discriminative performance even improved following doses causing a fall in response rate in the presence of S+.

As explained earlier (see *Schedules*) a schedule 4 series may be divided into 2 parts: an initial 4 periods in which the implication of the stimuli was conditional; and a final 2 periods in which the implication of the key color was unambiguous, as in schedule 1. The D.R. of each of these parts has been calculated separately for the after drug series following saline, pentobarbital and methamphetamine. Following saline alone, the D.R. for the conditional part was slightly, though consistently, lower than for the simple part (Table 5). Following the various doses of pentobarbital and methamphetamine studied the D.R. for the conditional part was always less than that for the simple part; the difference was usually large as can be seen from the averages shown in Table 5. It should be noted that the D.R. for the simple part did, on some occasions, fall to values lower than any seen with schedule 1.

Performance on schedules 2 and 3 and effect of drugs.   Performance on schedules 2 and 3 did not differ in any significant way from performance on schedule 1 (Tables 1 and 2). Doses of pentobarbital and methamphetamine which caused a fall in the D.R. of birds working on schedule 4 had no effect on the D.R. of birds working on schedules 2 and 3 (Table 6).

TABLE 5. Differential effect of pentobarbital and methamphetamine on performance of birds 6 and 7 in "conditional" and "simple" discrimination situations of schedule 4.

Pentobarbital			Methamphetamine		
Dose (mgm.)	DR (conditional)	DR (simple)	Dose (mgm.)	DR (conditional)	DR (simple)
0	0.95*	> .99	0	0.95*	> .99
1	0.79	> .99	0.3	0.55	0.76
3	0.20	> .99	0.52	0.88	0.98
5.2	<0	0.85	1.0	0.57	0.85

* S.E. = .037.

DISCUSSION. It has been shown that the discriminative performance of the pigeons based on either a difference in key color or the presence or absence of the house light was not disrupted by pentobarbital, methamphetamine or scopolamine in doses up to those causing complete cessation of pecking. On the other hand, pentobarbital and methamphetamine, but not scopolamine, interfered with the discriminative performance on schedule 4, a schedule which involved six different stimulus combinations and a conditional situation. These findings are clearly in agreement with the widely held view that "more complex" performance is more susceptible to drug effects than "simple" performance. However, the terms "complex" and "simple" are not easy to define in this context, and it would appear preferable to describe the differential sensitivity to drugs in terms of the operational difference between the schedules.

The analysis summarized in Table 5 makes it appear that it is the conditional feature of schedule 4 rather than simply the increased number of stimulus combinations involved, which determines this difference. However, the D.R. of the simple part of schedule 4 did fall on occasions, indicating that it was not altogether comparable to the completely simple schedules 1, 2, and 3. Moreover, the constant sequence of stimuli means that the effect of the conditional and simple parts of schedule 4 is confounded with time after drug. Further experimental analysis is required.

TABLE 6. Effect of pentobarbital and methamphetamine on performance on schedules 2 and 3 of birds 3 and 4.

Pentobarbital			Methamphetamine		
Dose	OR	DR	Dose	OR	DR
0	1.04	>0.99	0	1.04	>0.99
3	0.96	>0.99	0.3	0.81	>0.99
5.2	0.29	0.99	0.52	0.56	>0.99

Since the S+ and S− periods alternated, a change in stimuli always implied a change in contingencies. Hence the *changes* of stimuli, rather than the nature of the stimuli themselves may have played a part in the sudden changes in pecking rate shown in Figs. 2 and 3. It should be emphasized that schedule 4 did not differ from the other schedules in this regard.

No attempt was made to identify the specific feature or features of the stimuli on which the discriminations were based. The differences between the stimuli were made as gross as convenient; but it was not relevant to the present work to determine whether, for example, the discrimination of schedule 1 was based on the qualities of redness and blueness of the stimuli. There was, in fact, a distinct difference in brightness between the red and blue lights, and no attempt was made to balance them in this regard.

The absence of effect of scopolamine on the discriminations of schedule 4 has no obvious explanation. The pigeons ate freely when offered grain following doses of scopolamine abolishing pecking behavior in the Skinner box. Even a dose as large as 10 mgm. scopolamine (i.e. 100 times larger than the dose almost abolishing pecking behavior) caused no grossly observable change in behavior; 15 mgm. caused vomiting; 45 mgm. still caused only vomiting with no other unequivocal signs. From the point of view of the present work, the effects of scopolamine are of interest in showing that the effects of pentobarbital and methamphetamine on the D.R. were not entirely nonspecific.

At the appropriate dose level, both methamphetamine and pentobarbital caused a slight increase in the O.R. The very modest "stimulating" effect of methamphetamine seen in the present experiments is believed to be due to the nature of the schedule of reward. The rate of pecking is of the order of 1/sec. while rewards are set up only 1/min. on the average. A doubling in rate would mean that the rewards would be received at most only 0.5 secs. earlier, while 120 pecks/reward instead of 60 pecks/reward would be made. This decrease in "efficiency" with increase in rate probably tends to minimize any increase in rate above its already "inefficiently" high value.

The "S− renewing" procedure was used during training to prevent the change from S− to S+ (a rewarding event) from occurring shortly after a peck made in the presence of S−; such chance coincidences tend to maintain pecking in the presence of S−, increasing the probability of further coincidences of peck and change to S+ and thus starting a vicious circle.

SUMMARY.   Pigeons were rewarded with occasional access to food for 4–5 seconds for pecking a translucent plastic disc when certain environmental stimuli were present, but were never rewarded when other environmental stimuli were present. They came to peck at a steady rate of the order of 60/min. when the stimuli appropriate to rewards were present but at a rate of only about 1/min. or less when the stimuli appropriate to no rewards were present.

When the stimulus appropriate to rewards was a red light behind the translucent disc and the stimulus appropriate to no rewards was a blue light, then this differential performance was not disrupted by pentobarbital, methamphetamine or scopolamine, although as the dosage of any of the drugs was increased, pecking in the presence of the red light was progressively reduced.

When the stimuli appropriate to rewards were a red light, a blue light plus a differently located white light (the house light) or a yellow light plus the house light, and the stimuli appropriate to no rewards were a blue light alone, or a red or white light plus the house light, then the differential performance between the sets of stimuli was reduced by pentobarbital and methamphetamine, but not by scopolamine.

Preliminary analysis of the differences between the schedules determining this differential sensitivity to drugs is presented.

REFERENCES

Dews, P. B.: *J. Pharm. exp. Therap.,* 113: 393, 1955.
Skinner, B. F.: *The behavior of organisms.* New York, Appleton-Century-Crofts, p. 19, 1938.
Skinner, B. F.: *Science and human behavior.* New York, Macmillan, p. 102, 1953.

19

Influence of drugs on behavior controlled by internal and external stimuli [1]

VICTOR G. LATIES and BERNARD WEISS

In the fixed interval (FI) schedule, reinforcement is produced by the first response that occurs after a fixed period of time. Responses occurring earlier are ignored so far as reinforcement is concerned. Although no cues from the external environment are correlated with the passage of time, most organisms exposed to this schedule emit a distribution of responses in time which possesses a characteristic pattern: a pause at the beginning of the interval and, once responding starts, a rapid increase in rate to a value that remains fairly constant until the end of the interval (Skinner, 1938). This response distribution is extremely sensitive to the effects of drugs (*e.g.*, Bolotina and Popova, 1953; Boren and Navarro, 1959; Dews, 1955a, 1956, 1958a,b,c, 1962a, 1965; Ferster and Appel, 1963; Fry *et al.*, 1960; Herrnstein and Morse, 1956, 1957; Morse and Herrnstein, 1956; Smith, 1964; Verhave, 1959; Waller, 1961; Witoslawski *et al.*, 1963; Wurtman *et al.*, 1959).

Dews (1955a, 1958a,b) and Morse and Herrnstein (1956) have suggested that behavior controlled by internal stimuli may be more sensitive to modification by drugs than behavior controlled by external environmental stimuli. The present experiments examined this proposition in pigeons within the context of the FI schedule of reinforcement. Behavior on two different FI schedules was studied. One was a regular FI; the only discriminative stimuli available during the interval were those arising from within the pigeon's own body or those produced by its own behavior. Anger (1963) calls these "temporal stimuli" because their association with the passage of real time is presumed to give them some discriminative control over behavior. The other schedule was a FI schedule to which a "clock" had been added. The "clock" consisted of a sequence of external stimuli that varied systematically with time. Ferster and Skinner (1957, p. 277)

From *Journal of Pharmacology and Experimental Therapeutics*, 1966, **152**, 388–396. Copyright © 1966 by The Williams and Wilkins Co., Baltimore, Md.

[1] Supported in part by Grants MH-07498 and MH-11752 from the National Institute of Mental Health, National Institutes of Health, and in part by a contract between the Atomic Energy Commission and the University of Rochester Atomic Energy Project. Most of the statistical calculations were performed in the computing center of the Johns Hopkins University School of Medicine under NIH Grant FR-00004-03.

The authors gratefully acknowledge programming aid from Dr. Richard H. Shepard and Robert Burow, and the technical assistance of Ann B. Weiss.

have shown that such stimuli rapidly come to control FI responding. Thus, we varied the type of discriminative stimuli (internal *vs.* external) associated with responding on FI, keeping constant all other factors that affect this performance (Dews, 1962b, 1963; Ferster and Skinner, 1957). Once behavior was stable, we investigated the distribution of responses within the intervals, as modified by five drugs, all of which are known to interfere with regular FI performance. These were amphetamine, scopolamine, pentobarbital, chlorpromazine and promazine.

METHOD.   The subjects, three white Carneau pigeons kept at approximately 80% of their weight if fed *ad libitum,* were first trained to approach and eat from the grain feeder used to deliver the reinforcer. They then learned to peck an illuminated key (a 1-inch disk) to produce reinforcement. Next, they were given a few hours' experience on a fixed ratio schedule of reinforcement (FR100). Finally, the birds were trained on a three-component multiple schedule of reinforcement (Ferster and Skinner, 1957). While the transilluminated key was red, a regular FI schedule was in effect; the first peck made at least 5 min after the key became red operated the food magazine, giving the bird 3 sec assess to mixed grain. Other responses did not operate the magazine but were recorded. During the presentation of grain, the magazine opening was lighted and the key was not. The second component of the multiple schedule was also a FI schedule of reinforcement, but here the key, otherwise unlighted, had a different symbol projected onto it for each of the 5 min within the interval (triangle, multiplication sign, circle, plus sign, square). The last symbol, the square, remained on until the key peck that produced reinforcement. These symbols served as a "clock" and soon came to control responding (Ferster and Skinner, 1957; Segal, 1962); the subject usually started to respond only after the square had appeared. The third component was a time-out, during which the key was dark and no responses were reinforced. The time-out lasted 3 min, followed each reinforcement and was included to help minimize interaction between the two types of fixed intervals (Ferster and Skinner, 1957, p. 193). The FI components of the multiple schedule were presented in the sequence NC, NC, C, C, NC, NC, C, C, NC, NC, C, C, C, NC, C, NC where NC stands for FI5 (no clock) and C stands for FI5 (clock). Subjects were given between 410 and 650 hr of experience on the multiple schedule, exclusive of time spent in the time-out periods, before data collection was started.

The experimental space was a 1-foot cube made from ¼-inch Plexiglas. It was contained in a ¾-inch plywood external shell. Programming and recording equipment were located in a room adjacent to that containing the experimental chamber. White noise was also used to block extraneous sounds.

Data were gathered on the following drugs: amphetamine sulfate, scopolamine hydrobromide, pentobarbital sodium, chlorpromazine hydrochloride, and promazine hydrochloride. Most of the amphetamine data were collected first, all promazine data last, and doses of the other drugs (plus the 0.5 mg/kg dose of amphetamine) were intermixed irregularly during the middle portion of the 14 months over which these observations were made. Dilutions were made with normal saline; doses are in terms of the salts. At least 3, and usually 6 or 7, days intervened between experiments. Occasional sessions were run with saline injections. There were 10 such control sessions for bird 1, 13 for bird 2 and 7 for bird 3. With rare exceptions, at least duplicate and usually 3 or 4 experiments were performed at each dose level with amphetamine scopolamine, pentobarbital and chlorpromazine. The promazine data came from single experiments at each level with each subject.

The bird to be used as a subject on a particular day was put in the box at about 9:30 A.M. and predrug data obtained for at least 2 hr before an intramuscular injection of the drug (or saline) during a time-out. The experiment then continued until the next morning, although only 10 or 12 hr of this were actually analyzed. At the end of every minute, during the FI portions of the schedule, the total number of responses emitted during that period was recorded on a printing counter. Responses were also displayed on a cumulative recorder. The total number of responses made during time-outs was also recorded.

Our chief aim was to examine the differential effects of the drugs on the distribution of responses within the two types of FI schedule. We used the Index of Curvature developed by Fry et al. (1960) to characterize this distribution with a single number. This index varies between 0.80 and −0.80 if one divides the interval into fifths. A steady rate throughout the interval, a straight line on a cumulative record, yields a value of zero. A value of 0.80 reflects very pronounced positive curvative, meaning that the responding took place exclusively during the last fifth of the interval; and negative values reflect negative curvature, meaning that most of the responding occurred near the beginning of the interval. Intervals with fewer than 12 responses were ignored in calculating this index, since it then tends to be less reliable (Fry et al. 1960).

The response distributions of the three subjects had stabilized before any drug data were collected. The Index of Curvature of saline runs drifted slightly downward over the course of the study. The mean control values for the "clock" conditions were 0.76, 0.66 and 0.80 for birds 1, 2 and 3 respectively. These numbers derive from total performance over 2 hr before and 10 hr after the injection. "No clock" values were 0.34, 0.32 and 0.43. The latter values are lower than one would normally expect for the regular FI schedule. This may be due in part to induction from the "clock" component of the multiple schedule (cf., Waller, 1961). Exclusion of the rare intervals containing less than 12 responses also would tend to reduce the the Index; the responses in these intervals usually were concentrated near the end.

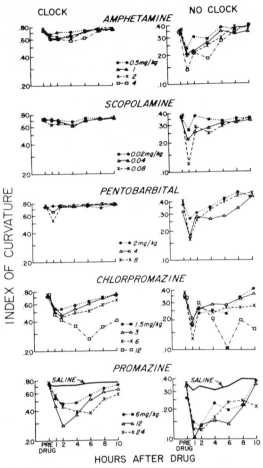

FIGURE 1.   Effects of drugs on the Index of Curvature during the F15 (clock) and F15 (no clock) components of the multiple schedule. Each of the points labeled predrug represents data gathered during eight intervals of one type ("clock" or "no clock") spread out over the slightly more than 2-hr period before the drug was given. Similarly, after drug, with the exception of the first 2 hr, each point represents performance during eight 5-min intervals spread out over a 2-hr period. The 1- and 2-hr points each represent performance during four 5-min intervals spread out over a single hour. The curves for saline are presented with the promazine data and, for clarity, have not been repeated with the other graphs. Ninety-five percent confidence limits around the saline curves vary in width over time from ±.02 to ±.06 for the "clock" conditions and between ±.06 and ±.08 for the "no clock" condition.

RESULTS.   The main results of the study are summarized in Fig. 1. The Index of Curvature is displayed for each of the drugs used and for each FI schedule. The plots show the arithmetic means of data from the three birds and are only for those dose levels at which each bird was used and at which no prolonged pausing was produced. Logarithmic scales on the ordinates are used to emphasize the relative nature of the changes from different pre-

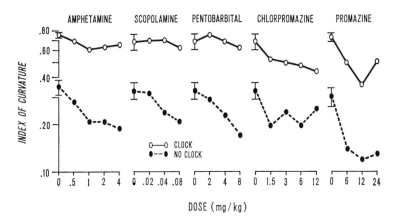

FIGURE 2.   Effects of drugs on the Index of Curvature during the first 2-hr period after treatment. Control values derive from the saline control data collected closest in time to that of a particular drug. The vertical lines indicate ±S.E. These values were estimated from the range of the 3 saline control means (one for each bird) according to the technique described by Wilcoxin and Wilcox (1964).

drug levels. It is apparent that for amphetamine, scopolamine and pentobarbital, proportionately greater changes in curvature occurred for FI5 (no clock) than for FI5 (clock). This difference is greatly attenuated for chlorpromazine and promazine; the two phenothiazines greatly altered response distribution even under the "clock" condition.

The 2-hr period directly after drug administration is considered in greater detail in Figs. 2, 3 and 4. The dose-effect curves for Index of Curvature (Fig. 2) show for this period taken as a whole the relative insensitivity of the FI5 (clock) response distribution to the effects of amphetamine, scopolamine and pentobarbital, and its sensitivity to the phenothiazines. Figures 3 and 4 show that the FI5 (clock) curvature changes induced by chlorpromazine and promazine were mainly the product of large increases in responding during the first 4 min of the interval. Changes in early responding under the "clock" condition were much smaller for the other drugs. With scopolamine, the changes in overall responding were due to changes in terminal rate, i.e., the rate at which the pigeons pecked the key during the last minute of the interval. With amphetamine and pentobarbital, changes in both early and terminal rate were responsible for the changes in overall rate.

The changes in overall rate for the regular FI were not remarkable. The slight increase with some doses of amphetmine (9% with 2 mg/kg), the decreases with all doses of scopolamine, the increases with pentobarbital, the small changes with chlorpromazine and the increases with promazine are similar to what has previously been shown, for example, by Dews (1955a, 1962a), Smith (1964) and Vaillant (1964).

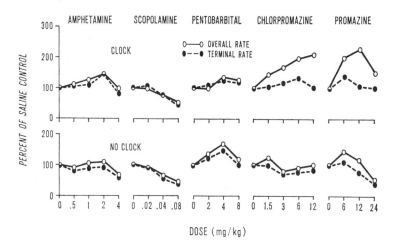

FIGURE 3.   Effects of drugs on *overall* and *terminal* response rates during the first 2-hr period after treatment. The rates are given as percentages of the comparable base-line rates during the saline control sessions run nearest in time to the particular drug sessions. The base-line overall response rates differed markedly for the two types of FI schedule. For example, during the 2-hr postdrug saline control sessions used as a base line for the amphetamine data, the overall rates were 13.7/min for the "clock" condition and 36.6/min for the "no clock" condition.

Performance under the "clock" condition stood up remarkably well to a dose level of amphetamine high enough (8 mg/kg) to produce a profound behavioral deficit for a significant length of time. Time-effect curves of the Index of Curvature are given in Fig. 5. This dose immediately abolished key pecking for all birds on each occasion it was used; the length of the pause before responding resumed varied from a little more than ½ to al-

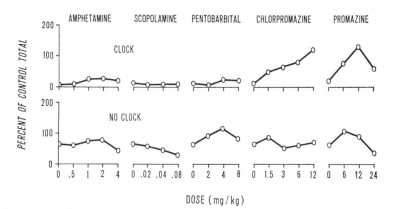

FIGURE 4.   Effects of drugs on response rate during the first 4 min of the interval, for the first 2 hr after treatment. Rates are given as percentages of the *overall* rates during the closest saline control sessions.

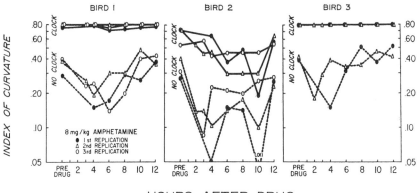

HOURS AFTER DRUG

FIGURE 5.   Effects of 8 mg/kg of amphetamine on the Index of Curvature during the F15 (clock) and F15 (no clock) components of the multiple schedule. Each of the points labeled predrug represents data gathered during eight intervals of one type ("clock" or "no clock") spread out over the slightly more than 2-hr period before the drug was given. The lines joining the predrug and first postdrug points do not imply possible interpolation. The first postdrug data points refer to performance between the end of the pause and the time given on the abscicca. (For instance, during the second replication, bird 1 paused 2 hr and 16 min after injection. Therefore, the points plotted at 3 hr postdrug refer to the intervals that occurred during the prior 44 min. Three of these were "no clock" and three were "clock" intervals, the rest of the 44 min being taken up by time-out periods.) The Index is given for 1-hr periods until the fourth hour and, thereafter, for 2-hr periods.

most 3½ hr. This renders average curves meaningless, since curvature cannot be measured in the absence of responses. Consequently, the individual sessions are presented, with the Index plotted only when the subjects emitted enough responses to make calculation possible. As soon as they resumed responding, birds 1 and 3 displayed hardly any effect of the amphetamine on "clock" curvature while showing considerable change in curvature during the "no clock" periods. Bird 2 showed changes in curvature under both conditions; however, the change was proportionately greater during the "no clock" component.

The differential effect of amphetamine is further illustrated by the cumulative records in Fig. 6. In the case of two birds, bird 1 and bird 3, the effects are quite straightforward; no change in curvature occurred for the "clock" condition, but drastic changes occurred while the birds worked without the additional stimuli present. For instance, for bird 3, the mean Index of Curvature for the three intervals shown for the predrug "clock" condition is 0.80 and it remains 0.80 at all times after the drug is given. However, the mean Index for the two end intervals that illustrate the predrug "no clock" condition is 0.66 and drops to 0.26 for the period 2 hr after drug administration, to 0.14 for the next time period and then to 0.21 and 0.48. This was produced by a dose of 8 mg/kg which caused a pause

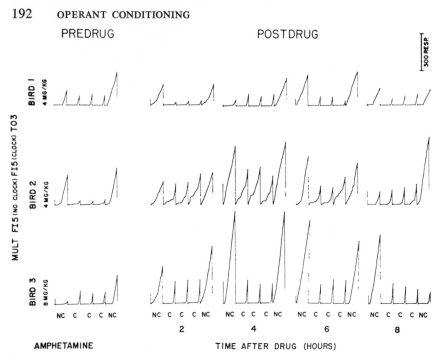

FIGURE 6. Cumulative records of performance after selected doses of amphetamine. In each sequence of five intervals, the middle three are F15 (clock) and the end two are F15 (no clock). The pen reset to the base line at reinforcement. A 3-min time-out, during which time the paper did not move, occurred after each reinforcement.

1 hr and 15 min in length immediately after the injection. A 4 mg/kg dose did interfere with the "clock" performance on bird 2. Here, while the "clock" Index changes from a mean of 0.65 predrug to 0.41, 0.30, 0.43 and 0.72 postdrug for the four time periods respectively, the "no clock" Index changes from 0.38 predrug to 0.14, 0, 0.26 and 0.44 for the postdrug time periods. Thus, the change in curvature, if expressed in terms of proportional change from predug performance, was greater for the "no clock" FI performance.

Figure 7 shows the effects of promazine on the performance of a single pigeon. A complete lack of discrimination between the two types of FI schedules can be seen in the bird's performance in the first several hours after a 12 mg/kg dose. However, it still stopped responding whenever the key was dark and also continued to feed at reinforcement, showing that some external stimuli were still exerting control over its behavior. At the highest dose used here, 24 mg/kg, some responding during the time-out can be seen on the record. The pen reset to the base line after reinforcement but did not reset at the end of the time-out. Since the paper drive was

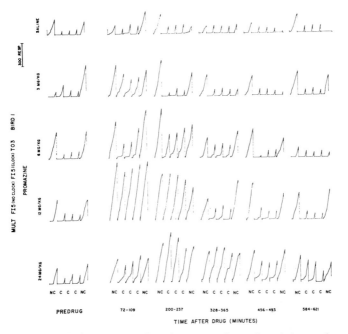

FIGURE 7. Cumulative records of performance after selected doses of promazine. In each sequence of five intervals, the middle three are F15 (clock) and the end two are F15 (no clock). The pen reset to the base-line upon reinforcement. A 3-min time-out, during which time the paper did not move, occurred after each reinforcement.

stopped during time-out, responding caused the pen to travel directly up-ward. The amount of responding during time-out, therefore, is revealed by the height at which the next interval begins.

With rare exceptions, such as the ones shown in Fig. 7, the birds made few responses during the time-out periods. Thus, bird 1 made a mean total of 8.4 time-out responses during saline control sessions (range, 0–42) and made large numbers of responses only after 24 mg/kg of promazine (1083), once after a dose of 6 mg/kg of chlorpromazine (456) and twice after doses of 12 mg/kg of chlorpromazine (667 and 1281). Bird 2 made a mean total of 10 responses during control sessions (range, 0–99). This bird made 100, 853 and 4415 responses during time-out after 6, 12 and 24 mg/kg of promazine, respectively. The only other occasions on which it responded much during time-out were once after receiving 0.04 mg/kg of scopolamine (469), once after receiving 6 mg/kg of chlorpromazine (242) and once after receiving 12 mg/kg of chlorpromazine (3002). Bird 3 never made more than 12 responses during the time-out of any drug session. During control sessions, it made between zero and 3 responses with its mean total being 0.6.

DISCUSSION.　All of the drugs used produced the expected large changes in FI response distribution when the pigeons had no special external "clock" available to them. Giving the birds a "clock" modified the response distribution greatly and decreased its sensitivity to amphetamine, scopolamine and pentobarbital; it left its sensitivity to chlorpromazine and promazine largely unchanged. The results indicate (1) that the source of the discriminative stimuli controlling the performance is important in determining the reaction to drugs, and (2) that it is relatively more important for some drugs than for others.

The dependence of drug effect on the source of stimulus control was especially striking for amphetamine, scopolamine and pentobarbital. The way the addition of the external "clock" lessened their effect on response distribution is congruent with most previous work. For instance, behavior under the control of two different lights in a multiple fixed interval, fixed ratio schedule remains distinctly under the control of the external stimuli after doses of d-amphetamine that produced profound changes in the interval component (Smith, 1964). On the same schedule, chlorpromazine can lead the pigeon to behave with less regard as to which light is present, an effect representing a loosening of external stimulus control (Dews, 1958a). Also, Blough (1958) has shown that chlorpromazine lengthens, whereas pentobarbital shortens, the time a pigeon can stand still when standing still is reinforced. Dews (1958a) has suggested, in explanation of Blough's finding, the possibility that chlorpromazine may reduce the tendency of external stimuli to provoke movement. Such an interpretation is in keeping with our results. On the other hand, control by external stimuli is not always disrupted by chlorpromazine or promazine (Cook and Kelleher, 1961; Kelleher et al., 1962; Terrace, 1963).

Why should the source of stimulation make such a difference? Location may be important only because of a correlation with another variable that is itself related to drug sensitivity. There are at least three such variables. Skinner (1957) has pointed out that discriminations based upon stimuli arising within the organism are likely to be imprecise because the controlling environment cannot easily reinforce the appropriate behavior, since it has no direct access to the controlling stimuli. A decrease in precision may act like an increase in the complexity of discriminative stimuli. The latter is known to lead to increased sensitivity to drug effects (Blough, 1956; Dews, 1955b; Waller, 1961). Related to the imprecision of discriminative control is the speed and manner in which the discrimination is originally acquired. A simple discrimination based upon external cues is more likely to be acquired rapidly and with a minimum of unreinforced responding as compared to a more complex, internally-based discrimination. Terrace (1963) has shown that a discrimination learned without errors is unaffected by doses of chlorpromazine that produce profound disruption of the same discrimination learned the usual way.

The third factor that co-varied with source of the discriminative stimuli was the response rate itself; as expected, the external stimuli that made up the "clock" came to control response rate, producing a low rate in the early parts of the interval. But base-line rate itself has been shown to be important in determining the effects of drugs, with low rates often rising and high rates falling in response to the same drug (Dews, 1958a, 1964; Smith, 1964). For amphetamine, scopolamine and pentobarbital, the base-line rates do not seem to have played an important role in determining the direction of change in overall rate; the drug-induced changes in rate early in the interval were, if anything, less important for the "clock" condition, when base-line rate was low, than for the "no clock" condition, when base-line rate was relatively high (Figs. 3 and 4). With chlorpromazine and promazine, the role of base-line rate was pronounced; for the "clock" condition, large increases in responding early in the interval accounted for much of the change in overall rate. We interpret this to mean that base-line rate is relatively unimportant when behavior is controlled by powerful discriminative stimuli. Conversely, base-line rate becomes more important in determining drug effects when the control exerted by these stimuli is lessened, as we believe it to be by chlorpromazine and promazine.

We have shown that the addition of systematically varying external discriminative stimuli makes the FI response distribution less sensitive to the effects of amphetamine, scopolamine and pentobarbital. The addition of such a "clock" did not modify, to the same extent, the effects on response distribution of chlorpromazine or promazine. We believe these results reflect the relative sensitivity to these five agents of external and internal discriminative stimuli. A corollary conclusion is that the distribution of responses on the FI schedule is altered by drugs in large measure because of its dependence upon internal stimuli.

SUMMARY.   Three pigeons were trained to peck an illuminated disk for a food reinforcer which was delivered according to a fixed interval (FI) schedule of reinforcement. Under one set of conditions, the stimulus projected on the disk remained constant during the 5-min FI. Under a second set of conditions, the symbol projected on the disk changed once per minute during the interval, thus providing the birds with a "clock." These two conditions were chosen to represent behavior controlled by internal and external stimuli respectively, and were presented to the bird in an irregular order. Greater changes in response distribution were produced by amphetamine, scopolamine and pentobarbital when no "clock" was available; with the added clock, the birds responded mostly near the end of the interval, and drug-induced changes in response rate were for the most part confined to the end of the interval. This confirms for these drugs the hypothesis that behavior largely controlled by externally based discriminative stimuli is more resistant to drugs than behavior controlled by internal stimuli. Chlorpromazine and promazine, however, did not display such a pronounced differential effect on response distribution.

REFERENCES

Anger, D.: The role of temporal discriminations in the reinforcement of Sidman avoidance behavior. *J. exp. Analysis Behav.* **6**:447–506, 1963.

Blough, D. S.: Technique for studying the effects of drugs on discrimination in the pigeon. *Ann. N.Y. Acad. Sci.* **65**:334–344, 1956.

Blough, D. S.: New test for tranquilizers. *Science, N.Y.* **127**:586–587, 1958.

Bolotina, O. P. and Popova, A. A.: Effect of phenamine on motor conditioned reflexes to time in the lower apes. *Proc. Pavlov Physiol. Inst.,* **2**:64–68, 1953. Cited in Dmitriev and Kochigina (1959).

Boren, J. J., and Navarro, A. P.: The action of atropine, benactyzine and scopolamine upon fixed-interval and fixed-ratio behavior. *J. exp. Analysis Behav.* **2**:107–115, 1959.

Cook, L., and Kelleher, R. T.: The interaction of drugs and behavior. In *Neuro-Psychopharmacology,* ed. by E. Rothlin, Vol. 2, Proceedings of the 2nd International Meeting of the Collegium Internationale Neuro-Psychopharmacologicum, Basle, pp. 77–92, Elsevier Pub. Co., Amsterdam, 1961.

Dews, P. B.: Studies on behavior. I. Differential sensitivity to pentobarbital of pecking performance in pigeons depending on the schedule of reward. *J. Pharmac. exp. Ther.* **113**:393–401, 1955a.

Dews, P. B.: Studies on behavior. II. The effects of pentobarbital, methamphetamine and scopolamine on performances in pigeons involving discriminations. *J. Pharmac. exp. Ther.* **115**:380–389, 1955b.

Dews, P. B. Modification by drugs of performance on simple schedules of positive reinforcement. *Ann. N.Y. Acad. Sci.* **65**:268–281, 1956.

Dews, P. B. Analysis of effects of psychopharmacological agents in behavioral terms. *Fedn Proc.,* Fedn Am. Socs exp. Biol. **17**:1024–1030, 1958a.

Dews, P. B.: Effects of chlorpromazine and promazine on performance on a mixed schedule of reinforcement. *J. exp. Analysis Behav.* **1**:73–82, 1958b.

Dews, P. B.: Studies on behavior. IV. Stimulant actions of methamphetamine. *J. Pharmac. exp. Ther.* **122**:137–147, 1958c.

Dews, P. B.: A behavioral output enhancing effect of imipramine in pigeons. *Int. J. Neuropharmac.* **1**:265–272, 1962a.

Dews, P. B.: The effect of multiple S^Δ periods on responding on a fixed-interval schedule. *J. exp. Analysis Behav.* **5**:369–374, 1962b.

Dews, P. B.: Behavioral effects of drugs. In *Conflict and creativity,* ed. by S. M. Farber and R. H. L. Wilson, pp. 138–153, McGraw-Hill Book Co., New York, 1963.

Dews, P. B.: A behavioral effect of amobarbital. *Arch. exp. Path. Pharmak.* **248**:296–307, 1964.

Dews, P. B.: Pharmacology of positive reinforcement and discrimination. In *Pharmacology of conditioning, learning and retention,* ed. by M. Ya. Mikhel'son and V. G. Longo, pp. 91–96, The Macmillan Co., New York, 1965.

Dmitriev, A. S., and Kochigina, A. M.: The importance of time as stimulus of conditioned reflex activity. *Psychol. Bull.* **56**:106–132, 1959.

Ferster, C. B., and Appel, J. B.: Interpreting drug-behavior effects with a functional analysis of behavior. In *Psychopharmacological methods,* ed. by Z. Votava, M. Horváth, and O. Vinař, pp. 170–181, Pergamon Press, New York, 1963.

Ferster, C. B., and Skinner, B. F.: Schedules of reinforcement, Appleton-Century-Crofts, New York, 1957.

Fry, W., Kelleher, R. T., and Cook, L.: A mathematical index of performance on fixed-interval schedules of reinforcement. *J. exp. Analysis Behav.* 3:193–199, 1960.

Herrnstein, R. J., and Morse, W. H.: Selective action of pentobarbital on component behaviors of a reinforcement schedule. *Science,* N.Y. 124:367–368, 1956.

Herrnstein, R. J., and Morse, W. H.: Effects of pentobarbital on intermittently reinforced behavior. *Science,* N.Y. 125:929–931, 1957.

Kelleher, R. T., Riddle, W. C., and Cook, L.: Observing behavior in pigeons. *J. exp. Analysis Behav.* 5:3–13, 1962.

Morse, W. H., and Herrnstein, R. J.: Effects of drugs on characteristics of behavior maintained by complex schedules of intermittent positive reinforcement. *Ann. N.Y. Acad. Sci.* 65:303–317, 1956.

Segal, E. F.: Exteroceptive control of fixed-interval responding. *J. exp. Analysis Behav.* 5:49–57, 1962.

Skinner, B. F.: *The behavior of organisms,* Appleton-Century-Crofts, New York, 1938.

Skinner, B. F.: Verbal behavior, Appleton-Century-Crofts, New York, 1957.

Smith, C. B.: Effects of d-amphetamine upon operant behavior of pigeons: Enhancement by reserpine. *J. Pharmac. exp. Ther.* 146:167–174, 1964.

Terrace, H. S.: Errorless discrimination learning in the pigeon: Effects of chlorpromazine and imipramine. *Science,* N.Y. 140:318–319, 1963.

Vaillant, G. E.: A comparison of chlorpromazine and imipramine on behavior in the pigeon. *J. Pharmac. exp. Ther.* 146:377–384, 1964.

Verhave, T.: The effect of secobarbital on a multiple schedule in the monkey. *J. exp. Analysis Behav.* 2:117–120, 1959.

Waller, M.: Effects of chronically administered chlorpromazine on multiple-schedule performance. *J. exp. Analysis Behav.* 4:351–359, 1961.

Weiss, B., and Laties, V. G.: Drug effects on the temporal patterning of behavior. *Fedn Proc.,* Fedn Am. Socs exp. Biol. 23:801–807, 1964.

Wilcoxin, F., and Wilcox, R. A.: *Some rapid approximate statistical procedures.* Lederle Laboratories, Pearl River, N.Y., 1964.

Witoslawski, J. J., Anderson, R. B., and Hanson, H. M.: Behavioral studies with a black vulture, *Coragyps atratus. J. exp. Analysis Behav.* 6:605–606, 1963.

Wurtman, R. J., Frank, M. M., Morse, W. H., and Dews, P. B.: Studies on behavior. V. Actions of l-epinephrine and related compounds. *J. Pharm. exp. Ther.* 127:281–287, 1959.

Section **D**   RESPONSE VARIABLES

Articles 20–24

While operants are not defined by their topographies, operationally defined operants frequently involve very different
topographies. Operationally defined operants may as well
have specific quantitative properties (e.g., force, duration,
position) distinguishing them from similar responses. Drugs
which affect one topography may profoundly alter one
operant while having little effect on another operant requiring a different topography (Article 20). Such effects
may be of particular importance when the probabilities of
given topographies vary according to the species (Article
24).

Perhaps less obvious but no less important are quantitative properties of a given response topography. A response
requiring excessive force may be readily affected by a drug
which produces slight motor incoordination. Similarly, depending on specified response position (Article 21) or duration (Article 22) or force (Article 23), drugs may have
quite different effects. Thus, not only are properties of a
response important in assessing behavioral actions of a
drug, but a carefully selected response can be a useful
tool in evaluating motor-acting drugs.

20

Immobility as an avoidance response, and its disruption by drugs [1]

DALBIR BINDRA and HARVEY ANCHEL

In a typical avoidance learning experiment, the animal is required to run from one side of a shuttle box to the other, or to press a bar, or to make some active response in order to terminate or avoid noxious stimulation (*e.g.,* electric shock). Much of the available literature on avoidance behavior deals with the characteristics of such active responses. The purpose of the present study was to determine whether animals can also learn to sit or stand motionless to escape or avoid electric shock. Blough (1958) has shown that pigeons can be trained to stand motionless in order to receive a food reinforcement; thus it appears not inconceivable that an immobility avoidance response can also be trained. In the present study, experimental rats were given escape-avoidance training, while control yoked animals received electric shocks without opportunity to escape or avoid them. The effects of shock intensity on the acquisition of the immobility response, as well as the influence of three drugs (chlorpromazine, imipramine, and methylphenidate) on the performance of the response, were studied.

EXPERIMENT I. The purpose of the first, preliminary, experiment was to determine whether immobility as an avoidance response to a specific stimulus situation could be learned by the rat.

Subjects. Ten naive adult male hooded rats, each weighing about 200 gm, were used. They were housed in small wire mesh cages, two to a cage. An experimental and a control animal comprised a cage pair.

Apparatus. The training was conducted in a wooden box, 38 in. long, 6 in. wide, and 20 in. deep. It was divided into two equal compartments, each 19 in. long. The box had a grid floor, through which a 0.75 ma (420 VAC) "scrambled" electric shock could be delivered. A single switch was used to turn the shock on or off simultaneously in both compartments.

Procedure and results. For training, the experimental animal of a pair was placed in one compartment and the control animal in the other. Each

From *Journal of the Experimental Analysis of Behavior,* 1963, 6, 213–218. Copyright 1963 by the Society for the Experimental Analysis of Behavior, Inc., Bloomington, Ind.

[1] This research was supported by a grant (MH-03238) from the United States Public Health Service. Chlorpromazine (Largactil) was supplied without charge by Poulenc, Ltd., imipramine (Tofranil) by Geigy (Canada), Ltd., and methylphenidate (Ritalin) by Ciba, Ltd.

animal of the pair was left in its respective compartment for a period of 10 min on each of 14 training sessions, one session per day. During a session, the experimenter observed the experimental animal and occasionally looked at the control animal. Shock was applied whenever the experimental animal walked, reared, sniffed, or was otherwise active in some way. The shock was terminated as soon as the animal stood or sat motionless; rats frequently sit motionless momentarily in the course of frantic jumping and running. Each time the experimental animal was shocked, the control animal also received the shock regardless of what it was doing; thus, the shocks received by the control animal were not consistently contingent on any specific behavior. The duration in seconds for which it was necessary to keep the shock on (*i.e.,* the time the experimental animal spent making any observable movements) was recorded by a running-time-meter connected to the shock switch; the time spent sitting motionless was calculated by subtracting this figure from 600 sec—the total duration of a session.

From the first to the second training session, there was a marked increase in immobility; both the experimental and the control animals remained motionless during more than 50% of the second session. On the third training session, it was noticed that, though the duration of immobility continued to increase in the experimental animals, the control animals began to move around. By the 14th session, all experimental animals had learned the response; each remained motionless for 9.99 min of the 10-min session. Clearly, like running or jumping, immobility can be trained as an avoidance response. In no case did the immobility represent lying flat on the grid, as rats sometimes do while they are being shocked; the observed immobility could more accurately be described as sitting rigidly motionless.

In order to determine how far the observed immobility was a response to the specific training situation, all animals were observed in four test sessions following training. One of the tests was given in the training situation and three in situations that differed from it in their stimulus characteristics. Each test was peceded and followed by a retraining session, using the original training procedure. During the retraining sessions all experimental animals maintained the 9.99/10-min performance level. During a test session, the experimenter recorded subject's action (*e.g.,* walking, rearing, grooming, sitting or standing motionless, *etc.*) at the end of each successive 6-sec interval; the click of a timer indicated each 6-sec interval. The reliability of this method has been discussed before (Bindra and Blond, 1958). All animals, experimental and control, were observed individually for a 10-min period, and the number of "motionless" entries was counted. No shock was given in any of the test sessions.

The results of the four test sessions are presented in Table 1. The figures describe the mean number of protocol entries (out of a total of 100) in which the animals were observed to be motionless. The results of Test Session 1, conducted in the training situation, clearly show the difference be-

TABLE 1.   Means and ranges of the frequencies of "motionless" entries in test sessions 1–4, and the significance level of differences between experimental and control groups.

Test Session No.	Experimental Condition	Experimental Animals	Control Animals	p-values (t-test; two-tailed)
1	Same as training	96.6 (93-100)	11.8 (0-32)	$<.001$
2	Square shallow box	70.2 (3-100)	21.8 (9-36)	$<.05$
3	Same as training but with a cardboard floor	62.2 (34-84)	12.4 (0-42)	$<.01$
4	Wire-mesh (living) cage	9.4 (1-15)	9.2 (2-21)	n.s.

tween the experimental and the control animals. Note that most of the experimental animals also displayed the immobility response in a square shallow box (Test Session 2), which had a grid floor similar to the one in the training situation, as well as in a situation in which the grid of the training box had been covered by a cardboard (Test Session 3). However, the response did not occur to any considerable extent in the wire-mesh cage (Test Session 4), which was identical to the ones in which the animals normally lived and was quite different from the training box.

Conclusion. The difference between control and experimental animals shows that immobility response in the experimental animals was not an unconditioned "freezing" response to electric shock. The differences in the incidence of immobility between Test Session 1 and the other test sessions, especially Sessions 3 and 4, indicate that the response was specifically associated with the situation in which it was trained.

EXPERIMENT II.   This experiment was designed to determine the relation between shock intensity and the acquisition of the immobility response.

Subjects and apparatus.   Thirty naive male hooded rats, each weighing about 200 gm, served. The apparatus described under Exp. I was used.

Procedure.   Twenty-four of the 30 rats were divided into four groups, A, B, C, and D. Each of Groups A, B, and D contained four animals; Group C contained 12. The remaining six rats, Group Y, served as yoked-control animals for six of the animals in Group C. Though the voltage of the shock generator was kept constant at 420 VAC, the shock intensity was different for the various groups: Group A, 0.50 ma; Group B, 0.75 ma; Groups C and Y, 2.00 ma, and Group D, 2.65 ma.

The training procedure for the six yoked pairs replicated that used in Exp. I. In the case of Groups A, B, D, and the six non-paired animals of Group C, only one compartment of the training box was used, but in every other respect the procedure was the same as in Exp. I. In the course of daily training sessions, when an animal remained motionless for 9.99 min in the 10-min session of a particular day, it was considered to have learned the immobility response.

The day after an animal reached the above learning criterion, it was given a test session. The time-sample method for recording the animal's behavior was the same as that used in Exp. I; the number of "motionless" and "rearing" entries during the test session was determined for each animal. No shock was given during the test session.

Results. Six of the 16 rats in Groups C and D failed to acquire the immobility response. All these non-learners managed to jump out of the training box when they were shocked during the first training session. Though they were immediately placed back into the box, each continued this jumping behavior and showed no signs of learning the required response even after 30 training sessions. The data from these non-learners are not included in the following analysis.

The general course of learning in the case of all learners, in Group A, B, C and D was the same as that observed in the first experiment. The duration of immobility increased rapidly during the first two sessions, and then continued to increase more slowly. There appeared to be no remarkable difference between Groups A and B, or between Groups C and D; therefore, the data for each of these two sets of groups were combined. The cumulative proportion of animals that reached the criterion of learning on each successive training session is shown in Fig. 1. It is clear that Groups A and B, which received a lower intensity of shock, did not learn the immo-

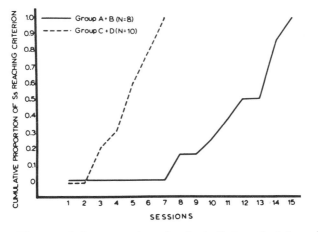

FIGURE 1. The cumulative proportion of animals that reached the criterion of learning (remaining motionless for 9.99 min out of 10 min) on each of the successive training sessions. Groups A and B (N = 8) were trained under low shock intensity; Groups C and D (N = 10) under high shock intensity.

bility response as readily as did the animals that received the two higher intensities of shock (Groups C and D). It also appeared that miscellaneous environmental disturbances were more likely to disrupt immobility in Groups A and B than in C and D; the higher intensities produced more stable responses.

Every animal in Groups A, B, C, and D that had reached the learning criterion remained motionless for at least 95% of the time (95% of the time-sample entries) during the test session. The yoked animals, Group Y, remained motionless significantly less than the paired animals in Group C (p < .01; two-tailed t-test). The yoked animals also reared significantly more than their paired experimental animals (p < .01). These results are shown in Table 2.

Conclusion. Considering only the animals that did not successfully escape the shock by jumping, the higher intensities of shock clearly produced quicker learning of the immobility response. However, shock intensity also seems to determine the probability of occurrence of the jumping response. Further, even at a high intensity of shock, the difference between the yoked-controlled animals and the experimental animals, in the case of which shock termination is contingent on their remaining motionless, is maintained; thus, a genuine learning of the immobility response is again demonstrated.

EXPERIMENT III. Active escape-avoidance responses, such as alley running, have been shown to be enhanced by stimulant drugs (Hamilton, 1960) and impaired by depressant drugs (Ader and Clink, 1957; Cook and Weidley, 1957; Irwin, 1961). The purpose of this experiment was to determine the effects of three commonly used drugs, methylphenidate, an amphetamine-like stimulant, chlorpromazine, a mild depressant or "tranquilizer," and imipramine, an "antidepressant" on the immobility avoidance response. Six dose levels of each of these drugs were used.

Subjects and apparatus. Thirteen naive adult male hooded rats, weighing about 200 gm each, served. The apparatus used is described under Exp. 1.

TABLE 2. Comparison of the frequency of "motionless" and "rearing" responses of the trained and the yoked-control animals at the end of training.

Responses	Experimental Animals Mean (Range)	Control Animals Mean (Range)	p
"Motionless"	96.1 (89-100)	53.7 (44-65)	< .01
"Rearing"	0.8 (0-4)	22.4 (17-70)	< .01

Procedure.   The training procedure was the same as employed in training Groups A, B, C and D of Exp. II, except that only one shock intensity, 0.75 ma, was used—the same intensity as was used in Exp. I. When all animals had learned the immobility avoidance response, they were divided into two groups, Group L, of five rats, and Group H, of eight rats. Group L was tested at the three lower drug doses, and Group H at the three higher drug doses.

All animals were tested in a series of sessions extending over about four weeks. Each test session was followed (and preceded) by a retraining session; the procedure for the retraining sessions was the same as that used in the original training. The retraining sessions ensured the maintenance of the avoidance response at a high performance level (9.99/10 min). The time-sample method used to record the occurrence of the motionless response in the test sessions has been described in Exp. I. No shocks were administered during the test sessions.

Every animal was given 11 test sessions; the first and the last of these were control tests (*i.e.,* no drug injections were given on these days). On the days of the other nine experimental test sessions, the animals in Group L and H were injected with the three drugs according to the schedule presented in Table 3. All animals in each group were given all the injections for that group in a scrambled order. The interval between the injection and the test was 30 min in the case of chlorpromazine and imipramine, and 15 min in the case of methylphenidate. All drugs were administered intraperitoneally.

Results.   As in Exp. I, in which the same shock intensity was used, all the animals reached the criterion of learning (remaining motionless for 9.99 min in 10 min) by the 17th training session. In the retraining sessions, all the animals maintained this criterion.

Figure 2 shows the mean frequencies of occurrence of the immobility response during the control session and under the influence of the six doses of each of the three drugs. The points for the three lower doses are based on Group L animals, and those for the three higher doses on Group H animals. It is clear that all three drugs produced a decrement in immobility. Within the limit of drug doses employed, this decrement was, roughly speaking, a direct monotonic function of dose in the case of methylphenidate, and an inverse monotonic function of dose in the case of chlorpromazine. Imipramine affected the response to about the same degree at all dose levels, except

TABLE 3.   Schedule of drug injections.

Group	Chlorpromazine Hydrochloride	Imipramine Hydrochloride	Methylphenidate Hydrochloride
L	2, 4, or 6 mg/kg	15, 20, or 25 mg/kg	4, 6, or 8 mg/kg
H	8, 10, or 12 mg/kg	30, 35, or 40 mg/kg	10, 12, or 14 mg/kg

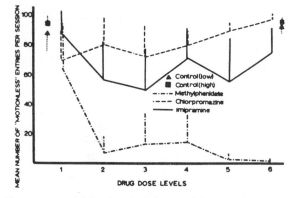

FIGURE 2. The mean and S.D. (vertical lines) of frequency of occurrence of the immobility response during the control sessions and under the influence of the six doses of each of the three drugs. The doses were as follows: chlorpromazine 2, 4, 6, 8, 10, or 12 mg/kg; imipramine 15, 20, 25, 30, 35, or 40 mg/kg methylphenidate 4, 6, 8, 10, 12, or 14 mg/kg. Group L was tested at the three lower doses of each drug, and Group H at the three higher doses of each drug. A control session was given at the beginning, and again at the end, of the test sessions.

the lowest. Correspondingly, the variability of immobility scores decreased markedly at the higher doses of chlorpromazine and methylphenidate, but remained large at the higher doses imipramine (see Fig. 2). Response decrement was significantly greater under the influence of the most potent dose of methylphenidate than under influence of the most potent dose of imipramine ($p < .01$) and of chlorpromazine ($p < .01$); under the influence of imipramine is was significantly greater than under the influence of chlorpromazine ($p < .06$). Every animal showed a marked decrement (compared to its own control score) in the avoidance response under the influence of chlorpromazine and of methylphenidate; only one animal in Group L failed to show a decrement under the influence of any of the three lower doses of imipramine.

Discussion. Methylphenidate is known to increase the level of spontaneous activity (Bindra and Baran, 1959); the decrement in the immobility response in the present experiment is most simply attributed to the hyperactivity induced by this drug.

Chlorpromazine is known to impair active avoidance responses (Ader and Clink, 1957); in general, the higher the dose, the greater the impairment. However, the present experiment shows that chlorpromazine reduces the occurrence of the immobility avoidance response only at extremely low doses. Irwin (1961) has shown that, in the case of an active avoidance response, the degree of impairment produced by phenothiazines is directly proportional to the extent to which they decrease spontaneous activity. Though the decrease in spontaneous activity produced by chlorpromazine is a direct function of the dose (Bindra and Baran, 1959), the impairment of the immobility avoidance response seems to be an inverse function of the dose.

Inasmuch as the effects of methylphenidate, as well as of chlorpromazine at certain doses, on the immobility avoidance response are opposite to the effects of these drugs on other, more active, avoidance responses, these effects must depend upon the exact behavioral components that make up different types of responses and on the effect that the drug has on each of those behavioral components (Bindra, 1961). In the light of this, the theoretical formulations, suggesting that drugs influence avoidance responding by modulating anxiety (Miller, Murphy, and Mirsky, 1957), must be re-examined.

Imipramine, which has been shown to resemble chlorpromazine in many of its behavioral effects (Herr, Stewart, and Charest, 1961), displayed a distinctive effect on the immobility avoidance response used in the present experiment. Though it is likely that at still higher doses imipramine, like chlorpromazine, may act as a sedative and have no decremental effect on the immobility response, the fact that it had this decremental effect over a wider range of doses than did chlorpromazine is notable and may have significance for drug screening (see Herr, Stewart and Charest, 1961). The usefulness of imipramine in the treatment of depressed patients (Kuhn, 1958) and the parallel between clinical depression and immobility as produced in the present experiment is also suggestive.

SUMMARY. Much of the available literature on avoidance behavior is based on responses which require the animal to run, lever-press, or to make some active response to avoid noxious stimulation. The purpose of Exp. I was to determine whether animals can learn to sit or stand motionless in order to escape or avoid electric shock. Five experimental rats were given escape-avoidance training, while five yoked control animals received electric shocks without any response-related contingency. It was shown that an immobility avoidance response, as distinct from the unconditioned "freezing" response to shock, can be trained. The results of Exp. II (30 rats) revealed that this response is more readily acquired at higher shock intensities than at lower ones, provided escape by jumping is prevented at the high shock intensities. The effects of six doses of each of three drugs on the immobility avoidance response were studied in Exp. III (13 rats). Methylphenidate, chlorpromazine, and imipramine all produced a decrement in the immobility response, but the pattern and amount of the effects of the three drugs were quite different, one from the other. The implications of these findings for a general theory of avoidance behavior and for drug screening are discussed.

REFERENCES

Ader, R., and Clink, D. W. Effects of chlorpromazine on the acquisition and extinction of an avoidance response in the rat. *J. Pharmacol. exp. Therap.*, 1957, **121**, 144–148.

Bindra, D. Components of general activity and the analysis of behavior. *Psychol. Rev.*, 1961, **68**, 205–215.

Bindra, D., and Baran, D. Effects of methylphenidylacetate and chlorpromazine on certain components of general activity. *J. exp. Anal. Behav.*, 1959, **2**, 343–350.

Bindra, D., and Blond, Joyce. A time-sample method for measuring general activity and its components. *Canadian J. Psychol.*, 1958, **12**, 74–76.

Blough, D. S. New test for tranquilizers. *Science*, 1958, **127**, 586–587.

Cook, C., and Weidley, E. Behavioral effects of some psychopharmacological agents. *Ann. N.Y. Acad. Sci.*, 1957, **66**, 740–752.

Herr, F., Stewart, Jane, and Charest, Marie-Paule. Tranquilizers and antidepressants: A pharmacological comparison. *Arch. int. Pharmacodyn.*, 1961, **134**, 328–342.

Hamilton, C. L. Effects of LSD-25 and amphetamine on a running response in the rat. *Am. Med. Assn. Archiv.*, 1960, **2**, 104–109.

Irwin, S. Correlation in rats between the locomotor and avoidance-suppressant potencies of eight phenothiazine tranquilizers. *Arch. int. Pharmacodyn.*, 1961, **132**, 279–286.

Kuhn, R. The treatment of depressive states with G22355 (Imipramine hydrochloride). *Am. J. Psychiat.*, 1958, **115**, 459–464.

Miller, R. E., Murphy, J. V., and Mirsky, I. A. The effects of chlorpromazine on fear-motivated behavior in rats. *J. Pharmacol. exp. Therap.*, 1957, **120**, 379–387.

21

Drug effects on lever positioning behavior

ROBERT CLARK, JAMES A. JACKSON, and JOSEPH V. BRADY

As part of a research program concerned with the development of an automated motor assessment test battery for use with primate subjects, we have devised a technique for generating a lever positioning response in the rhesus monkey. Our aim was to obtain a quantitative index of muscle steadiness and fatigue that would perhaps be sensitive to the effects of drugs, ionizing radiations, and other biologically effective variables. Also, we felt that some of the properties of lever positioning were of interest in their own right, since the continuous nature of this behavior distinguishes it from such discrete responses as lever pressing and key pecking, and such discrete response measures as rate, latency, and duration.

The subjects for the initial phase of this experiment were three rhesus monkeys maintained in restraining chairs. Crackers and water were continually available to them. Each chair was fitted with a lever positioning device placed at waist level within easy reach of the animal's outstretched arm. The lever was an aluminum rod, ¾ inch in diameter and 4½ inches long. It could be moved through an arc of 72° along the animal's midline. The lever housing (a 3- by 5-inch aluminum chassis) was continually electrified to prevent the subject from resting or bracing its arm or paw during test sessions.

In the experiments to be described, each subject was tested for 1 hour each day. A red flashing light was on during test sessions and off at all other times. By means of a 0.25-megohm potentiometer connected to the lever, and a Varian recorder, a continuous record of the lever position through time was obtained.

During the first 10 days of training, each monkey was continually shocked as long as the lever was located within 24° of the resting position. (The lever was closest to the animal when in its resting position.) If the subject moved the lever to any point more than 24° away from the resting position, that is, between 24° and 72°, the shock was turned off and remained off as long as the lever was held within this region. By means of a cable, pulley, and weight (0.9 kg) system, the lever, when released, would return to its resting position. Thus, the subject could avoid shock only as long as it held the lever within the 24° to 72° region. Each subject learned to correctly position and hold the lever within the first 30 to 60 minutes of

From *Science*, 1962, 135, 1132–1133. Copyright 1962 by the American Association for the Advancement of Science, Washington, D.C.

training and each remained virtually shock-free throughout the next 10 sessions. The contingencies for shock avoidance were then changed. During the next 3 months of training, the subjects could avoid shock only by positioning the lever more than 24° but less than 48° from the resting position: that is, between 24° and 48°. Movement of the lever into either the 0° to 24° or the 24° to 72° regions now produced shock. The subjects again learned to correctly position and hold the lever within the first two or three training sessions and each remained virtually shock-free thereafter. A typical record from this base-line determination period is shown in Fig. 1. Fluctuations in the base-line curves were generally negligible, and each subject usually held the lever within 2° to 3° of the center position throughout the hour-long session. (A point 32° from the resting position was taken

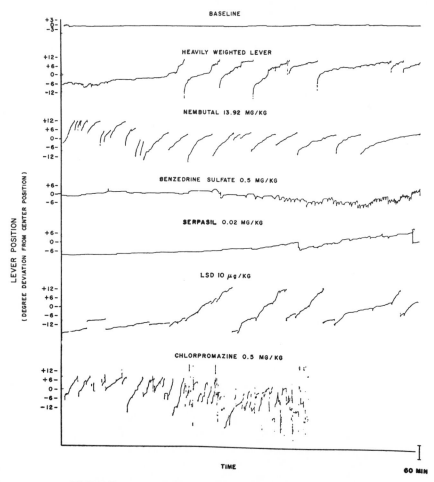

FIGURE 1.   Drug effects on lever positioning. (U.S. Army)

as the center or "zero" position. The subject was thus shocked whenever the curve exceeded ± 12°.)

The following data were obtained from a single subject. By increasing the weight load on the lever to 4 kg, the "heavily weighted lever" curve of Fig. 1 was obtained. A recurrent pattern of slow release of the lever to the point where shock was received, followed by a rapid recovery to a "safe" position can be seen. Similar effects were obtained after intramuscular (IM) injections of either Nembutal or lysergic acid diethylamide (LSD). These curves differ mainly in the rate of recurrence of the release and recovery pattern, although it is possible that such differences are due mainly to the particular dosage values used. An IM administration of Benzedrine produced a series of spindly curves toward the end of the session, which are interpreted as an increase in muscular tremor. The slow drift in the Serpasil (IM) curve may indicate a fatigue effect or perhaps a partial extinction of the avoidance response due to the tranquilizing properties of this drug. The chlorpromazine (IM) run, which was characterized by an extremely rapid rate of release and recovery, was stopped after approximately 45 minutes because of the large number of shocks the animal was receiving. Each curve was obtained approximately 15 minutes after drug administration, and at least 2 weeks intervened between drug administrations. The curves shown here represent the second or third determination for each drug. Good reproducibility of each drug effect was obtained in all cases.

It is clear, then, from the data for three subjects, that the lever positioning response is easily conditioned and quite stable. The data from one subject indicates that this measure is at least partially sensitive to factors known to produce fatigue and tremor, and appears to differentiate among several classes of drugs. In addition to exploring the effects of other drugs on lever positioning, future research will focus on dose-response relations and drug interactions with such behavioral variables as the orientation and physical characteristics of the lever, the width of the "safe" region, and the probability of being shocked for incorrect positioning.

SUMMARY.   A technique is described for generating a continuous lever positioning response in the rhesus monkey. The effects of several drugs on this behavior were studied.

22

Effects of amphetamine, chlorpromazine, pentobarbital, and ethanol on operant response duration [1]

BERNARD WEISS and VICTOR G. LATIES

One way to study the behavioral effects of drugs is to observe the changes that they produce in the temporal distribution of behavior. Certain reinforcement schedules generate reliable and recognizable temporal patterns in behavior that reflect specific temporal contingencies in the schedule. For example, the DRL (Differential Reinforcement of Low Rate) schedule specifies that only responses separated from the immediately preceding response by more than a stated interval will be reinforced. Such a contingency tends to produce an interresponse time distribution with a mode near the minimum reinforced interval (Skinner, 1938; Wilson and Keller, 1953; Ferster and Skinner, 1957).

The behavior that we studied in the present experiments was maintained by a reinforcement schedule with a temporal contingency different from those typically used. Dogs were trained to push a button with their noses. They were reinforced when they accumulated a specified duration of nose-pressing. No temporal constraints limited the possible distribution of response durations except the length of the interval that had to be accumulated. Such an arrangement permits great variation in the temporal characteristics of the behavior that can produce reinforcement but still retains a temporal contingency. It seemed possible that it would illuminate the action of certain drugs observed to produce changes in the temporal character of the behavior arising from other schedules of reinforcement.

METHODS. Figure 1 illustrates the way in which the present experiments were arranged. Whenever the dog pressed his nose against the response button [2] with a pressure exceeding 15 grams, the tape drive moved the tape. A tone sounded at the same time and remained on as long as the response button remained pressed. Holes were punched in the tape to cor-

From *Journal of Pharmacology and Experimental Therapeutics,* 1964, **144**, 17–23. Copyright © 1964 by The Williams and Wilkins Co., Baltimore, Md.

[1] Supported by USPHS Research Grants MH-03229 from the National Institute of Mental Health and B-865 from the National Institute of Neurological Diseases and Blindness. The authors are grateful to Barbara Folderauer for technical assistance and to Dr. Walter C. Stanley and the Roscoe B. Jackson Laboratories for providing the Basenji dogs.

[2] Nose-pressing has been used as an operant in dogs by Waller (1961) and by Lindsley (1957).

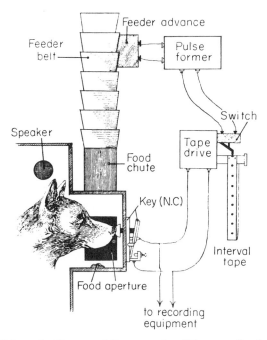

FIGURE 1.   Schematic diagram of the apparatus. Whenever the dog pressed the key enough to break the circuit, the tape drive moved the punched tape. After the tape moved a distance corresponding to 60 seconds of nose-pressing, the microswitch arm closed a circuit and delivered the food to the dog.

respond to 1-minute intervals. When a hole moved past the microswitch, the switch arm dropped and closed a circuit that advanced the belt feeder. This operation dumped about 5 grams of dry dog food pellets (Kasco or Hunt Club) into the small subchamber that contained the response key. Each reinforcement, therefore, represented a total of 1 minute of key-pressing. Such a schedule might be termed a *cumulative response duration* (CRD) schedule.

The subchamber was a 13-cm cube. The experimental chamber proper was a 60-cm cube. The recording and programming equipment was located in an adjoining room. A noise generator connected to a loudspeaker near the chamber helped to mask extraneous noises. Water was available in the chamber.

The distribution of response durations was obtained by allocating durations between specified limits to particular counters by means of a timer and stepping switch. These categories were each 1 second wide for responses lasting less than 10 seconds. Responses longer than 10 seconds were all allocated to an eleventh category. Response onsets were recorded on a cumulative recorder.

The subjects were 4 adult male Basenji dogs originally from the Roscoe

B. Jackson Memorial Laboratories. Basenjis proved to be a useful laboratory animal. They were quiet, tractable, not easily disturbed, and readily adapted to the situation. The dogs were first trained to press the button on a continuous reinforcement schedule; *i.e.,* each press, regardless of its duration, produced a reinforcement. Once this behavior was acquired, a minimum response duration of 0.5 second was specified for reinforcement. This requirement was gradually raised until the minimum duration equaled 3 seconds. The next step in training was to require the dogs to accumulate a total of 30 seconds of key-pressing in order to obtain reinforcement. The minimum duration of a single response remained 3 seconds and time could therefore be accumulated only in 3-second blocks.

Under these conditions, as well as the previous ones in this training sequence, most of the responses tended to be of short duration (less than 1 second long). Since this meant that only a relatively small proportion of responses would be eligible for reinforcement—a factor that we believed might make drug effects less visible—the schedule was modified.

We decided to study changes in response duration when no constraints on minimum duration were imposed. The arrangement illustrated in Fig. 1 was then devised. This allowed the dogs to accumulate 60 seconds of nose-pressing with each response, no matter how short, contributing to the sum. Note, however, that long responses are differentially reinforced because they are more likely than short ones to terminate in reinforcement. This is the reason that a substantial incidence of long responses is maintained. The dogs were then exposed to this set of conditions until the number of responses per reinforcement showed no definite trend from session to session. This required a total of 6 sessions during each of which 66 reinforcements were dispensed. During the last 3 of these sessions, the mean proportion of responses less than 1 second long varied between 0.55 and 0.57 and the number of responses per reinforcement between 10.6 and 12.6. The drug experiments then began.

For a particular drug, the sequence of doses was counterbalanced among dogs. The ethanol was administered *via* stomach tube in 150 ml of water. The other agents were administered subcutaneously. Amphetamine-pentobarbital and amphetamine-ethanol combinations were studied after the data on the effects of the individual drugs had been gathered. No less than 3 days separated successive drug administrations. During the experiments the dogs were maintained at approximately 80% of the free-feeding weight on a dry dog food diet and were given no food for 24 hours before a session.

An experimental session began with a control period during which the dog was permitted to obtain 16 reinforcements. The control session lasted a maximum of 1 hour. The drug was then administered. After amphetamine, chlorpromazine, and pentobarbital, 30 minutes elapsed before the experiment proceeded. This period was reduced to 10 minutes for ethanol. The experimental period lasted 3 hours or until 50 reinforcements had been obtained. Isotonic saline was used as the control injection and tap water as the control for ethanol.

RESULTS. The distribution of response durations emitted under the CRD schedule approximates an exponential function. The incidence of short responses is high. Frequency falls in an exponential fashion as duration increases. This is the kind of distribution that would be expected were response durations generated by a Poisson process, as would be predicted from the holding-time model discussed by Feller (1957) except that the proportion of very short responses is slightly excessive for this model.

Amphetamine, pentobarbital, and ethanol all shortened response duration. Chlorpromazine had no discernible effect. Combinations of amphetamine with pentobarbital and with ethanol reduced response duration even more. These results will be described mainly in two ways. One is the number of responses per reinforcement, *i.e.,* the number of responses required to accumulate 60 seconds. These values are inversely related to mean response duration and are easily convertible to the latter by inspection. Mean duration, however, does not reflect the results adequately because the distribution of response durations is quite skewed.

The results will also be described in terms of the proportion of responses lasting less than 1 second. The changes that took place in the frequency of these short responses represent a better index of the drug effects than the distribution of response durations because the most substantial and reliable effects were observed in this frequency. Drug treatments also produced great changes in the proportion of responses lasting more than 10 seconds. Since, however, several treatments reduced the number of responses of this duration nearly to zero, estimates of the proportion could be less reliably computed.

Figure 2 presents the mean responses per reinforcement and Fig. 3 the proportion of responses less than 1 second long. Both of these criteria, which are necessarily correlated, show similar changes for each of the drugs and dose levels studied.

Amphetamine sulfate produced a progressive increase in the number of responses per reinforcement and in the proportion of responses less than 1 second long as dose was increased. The higher doses of sodium pentobarbital (8 and 16 mg/kg) also produced effects similar to those observed after amphetamine. The dose-response function for ethanol was less steep than that for either amphetamine or pentobarbital. At the highest dose, however, there was a clear increase in the number of responses per reinforcement and in the incidence of very short responses.

Chlorpromazine hydrochloride, up to 2 mg/kg, a dose level that made the dogs quite lethargic, did not produce any change in the criteria shown in the figures. In fact, a second chlorpromazine study conducted with a dose of 4 mg/kg (the reason for the second control treatment shown in

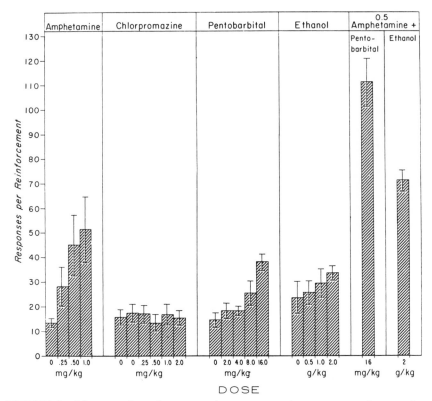

FIGURE 2. Mean number of nose-pressing responses (response onsets) per reinforcement as a function of drug treatment (N = 4). Each bar represents the number of responses required to accumulate a total of 60 seconds of nose-pressing. The standard errors for each condition are shown as vertical lines.

the figures) completely eliminated all relevant behavior; the dogs simply went to sleep.

Two other observations deserve mention. One is that at the highest doses used, both pentobarbital and ethanol made the dogs observably ataxic. This was one reason for not using higher dose levels of these drugs. The other observation is that at no time did the dogs fail to eat the food delivered at reinforcement, even after the high dose of amphetamine. After this dose, however, three of the four dogs did not immediately resume responding when the apparatus was turned on following the 30-minute waiting period after administration. They waited a mean of 33 minutes more before beginning to respond. In a later experiment 2 mg/kg of amphetamine eliminated responding for the full 3-hour period.

The combinations of amphetamine with pentobarbital and amphetamine with ethanol produced striking increases in the effect produced by these drugs individually. The number of responses per reinforcement evoked by

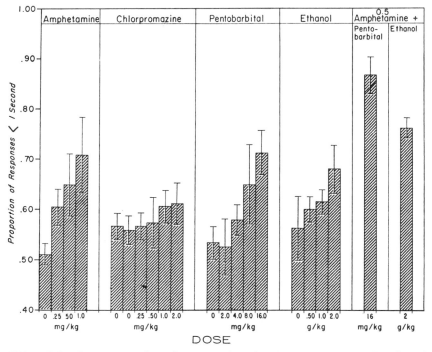

FIGURE 3.   Mean proportion of responses less than 1 second long as a function of drug treatment (N = 4). These were obtained from the counters that registered response duration in 1-second blocks. The standard errors for each condition are shown as vertical lines.

the amphetamine-barbiturate mixture was 34% greater than the sum of the numbers of the responses following the individual doses and close to 10 times as great as the number following saline. Gross behavior was also affected in a striking way. Instead of displaying their usual docility, the dogs, despite signs of ataxia (presumably attributable to the pentobarbital and ethanol), became extremely hyperactive, howling, whining, and struggling against the leash.

Treatments that increased the number of responses per reinforcement shifted the entire distribution of durations toward the shorter durations, as can be seen in Table 1, which presents, as an example, the response duration distributions for amphetamine. As the proportion in the first interval climbed from 0.510 after saline to 0.708 after 1 mg/kg of amphetamine, the proportion of responses lasting more than 10 seconds fell from 0.126 to 0.010. After administration of the amphetamine-barbiturate combinations, which placed 0.867 of the total responses in the first category, less than 0.001 of the total was found in all the categories past 4 seconds. Another aspect of these results is reflected in the mean duration of re-

TABLE 1.   Distribution of the duration of nose-pressing responses of dogs after the subcutaneous administration of amphetamine sulfate; each entry represents the mean of 4 dogs.

Dose of Amphetamine (mg/kg)	Response Duration in Seconds										
	0–1	1–2	2–3	3–4	4–5	5–6	6–7	7–8	8–9	9–10	10+
0	0.510	0.134	0.066	0.044	0.036	0.029	0.014	0.016	0.011	0.012	0.126
0.25	0.617	0.135	0.044	0.036	0.030	0.026	0.020	0.012	0.008	0.010	0.062
0.50	0.649	0.152	0.064	0.034	0.026	0.018	0.012	0.009	0.006	0.004	0.020
1.00	0.708	0.132	0.066	0.035	0.022	0.011	0.007	0.004	0.003	0.002	0.010

sponses lasting more than 10 seconds. Those made during drug sessions were shorter than those made during saline sessions. The mean length of responses lasting more than 10 seconds was 27.21 seconds after saline. The mean duration of these long responses fell progressively to 17.11, 13.51, and 13.48 seconds as the dose of amphetamine went from 0.25 to 0.50 to 1.0 mg/kg.

Figures 4 and 5 show sample cumulative records from various sections of these experiments. The data from the other two dogs are similar. These demonstrate that the decreases in response duration displayed in Figs. 2 and 3 were accompanied by increases in response rate, which means that interresponse times were simultaneously shortened. Note that the two measures are not necessarily related; an animal could maintain a constant rate even while decreasing response duration by increasing the interresponse times. Another interesting feature of these records is the tendency for post-reinforcement pauses to occur, particularly in the case of Dog 2. These produced discontinuities in the cumulative record reminiscent of both fixed-interval and fixed-ratio reinforcement schedules.

DISCUSSION.   Amphetamine, pentobarbital, and ethanol all produced similar effects on behavior controlled by the CRD schedule, increasing the number of responses per reinforcement as dose was increased. Chlorpromazine had no effect on this type of behavior. On other schedules of reinforcement that are comparable in some respect to the CRD schedule, the same pattern of drug response does not appear to prevail, although data from the dog are scarce.

With rats on DRL schedules, for example, amphetamine shifts the modal interresponse time toward the shorter intervals (Sidman, 1955; Kelleher *et al.*, 1961; Segal, 1962). Barbiturates do not seem to affect DRL distributions except at dose levels that produce erratic behavior characterized by bursts of responses alternating with long pauses (Sidman, 1956; Kelleher *et al.*, 1961). Ethanol seems to produce little change in DRL distributions

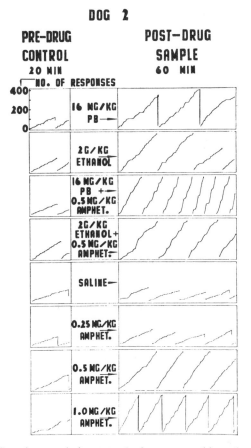

FIGURE 4. Sample cumulative records from one subject showing the effects of various drug treatments on rate of response onsets. A 20-minute segment from the control period is shown for comparison with a 1-hour segment obtained during the period following drug administration. Resets of the recording pen to the baseline seen on those segments with low rates resulted from the fact that this recorder was connected in parallel with a second recorder that counted seconds.

except to lower the overall response rate (Sidman, 1955; Laties and Weiss, 1962). Chlorpromazine tends to produce a similar effect (Kelleher et al., 1961).

Fixed-interval reinforcement schedules also produce recognizable temporal patterns in behavior. In pigeons and rats, the typical pattern can be disrupted by amphetamine, barbiturates, and chlorpromazine. The disruption consists of the production of a uniform rate of responding through the interval between reinforcements rather than a preponderance of responses toward the end (Dews, 1958; Herrnstein and Morse, 1957). Similar kinds

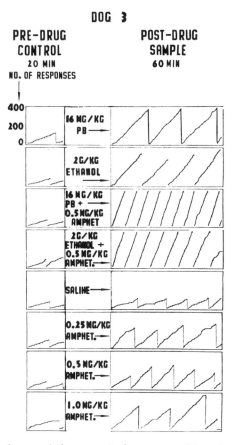

FIGURE 5. Sample cumulative records from one subject showing the effects of various drug treatments on rate of response onsets. A 20-minute segment from the control period is shown for comparison with a 1-hour segment obtained during the period following drug administration. Resets of the recording pen to the baseline seen on those segments with low rates resulted from the fact that this recorder was connected in parallel with a second recorder that counted seconds.

of disruption occur in the dog after oral doses of chlorpromazine in the range of 4 to 8 mg/kg (Waller, 1961). This sort of action in dogs contrasts greatly with the total lack of effect that we observed on the CRD schedule after chlorpromazine.

In one of the rare studies performed on dogs, Lindsley (1957) found that the intravenous administration of 8 mg/kg of pentobarbital produced a reliable increase in response rate on a variable-interval schedule of reinforcement. The same dose also increased responding during periods of extinction signaled by a visual stimulus. In an earlier publication (Jetter *et al.,* 1953) the same author described similar effects in dogs immediately after an intramuscular injection of 1 mg/kg of amphetamine. An hour after injection, however, response rate fell below the control level. Chlorpromazine given to dogs on a variable-interval schedule decreases response rate as dose is increased (Waller and Waller, 1962).

Hefferline's holding schedule (1950) is similar to the CRD schedule in specifying a holding response, but it does not involve any temporal contingency. Instead, an aversive stimulus is occluded as long as the subject holds down a lever or a panel. Harrison and Abelson (1959), using intense noise as the aversive stimulus, found that 2 mg/kg of amphetamine to rats shortened both the duration of a similar holding response and the interresponse times, a result similar to that shown in Figs. 4 and 5.

Blough (1958) differentially reinforced pigeons for maintaining a stationary posture. The required duration was programmed by an adjusting schedule. Chlorpromazine increased and pentobarbital decreased the lengths of time that the birds stood still. The effect of pentobarbital is congruent with the present results.

Amphetamine-barbiturate synergism has been observed both in rats (Steinberg *et al.,* 1961; Rushton *et al.,* 1963; Rushton and Steinberg, 1963) and humans (Legge and Steinberg, 1962). Doses that individually produced little change in the exploratory behavior of rats produced great changes when combined. The combinations producing peak enhancement consisted of 0.75 mg/kg of amphetamine + 15 mg/kg of sodium amytal, and 1.18 mg/kg of dextro-amphetamine + 7.5 mg/kg of sodium amytal. The former combination approximated the ratio used in the present experiment. The data reported in the literature plus our own suggest that such synergism extends over a wide range of behavior and species.

In conclusion, we should like to point out, first, that we expected to find differences among the drugs used rather than similarities, and, second, that we combined amphetamine with pentobarbital in an attempt to counteract one with the other. Both premises were wrong. Our results demonstrate once again how misleading it can be to accept the traditional categories of "stimulant" and "depressant" drugs and also emphasize the central role than reinforcement schedules occupy in determining the effect a given drug will have on behavior (Dews and Morse, 1961).

SUMMARY.   Dogs were trained to press against a response button with their noses. Whenever a dog accumulated 1 minute of nose-pressing, a food reinforcement was delivered. No restriction was placed on the number of individual responses needed to accumulate the 1-minute total. Amphetamine, pentobarbital, and ethanol all produced increases in the number of responses per reinforcement as dose was increased. Chlorpromazine had no effect up to a dose that caused the dogs to sleep. Combinations of amphetamine and ethanol, or amphetamine and pentobarbital produced substantial increases in the effects observed with the individual doses.

REFERENCES

Blough, D. S.: *Science* **127**:586, 1958.

Dews, P. B.: *Fed. Proc.* **17**:1024, 1958.

Dews, P. B., and Morse, W. H.: *Annu. Rev. Pharmacol.* **1**:145, 1961.

Feller, W.: *An introduction to probability theory and its applications,* 2nd ed., John Wiley & Sons, New York, 1957.

Ferster, C. B., and Skinner, B. F.: *Schedules of reinforcement,* Appleton-Century-Crofts, New York, 1957.

Harrison, J. M., and Abelson, R. B.: *J. exp. Anal. Behav.* **2**:23, 1959.

Hefferline, R. F.: *Genet. Psychol. Monogr.* **42**:213, 1950.

Herrnstein, R. J., and Morse, W. H.: *Science* **125**:929, 1957.

Jetter, W. W., Lindsley, O. R., and Wohlwill, F. J.: The effects of X-irradiation on physical exercise and behavior in the dog; related hematological and pathological control studies, Boston University, 1953. (Abstr., *Nuc. Sci. Abstr.* **8**:384, 1953.)

Kelleher, R. T., Fry, W., Deegan, J., and Cook, L.: *J. Pharmacol.* **133**:271, 1961.

Laties, V. G., and Weiss, B.: *J. comp. Physiol. Psychol.* **55**:85, 1962.

Legge, D., and Steinberg, H.: *Brit. J. Pharmacol.* **18**:490, 1962.

Lindsley, O. R.: Conditioned suppression of behavior in the dog and some sodium pentobarbital effects, Ph.D. thesis, Harvard University, 1957.

Rushton, R., and Steinberg, H.: *Nature,* Lond. **197**:1017, 1963.

Rushton, R., Steinberg, H., and Tinson, C.: *Brit. J. Pharmacol.* **20**:99, 1963.

Segal, E. F.: *J. exp. Anal. Behav.* **5**:105, 1962.

Sidman, M.: *Science* **122**:925, 1955.

Sidman, M.: *Ann. N.Y. Acad. Sci.* **65**:282, 1956.

Skinner, B. F.: *The behavior of organisms,* Appleton-Century-Crofts, New York, 1938.

Steinberg, H., Rushton, R., and Tinson, C.: *Nature,* Lond. **192**:533, 1961.

Waller, M. B.: *J. exp. Anal. Behav.* **4**:351, 1961.

Waller, M. B., and Waller, P. F.: *J. exp. Anal. Behav.* **5**:259, 1962.

Wilson, M. P., and Keller, F. S.: *J. comp. Physiol. Psychol.* **46**:190, 1953.

23

The behavioral measurement of fine motor control: Effects of pharmacological agents [1]

JOHN L. FALK

The aim of the present research was to develop an objective, quantitative method for studying fine motor control, and to evaluate a few commonly used drugs with this method. Investigations in neurology, neuropharmacology, and physiology have typically attempted to measure tremor in restrained, anesthetized, or statically resting subjects. Often a small transducer or accelerometer is fastened to some extremity, and the consequences of experimental brain lesions (Wachs, 1964), neural interventions to alleviate Parkinson's disease (Webster, 1960), or pharmacological agents (Connor, Rossi, and Baker, 1966; George, Haslett, and Jenden, 1966) are evaluated. However, this general approach to tremor evaluation is unsatisfactory in the unrestrained animal, and a variation of it "produces qualitative characterizations of the tremor rather than quantitative ones" (Dill, Dorman, and Nickey, 1968). Furthermore, quantitative measurement of motor states more complicated than resting or postural tremors, such as action tremor and dyskinesia, poses such difficulties that frame-by-frame analysis of motion pictures or simply clinical impressions are relied on (Carpenter, Whittier, and Mettler, 1950; Vernier and Unna, 1963; Growdon, Chambers, and Liu, 1967).

The present undertaking was encouraged by the pioneering findings of Notterman and Mintz (1962) that a rather fine aspect of an operant response, the peak force, could be brought under behavioral control. Also, Clark, Jackson, and Brady (1962) had demonstrated that a related motor task, lever positioning, was sensitive to the effects of drugs. Our approach is similar to one developed independently by Carrie (1965) for use with human subjects.

In the evaluation of the behavioral effects of drugs, the investigator is usually not primarily interested in motor effects *per se* and, in fact, attempts to experiment at dose levels less than those resulting in ataxia. The literature is replete with asides such as: "No gross motor deficit was observed." Sometimes it is demonstrated that, under the influence of a particular drug, fixed-ratio behavior can nevertheless be elicited. This demonstrates that any interference with more complex schedules of reinforcement by this drug

[1] This work was supported by Project THEMIS, ONR (DOD) Contract N00014-68-A-0150; USPHS Grant B3861 and Atomic Energy Commission Contract AT(11-1)-1201.

dose is not primarily due to motor effects which directly limit the rate of responding. But it does not preclude the possibility that this drug dose might still have profound motor effects not measured by the usual microswitch-pulse former interface with the organism, or the absence of grossly observable ataxia.

METHOD

SUBJECTS AND EXPERIMENTAL SPACE.   The animals were five Irish female rats, 13–16 weeks old at the start of the experiment. They were a first-generation cross between two inbred strains, brother-sister mated: an albino line and a black, non-agouti, selfed line. They were individually housed in a temperature-controlled, constantly illuminated room.

The experimental space was a picnic ice chest fitted with an air exhaust system and enclosed in a larger plywood acoustic tile-clad, fiberglass-lined, sound-attenuating box. The chest was partitioned so that one side contained a food-pellet magazine (Ralph Gerbrands Co.), a loudspeaker, two GE 1224 DC lights for illumination, and a force transducer rigidly mounted. On the other side, the free-moving animal, standing on a floor of spaced, stainless-steel rods, had access to a food-pellet receptacle and a lever. The back leaf of this lever was in contact with the force-transducer drive rod. The lever surface available to the animal was 13 mm wide. The electronic apparatus for programming and recording the animals' motor behavior has been described in more detail in a previous publication (Falk and Haas, 1965).

PROCEDURE.   *Training.*   Animals were placed on food deprivation for one day, and daily training in the experimental apparatus was then started. During the training period, the animals were permitted to earn up to 100 food pellets (45-mg Lab Rat Food Pellets, P. J. Noyes Company) per daily training session. Little or no food supplement was allowed when animals were returned to their respective individual living cages after each daily session until their pre-session body weight reached 80 percent of their free-feeding weight. They were then allowed an amount of food (Purina Mouse Breeder Chow) post-session each day which was sufficient to maintain their weight at this 80 percent point for the remainder of the experiment. Water was available in the home cage but not in the experimental space.

Animals were trained to press the lever with their paw by the method of successive approximation (Ferster and Skinner, 1957). The apparatus was adjusted so that any response force greater than 5 grams operated the pellet magazine once, a pellet being thereupon delivered into the pellet receptacle. By about the third daily session, all animals were earning 100 pellets in rapid succession. To complete the remaining steps in training, the animals required from 5 to 11 sessions. The steps essentially involved shaping the intensive dimensions of the lever-pressing behavior so that the animals held the transducer operated within the limits of a narrow force band (15–20 grams) continuously for at least 1.5 seconds. This was accomplished by first requiring that the response operating the pellet magazine be greater that 15 grams, rather than 5 grams. In other words, only 15-gram-or-greater response-force peaks were reinforced (strengthened) by delivery of a food pellet. Next, reinforcement was withheld until this 15-gram-or-greater criterion was met and held for a certain period of time. This period of time was gradually increased up to approximately one second. Whenever an adequate force criterion was being met (force on the lever greater than 15 grams), a continuous buzzer sounded. This feedback sound was 300 clicks/second, 90 dB re 0.0002 dynes/cm² (Malis and Curran, 1960). The provision of the feedback sound whenever the response force lay within the limits required remained a feature of the rest of the experiment. Next, the response force was required not only to lie over 15 grams but also to be less than 30 grams. The reinforced response band was then narrowed to 15–20 grams, and the holding time within this band was increased to 1.5 seconds. The task required, then, a continuous application of force within a 15–20-gram force band for not less than 1.5 seconds. Each fulfillment of this requirement yielded a food pellet. An excursion of force outside the band for longer than 60 milliseconds reset the 1.5-second timer.

Each animal worked daily in the experimental space and was allowed to earn 100 food pellets. The termination of the session was signaled to the animal by the cessation of illumination in the box when the one hundredth pellet was earned. When the day-to-day session performance reached a stable baseline state for each animal, it was adapted to restraint for several seconds within a plastic holding device 45 minutes before its experimental session. This was in preparation for later drug injections. Ten consecutive days were run under these baseline conditions.

Motor performance measures. Several measures of motor behavior were calculated from the overall session performance each day. These measures were derived from the values accumulated on three running time meters and two impulse counters over the session. One time meter simply recorded the total elapsed time from the initiation of the session to its end, when 100 pellets had been earned. This value is called *session time.* Another time meter accumulated *total response time.* This is the amount of session time that the animal spent actually responding on the force lever. The meter was started whenever the response force on the lever exceeded a response threshold value defined as 5 grams. A third time meter accumulated the total *in-band time* for the session. This meter operated as long as the force applied to the lever remained within the reinforced band (15–20 grams), ceasing when the force either dropped below 15 or increased above 20 grams. From these three time values accumulated over the session, the first three motor performance measures were calculated, as shown in Table 1.

Some comments on these measures are in order before the remaining measures are described. Since the number of pellets per session was fixed at 100, and the continuous in-band time to earn each pellet was fixed at 1.5 seconds, the minimum possible in-band time for a session was 150 seconds. If this number is divided by the in-band time which was actually accumulated over the session, the result is an efficiency measure. For example, the denominator would accumulate a relatively large number if the force repeatedly went outside the reinforced band after driving the clock almost to 1.5 seconds.

The *tonic accuracy* measure gives the proportion of the total response time that the responding was in the required band. This is independent of whether the organism can remain in the band for the required continuous holding time. The applied force would exit repeatedly from the band if, for example, a postural tremor were superimposed upon an accurate tonic contraction pattern. In such a case, the tonic accuracy measure would be high (relatively little time is spent outside the band), but the in-band efficiency would be low.

Work rate is simply the proportion of the session time in which the animal was engaged in responding on the lever over the 5-gram threshold.

An electromechanical impulse counter operated each time the applied force entered the band, whether this entrance was from the bottom or the top of the band. This is designated as the *dyskinesia score*. An organism

TABLE 1.   Motor performance measures.

Measure	Derivation of the measure
Efficiency in-band	$\dfrac{\text{Minimum possible in-band time}}{\text{In-band time}}$
Tonic accuracy	$\dfrac{\text{In-band time}}{\text{Total response time}}$
Work rate	$\dfrac{\text{Total response time}}{\text{Session time}}$
Dyskinesia score	Total number of entrances into band
Mean in-band time	$\dfrac{\text{In-band time}}{\text{Dyskinesia score}}$
Pellets as multiples	Total number of pellets earned in lots of two or more, where applied force remains above 5 grams after the first of the series is earned.

with an action tremor, for example, which rapidly transected the band many times would accumulate relatively little time on the in-band timer and thus not seriously lower its in-band efficiency. But such a bout of dyskinesia would be reflected in the dyskinesia score.

The *mean in-band time* is calculated by simply dividing in-band time by the number of times the animal was in the band, i.e., by the dyskinesia score.

In previous experiments, it was noted that some animals preferred to remain holding the lever within the band until two, or even as many as six, pellets had been delivered, before approaching the tray to eat. Oscillographic records showed that the animals either remained steadily within the band or were momentarily startled out of the band by the operation of the magazine, but re-entered it quickly. Because of the startle response, it was felt that a measure of the number of pellets earned as multiples without leaving the band would be too stringent a criterion to reflect adequately the phenomenon of multiple pellet earning. Consequently, the delivered pellet is considered a member of a multiple-pellet group as long as the response force does not go below the defined response threshold of 5 grams (see Table 1).

The first three motor performance measures could, theoretically, take on values approaching zero as a minimum and one as a maximum. *Pellets as multiples* must lie between zero and 100 inclusive.

Drug administration.   After steady baseline daily performance had been attained, four of the animals were given doses of *d*-amphetamine sulphate dissolved in saline. Drug doses or a saline placebo were administered subcutaneously 45 minutes before an animal's session. At least two non-injection sessions separated each drug or saline session. Saline and four dose levels of *d*-amphetamine were given, each three times (0.125, 0.25, 0.5, and 1.0 mg/kg *d*-amphetamine sulphate). Saline and the first three drug dosage levels given to rats I-96, I-99, and I-100 in random order. This was followed by completion of the dose-effect curve for the highest dosage level (1.0 mg/kg). Rat I-101 received all treatments in random order.

Following the above, two of these animals (I-100, I-101) were used to study the effects of chlorpromazine hydrochloride and *d*-amphetamine-chlorpromazine antagonism. Chlorpromazine dosages were 1.0, 2.0, and 4.0 mg/kg given 45 minutes before the session. The *d*-amphetamine-chlorpromazine combinations were administered in two injections 45 minutes before the session. In the combination, the *d*-amphetamine dosage was always 1.0 mg/kg and the chlorpromazine was either 1.0 or 2.0 mg/kg. All doses, both chlorpromazine alone and the combination, were administered in random order except the 4.0 mg/kg chlorpromazine doses. These were administered last. All drug dosages and placebo treatments were repeated either two or three times. As before, at least two non-injection sessions separated each drug or saline session. A third animal (I-103) was given only chlorpromazine at 1.0 and 2.0 mg/kg dosages in the order 1.0, 2.0, 1.0, and 2.0 mg/kg.

All five animals were given 4.0, 8.0, and 16.0 mg/kg pentobarbital sodium 45 minutes before the session. Dosages were administered in random order and given twice. Again, at least two non-injection sessions separated each drug or saline session.

Prefeeding control. Two animals (I-96, I-99) were given food (Purina Mouse Breeder Chow) 45 minutes before certain sessions. Both animals received 2.25, 4.50, and 9.0 grams of food in an ascending order. At least two normal control sessions intervened between each food treatment.

RESULTS

The results are presented as means of baseline performances (± standard error) and drug dosages for each animal. The baseline was taken as the mean of all the sessions just prior to each drug session, as well as

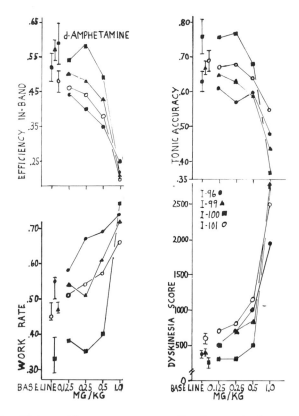

FIGURE 1. Motor performance measures for four animals as a function of *d*-amphetamine dosage.

the saline treatments, within a particular dose-effect relation. Saline administration revealed no effects different from the pre-drug sessions. For work rate, however, medians (with baseline interquartile range) are presented, since occasional long pauses with the highest dosage of *d*-amphetamine would have made the mean an unrepresentative measure of central tendency.

d-Amphetamine (see Figs. 1 and 2).   While absolute sensitivity to the effects of *d*-amphetamine varied among the animals, all showed a clear impairment of performance at 0.5 mg/kg with respect to efficiency in-band and dyskinesia score. At 1.0 mg, tonic accuracy, as well as the other measures, was severely affected in all animals. Work rate increased as a function of dosage level, although I-100 was rather resistant to this effect at doses below 1.0 mg/kg. With the decrease in fine motor control, those animals which earned pellets as multiples also began earning more pellets as singles as a function of dosage. The decreasing motor efficiency was also reflected in a progressive shortening of mean in-band time as a function of dosage. There was no evidence of anorexia. Food pellets were consumed with alacrity at all dosage levels.

Chlorpromazine (see Fig. 3).   The effects of chlorpromazine varied with different animals. Even the 2.0 mg/kg dose did not produce the adverse effects on performance that 1.0 mg/kg *d*-amphetamine did. In two of the three animals, all the measures were adversely affected by chlorpromazine, except pellets as multiples. Rat I-103 was not greatly affected by doses of chlorpromazine up to 2.0 mg/kg, except on the pellets as multiples and

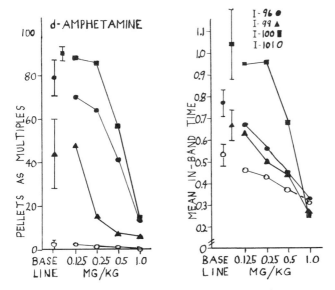

FIGURE 2. Motor performance measures for four animals as a function of *d*-amphetamine dosage.

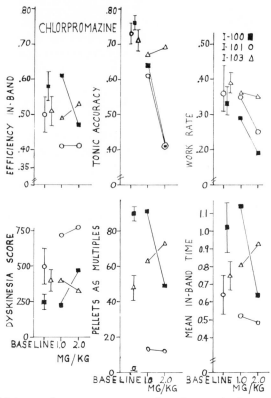

FIGURE 3. Motor performance measures for three animals as a function of chlorpromazine dosage.

mean in-band time measures. No results for 4.0 mg/kg are shown, since at this dose little behavior occurred, and protracted pauses of more than 2 hours' duration resulted.

Certain features of the chlorpromazine results should be noted. While tonic accuracy was severely decreased for rats I-100 and I-101, pellets as multiples decreased at 2.0 mg/kg for the animal with the high baseline level (I-100), whereas for I-101 this measure increased markedly over a baseline level close to zero under both 1.0 and 2.0 mg/kg dosage levels. A similar increase occurred for rat I-103, and was also noticeable in the mean in-band time at 2.0 mg/kg.

d-Amphetamine-chlorpromazine antagonism. Figure 4 shows the non-drug baseline, the effects of 1.0 mg/kg *d*-amphetamine alone, and 1.0 mg/kg *d*-amphetamine combined with 1.0 and 2.0 mg/kg chlorpromazine. Increasing the chlorpromazine dose had salutary effects on efficiency in-band, dyskinesia score, work rate, and mean in-band time. The deficits in tonic accuracy produced by 1.0 mg/kg *d*-amphetamine, however, seemed

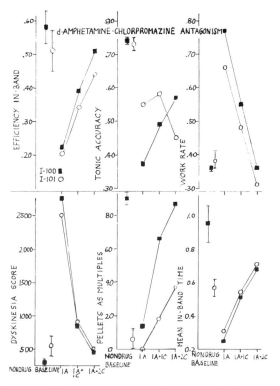

FIGURE 4. Motor performance measures for two animals as a function of combined *d*-amphetamine-chlorpromazine dose. 1A = 1.0 mg/kg *d*-amphetamine; 1C = 1.0 mg/kg chlorpromazine.

less successfully antagonized by chlorpromazine, perhaps owing to the impairment of tonic accuracy produced when chlorpromazine was given alone (cf. Fig. 3). The measure of pellets as multiples presents an interesting case. The performance of I-100 on this measure was severely impaired by both 1.0 mg/kg *d*-amphetamine and 2.0 mg/kg chlorpromazine when these were given alone, but when they were given in combination the behavior was brought back up to the baseline performance. For rat I-101, which had a low baseline level, the largest drug combination elicited a performance not only in excess of the baseline, but over twice as great as that produced by 2.0 mg/kg chlorpromazine alone.

Pentobarbital (see Fig. 5). The effects of pentobarbital at the highest dose level (16 mg/kg) were not as severe as those of 1.0 mg/kg *d*-amphetamine on either efficiency in-band or dyskinesia score. The effect on tonic accuracy was about the same at the high dosage end for both drugs. The work rate effects were opposite. In general, all measures showed a deterioration in performance as a function of dosage. At 4.0 mg/kg, most of the

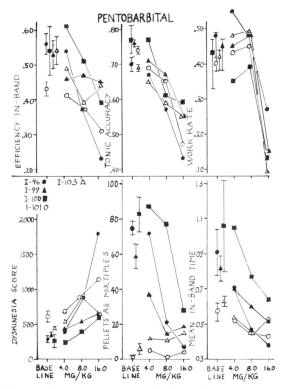

FIGURE 5.   Motor performance measures for five animals as a function of pento-barbital dosage.

animals' tonic accuracies were affected, but the other measures revealed little. The 8.0 mg/kg dose affected all measures except the work rate. At 16.0 mg/kg, the low work rate made it impractical to explore higher doses. At this dosage, considerable postural ataxia was evident.

PREFEEDING CONTROL.   None of the measures were affected by the prefeeding control procedures at either 2.25 or 4.50 grams. At 9.0 grams, protracted pauses occurred which lengthened session time to as much as 1.5 hours. This, of course, led to a lowered work rate, but all other measures remained unaffected.

DISCUSSION

The present research attempted to apply a direct approach to the measurement of motor steadiness under specific conditions of load and force-band width. The goal was to go beyond ataxia scores, righting reflex descriptions, and locomotory activity measures in evaluating the motor effects of drugs. It is important to note that there is no *a priori* reason to believe that attaching an accelerometer to the paw of a restrained or anesthetized animal would yield results similar to those of the present study. Training to the point of steady-state baseline behavior on a quantified task is a necessity if one wishes to evaluate the operant aspects of motor control as opposed to resting or postural effects which may or may not have consequences with respect to skilled movement.

d-Amphetamine. While amphetamines are known to increase general activity, tremor is not usually noted until toxic dosage levels. However, a recent report outlined four cases of dystonic or choreoathetoid movements induced by small doses of *d*-amphetamine given in the normal course of treatment (Mattson and Calverley, 1968). Grossly observable dyskinesia is not seen in animals until a dosage level of 5–20 mg/kg is administered (Randrup and Mundvak, 1967). Using high doses (4, 8, and 16 mg/kg) of *d*-amphetamine in mice, Watzman and Barry (1968) found improved rotarod balancing performances at all three dose levels. Perhaps animals are aided by amphetamines when the behavior requirement is one of rapid postural movement, whereas the present task required dynamic steadiness. Using dogs, Weiss and Laties (1964) found that in a task requiring continuous pressure with the nose on a microswitch, amphetamine (0.25–1.0 mg/kg) produced a higher frequency of closures (less holding) and particularly more responses lasting less than one second. This is congruent with the present findings.

Chlorpromazine. Chlorpromazine was found to impair rotarod performance, but the range of doses used was higher than in the present experiment, 4, 8, and 16 mg/kg (Watzman and Barry, 1968). Weiss and Laties (1964) found no change in their microswitch holding task over a chlorpromazine dose range (0.5–2.0 mg/kg) similar to the present one. However, Blough (1958) found that 5 and 10 mg/kg chlorpromazine improved an operant performance in pigeons which required them to stand still with their heads in one position. This effect is perhaps related to the improvement seen in the pellets-as-multiples measure when the baseline performance was in the low or middle range of possible values. The general picture of the present chlorpromazine results, however, was not one of improved performance. The markedly lower tonic accuracy measure in two of the three animals indicates that a good deal of the holding was outside the force band. The unimpressive efficiency in-band and dyskinesia measures indicate that overall in-band performance was less steady than under the non-drug condition.

d-Amphetamine-chlorpromazine antagonism. A considerable amount of research has accumulated on the *d*-amphetamine-chlorpromazine antagonism relation. Lasagna and McCann (1957) showed that chlorpromazine antagonized amphetamine toxicity in aggregated mice. Clinically, Espelin and Done (1968) have found that chlorpromazine doses of approximately 1–2 mg/kg quite successfully antagonized amphetamine poisoning. Using rats trained on a fixed-ratio-10 schedule for food, Brown (1963) found that 2.5 mg/kg d-amphetamine suppressed responding for at least an hour and that a 1.5 mg/kg dose of chlorpromazine given concomitantly produced maximal antagonism of this effect. Similar results have been obtained in the pigeon (Davis, 1965). The present findings indicate that while chlorpromazine antagonized the effects of d-amphetamine with respect to most of the measures used, its specific effects were probably instrumental in preventing a complete titration back to baseline performance.

Pentobarbital. Working within the dose range of the present experiment, Waller and Morse (1963) found that low doses of pentobarbital increased response rates in pigeons working on a fixed-ratio food schedule, while higher doses decreased the rate. There is the suggestion of a similar effect in two of the five animals at 4.0 mg/kg. The general picture of decreasing competence with increasing dosage contrasts with findings on the rotarod test indicating improved performance at 20 and 40 mg/kg and decreased performance at 80 mg/kg pentobarbital (Watzman and Barry, 1968). Again, these two approaches to motor coordination probably measure rather different processes. Weiss and Laties (1964) found a progressive increase in response rate in their microswitch holding task from 4.0 through 16.0 mg/kg pentobarbital. They found that the proportion of responses less than one second in duration at 16.0 mg/kg was quite similar to the value for 1.0 mg/kg d-amphetamine. The present results indicate rather more performance impairment at these dosages for d-amphetamine than in the case of pentobarbital (cf. the dyskinesia scores).

PREFEEDING CONTROL. When prefeeding food doses were increased to the point of producing sharp decrements in work rate, other measures remained unaffected. The prefeeding results do not mimic the effects of any of the drugs used. It may be inferred, then, that the drug effects noted were not attributable to anorexia or a loss of control of food over the operant.

SUMMARY

A behavioral method was used to study fine motor control in rats. Trained, unrestrained animals responding in a relatively unstressful, free-operant situation were required to hold a force-transducer lever within the limits of a 15–20-gram force band continuously for 1.5 seconds for each food pellet. Dose-effect relationships were explored with this behavior for d-amphetamine, chlorpromazine, pentobarbital, and d-amphetamine-chlorpromazine antagonism.

REFERENCES

Blough, D. S. New test for tranquilizers. *Science,* 1958, **127**, 586–587.

Brown, H. *d*-Amphetamine-chlorpromazine antagonism in a food reinforced operant. *J. exp. Anal. Behav.,* 1963, **6**, 395–398.

Carpenter, M. B., Whittier, J. R., and Mettler, F. A. Tremor in the rhesus monkey produced by diencephalic lesions and studied by a graphic method. *J. comp. Neurol.,* 1950, **93**, 1–12.

Carrie, J. R. G. Visual effects on finger tremor in normal subjects and anxious patients. *Brit. J. Psychiat.,* 1965, **111**, 1181–1184.

Clark, R., Jackson, J. A., and Brady, J. V. Drug effects on lever positioning behavior. *Science,* 1962, **135**, 1132–1133.

Connor, J. D., Rossi, G. V., and Baker, W. W. Characteristics of tremor in cats following injections of carbachol into the caudate nucleus. *Exp. Neurol.,* 1966, **14**, 371–382.

Davis, J. L. Antagonism of a behavioral effect of *d*-amphetamine by chlorpromazine in the pigeon. *J. exp. Anal. Behav.,* 1965, **8**, 325–327.

Dill, R. E., Dorman, H. L., and Nickey, W. M. A simple method for recording tremors in small animals. *J. appl. Physiol.* 1968, **24**, 598–599.

Espelin, D. E., and Done, A. K. Amphetamine poisoning: Effectiveness of chlorpromazine. *New England J. Med.,* 1968, **278**, 1361–1365.

Falk, J. L., and Haas, W. O., III. The control and recording of response force. *J. exp. Anal. Behav.,* 1965, **8**, 195–197.

Ferster, C. B., and Skinner, B. F. *Schedules of reinforcement.* New York: Appleton-Century-Crofts, 1957.

George, R., Haslett, W. L., and Jenden, D. J. The production of tremor by cholinergic drugs: Central sites of action. *Int. J. Neuropharmac.,* 1966, **5**, 27–34.

Growdon, J. H., Chambers, W. W., and Liu, C. N. An experimental study of cerebellar dyskinesia in the rhesus monkey. *Brain,* 1967, **90**, 603–632.

Lasagna, L., and McCann, W. P. Effect of "tranquilizing" drugs on amphetamine toxicity in aggregated mice. *Science,* 1957, **125**, 1241–1242.

Malis, J. L., and Curran, C. S. A reliable, low-cost generator for audio stimuli. *J. exp. Anal. Behav.,* 1960, **3**, 200.

Mattson, R. H., and Calverley, J. R. Dextroamphetamine-sulphate-induced dyskinesias. *J. Amer. Med. Assn.,* 1968, **204**, 400–402.

Notterman, J. M., and Mintz, D. E. Exteroceptive cueing of response force. *Science,* 1962, **135**, 1070–1071.

Randrup, A., and Mundvak, I. Stereotyped activities produced by amphetamine in several animal species and man. *Psychopharmacologia,* 1967, **11**, 300–310.

Vernier, V. G., and Unna, K. R. The central nervous system effects of drugs in monkeys with surgically-induced tremor: Atropine and other antitremor agents. *Archives Internationales de Pharmacodynamie et de Thérapie,* 1963, **141**, 30–53.

Wachs, H. Studies of physiologic tremor in the dog. *Neurology,* 1964, **14**, 50–61.

Waller, M. B., and Morse, W. H. Effects of pentobarbital on fixed-ratio reinforcement. *J. exp. Anal. Behav.,* 1963, **6**, 125–130.

Watzman, N., and Barry, H. III. Drug effects on motor coordination. *Psychopharmacologia,* 1968, **12**, 414–423.

Webster, D. D. Dynamic measurement of rigidity, strength, and tremor in Parkinson patients before and after destruction of mesial globus pallidus. *Neurology,* 1960, 10, 157–163.

Weiss, B., and Laties, V. G. Effects of amphetamine, chlorpromazine, pentobarbital, and ethanol on operant response duration. *J. Pharmacol. exp. Therap.,* 1964, **144,** 17–23.

24

The differential effects of chlorpromazine and
pentobarbital on two forms of conditioned avoidance
behavior in *Peromyscus maniculatus gracilis* *

HAROLD H. WOLF, EWART A. SWINYARD, and
LINCOLN D. CLARK

There are numerous studies in the literature on the rate of acquisition
and extinction of conditioned avoidance responses in laboratory animals
(Osgood, 1953; Woodworth and Schlosberg, 1954; Hilgard and Marquis,
1961) and on the relative effectiveness of drugs in altering such responses
(Miller *et al.,* 1957; Ader and Clink, 1957; Cook and Weidley, 1957;
Denenberg *et al.,* 1959; and others). Most of these studies are based on a
conditioned response which is not part of the experimental animal's usual
behavior repertoire. Indeed, we are not aware of any studies which compare
a conditional avoidance response analogous to that which the animal
habitually employs with a conditioned response based on behavior not
usually exhibited by the animal. Therefore, it was thought important to
compare these two forms of conditioned avoidance behavior and to study
the differential effects of drugs upon them.

Peromyscus maniculatus gracilis is a subspecies of deermouse that spends
part of its life on the trunks and branches of trees and shrubs. Several
studies have shown that it is well-adapted to a semi-arboreal habitat (Horner,
1954; King, 1958; King and Shea, 1959). Therefore, it is not unreasonable
to assume that this animal may seek an arboreal means of escape when
threatened by predators. In order to test this assumption, a series of experiments was designed to compare the acquisition and extinction of, as well
as the acute effects of chlorpromazine and pentobarbital on, two types of
conditioned responses elicited in this animal: (1) avoidance of shock by
climbing a vertical pole (arboreal response), and (2) avoidance of shock
by sitting on a non-electrified pan located at grid level (terrestrial response). It was hypothesized that, in this subspecies, the phenotypically
predisposed conditioned arboreal response would be more readily acquired,
less readily extinguished, and less susceptible to drug effects than would be

From *Psychopharmacologia* (Berl.), 1962, 3, 438–448. Copyright 1962 by Springer-
Verlag, Heidelberg, Germany.

    * Supported by a research grant from the National Institute of Neurological Dis-
eases and Blindness (B-381), National Institutes of Health, U.S. Public Health
Service.

the conditioned terrestrial response. The results obtained provide the basis for this report.

METHODS.   The experimental subjects were 48 adult male and female mice of the subspecies *Peromyscus maniculatus gracilis*. All animals were allowed free access to food (Rockland Rat Diet supplemented with wheat) and water except during actual test procedures. The animals were randomly divided into two experimental groups of 24 animals each (12 males and 12 females). One group, hereafter referred to as Group A, was trained to exhibit a terrestrial conditioned avoidance response, which consisted of finding and remaining on a "safe area" pan, whereas the other group, hereafter referred to as Group B, was trained to exhibit an arboreal conditioned avoidance response, which consisted of finding and climbing a vertical pole.

The apparatus employed to evaluate the terrestrial (pan) response consisted of a shuttle box (71.1 × 10.2 × 20.3 cm high) with a starting section at one end and a "safe area" pan close to the opposite end. The shuttle box, made of clear Plexiglas, was closed at the top in order to retain the animal in the apparatus and had a stainless steel grid floor through which an electric shock (60-cycle alternating current; 25 volts, delivered through a grid scrambler) could be applied to the feet of the mouse. An electric buzzer was placed beneath the grid floor and served as the source for the conditioned stimulus. The onset of both buzzer and shock was manually controlled. This same apparatus was used to evaluate the arboreal (pole) response except that the pan area was blocked off with an opaque gate, and an aluminium pole (1.27 cm diameter; grooved at 1.27 cm intervals) was suspended from the cover of the box to 2.54 cm above the grid floor. This pole, located 45.72 cm from the starting section, offered the only route of escape from the electrified grid floor.

The mice were trained to respond to the buzzer and thus avoid shock (unconditioned stimulus) by finding and remaining on either the pan or the pole for a period of at least 5 sec. In both response situations, the following conditioning scheme was employed: a mouse was placed in the starting area and an electric timer started. At the end of 5 sec, the door separating the starting area from the rest of the shuttle box was elevated, and the mouse was given 5 sec of exposure to the environment. Following this, the buzzer was activated for 15 sec. If an avoidance response was not made within this interval, the buzzer remained on and an electric shock was applied to the feet of the animal through the grid floor until the animal made the appropriate response or until 35 sec had elapsed. Thus, one training trial consisted of 5 sec in the start box, 5 sec exposure to the environment, 15 sec of buzzer, and up to 35 sec of buzzer and shock. Each animal received 8 such trials per day at the rate of 4 trials per 5 min.

To determine the rate of acquisition of the two avoidance responses, both experimental groups were subjected to 48 conditioning trials (8 per day for 6 days). All animals were required to exhibit more than one avoidance response in 8 trials and at least 6 consecutive avoidance responses in 32 trials. Two animals failed to meet these criteria and were dropped from the study. Two other animals died during the course of the study. Thus, the total population of the sample was reduced to 44.

The total number of conditioned responses which occurred during the 48 conditioning trials was recorded and the results obtained were analyzed for avoidance, sex, and avoidance-sex interaction with a 2×2 factorial analysis of variance.

To determine rate of extinction of the two avoidance responses, 12 mice from each of the two experimental groups (Group A and Group B) were randomly chosen from animals which exhibited at least 6 consecutive avoidance responses in their last 8 trials. To ensure that both experimental groups started the study at the same conditioning level, all mice were conditioned to a criterion of 8 consecutive avoidance responses (100%). Extinction trials were begun on the day after an animal demonstrated that it had reached requisite conditioning criterion.

The procedure during extinction was similar to that during conditioning except that the shock was eliminated. The animals were given extinction trials over a 15-day period, in blocks of 8 per day; the first 3 blocks of trials were conducted daily, whereas 48 hours was allowed to elapse between the remaining blocks. The measure recorded during extinction was the number of responses to the buzzer. In order to determine if true differences existed in the extinction rates of Group A and Group B, the results obtained were analyzed by means of a group comparison "t" test.

In the drug studies, chlorpromazine and pentobarbital were administered intraperitoneally in aqueous solution in such concentration that 1.0 ml/100 g body weight of the solution contained the appropriate dose. All tests were conducted at the time of peak effect for each drug. The time of peak effect was determined as follows: at 15, 30, 60, 90, and 120 min after drug administration, all animals were examined for loss of righting reflex, loss of placing reflex, abnormal body posture, ataxia, and ability to maintain equilibrium for 1 min on a horizontal plastic rod rotating at 6 revolutions per minute. The time of greatest neurological deficit as indicated by these tests was taken as the time of peak drug effect. The dose of each drug which produced overt evidence of minimal neurotoxicity in 50% of mice (TD50) was calculated by the method of Litchfield and Wilcoxon (1949). The time of peak effect and TD50 were found to be 60 min and 16.0 mg/kg, respectively, for chlorpromazine, and 10 min and 14.6 mg/kg, respectively, for pentobarbital.

It was observed during the acquisition studies that many of the mice were readily trained to a point where they exhibited an appropriate conditioned avoidance response before the presentation of the conditioned stimulus, *i.e.,* they developed a secondary conditioned response (Maffii, 1959) induced by the experimental environment. It was also observed that this response underwent extinction more rapidly than did the response to the buzzer. To take advantage of these differential levels of conditioning, and as an aid in evaluating the effects of the two drugs, a scoring system was devised which arbitrarily rated each animal's behavior as follows: a mouse exhibiting a secondary conditioned response (to 5 sec of environment) was assigned 4 points; one exhibiting a conditioned response (to 5 sec of environment and up to 15 sec of buzzer) was assigned 3 points; one exhibiting an unconditioned response (to 5 sec of environment, 15 sec of buzzer, and up to 35 sec of shock associated with the buzzer) was assigned 2 points; and non-responders were assigned 1 point.

For the determination of the behavioral effects of chlorpromazine, the 24 animals used in the extinction study cited above were reconditioned to a criterion of 6 consecutive conditioned responses in 8 trials and the two experimental groups (Group A and Group B) were each randomly divided into two treatment groups: 6 chlorpromazine-treated animals and 6 saline-treated animals (controls). Each drug-treated group was given 2.0 mg/kg (⅛ TD50) chlorpromazine and each control group was given the requisite volume of 0.9% saline solution. At the time of peak drug activity, all mice were subjected to 4 conditioned avoidance trials, the response was noted, and the behavior was rated according to the scale described above. In this manner, a fully-conditioned, saline-treated mouse would score 16 points for a block of 4 trials. Forty-eight hours later, all animals in both experimental groups were again reconditioned to criterion. The treatment assignments were then reversed, *i.e.,* the animals previously given chlorpromazine were given 0.9% saline solution and those previously serving as controls were given 2.0 mg/kg chlorpromazine. Thus, each mouse served as its own control. This entire experimental procedure was repeated three additional times, with the following drugs and doses: 4.0 mg/kg (¼ TD50) chlorpromazine, 7.3 mg/kg (½ TD50) pentobarbital, and 14.6 mg/kg (TD50) pentobarbital in the drug-treated group, and the requisite volume of 0.9% saline solution in the control group.

The data concerned with the behavioral effect of drug vs. saline were statistically analyzed by the Wilcoxon Matched-Pairs Signed-Ranks Test (Siegal, 1956), whereas the data dealing with the differential effects of drug on arboreal vs. terrestrial types of avoidance were statistically analyzed by the Mann-Whitney U Test (Siegal, 1956).

RESULTS.   The acquistion of the two avoidance responses, as a function of time and trials, is shown in Fig. 1. As can be seen in the figure, the *total* population of pole-escape animals (Group B) exhibited a higher level of conditioning throughout the experiment than did the *total* population of pan-escape animals (Group A). At the end of 48 trials, both experimental groups apparently reached a plateau, at which time Group B performed at

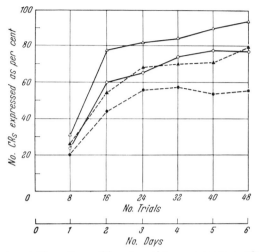

FIGURE 1. Acquisition of conditioned avoidance responses (CRs) in *Peromyscus maniculatus gracilis*. Black circles: total population of pan-trained Animals (Group A); white circles: total population of pole-trained animals (Group B); black triangles: selected population from Group A; white triangles: selected population from Group B.

a level of 78% conditioned responses and Group A performed at a level of 56% conditioned responses.

For comparative purposes, the acquisition cuves of the 24 animals later used in the extinction study (*selected* population) are also included in Fig. 1. The curves for the *selected* population were qualitatively similar to those representing the *total* population, but a higher level of conditioning existed in the former. Thus, at the end of 48 trials, the *selected* populations of Group B and Group A animals exhibited the appropriate conditioned responses 94% and 80% of the time, respectively.

Over-all analyses of variance revealed that the total number of conditioned responses achieved by the two experimental groups (Group A vs. Group B) differed significantly ($P<.01$) for the *selected* as well as the *total* population. The sex of the animal had only a negligible effect on the results; likewise, the interaction of sex and type of avoidance was also insignificant.

The results of the extinction study are illustrated in Fig. 2 from which it can be seen that the rate of extinction was essentially the same in both groups subjected to daily trials for 3 days. However, a difference in the extinction rates appeared by day 5, when the interval between trials was extended to 48 hours, and reached a maximum by day 15. Thus, at the end of 24 extinction trials, the mean level of conditioned responses was 91% for Group B and 93% for Group A, whereas, after 32 extinction trials, the mean level of conditioned responses for Group B was 93% and the corresponding value for Group A was 85%. This divergence continued until, at

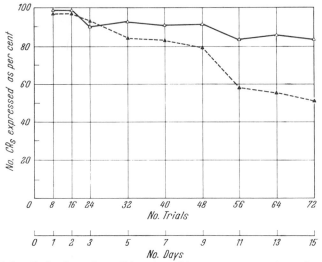

FIGURE 2. Extinction of conditioned avoidance responses (CRs) in *Peromyscus maniculatus gracilis*. Black triangles: pan-trained animals (Group A); white triangles: pole-trained animals (Group B).

the end of 72 trials, Group B exhibited conditioned responses 84% of the time, whereas Group A displayed conditioned responses only slightly more than half the time (52%). A statistical comparison of the last 48 extinction trials revealed that Group A had undergone significantly more extinction than had Group B ($P<.05$).

The effect of chlorpromazine and pentobarbital on the two conditioned avoidance responses is illustrated in the Table. The numbers in the second and third columns represent the per cent difference in the average scores of drug-treated vs. saline-treated (control) animals. The results of a statistical comparison of the magnitude of drug interference with avoidance by means of pan vs. pole are given in the last column.

It may be seen that chlorpromazine (2.0 mg/kg) significantly depressed the avoidance behavior of Group A (pan-escape mice) but had no significant effect on that of Group B (pole-escape mice). Moreover, the extent to which this dose of chlorpromazine interfered with avoidance behavior was significantly greater in pan-trained animals than in pole-trained animals (Δ_1 vs. Δ_2; $P<.025$).

A 4.0 mg/kg dose of chlorpromazine significantly reduced both the pan and the pole response. However, the magnitude of this reduction was still significantly greater for Group A than it was for Group B (Δ_1 vs. Δ_2; $P<.025$).

The effect of pentobarbital in doses of 7.3 mg/kg and 14.6 mg/kg is also recorded in the Table. At both dose levels the drug had a negligible effect ($P>.05$) on the phenotypically predisposed means of avoidance (pole response; Group B). On the other hand, the avoidance behavior in Group A

TABLE. The effect of chlorpromazine and pentobarbital on two types of conditioned avoidance behavior in *Peromyscus maniculatus gracilis*.

Treatment	Avoidance behavior		Δ_1 vs. Δ_2
	Group A Δ_1**	Group B Δ_2	
Chlorpromazine			
2.0 mg/kg ($\frac{1}{8}$ TD 50)	− 13.5*	− 3.9	$P < 0.05$
4.0 mg/kg ($\frac{1}{4}$ TD 50)	− 20.4*	− 11.4*	$P < 0.025$
Pentobarbital			
7.3 mg/kg ($\frac{1}{2}$ TD 50)	− 8.7	+ 1.2	$P < 0.025$
14.6 mg/kg (TD 50)	− 19.4*	+ 1.8	$P < 0.001$

Group A — Animals conditioned to a terrestrial means of avoidance (pan-trained).

Group B — Animals conditioned to an arboreal means of avoidance (pole-trained).

* Significant drug effect: $P < .01$.

** Δ = The per cent difference in the average scores of drug-treated vs. saline-treated (control) animals.

was considerably more susceptible to the effects of pentobarbital in that the smaller dose tended to depress the response and the larger dose significantly depressed it. Moreover, at both dose levels, the magnitude of drug interference with avoidance behavior (Δ_1 vs. Δ_2) was significantly greater in Group A than in Group B.

The results obtained reveal several quantitative differences between the two types of conditioned avoidance behaviors which were examined. For example, at the end of an equivalent amount of training (48 trials), the *total* population of pole-escape mice (Group B) demonstrated a significantly higher level of conditioning than did the *total* population of pan-escape mice (Group A), 87% vs. 56% of the total possible conditioned responses, respectively. During these training trials it was often observed that several of the animals being conditioned to produce a terrestrial means of avoidance would repeatedly leap from the escape pan back onto the electrified grid. This observation is in agreement with that reported by King and Shea (1958), and such behavior may undoubtedly contribute to the comparatively low level of conditioning in the *total* population of Group A. However, a similar difference in level of avoidance conditioning can also be seen when such animals are excluded from the study and an examination is made of the acquisition curves which represent only the best responders in each experimental group (*selected* population). In this situation the difference between the two groups was not as marked, but Group B still made significantly more conditioned responses than Group A. Consequently, it is apparent that, in this subspecies, conditioned avoidance behavior is more readily acquired when a technic is employed which takes into consideration the natural escape pattern of the experimental animal.

A second difference between the two conditioned avoidance behaviors is the rate at which they underwent extinction. As shown by the results (Fig. 2), the avoidance behavior of Group B was considerably more resistant to extinction than was that of Group A. Although both experimental groups started the study at the same level of conditioning (100% conditioned responses), at its termination the pole-trained (Group B) animals were exhibiting 32% more conditioned responses than were the pan-trained (Group A) animals. Therefore, with respect to extinction, the phenotypically predisposed behavior is the more stable of the two conditioned avoidance behaviors investigated.

It was considered possible that the rates of acquisition and extinction in the two groups of mice might be affected by intrinsic properties of the experimental environment. In other words, there might be a difference in the relative strength of the perceptual and motor cues. Thus, if the pole-avoidance response was more strongly "cued" than the pan-avoidance response, one would expect the former to be more easily acquired and more resistant to extinction. The fact that laboratory mice (CF no. 1 strain) are readily trained to avoid shock by the pan technic but are hard to train to avoid shock by the pole technic suggests that the results obtained were not affected by the properties of the experimental environment and lends support to the concept that the observed differences in the rates of acquisition and extinction by the two groups of mice are due to genetic factors.

A third quantitative difference was the degree to which the behavior in each experimental group could be altered by chlorpromazine and pentobarbital. From the results obtained (Table), it is manifest that small, nontoxic doses of chlorpromazine can interfere with both types of avoidance response. It is also evident that, as the dose of chlorpromazine was increased, the drug produced a greater suppression of avoidance behavior in both groups of mice. These results are not unexpected and agree with many reports relative to the effects of chlorpromazine on conditioned avoidance behavior. It is interesting to note, however, that twice as much chlorpromazine (4.0 mg/kg) was required to depress significantly the avoidance behavior of Group B as was necessary to produce a similar effect on the behavior of Group A. Furthermore, at both the 2.0 mg/kg and 4.0 mg/kg dose levels, the magnitude of drug interference with avoidance behavior was significantly greater in Group A than in Group B. This provides additional evidence for the greater stability of avoidance behavior based on an innate response.

When a comparison is made between the effect of chlorpromazine and pentobarbital (Table) on the two avoidance behaviors, it is evident that the phenothiazine contrasts sharply with the barbiturate. Chlorpromazine effectively interferes with both pan- and pole-conditioned avoidance responses in non-toxic doses of ⅛ and ¼ TD50, respectively. In order to obtain similar effects with pentobarbital, a dose of the drug equivalent to the

TD50 is required to interfere with the pan-conditioned avoidance response (Group A), and a dose larger than the TD50 would be required to interfere with the pole-conditioned avoidance response (Group B). Since the TD50 of pentobarbital produces ataxia in many of the animals, it is clear that the avoidance behavior of the pole-trained animals persists even when motor coordination is slightly impaired. Furthermore, since non-toxic doses of pentobarbital had little effect on either conditioned avoidance response, it is obvious that pentobarbital is less selective than chlorpromazine on this type of behavior. This is in agreement with the observations of others (Cook and Weidley, 1957; Verhave *et al.*, 1958; Maffii, 1959).

It appears that the naturally-occurring arboreal escape response of *Peromyscus maniculatus gracilis* represents a phenomenon which can be easily replicated in the laboratory. The avoidance behavior which results from the conditioning of this response is more readily acquired, less readily extinguished, and less susceptible to the effects of CNS depressant drugs than is a conditioned avoidance behavior based on a response which is not a part of this animal's usual behavioral repertoire. Moreover, it would appear that pentobarbital can be distinguished from chlorpromazine by means of laboratory technics which employ this species of rodent.

SUMMARY.   A series of experiments was designed to compare the conditioned behavior of a subspecies of deermouse (*Peromyscus maniculatus gracilis*) in two response situations: (1) avoidance of shock by climbing a pole, and (2) avoidance of shock by remaining on a non-electrified pan located at grid level. This subspecies is semi-arboreal in its natural habitat. As was expected, an experimentally-induced response analogous to those to which the animal is phenotypically predisposed is rapidly acquired and resistant to spontaneous extinction. Thus, the pole response was acquired more rapidly, was more resistant to extinction, and was less susceptible to suppression by drugs. The stability of such behavior makes mice exhibiting this type of response advantageous for testing the effects of psychotropic drugs. The fact that chlorpromazine may be differentiated from pentobarbital by means of these technics supports this conclusion.

REFERENCES

Ader, R., and Clink, D. W.: Effects of chlorpromazine on the acquisition and extinction of an avoidance response in the rat. *J. Pharmacol. exp. Ther.* **121**, 144–148 (1957).

Cook, L., and Weidley, E.: Behavioral effects of some psychopharmacological agents. *Ann. N.Y. Acad. Sci.* **66**, 740–752 (1957).

Denenberg, V. H., Ross, S., and Ellsworth, J.: Effects of chlorpromazine on acquisition and extinction of a conditioned response in mice. *Psychopharmacologia* (Berl.) **1**, 59–64 (1959).

Hilgard, E. R., and Marquis, D. G.: *Conditioning and learning,* 2nd ed. New York: Appleton-Century-Crofts 1961.

Horner, B. E.: Arboreal adaptations of *Peromyscus,* with special reference to use of the tail. *Contr. Lab. Vert. Biol.,* Univ. of Mich. **61**, 1–85 (1954).

King, J. A.: Maternal behavior and behavioral development in two subspecies of *Peromyscus maniculatus. J. Mammal.* **39**, 177–190 (1958).

King, J. A., and Shea, N. J.: Behavioral development in two subspecies of *Peromyscus maniculatus. Anat. Rec.* **131**, 571–572 (1958).

King, J. A., and Shea, N. J.: Subspecific differences in the responses of young deermice on an elevated maze. *J. Hered.* **50**, 14–18 (1959).

Litchfield, J. T., Jr., and Wilcoxon, F.: A simplified method of evaluating dose-effect experiments. *J. Pharmacol. exp. Ther.* **96**, 99–113 (1949).

Maffii, G.: The secondary conditioned response of rats and the effects of some psychopharmacological agents. *J. Pharm. Pharmacol.* **11**, 129–139 (1959).

Miller, R. E., Murphy, J. V., and Mirsky, I. A.: The effect of chlorpromazine on fear-motivated behavior in rats. *J. Pharmacol. exp. Ther.* **120**, 379–387 (1957).

Osgood, C. E.: *Method and theory in experimental psychology.* New York: Oxford University Press 1953.

Siegal, S.: *Nonparametric statistics for the behavioral sciences.* New York: McGraw-Hill 1956.

Verhave, T., Owen, J. E., Jr., and Robbins, E. B.: Effects of chlorpromazine and secobarbital on avoidance and escape behavior. *Arch. int. Pharmacodyn.* **116**, 45–53 (1958).

Woodworth, R. S., and Schlosberg, H.: *Experimental psychology,* Rev. ed. New York: Holt & Co. 1954.

Section **E**   CONSEQUENCE VARIABLES: TYPES
                  AND PARAMETERS OF CONSEQUENCES

Operants are defined by the covariation of an aspect of behavior and some consequent event. Consequences which increase the probability of recurrence of the response are called *reinforcers,* whereas consequences which decrease response probability are called *punishers.* Reinforcing consequences can involve either presentation of some stimulus (i.e., a *positive reinforcer*) or removal of a stimulus (i.e., a *negative reinforcer*). Some reinforcers are effective on their first presentation (e.g., water) or removal (e.g., painful electric shock), while others require repeated presentation in close temporal proximity to another reinforcer to gain reinforcing properties. Stimuli effective as reinforcers without prior experience are called *unconditioned reinforcers,* while those which gain reinforcing properties through pairing with a known reinforcer are called *conditioned reinforcers.* Among the most important reinforcement variables controlling operant behaviors are the contingencies for reinforcement, i.e., the conditions under which responses will be reinforced. A formal statement of the contingencies for reinforcement is called a *reinforcement schedule.* Reinforcement schedules can be subdivided according to the numbers of responses and/or elapsed time intervals for reinforcement to be forthcoming. According to this classification, reinforcement schedules may be simple, compound, or complex. These further subdivisions will be discussed below.

It would seem obvious that the type of reinforcer maintaining an operant might influence the effect of a drug on behavior. Commonly used reinforcers, such as painful shock (Article 25), food and water (Article 26), brain stimulation (Article 27), sugar (Article 28), and heat (Article 29), all yield different behavioral baselines and interact differently with drugs. Less commonly, drugs themselves can serve as reinforcers. For example, it has been reported that histamine (Article 31) can serve as an unconditioned negative reinforcer. Cocaine (Article 30) and morphine (Articles 32 and 33) can serve as effective unconditioned positive reinforcers.

Perhaps the greatest differences in drug effects on behaviors maintained by different reinforcers would be expected in cases involving positive as opposed to negative reinforcement. This comparison has been of consistent interest since the beginning of drug-behavior research, but poses many complex problems. Two approaches to teasing apart these effects are represented in Articles 34 and 45 with food-reinforced and shock avoidance behaviors. These studies do not answer all of the questions involved in separating type-of-reinforcement effects from other variables, as we shall see below.

Not only the kind but the amount of reinforcement can significantly influence the behavioral action of a drug. The length of presentation of a pre-shock stimulus in an avoidance situation was found to alter the effect of chlorpromazine, whereas altering the intensity of the shock reinforcer had little effect (Article 36). Using hypothalamic brain stimulation as a reinforcer, other investigators found that the magnitude of electrical stimulation which would effectively serve as a positive reinforcer was raised following chlorpromazine administration (Article 37). By use of a similar technique, the value of a painful shock which was tolerated was changed following treatment with several drugs (Article 38).

As indicated above, consequences which suppress responding are called punishers, while those which increase responding are called reinforcers. While it may seem that shock presentation and removal have to do with the same "motivational state," it is clear that shock escape and avoidance and shock punishment do not have the same behavioral properties. Further, different chemical compounds have quite different effects on punished responding, though they generally fall within the family of sedative-tranquilizing drugs. For example, amobarbital diminishes the suppressing effect of punishing shock, but chlorpromazine has little or no effect on behavior suppressed in this way (Article 40). Punishment can involve manipulations other than pain-shock. For example, time-out from positive reinforcement also has properties of punishment (i.e., it suppresses antecedent behavior). Drugs differentially affect behavior suppressed by time-out from positive reinforcement, depending on parameters of the schedule and drug dosage (Article 39).

A less obvious behavioral mechanism of drug action involves alteration of the effectiveness of conditioned reinforcers. This line of research has received little attention, but is of potentially great importance in understanding the effect of drugs on complex behavior. The differential effects of drugs on stimulus-producing and food-producing responses were first reported using an "observing-response" technique (Article 41) and more recently using chained and tandem schedules (Article 42).

25

Augmentation of the behavioral effects of amphetamine by atropine [1]

PETER L. CARLTON and PAULINE DIDAMO

The experiments reported herein are a part of a series on the effects of parasympatholytic and sympathomimetic drugs on learned behavior. In particular, doses of atropine, ineffective in themselves, were studied in combination with amphetamine. In a series of subsidiary experiments methyl atropine was also studied in combination with amphetamine.

Tripod (1957) has reported that the increase in random, motor activity in mice produced by amphetamine was enhanced by the concurrent administration of atropine. The present study constitutes, in part, an extension of this finding to the learned, operant behavior of rats.

MATERIALS AND METHODS. *Subjects.* Five adult, male, albino rats were used. The animals had continuous access to food and water except during experimental sessions. Each rat had had extensive training in the avoidance schedule to be described and had been used in a study of the behavioral effects of atropine (Carlton, unpublished experiment). On the basis of this study it was possible to estimate, for each rat, the doses of atropine used throughout the present study.

Apparatus. The animals worked in a standard, sound-insulated response chamber which contained two lever-operated switches and a grid floor through which brief electric shocks could be delivered. The general features of this type of apparatus have been described elsewhere (Ferster and Skinner, 1957). A system of relays, timers, and counters automatically programmed the experiments and recorded depressions of the levers and the delivery of shocks. In addition, a Gerbrands cumulative recorder provided a continuous record of the animals' lever-pressing behavior.

Avoidance procedure. The shock-avoidance schedule used has been detailed previously (Sidman, 1953). The essential component of the schedule was a recycling timer set to deliver an inescapable shock of about 1.5 mA intensity and 0.25-second duration every 20 seconds. The circuit was arranged so that each depression of one of the levers in the response chamber reset the timer. After each reset, the timer started again and, in the absence

From *Journal of Pharmacology and Experimental Therapeutics,* 1961, 134, 91–96. Copyright © 1961 by The Williams and Wilkins Co., Baltimore, Md.

[1] The authors are indebted to Dr. B. N. Carver for his generous advice on the course of the experiments and the preparation of the manuscript.

of a subsequent response, delivered the shock at the end of 20 seconds. Thus, any 20-second period in which a lever depression did not occur terminated with delivery of shock, whereas each response reset the timer and thereby postponed the shock. An animal that depressed the lever at a rate no lower than 1 per 20 seconds never received a shock; one that never pressed the lever was shocked every 20 seconds. Each of the animals developed a stable response rate between these two extremes. Depression of the second lever in no way influenced the delivery of shock.

General procedure. Each animal underwent two experimental sessions per week. The experimental session began immediately after the animal had been placed in the response chamber. After 1 hour the animal was removed, given either saline or drug injections, and replaced in the apparatus for 5 hours or, in the case of one rat, for 1 hour. Each animal received one control and one drug session per week. A drug was not given more often than once a week.

The drugs, atropine sulfate, methyl atropine nitrate, and *d*-amphetamine sulfate, were dissolved in normal saline and so diluted that the required dose per kg was contained in 1 ml. In each session the rats were given two intraperitoneal injections no more than 1 minute apart. In the main experimental series the following pairs of doses were given: saline-saline (control), atropine-amphetamine, saline-amphetamine, and atropine-saline. For each animal the atropine dose was constant throughout the experiment, whereas two or three amphetamine dosages were used. The various drug combinations were given in an irregular order. All doses have been given in terms of the weight of the salts.

From one to four, in most cases two, determinations of the effects of each of the drug combinations were made for each animal; each rat received ten to fourteen saline-saline (control) sessions. Except as noted, all data are averages.

In a subsidiary experimental series three animals (two sessions each) were given injections of methyl atropine nitrate in combination with amphetamine at dose levels approximately equimolar to the atropine doses. In a subsequent series, two of the animals were given higher methyl atropine doses in combination with amphetamine.

RESULTS.   *Atropine effects.*   Atropine, with one exception, was uniformly ineffective in increasing the rate of avoidance responding and had, in fact, a slight tendency to depress responding. The single exception was one animal in which atropine, in the last two of four determinations, produced a moderate, transient increase in avoidance responding.

Atropine-amphetamine interactions.   Figure 1 shows a representative set of cumulative response records from single sessions for I-12, the one animal given 2-hour sessions. The recording pen was reset to the base line after each 20-minute period and after the accumulation of 500 responses. Only

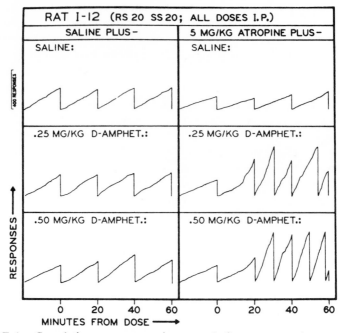

FIGURE 1.   Cumulative response *vs.* time records for one rat under control, atropine, and atropine plus amphetamine conditions. The recording pen reset to the baseline after each 20-minute period and after 500 responses had been cumulated. Only the last 20 minutes of each of the 1-hour pre-dose periods have been shown. The response scale is at the upper left; the slope of the response record is proportional to rate of response. The rat was given two injections in each session: the first dose was saline for the records in the left-hand column and atropine for those in the right. The second dose of each of the dose-pairs is given at the top of each record.

the last 20 minutes of the pre-dose period have been shown. The figure demonstrates (1) that neither saline plus saline nor atropine plus saline altered the rate of responding that had characterized the pre-dose period, (2) that saline plus 0.25 mg/kg amphetamine did not produce an effect, whereas 0.5 mg/kg amphetamine was followed by a slight increase in response rate, and (3) that atropine plus either dose of amphetamine produced marked increases in responding. Following atropine plus 0.5 mg/kg amphetamine, for example, the animal emitted over 1000 responses in the 40- to 60-minute post-dose period, whereas the maximum number emitted after the same dose of amphetamine without atropine was about 270. A lesser augmentation was apparent at the lower dose of amphetamine. These data were essenially replicated in subsequent sessions.

The data from the rats given 6-hour sessions indicated that atropine combined with amphetamine not only increased the maximum output of responses seen after amphetamine alone, but also that it markedly prolonged the period of increased responding.

Figure 2 shows the mean number of responses emitted in each of the successive 20-minute periods of the 5-hour post-dose periods for Rat I-22 following saline-amphetamine and atropine-amphetamine at three levels of amphetamine. The points plotted at 0 were taken from the last 20 minutes of the pre-dose period. With each of the three amphetamine doses, atropine increased, relative to the saline-amphetamine sessions, both the maximum number of responses recorded in any 20-minute period (the "peak" response output) and also the duration of the increase in responding.

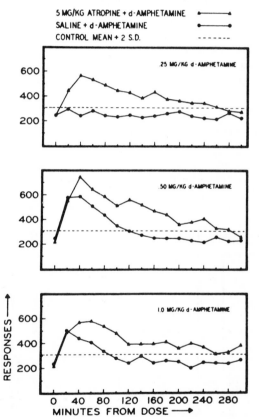

FIGURE 2. The mean number of responses in each 20-minute interval of the 5-hour post-dose period for one animal at three levels of amphetamine and atropine plus amphetamine. The legend is given at the top; amphetamine doses are given in each graph. The atropine dose was constant throughout the three dose combinations. The points plotted at 0 are from the last 20 minutes of the pre-dose period. The vertical dashed line in each graph was computed from the control data (see text) and estimates the maximum response value to be expected on the basis of random variations in these data. In each of the comparisons, the upper curve is a plot of the response values obtained after atropine plus amphetamine, whereas the lower curve is a plot of those obtained after saline plus an equivalent dose of amphetamine.

The horizontal line at about 300 responses in each graph of Fig. 2 equals the control mean plus 2 S.D. This animal underwent thirteen control (saline plus saline) sessions. The mean and S.D. computed from each of the fifteen 20-minute periods for all thirteen sessions (*i.e.,* 195 numbers entered into the computations) were 236 and 33.5, respectively. Thus, any response value for a 20-minute period greater than 303 (236 plus 67) could reasonably be attributed to the drugs and not to random variations in responding.

The duration of increased responding was arbitrarily defined as terminated at the first 20-minute period in which the number of responses was equal to or less than the control mean plus 2 S.D. Thus rat I-22 was assigned a duration value of 280 minutes for atropine plus 0.25 mg/kg amphetamine and one of 300 minutes for atropine plus 0.25 mg/kg amphetamine. Following saline plus 0.25 mg/kg amphetamine, on the other hand, no response value was greater than 303; accordingly, the assigned duration value was 0. Similarly, all duration values for the control data were by definition equal to 0.

It should be noted that the duration criterion tends to err in a conservative direction. In Fig. 2, for example, the rise in responses in the last 40 minutes of the session suggests that the assigned duration value of 260 minutes for atropine plus 1.0 mg/kg amphetamine may have underestimated the true duration.

In Fig. 3, the maximum number of responses (in any 20-minute interval) and the duration values, for each of the rats given 6-hour sessions, at

MAXIMUM RESPONSE AND DURATION EFFECTS

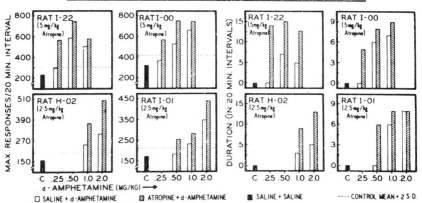

FIGURE 3. Maximum number of responses in any 20-minute interval and estimated durations of supernormal responding (see text) for four animals. The values on the abscissa are the various amphetamine doses (C denotes control); the atropine doses, which were constant for each rat, are given at the top of each graph. The legend is at the bottom of the figure. The vertical dashed line in each of the maximum response graphs is an estimate of the maximum response value to be expected on the basis of random variations in the control data (see text).

the various amphetamine and atropine plus amphetamine doses, were obtained from sets of data similar to the one shown in Fig. 2.

In virtually all instances both maximum response and duration values were greater for the atropine plus amphetamine doses than for the corresponding saline plus amphetamine doses. The exceptions to this generality were at the higher amphetamine doses at which there was a tendency for the saline plus amphetamine and the atropine plus amphetamine values to converge. This finding presumably reflects a maximum beyond which response output could not increase. A similar "ceiling effect" has been obtained with amphetamine in other studies of operant behavior (Carlton, unpublished data; Weissman, 1959).

The differences in the maximum response values afforded by saline plus amphetamine (S-A) and by atropine plus amphetamine (A-A) were statistically evaluated by (1) subtracting, for each dose of amphetamine, the S-A maximum response value from the corresponding A-A value for each rat and (2) taking the mean of these differences. Thus, each rat was given an average difference score. These differences, for all animals, were then evaluated by a t test under the hypothesis that the mean difference in the population equalled zero (Lewis, 1960). The resultant t value was 6.21 ($P < 0.01$, using a two-tailed test). An analogous t computed from the average differences in duration value was 3.27 ($P < 0.05$).

A third measure which can be used in describing response data of the type shown in Fig. 2 is the total number of responses made in the 5-hour post-dose period. These totals, for each rat at each dose combination, have been given in Table 1. Two features of the data in Table 1 deserve comment. First, with the exception of one animal, atropine-saline produced a

TABLE 1.   Average total post-dose responses (in thousands of responses).

Rat	First Injection	Second Injection					
		Saline	Amphetamine (mg/kg)				
			0.25	0.5	1.0	2.0
H-02	Saline	2.4 (0.24)*	—	—	2.4	3.1
	Atropine (2.5)†	2.1	—	—	3.7	4.9
I-00	Saline	4.9 (0.35)	5.2	5.5	6.3	—
	Atropine (5.0)	4.5	5.9	7.1	7.1	—
I-01	Saline	2.6 (0.22)	—	2.5	2.6	3.2
	Atropine (2.5)	1.9	—	3.0	3.0	3.6
I-22	Saline	3.5 (0.36)	3.7	4.9	4.4	—
	Atropine (5.0)	4.1	6.0	7.1	6.4	—

* S.D. of saline-saline (control) sessions.
† Atropine dose (in mg/kg) used in all determinations involving atropine.

slight decrease in response output. The increase noted for I-22 reflects the fact that atropine produced a moderate increase in responding in the last two of the four determinations. Second, it should be noted that the atropine-amphetamine values were, without exception, greater than the corresponding saline-amphetamine values.

Methyl atropine effects. The effects of methyl atropine or atropine, each in combination with amphetamine, are shown in Table 2. In the case of Rat H-02, 2.5 mg/kg of either atropine or methyl atropine produced an augmentation of the effects of 1.0 mg/kg amphetamine (the amphetamine-saline values from Table 1 have been entered for purposes of comparison); the augmentation produced by methyl atropine was, however, less than that produced by atropine. In Rat I-01 a slight augmentation was not observed until the dose of methyl atropine had been increased to 10.0 mg/kg and the amphetamine dose to 1.0 mg/kg.

The data for Rat I-22 are in essential agreement with those for the other animals; approximately equimolar doses of either atropine or methyl atropine augmented the effects of amphetamine. The augmentation observed with methyl atropine was, however, less than that observed with atropine. Further, after the dose of methyl atropine had been doubled, an augmentation greater than that produced by 5.0 mg/kg, but less than that produced by 5.0 mg/kg atropine, was recorded. This differential action was also reflected in the maximum response and duration values for each animal. In general, then, methyl atropine was found to augment the effects of amphetamine but in this action was consistently less potent than atropine.

TABLE 2.   Comparisons of methyl atropine or atropine in combination with amphetamine.

Rat	Second Injec- tion	First Injection (mg/kg)					
	Amphe- tamine (mg/ kg)	Saline	Methyl atropine			Atropine	
			2.5	5.0	10.0	2.5	5.0
H-02	1.00	2.4*	3.3	—	—	3.7	—
I-01	0.50	2.5	2.3	2.1	2.2	3.0	—
	1.00	2.6	—	—	2.8	3.0	—
I-22	0.25	3.7	—	3.8	4.1	—	6.0

* Thousands of responses.

DISCUSSION.   As previously noted, the avoidance responding of one animal when given atropine alone was moderately increased in the third and fourth of the series of determinations. Even if the data from only these sessions were to be used in estimating the effects of atropine, however, the marked increases in responding observed following atropine plus amphetamine would far exceed the sum of the effects of these two drugs given separately.

There are undoubtedly several hypotheses which could be offered to account for the augmentation of the effects of amphetamine by atropine; the data presented herein are not, however, sufficient to suggest which of the several might be correct. Nevertheless, the differential effects of atropine and methyl atropine do suggest that these two drugs interact on the central, rather than peripheral, nervous system.

Since (1) both drugs are potent parasympatholytics and (2) methyl atropine is *more* potent than atropine with respect to certain peripheral actions (inhibition of salivary secretion and of parasympathomimetic intestinal and cardiac responses (Graham and Lazarus, 1940; Bülbring and Dawes, 1945) it seems to us reasonable to suppose that the locus of the interaction was primarily central rather than peripheral. If the interaction had been primarily peripheral it would have been expected that methyl atropine would have been at least as potent as atropine in augmenting the effects of amphetamine.

If it is tentatively assumed that the effects of atropine combined with amphetamine reflect a central action, it would follow that methyl atropine, which produced a slight augmentation, could be shown to have central effects by some direct measure of central activity. Recent studies (Paul-David *et al.*, 1960; Horovitz, unpublished data) have indicated that this is indeed the case; in general, methyl atropine produced atropine-like slowing of the cortical EEG, but only at doses 4 to 5 times greater than the doses of atropine.

It may be, of course, that the data presented here are peculiar either to (a) behavioral situations involving shock-avoidance or (b) the particular drugs employed. These possibilities are rendered somewhat less likely by two considerations: (a) studies currently in progress indicate that the action of amphetamine in *depressing* one variety of *food*-rewarded behavior is accentuated by atropine; and (b) at least two other compounds (scopolamine and imipramine) have been found to augment the behavioral effects of amphetamine (Carlton, unpublished data). Studies on the interactions of various parasympatholytics with sympathomimetics other than amphetamine are indicated.

SUMMARY.   Amphetamine, intraperitoneally administered in doses from 0.25 to 2.0 mg/kg, increased the rate of lever-pressing of rats working in an operant, shock-avoidance situation. Doses of atropine, ineffective in themselves, markedly augmented the increases in rate observed after amphetamine as well as the duration of these increases. In a subsidiary series of experiments methyl atropine was found to be much less potent than atropine in augmenting the effects of amphetamine on responding.

REFERENCES

Bülbring, E., and Dawes, G. S.: *J. Pharmacol. exp. Ther.* **84**:177, 1945.

Ferster, C. B., and Skinner, B. F.: *Schedules of reinforcement,* Appleton-Century-Crofts, New York, 1957.

Graham, J. D., and Lazarus, S.: *J. Pharmacol. exp. Ther.* **70**:165, 1940.

Lewis, D.: *Quantitative methods in psychology,* McGraw-Hill, New York, 1960.

Paul-David, J., Riehl, J. L., and Unna, K. R.: *J. Pharmacol. exp. Ther.* **129**:69, 1960.

Sidman, M.: *Science* **118**:157, 1953.

Tripod, J.: *Int. Symposium on Psychotropic Drugs,* p. 437, Milan, 1957.

Weissman, A.: *J. exp. Anal. Behav.* **2**:271, 1959.

26

Effects of *d*-amphetamine on behavior reinforced by food and water [1]

ELIOT HEARST

The depressive effects of amphetamine on food and water intake are well-known (Harris, Ivy, and Searle, 1947; Andersson and Larsson, 1957). There are, however, some conflicting data as to the effects of this sympathomimetic drug on behavior which is maintained by food or water reward.

Wentink (1938) found that amphetamine increased the rate at which rats worked on a fixed-interval reward schedule for food, and Brady (1956) obtained a similar excitatory effect in *S*s responding on variable-interval schedules with superimposed "anxiety." Large increases in response output under amphetamine have also consistently been observed on schedules in which low rates of response are differentially rewarded (e.g., Sidman, 1956) and under extinction conditions where responding is no longer rewarded (Skinner and Heron, 1937; Miller, 1956). *S*s on shock-avoidance procedures, too, have uniformly shown increased response rates under amphetamine (Verhave, 1958; Teitelbaum and Derks, 1958). Citing some of the above studies, Epstein (1959) provisionally described the behavioral effects of amphetamine as "an increase in either learned or unlearned motor activity and a suppression of consummatory response."

A few recent papers have reported findings which do not justify such a general conclusion. For example, Miller (1956) reported reliable decreases in food-rewarded variable-interval performance after injection of amphetamine, as did Kelleher and Cook (1959) and Owen (1960) on fixed-ratio reward schedules.

In the present experiment rats were taught to make two different lever-responses to obtain food and water, respectively. Injections of *d*-amphetamine sulfate were then given over a range of dosages to observe the drug's general effects on lever-rsponding and to see if the drug had any differential effects on food-maintained and water-maintained behavior.

METHOD. *Subjects.* *S*s were six male Sprague-Dawley albino rats, approximately 3 mo. old at the start of experimentation. For several weeks

From *Psychological Reports,* 1961, 8, 301–309. Copyright 1961 by Southern Universities Press, Missoula, Mont.

[1] The help of Mrs. Yvonne Leacock in the running of the experiment and in the analysis of data is gratefully acknowledged.

prior to training the animals were accustomed to a food and water rhythm in which they were given access to Purina Chow pellets and ordinary tap water for only 1 hr. daily (12:30 to 1:30 PM), seven days per week.

Apparatus.   A commercially-produced (Foringer) experimental box was used, the details of which have been described elsewhere (Herrnstein and Brady, 1958). Two telegraph-key levers, adjusted for approximately equal force requirements, were mounted at opposite corners of the front panel of the box. Food reinforcements consisted of single Animal Feed pellets (P. J. Noyes Co., 4.8 mm. × 4.9 mm. × 97 mg.), delivered by means of an automatic feeder (Davis) to a food hopper near the left-hand lever (the "food lever"). Water rewards, 0.1 ml. available for 3 sec., were presented by means of a dipper located below and midway between the two levers. The right-hand lever ("water lever") was instrumental in the production of water reinforcements. Programming of food and water reinforcements, reward schedules, etc., was accomplished automatically through a system of timers and relays. Sodeco counters and two Gerbrands cumulative recorders provided records of performance on each lever.

Procedure.   Animals were first trained to approach the food hopper for pellets whenever the feeder mechanism was operated and to drink from the water dipper. Ss were next given lever-pressing training, during which presses on the food lever produced food pellets and presses on the water lever produced water reinforcements on a continuous reinforcement schedule, i.e., every response was rewarded (Ferster and Skinner, 1957).

After the rats were lever-pressing regularly on both levers, variable-interval (VI) schedules (Ferster and Skinner, 1957) were substituted for the continuous reinforcement schedules. Reinforcement opportunities were programmed on the average every 2 min. (VI 2′) on each lever. The two punched tapes which controlled the separate VI 2′ schedules for food and water ran independently of each other.

Experimental sessions were 4 hours long. Since only three animals could be tested per day, each animal was used on alternate weekdays, Monday through Friday. On non-test days and weekdays Ss were fed and watered for 1 hr. (at 12:30 PM), as in the preliminary phases of the experiment. Animals AA-7 and AA-10 were tested from 8:30 AM to 12:30 PM, AA-27 and AA-28 from 12:30 PM to 4:30 PM, and AA-9 and AA-12 from 4:30 PM to 8:30 PM. As a result of this test and food-water schedule, morning Ss were tested when approximatey 19 hr. deprived, afternoon Ss 23 hr. deprived and night Ss 27 hr. deprived.

After 25 sessions on this procedure Ss displayed very reliable and stable performances on both levers. Administration of *d*-amphetamine was then initiated. *d*-Amphetamine sulfate (Dextromine, Tech Bio-Chemical Co.) was dissolved in physiological saline solution and injected intraperitoneally 2 to 3 min. before the start of selected test sessions. Drug sessions were never scheduled on Mondays or Tuesdays (following the weekend break) and at least one control (no drug) session intervened between drug test sessions.

d-Amphetamine doses of 1, 2, 3, and 5 mg./kg. were tested in a mixed order until three sets of data had been collected at each of the four dose levels. Several control saline injections were given at random intervals to check on whether the injection itself had any appreciable behavioral effects. On no occasion was there any evidence of such a placebo effect.

RESULTS. The effects of *d*-amphetamine on total response output are shown in Fig. 1. Three determinations entered each mean for the four dose levels, while the control value, plotted on the abscissa as 0 mg./kg., is the mean of 10 randomly selected sessions on which either a placebo ($N = 2$ or 3 sessions) or no drug ($N = 8$ or 7 sessions) was injected. In general, increasing doses of *d*-amphetamine have a suppressive effect on the conditioned responses for both food and water; the highest dose, 5 mg./kg.,

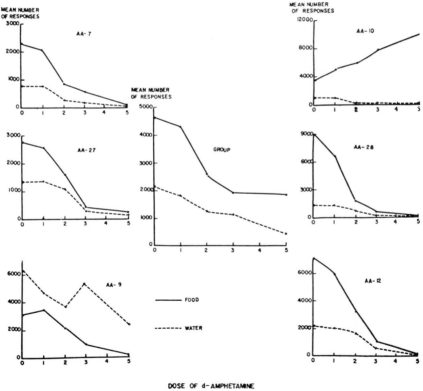

FIGURE 1. Total response output on food and water levers as a function of *d*-amphetamine dose. In addition to the group function (center), functions for all six individual *S*s are included.

results in an almost complete suppression on both levers throughout the greater part of the 4-hr. test for most Ss.

The group curve depicts the inhibitory effect of d-amphetamine on response output, but masks certain individual eccentricities, especially revealed in the data of AA-10. This animal showed a differential effect on the food and water levers. Its response rate actually increased on the food-lever with increments in the d-amphetamine dose, even though its water-lever responses reflect the suppressive effect of d-amphetamine characteristic of the other Ss.

Visual observation of AA-10 indicated that this S did not eat many of the food pellets obtained as a result of the very high response output under the larger d-amphetamine doses.

Figure 2 presents data concerning the time duration of the drug's suppressive effect. Plotted on the ordinate for each S, and for the grouped data, is the mean time elapsed from the beginning of each session until the time when Ss had emitted ¼ of the total number of responses made during the entire session. This "quarter-life" measure (see Herrnstein and

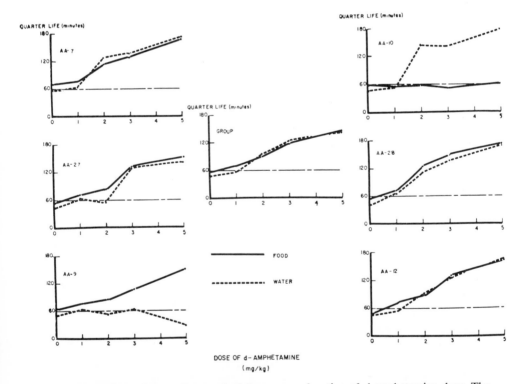

FIGURE 2. Quarter-lives on both levers as a function of d-amphetamine dose. The 60-min. baseline was drawn to indicate the value to be obtained if response rate were constant throughout a session.

Morse, 1957) is an index of the stability of responding throughout a session; if response rate were maintained at a steady pace over a 4-hr. session, ¼ of the total response output would be emitted after approximately 60 min. had elapsed, which is the case for the days on which no drug was injected (0 mg./kg. on the Fig. 2 abscissa). Increases in the quarter-life reflect a relatively greater occurrence of responses toward the end of a session, or conversely, a greater suppression of responding at the beginning of a session, shortly after drug injection.

In general, increases in the d-amphetamine dose result in increased quarter-lives on both the food and water levers. The only exceptions to this direct relationship are the data of AA-9 and AA-10 on only one of the two levers. Even at high drug doses, responding was maintained at a fairly constant rate throughout the session (quarter-life approximately 60 min.) on AA-9's water lever and AA-10's food lever.

Figures 3A and 3B present typical cumulative response curves for rat AA-7 under control conditions and the four different d-amphetamine doses. A 1 mg./kg. dose had much greater suppressive effect (compared to control levels) on food-lever responding than on water-lever responding. Successively higher does result in longer and longer periods of complete response suppression, which sometimes last over 2 hr. (e.g., for the 5 mg./kg. dose). Rats AA-27, 28, and 12 showed cumulative curves which closely parallel those of AA-7. The more or less atypical results for AA-9 and AA-10 have already been noted in the presentation of Figs. 1 and 2.

Observation of the drugged animals during periods of very low response rate indicated that Ss were not rendered unconscious by the drug. Rather, the rats characteristically stood in one corner of the experimental box and displayed vigorous head and body movements, typical sympathomimetic effects of the drug.

DISCUSSION. The results indicate a general suppressive effect of d-amphetamine on responses which produce food and water. This effect on instrumental behavior parallels the inhibitory effects of the drug on the consummatory responses of eating and drinking, and thus does not confirm the generalization offered by Epstein (1959) to the effect that amphetamine has opposite effects on consummatory and learned behavior. Since other forms of food-rewarded behavior have been reported to be stimulated by amphetamine, the drug's effects are apparently quite dependent on the type of baseline behavior being studied.

Rewarded behavior occurring at a relatively low rate (e.g., schedules of spaced responding, long fixed-interval schedules) seems much more likely to be stimulated by the administration of amphetamine (Sidman, 1956; Wentink, 1938) than schedules on which relatively high rates of response are emitted [variable-interval in the present experiment, or fixed ratio as in Kelleher and Cook's work (1959) or Owen's (1960)]. A high response

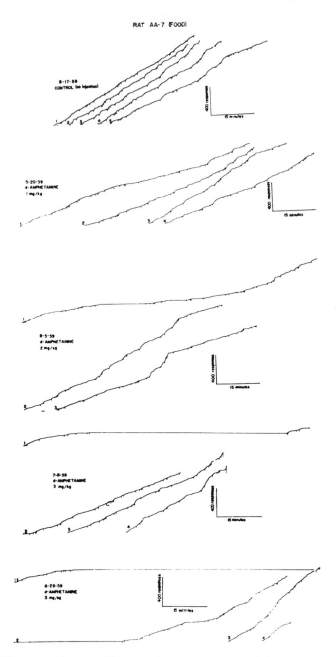

FIGURE 3A. Typical cumulative response curves for Rat AA-7 on the food lever. Samples of control performance and performance under the four different *d*-amphetamine doses are included. Successive segments of each cumulative record are numbered consecutively; the records are "telescoped" to conserve space. Downward deflections in the records indicate reinforcements.

RAT AA-7 (WATER)

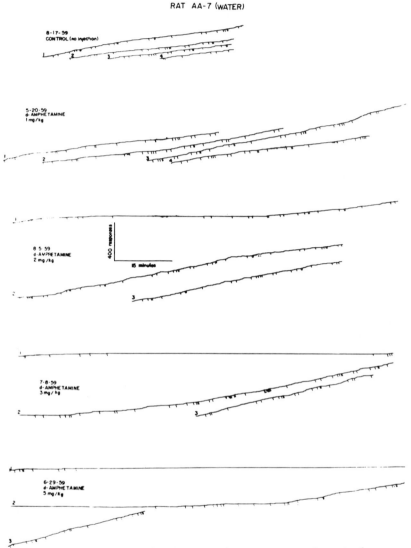

FIGURE 3B.   The same as Fig. 3A, except that responses on the water lever are re-corded.

rate in itself, however, does not seem to make a particular type of be-havior susceptible to the suppressive effects of amphetamine, since very rapid response rates on shock avoidance schedules are ordinarily increased even further by *dl*- and *d*-amphetamine in doses comparable to those used in the present experiment (e.g., see Sidman, 1956; Teitelbaum and Derks, 1958). With regard to the dependence of amphetamine's effects on the type of baseline behavior, Sidman's remark that the "relations between drugs and behavior are a function not only of the drug but also of the conditions under which the behavior is generated" is applicable here.

d-Amphetamine was not found to exert a differential effect on food-maintained and water-maintained behavior. Other (Heise *et al.*, 1960) have shown a selective effect of *d*-amphetamine on two types of behavior (food-reinforced and shock-avoidance) sampled in one experimental session in the same organism, so that the concurrent suppression of both performances in the present experiment is probably not due to an "all-or-none" inhibitory action of the drug on all ongoing behavior.

The long pauses in behavior under amphetamine, during which not a single response occurs on either lever (as in Fig. 3), were reported by Owen (1960) to be characteristic of amphetamine's effects on fixed-ratio responding, where animals are rewarded for emitting a fixed *number* of responses. Apparently this type of effect can be obtained not only with ratio schedules, but on interval schedules as well.

SUMMARY.   Six albino rats were trained to make two different lever-responses to obtain food and water. When variable-interval response rates had stabilized on both levers, *d*-amphetamine in doses from 1 mg./kg. up to 5 mg./kg. was administered before the start of a number of test sessions. For a majority of *S*s an inverse relation was found between dose of *d*-amphetamine and response output. The time duration of the drug's inhibitory effects increased with increasing dosage. *d*-amphetamine did not appear to have differential effects on food-controlled and water-controlled behavior. These inhibitory effects of *d*-amphetamine on behavior instrumental in procuring food and water are congruent with other results which indicate a suppressive effect of the drug on the consummatory responses of eating and drinking. The suppressive effects of amphetamine in the present instrumental situation were compared with its differential effects on other types of rewarded and punished behavior.

REFERENCES

Andersson, B., and Larsson, S. Water and food intake and the inhibitory effect of amphetamine on drinking and eating before and after "prefrontal lobotomy" in dogs. *Acta physiol. Scand.*, 1956, 38, 22–30.

Brady, J. V. Assessment of drug effects on emotional behavior. *Science*, 1956, 123, 1033–1034.

Epstein, A. N. Suppression of eating and drinking by amphetamine and other drugs in normal and hyperphagic rats. *J. comp. physiol. Psychol.*, 1959, 52, 37–45.

Ferster, C. B., and Skinner, B. F. *Schedules of reinforcement*. New York: Appleton-Century-Crofts, 1957.

Harns, S. C., Ivy, A. C., and Searle, L. M. The mechanism of amphetamine loss of weight. *J. Amer. Med. Assn,* 1947, 134, 1468-1475.

Heise, G. A., Walker, E., and Scheckel, C. Concurrent measurements of food-rewarded behavior and stimulation or depressant action of *d*-amphetamine and other drugs. Paper presented at meetings of Eastern Psychol. Assn, New York, May, 1960.

Herrnstein, R. J., and Morse, W. H. Effects of pentobarbital on intermittently reinforced behavior. *Science,* 1957, 125, 929–931.

Herrnstein, R. J., and Brady, J. V. Interaction among components of a multiple schedule. *J. exper. anal. Behav.,* 1958, 1, 293–300.

Kelleher, R. T., and Cook, L. Effects of *d*-amphetamine, meprobamate, phenobarbital mephenesin, or chlorpromazine on DRL and FR schedules of reinforcement with rats. *J. exp. anal. Behav.,* 1959, 2, 267. (Abstract)

Miller, N. E. Effects of drugs on motivation: The value of using a variety of measures. *Ann. N.Y. Acad. Sci.,* 1956, 65, 318–333.

Owen, J. E. The influence of *dl-, d-* and *l*-amphetamine and *d*-methamphetamine on a fixed-ratio schedule. *J. exp. anal. Behav.,* 1960, 3, 293–310.

Sidman, M. Drug-behavior interaction. *Ann. N.Y. Acad. Sci.,* 1956, 65, 282–302.

Skinner, B. F., and Heron, W. T. Effects of caffeine and benzedrine upon conditioning and extinction. *Psychol. Rec.,* 1937, 1, 340–346.

Teitelbaum, P., and Derks, P. The effect of amphetamine on forced drinking in the rat. *J. comp. physiol. Psychol.,* 1958, 51, 801–810.

Verhave, T. The effect of methamphetamine on operant level and avoidance behavior. *J. exp. anal. Behav.,* 1958, 1, 207–219.

Wentink, E. A. The effects of certain drugs and hormones upon conditioning. *J. exp. Psychol.,* 1938, 22, 150–163.

27

Self-stimulation of the brain by cats: Effects of imipramine, amphetamine, and chlorpromazine *

ZOLA P. HOROVITZ, MAY-I CHOW, and PETER L. CARLTON

In general, the behavior of cats is stimulated by amphetamine (e.g., Bradley and Elkes, 1957) and depressed by chlorpromazine (e.g., Killam and Killam, 1959; Bradley and Elkes). Imipramine, a clinical antidepressant having a structure similar to chlorpromazine, presents a more confusing picture. Most reports indicate that imipramine produces manifestations of depression in both the cat and other laboratory animals (e.g., Sigg, 1959; Horovitz and Chow, 1962). Maxwell and Palmer (1961) have reported, however, that, with certain techniques, imipramine (5.0–10.0 mg/kg, orally) produce indirect signs of stimulation. Further, Vernier (1961) showed that imipramine (0.1 to 3.5 mg/kg, i.v.) as well as its congener, amitryptyline, produced moderate increases in the lever pressing of monkeys trained on an avoidance schedule. Further, Penaloza-Rojas *et al.* (1961) have reported a lowering of the threshold for producing hypothalamic rage after intraperitoneal injection of 2.0–5.0 mg/kg of imipramine in the cat.

These data and a previously demonstrated sensitivity to drugs of the behavior of cats maintained by "rewarding" self stimulation (Horovitz *et al.,* 1962), prompted detailed investigation of the effects of imipramine, chlorpromazine and amphetamine upon this self-stimulation behavior.

METHODS.   Cats with electrodes in the lateral hypothalamus or caudate nucleus were trained to respond for electrical stimulation in these areas. The self-stimulation procedure has been described in detail by Horovitz *et al.* (1962).

The animals were tested three time a week at approximately the same time of day and were given intraperitoneal injections of saline immediately before each 1-hour session. When administered, various doses of imipramine hydrochloride, *d*-amphetamine sulfate or chlorpromazine hydrochloride were substituted for the saline before the second session of each week.

From *Psychopharmacologia* (Berl.), 1962, 3, 455–462. Copyright 1962 by Springer-Verlag, Heidelberg, Germany.

* The generous advice and encouragement of Dr. B. N. Craver and the invaluable technical assistance of Mr. T. Waldron are gratefully acknowledged. The authors thank the Geigy Pharmaceutical Company, Ardsley, New York, for supplying the imipramine used in these experiments and Smith, Kline & French Laboratories, Philadelphia, Pennsylvania, for the chlorpromazine and amphetamine.

All doses were in terms of the salt and were given in random order. At least one week intervened between drug injections.

In all instances the stimulating current was adjusted to a low level that maintained a low, erratic rate of responding. These reduced currents were used because they were found to control behavior optimally sensitive to drugs that tended to increase responding (cf. Stein and Seifter, 1961; Dews, 1958). In some of the instances in which responding was found to be *decreased* by a drug, however, the current was subsequently increased to a level that normally maintained high, stable rates of responding. The higher currents were used to determine whether the decrease in responding was related to the low currents usually used or to a simple debilitation of the animal such that responding would not be maintained, regardless of current.

RESULTS. The effects of imipramine on behavior maintained by lateral hypothalamic self-stimulation are given in Table 1. None of the 4 cats showed appreciably increased rates of responding after a dose of 1.0 mg/kg, whereas the rates of all the animals were more than doubled after 2.0

TABLE 1. Self-stimulation rates (responses/minute) of cats following imipramine hydrochloride or saline.

Cat	Location	I.p. dose mg/kg, in order administered	Current (mamps.)	Pre-drug day (Saline)	Drug day	Post-drug day (Saline)
2	Lateral hypothalamus	1	0.6	28.3	39.7	25.7
		2	0.6	35.5	71.0	32.4
		3	0.6	39.3	56.3	26.7
		4	0.6	26.0	30.8	32.3
3	Lateral hypothalamus	2	0.5	24.5	49.2	23.3
		1	0.45	16.9	15.7	14.0
		3	0.45	13.6	28.7	12.3
		4	0.5	23.6	51.5	19.7
8	Lateral hypothalamus	3	0.25	25.3	47.8	27.6
		2	0.25	16.3	44.4	21.1
		1	0.25	22.4	26.4	19.8
		4	0.25	19.9	34.2	24.2
9	Lateral hypothalamus	4	0.3	13.3	12.8	14.0
		2	0.3	13.5	35.5	15.3
		1	0.3	15.1	15.7	13.0
11	Caudate nucleus	2	0.5	26.8	23.7	23.6
		3	0.5	26.9	26.1	24.6
		1	0.5	26.1	27.5	25.0
12	Caudate nucleus	3	0.6	30.1	33.7	35.6
		1	0.6	34.0	34.7	40.1
		2	0.6	33.8	35.0	34.0
13	Caudate nucleus	1	1.0	23.1	21.7	24.8
		2	1.0	22.8	25.1	25.0
		3	1.0	24.7	25.2	22.8

mg/kg. Four mg/kg did not increase rates in 2 of the 4 animals. A related biphasic action has been reported by Vernier and by Penaloza-Rojas *et al.* Two cats were also given 5.0 mg/kg and 7.5 mg/kg; responding ceased entirely after about fifteen minutes.

Figure 1 illustrates the cumulative records of responding for the first and last saline sessions and all of the imipramine sessions for cat No. 2.

Three cats working for stimulation of the caudate nucleus were given doses of 1.0, 2.0 and 3.0 mg/kg of imipramine hydrochloride. None of these animals showed reliable changes in response rates (see Table 1.)

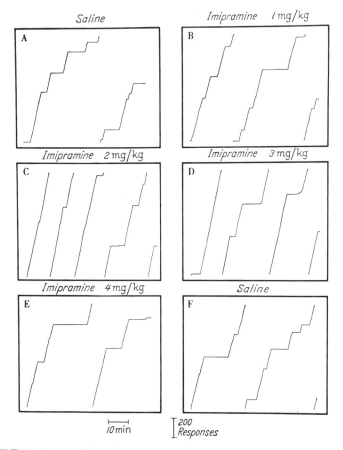

FIGURE 1. Cumulative records of the effects of intraperitoneal pre-session injections and imipramine hydrochloride on a cat responding for stimulation of the lateral hypothalamus. Imipramine sessions were one week apart. The saline sessions depicted are: A, the day before B; F, the day after E. Because responses are plotted cumulatively, the slope of each record is proportional to rate of responding. The recording pen was reset to the baseline when 1000 responses had been cumulated. Each session lasted for 1 hour.

Initial results from larger doses indicate the depressant effect on responding is also present in the caudate nucleus.

Table 2 summarizes the effects of amphetamine on cats working for self-stimulation of the lateral hypothalamus or caudate nucleus. The dose of 0.1 mg/kg had a slight stimulatory effect on responding for self-stimulation of the lateral hypothalamus; grossly observable behavioral "stimulation" was not, however, noted after this dose. Doses of 0.25 and 0.5 mg/kg caused increases in responding rates at both placements greater than those obtained following saline.

In a few cats amphetamine injections at 2.5 mg/kg decreased rates. This effect was apparently due to an "overstimulation" (piloerection and dilated pupils associated with general immobility) that interfered with self-stimulation behavior.

The effects of 2.5, 3.75 and 5.0 mg/kg of chlorpromazine hydrochloride on cats working for self-stimulation of the lateral hypothalamus and caudate nucleus are given in Table 3. All of these doses produced rates lower than saline. Doses of 0.5 and 1.0 mg/kg, tested in two cats with each placement, did not affect responding.

A representative set of cumulative records for one cat working for stimulation of the lateral hypothalamus has been presented in Fig. 2. That amphetamine produced a marked increase in the normally low, irregular rates of responding (due to the low current) is apparent in the

TABLE 2. Self-stimulation rates (responses/minute) of cats following amphetamine or saline.

Cat	Location	I.p. dose mg/kg, in order administered	Current (mamps.)	Pre-drug day (Saline)	Drug day	Post-drug day (Saline)
1	Lateral hypothalamus	0.1	0.25	29.1	33.5	30.2
		0.25	0.30	25.8	52.1	28.3
		0.5	0.25	14.4	61.3	13.6
2	Lateral hypothalamus	0.1	0.75	28.4	32.8	23.2
		0.5	0.75	22.4	52.8	21.9
		0.25	0.75	25.8	38.4	23.0
3	Lateral hypothalamus	0.5	0.5	18.4	36.0	15.8
		0.1	0.5	18.2	29.1	19.0
		0.25	0.5	22.2	35.4	18.6
4	Lateral hypothalamus	0.25	0.43	21.3	34.1	17.2
		0.1	0.43	18.4	21.3	16.9
		0.5	0.43	18.7	42.3	20.4
10	Caudate nucleus	0.25	1.0	17.2	25.2	17.1
		0.5	1.0	17.9	31.4	18.6
11	Caudate nucleus	0.5	0.5	24.2	37.7	26.1
		0.25	0.5	25.0	30.1	24.6
12	Caudate nucleus	0.25	0.6	33.8	35.0	30.1
		0.5	0.6	30.1	42.0	26.0

TABLE 3. Self-stimulation rates (responses/minute) of cats following chlorpromazine hydrochloride or saline.

Cat	Location	I.p. dose mg/kg, in order administered	Current (mamps.)	Pre-drug day (Saline)	Drug day	Post-drug day (Saline)
1	Lateral hypothalamus	5.0	0.25	15.4	5.0	18.8
		2.5	0.25	10.5	13.3	15.5
		3.75	0.25	15.0	7.9	14.1
5	Lateral hypothalamus	2.5	0.5	46.2	40.1	49.2
		3.75	0.5	43.0	21.8	39.4
		5.0	0.5	44.4	26.6	50.4
6	Lateral hypothalamus	3.75	0.35	42.9	28.7	48.1
		2.5	0.35	43.1	39.5	44.4
		5.0	0.35	51.8	18.4	43.2
7	Lateral hypothalamus	2.5	0.53	34.1	20.4	27.2
		5.0	0.53	28.5	16.0	29.5
		3.75	0.53	26.3	16.2	29.8
11	Caudate nucleus	5.0	0.5	23.7	12.5	26.1
		2.5	0.5	23.6	18.7	24.0
12	Caudate nucleus	5.0	0.6	32.1	17.1	32.9
		2.5	0.6	33.7	22.0	30.2
13	Caudate nucleus	2.5	1.0	24.5	19.4	23.6
		5.0	1.0	23.1	6.0	21.4

middle record at the left. Data taken from the control sessions immediately preceding and following the drug session have been entered for comparison. The effect of chlorpromazine is shown at the right. Note the prompt resumption of responding when the current was increased. The rate at this higher current was, however, less (63.9 responses/min.) than that obtained at the same amperage in the preceding and following control sessions (89.0 responses/min. and 94.2 responses/min., respectively).

The complex series of effects presented in the tables is more conveniently summarized in Fig. 3. In preparing the figure, the rates obtained in sessions before and after each drug session were averaged for each cat. The rate obtained in the drug session was then divided by this average to provide a "drug to control" ratio. The ratios obtained following each dose of each drug were then averaged for all cats having a common electrode placement. These values have been plotted in Fig. 3. The general reliability of the effects described by these averages is apparent from inspection of the data for individual animals in Tables 1, 2 and 3.

DISCUSSION.   The effects of the drugs on self-stimulation of the caudate tended to be smaller than those on responding maintained by lateral hypothalamic stimulation. This relative insensitivity may reflect a corresponding insensitivity of the caudate areas to the particular drugs studied. It is more likely, however, that this finding is related to (1) the rather high

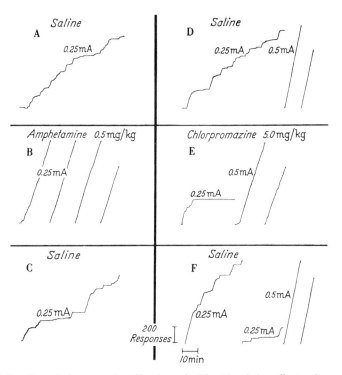

FIGURE 2. Cumulative records (like those in Fig. 1) of the effects of pre-session injections of amphetamine sulfate and chlorpromazine hydrochloride on a cat responding for stimulation of the lateral hypothalamus. A, B, C and D, E, F each represent records of three consecutive days, with two weeks between the two groups.

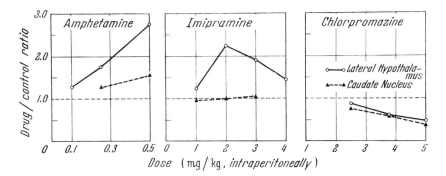

FIGURE 3. Average drug/control ratios (see text) for amphetamine, imipramine and chlorpormazine. Ratios have been averaged for all cats having common electrode placements (caudate nucleus or lateral hypothalamus). The vertical dashed line in each graph indicates a ratio of 1.0, i.e., no effect.

currents required to maintain responding, and, especially (2), the fact that large increases in current produced only small increases in the responding of normal cats (also see Horovitz *et al.,* 1962).

Thus, the effective current-range for caudate stimulation was a sharply restricted one. Accordingly, the increase in self-stimulation of the caudate that a drug *could* produce may have been restricted by a "ceiling" beyond which responding could not be increased. It should be noted, however, that doses of amphetamine that increased hypothalamic self-stimulation also increased, to a smaller degree, caudate stimulation; a comparable parallelism was not obtained with imipramine.

All three of the drugs studied altered rates of responding maintained by lateral hypothalamic stimulation, whereas only amphetamine and chlorpromazine produced comparable effects on self-stimulation of *both* sites. Thus, there is a suggestion that the action of imipramine may be a rather restricted one. In contrast, the action of amphetamine and chlorpromazine appears to be more general. That is, *both* caudate and hypothalamic areas may be affected by amphetamine and chlorpromazine, whereas the action of imipramine may be restricted to the hypothalamic area. Alternatively, the actions of chlorpromazine and amphetamine may be primarily on some third area (e.g., the reticular formation) that has a general modulating influence on all rewarded behavior.

Although the extent of imipramine's specificity cannot be assessed in the absence of information on its effects elsewhere in the brain, the present data do suggest that the site of action of imipramine is, first, different from that of chlorpromazine and amphetamine and, second, may be restricted to hypothalamic structures. These speculations are commensurate with the distribution of "sympathin" in the cat brain (Vogt, 1954) and with the suggestion (Sigg) that imipramine may "sensitize" adrenergic systems in the brain.

Other considerations suggest that this specificity may also extend to the species studied. For example, Carlton (1961) found that the operant, shock-avoidance responding of rats after amphetamine was markedly potentiated by imipramine in doses that, when given alone, either did not affect or slightly depressed responding. In contrast, Vernier reported that the responding of monkeys working in a similar avoidance situation was increased by imipramine. Still a third line of evidence indicates that, although imipramine is evidently a moderate depressant of the operant behavior of rats, the responding of pigeons is, under certain contingencies at least, markedly increased by imipramine (W. H. Morse, personal communication; Cook and Kelleher, 1962).

Stein and Seifter have reported that the effects of amphetamine on the self-stimulation responding of rats was, like the avoidance responding studied by Carlton, potentiated by doses of imipramine that were non-effective or slightly depressant when given alone. They did not report on a lateral hypothalamic placement; detailed evaluation of the effects of imipramine on lateral hypothalamic self-stimulation in rats evidently remains to be done.

SUMMARY

The effects of imipramine, chlorpromazine and amphetamine were evaluated in terms of their effects on the self-stimulation responding of cats. Amphetamine increased the responding of cats working for stimulation of the caudate nucleus and lateral hypothalamus. Chlorpromazine decreased responding in cats working for stimulation of these two areas. In contrast, imipramine increased responding maintained by stimulation of lateral hypothalamic sites, but did not have a comparable effect on self-stimulation of the caudate.

REFERENCES

Bradley, P. B., and Elkes, J.: The effect of some drugs on the electrical activity of the brain. *Brain* 80, 77–117 (1957).

Carlton, P. L.: Potentiation of the behavioral effects of amphetamine by imipramine. *Psychopharmacologia* (Berl.) 2, 364–376 (1961).

Cook, L., and Kelleher, R. T.: Drug effects on the behavior of animals. *Ann. N.Y. Acad. Sci.* 96, 315–335 (1962).

Dews, P. B.: Studies on behavior. IV Stimulant actions of methamphetamine. *J. Pharmacol. exp. Ther.* 122, 137–147 (1958).

Horovitz, Z. P., and Chow, M.: Effects of centrally acting drugs on the correlation of electrocortical activity and wakefulness in cats. *J. Pharmacol. exp. Ther.* 137, 127–132 (1962).

Horovitz, Z. P., Chow, M., and Carlton, P. L.: Self-stimulation of the brain by cats: Techniques and preliminary drug effects. *Psychopharmacologia* (Berl.) 3, 449–454 (1962).

Killam, E. K., and Killam, K. F.: Phenothiazine-pharmacologic studies. In F. J. Braceland, ed., *The effects of pharmacologic agents on the nervous system,* pp. 245–265. Baltimore: Williams & Wilkins 1959.

Maxwell, D. R., and Palmer, H. T.: Demonstration of anti-depressant or stimulant properties of imipramine in experimental animals. *Nature* (Lond.) 191, 84–85 (1961).

Penaloza-Rojas, J. H., Bach-y-Rita, G., Rubio-Chevannier, H. F., and Hernandez-Peon, R.: Effects of imipramine upon hypothalamic and amygdaloid excitability. *Exp. Neurol.* 4, 205–213 (1961).

Sigg, E. G.: Pharmacological studies with Tofranil. *Canad. psychiat. Ass. J.* 4, Special Suppl. 75–85 (1959).

Stein, L., and Seifter, J.: Possible mode of antidepressive action of imipramine. *Science* 134, 286–287 (1961).

Vernier, V. G.: Pharmacology of antidepressant agents. *Dis. nerv. Syst.* 22, 7–14 (1961).

Vogt, M.: The concentration of sympathin in different paths of the central nervous system under normal conditions and after administration of drugs. *J. Physiol.* (Lond.) 123, 451–481 (1954).

28

Studies on sugar preference: The preference for
glucose solutions and its modification by injections of
insulin [1]

HARRY L. JACOBS

This report summarizes the first of a series of studies on the motivation
of sugar preference. The present study was designed to investigate some
of the factors producing glucose preference under normal dietary conditions and under an experimentally induced need for glucose.

A very specific organic need for glucose can be induced by producing
hypoglycemia with injections of insulin. Since the central nervous system
uses glucose as a primary source for energy utilization, profound hypoglycemia can cause coma, convulsions, and death. Only glucose will raise
the blood-sugar level quickly; thus, exogenous glucose becomes absolutely
necessary for survival (8, Chap. 1).

There have been three studies in which insulin-produced hypoglycemia
has been related to sugar appetite. Richter (5) and Soulairac (9) have
demonstrated a specific hunger for glucose in hypoglycemic rats given a
choice among glucose in solution, water, and food. The third study, by
Mayer-Gross and Walker (4), suggests that the specificity of hypoglycemia-
induced sugar hunger extends to preference between solutions of different
concentration. Using schizophrenics who were receiving insulin shock
therapy, they found that hypoglycemia induced a switch from a 5%
sucrose solution to a 30% solution, previously rejected as too sweet.
Preference was measured by allowing Ss to taste the solutions and then
asking them which they would prefer for a long drink. An additional
reason for doing the present study was to obtain more precise information
on hypoglycemia-induced preference by using consummatory responses
rather than verbal report.

METHOD [2]

SUBJECTS. The Ss were 50 male albino rats of the Wistar strain. They
were about three and one-half months old at the start of the experiment,

From *Journal of Comparative and Physiological Psychology,* 1958, **51**, 304–310.
Copyright 1958 by the American Psychological Association, Washington, D.C.

[1] The second experiment was performed at Bucknell University under the support
of a grant from the National Science Foundation.

[2] The glucose used in these experiments was supplied by J. M. Krno and David
Linn of the Corn Products Sales Company. Insulin was supplied by W. R. Kirtley of
the Eli Lilly Company.

with a maximum age difference of one week. None of them had tasted sugar solutions prior to the experiment.

Maintenance. The animals were housed in single cages in an experimental room with a 12-hr. light-dark cycle and a temperature range of 75° to 84° F. Food cups were firmly mounted at the rear of each cage, and liquids were presented for choice in inverted graduate cylinders containing a Pyrex drinking tube mounted in a rubber stopper. Position habits were corrected for by shifting the choice bottles each day. The order of presentation was chosen so that position habits could be factored out of the data by using two-day averages for a two-choice situation and three-day averages for a three-choice situation. The glucose solutions were made with distilled water and were mixed in weight/volume ratios, i.e., a 10% solution contained 10 gm. of solute per 100 cc. of solution. The glucose solutions were left standing 12 hr. after mixing to allow stabilization of mutarotation. They were periodically inspected for fermentation and immediately changed if any was noted. All unused solutions were discarded every 72 hr. Big Red Dog Food, a dry mash obtained from the G. L. F. Marketing Service, was used as the stock diet.

Injections. Protamine-Zinc Insulin (40 U/cc) was administered subcutaneously twice daily, at 12-hr. intervals. A schedule of increasing daily dosages was used, consisting of 2, 3, 4, 6, 8, 10, 10, 12, and 12 units per day. All control injections were of physiological saline. Alternate sides of the animal were used for successive injections. A 23-gauge needle was inserted beneath the loose folds of skin around the groin. Care was taken to avoid autonomic involvement, which might have affected the blood-sugar level. The animals were allowed to remain in a standing position during injection, the *E* pinching the skin fold and stroking the *S* with one hand, while holding the syringe with the other. This method produced little emotional disturbance; no defecation or urination was observed after the first injection. Zepharin (1:1000) and ethanol (95:100) were used to prevent contamination of the needles, syringes, and insulin, although the injections themselves were not carried out under aseptic conditions.

EXPERIMENTAL PROCEDURE. *Experiment I.* All *S*s were given a seven-day adaptation period in which they had access to food and water. The food and water intake for the last three days of this period was used as a baseline to evaluate appetite. This was followed by a nine-day experimental period in which all *S*s were presented with a four-choice self-selection diet, consisting of food, water, a 10% glucose solution, and a 35% glucose solution. In keeping with Mayer-Gross and Walker (4), salt licks were put in each cage. It was assumed that this would allow independent satisfaction of any salt need engendered by insulin-produce electrolyte shifts and concomitant upsets in water balance.

During the experimental period *S*s were split into two groups ($N = 11$ in each group), an insulin group receiving insulin injections and a control group receiving saline injections. Daily records were made of weight and of food, water, and solution intake. Salt intake was recorded at the end of the experiment.

Experiment II.   Except for the number of sugar solutions in each cage, the conditions of this experiment were identical to those for the control group in Experiment I. Two groups of *S*s (*N* = 14 in each group) were given 22 days' access to food, water, and *one* glucose solution. One group was given a 10% glucose solution, the other a 30% glucose solution. These groups will be designated as the 10-W group and the 30-W group, according to the solution presented.

RESULTS

The major results will be presented without special reference to analytic details. Significance levels will be noted where relevant. Complete tables and rationale for all analyses of variance, sets of *t* tests, and linear and quadratic tests for trend can be found elsewhere (2).

EXPERIMENT I.   *Salt intake.*   No significant difference was found in the salt intake of the two groups (*df* = 21; *t* = .82). Thus, insulin had no demonstrable effect on salt intake.

Weight.   The increase in weight for the experimental period was 10.64% for the control group and 16.49% for the insulin group. The difference was significant ($p < .01$), showing that insulin produced a greater weight gain.

Caloric intake.   Figure 1 shows the results on caloric intake; combined intake (food plus glucose) is plotted on the upper graph, food intake on the middle graph, and total glucose intake on the lower graph.

1. Combined intake: Although combined intake rose significantly for both groups during the first three days ($p < .01$), there was no demonstrable difference between groups. An analysis of variance for the full experimental period showed significant between-treatments and between-days effects ($p < .001$ in both cases). Thus, the initial increase in combined intake reflected the introduction of sugar choices to both groups. Insulin did not take effect until the last six days of the experimental period.

2. Food intake: Although the food intake of both groups dropped significantly during the first three days ($p < .01$ in both cases), the difference between groups was not significant. Thus, the introduction of the glucose choices at the beginning of the experimental period would appear to be the only factor mediating the initial decrease in food intake.

An over-all analysis of variance showed that the between-treatments, between-days, and the interaction (treatments × days) effects were significant ($p < .001$ in all three cases). As was the case with the combined intake, the insulin-mediated increase in food intake was limited to the last two

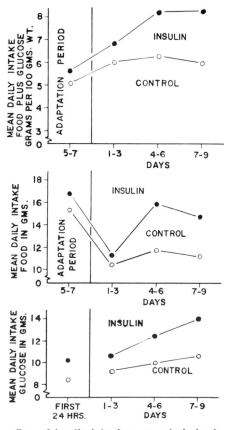

FIGURE 1. The effect of insulin injections on caloric intake. The approximate intake in cal/100 gm wt may be obtained by multiplying the ordinate values on the
upper graph by a factor of 4.

three-day periods. This increase in food intake raised it to the baseline level,
compensating for the initial decrease which occurred when the sugar solutions were introduced.

3. Total glucose intake: The insulin group ingested significantly more
glucose during the first 24 hr. of the experiment ($p < .01$). An analysis of
variance for the full experimental period showed between-treatments and
between-days effects to be significant ($p < .001$ in both cases) as well as
their interaction ($p < .05$). A trend analysis of the linear and quadratic
components of each curve showed the linear component to be significant for
the insulin group ($p < .001$) and the control group ($p < .01$). Thus, insulin consistently increased glucose intake throughout the experimental
period.

Solution preferences. Figure 2 shows the average volume consumed for
each of the three choices during the experimental period. The water intake

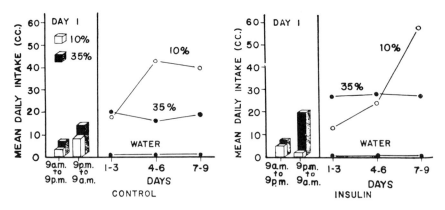

FIGURE 2.   The relationship between insulin administration and the preference for a 10% and a 35% glucose solution.

was less than 1 cc. per day for both groups throughout the experiment. Since the water intake was negligible, further data analysis was limited to the two glucose solutions.

Inspection of the over-all intake of the 35% solution and its relative intake compared to the 10% solution shows the effect of insulin quite clearly. The over-all intake of the 35% solution will be considered first. The only effect of insulin was to increase this intake for the period as a whole ($p < .01$).

Preference was evaluated by comparison of the intake of the two solutions. The data for the first 24 hr. of the experimental period are shown on the left of each graph in Figure 2. Although both groups ingested more of the 35% solution throughout the first day, the only significant preference was that shown by the insulin group during the second 12-hr. interval ($p < .001$).

The results for the full period followed this pattern. The insulin group significantly preferred the 35% solution for the first three-day period ($p < .001$). Although the intake of the 10% solution showed a significant linear increase ($p < .01$) for the rest of the experiment, it was never significantly preferred. During the last three-day period, when the 10% solution intake of the insulin group reached its peak, 5 of the 11 animals still preferred the 35% solution.

Unlike the consistent rise in 10% intake shown in the curve of the group under insulin treatment, the control group's curve had significant linear ($p < .01$) and quadratic components ($p < .001$), leveling off during the last three days. Although no preference was demonstrated during the first three days, this group showed a significant preference for the 10% solution for the second ($p < .01$) and third ($p < .05$) three-day period.

The preference results may be summarized by noting three general effects

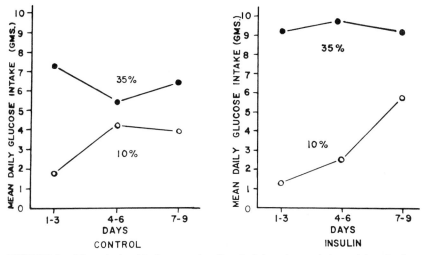

FIGURE 3. The relationship between insulin administration and the weight of solute obtained from the intake of the two glucose solutions.

of insulin: (*a*) It delayed the rapid rise in the intake of the 10% solution shown by the control group. (*b*) It increased the over-all intake of the 35% solution. (*c*) It produced a preference for the 35% solution for the first three-day period.

Glucose intake from individual solutions. Figure 3 shows that both groups ingested more glucose from the 35% solution that from the 10% solution throughout the experimental period. The over-all difference in favor of the 35% solution was significant for both groups ($p < .001$ in both cases). Thus, even though the control group preferred the 10% solution, it received more glucose from the 35% solution.

EXPERIMENT II. Figure 4 presents the volume-intake results for Experiment II. The relative intake of the glucose solutions is in accord with the results obtained when simultaneous sugar choices were available (see Fig. 2). In Experiment I the control group preferred the 10% solution; in this experiment the intake of the 10% solution was three times that of the 30% solution.

The total glucose and water intake for this experiment and for the control group in Experiment I are summarized in Table 1. The total glucose intake and the liquid intake from the water bottle were very stable. Total water intake was the only dependent variable which varied as a function of the choice situation. The control group and the 10-W group both ingested more water than the 30-W group. In both cases, most of the extra water was obtained from the 10% solution. The control group's water in-

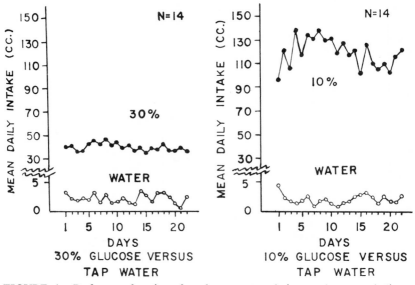

FIGURE 4. Preference functions for glucose-water choices under normal dietary conditions in Experiment II.

TABLE 1. Average daily glucose and water intake.

Experiment	Group	Total Glucose Intake (gm.)	Water[a] Intake (cc.)	Total Water Intake (cc.)
I	Control	10.23	0.6	49.9
II	30-W	11.73	2.2	30.2
	10-W	12.04	2.1	109.0

[a] From the water bottle.

take from the 10% solution alone (37.7 cc.) was 25% greater than the total intake of the 30-W group.

DISCUSSION

TOTAL CALORIC INTAKE. Although insulin increased both food and glucose intake in Experiment I, the food shifts were delayed and well within the normal intake range. The major effect of insulin was to produce a specific hunger for glucose. This is in agreement with the results of Richter (5) and Soulairac (9).

THE INSULIN-INDUCED PREFERENCES. The insulin-induced preference for the 35% glucose solution found in Experiment I is consistent with the work of Mayer-Gross and Walker (4). This shows that the glucose hunger which is engendered by insulin is specific enough to make the organism prefer the sweeter solution, thus allowing more efficient need reduction.

There are two ways of explaining these facts. Homeostatic physiological mechanisms such as those postulated by Richter (6) in similar cases may underlie the preference change. The relation between need and choice could also be learned, the sweeter taste developing secondary reinforcing properties through association with primary need reduction (1). One prediction which differentiates these two explanations relates to the delay between organic need induction and the preference change. An immediate shift in preference could be produced by homeostatic mechanisms; a delayed shift would imply learning.

In Experiment I the preference change appeared during the second 12-hr. period after insulin administration. The peak effect of the Protamine-Zinc Insulin used in this experiment would also be expected to occur during the same interval. This suggests that any assumed association between need and the stimulus characteristics of the 35% solution would have had to occur very quickly. A detailed record of the changes in blood-sugar level and consummatory response would have to be obtained before this delay could be unequivocally interpreted.

In conclusion, the preference for the sweeter solution is interpreted to be a function of the increased need for glucose resulting from insulin injections. The design of this experiment did not allow clear separation of learning from homeostatic factors in explaining the results.

THE NORMAL PREFERENCE.   The control group's preference for the 10% solution in Experiment I presents an interesting problem in interpretation. This solution contained three potential reinforcers: glucose, water, and taste.

Glucose.   Although the control group preferred the 10% solution, it obtained more glucose from the nonpreferred solution. If glucose was acting as a differential reinforcer, these animals were receiving more of it from the nonpreferred solution. Thus, glucose could not have been a positive reinforcer for the 10% solution preference.

Water and taste.   The postingestinal hypothesis of McCleary (3) and Steller *et al.* (10) may be applied to explain the water intake. This states that the ingestion of hypertonic solutions dehydrates the organism, making it thirsty. Thus, as the hypertonic 35% solution was ingested, postingestinal factors drove the Ss to take the 10% solution in larger amounts to satisfy the need for water. The fact that the 10% solution actually provided 75% of the control group's total water intake is consistent with this approach.

There are three other findings, however, that are not in agreement with predictions from the postingestinal hypothesis:

1. If ingestion of the hypertonic solution forced the Ss to the 10% solu-

tion to obtain water, removal of this choice should force them to the water bottle or result in avoidance of the sugar solution. In Experiment II the 30-W group did not avoid the hypertonic solution and still ingested very little from the water bottle.

2. The operation of postingestinal factors should also have increased the total water intake of the 30-W group. Before the experiment started, these animals obtained 27.1 cc. of liquid per day from the water bottle. The addition of the 30% solution increased the total water intake 3.1 cc. per day. This rise was not significant.

3. If dehydration were the only factor mediating the control group's liquid intake in Experiment I, the water bottle would have been the most efficient choice. The control group ignored the water bottle, preferring the 10% solution, which provided sweetness as well as water. Since the extra water could have been provided by either choice, this shows that taste served as the differential reinforcer for the 10% solution preference.

The difficulties in applying the postingestinal hypothesis in this study may be related to the fact that most of the data on which this hypothesis is based have been collected during 1-hr. intake tests following hypertonic stomach loads (3, 10). Smith (7) has found discrepancies between the short- and long-term effects of hypertonic loads. It may be that short-term postingestinal effects may not be as important in the ad libitum situation using 24-hr. intake measures.

On the basis of this discussion, it is concluded that glucose was not a factor in the control group's preference for the 10% solution, and that reinforcement was provided by the intrinsic acceptability of the taste itself (11).

SUMMARY

Rats were given a choice between a 10% glucose solution and a 35% solution. The 10% solution was preferred. Glucose, water, and taste were evaluated as possible reinforcers. Glucose and water were eliminated, leaving taste. The possible operation of postingestinal factors is discussed. It was concluded that taste factors mediated the preference for the 10% solution.

When insulin was administered, the preference shifted to the 35% solution. Glucose was shown to be the reinforcer. Learning or homeostatic mechanisms are considered as alternate explanations of the results. Either factor could explain the results of the insulin-induced choice.

REFERENCES

1. Hull, C. L. *Principles of behavior*. New York: Appleton-Century-Crofts, 1943.
2. Jacobs, H. L. The motivation of sugar preferences in the albino rat. Unpublished doctoral dissertation, Cornell Univer., 1955.
3. McCleary, R. A. Taste and postingestinal factors in specific-hunger behavior. *J. comp. physiol. Psychol.*, 1953, 46, 411–421.
4. Mayer-Gross, W., and Walker, J. Taste and selection of food in hypoglycaemia. *Brit. J. exp. Pathol.*, 1946, 27, 297–305.
5. Richter, C. Increased dextrose appetite of normal rats treated with insulin. *Amer. J. Physiol.*, 1942, 135, 781–787.
6. Richter, C. Behavioral regulations of carbohydrate homeostasis. *Acta neurovegetativa*, 1954, 9, 247–259.
7. Smith, M. Tonicity of stomach contents and hunger. Paper read at A.P.A., New York, September, 1957.
8. Soskin, S., and Levine, L. *Carbohydrate metabolism*. Chicago: Univer. Chicago Press, 1952.
9. Soulairac, A. Le rôle de l'estomac dans le mécanisme physiologique de l'appétit pour les glucides. *C.R. Acad. Sci.*, Paris, 1950, 231, 73–75. (Abstract)
10. Stellar, E., Hyman, R., and Samet, S. Gastric factors controlling water and salt-solution drinking. *J. comp. physiol. Psychol.*, 1954, 47, 220–226.
11. Young, P. T. Appetite, palatability and feeding habit: A critical review. *Psychol. Bull.*, 1948, 45, 289–320.

29

Effects of amphetamine, chlorpromazine, and pentobarbital on behavioral thermoregulation [1]

Bernard Weiss and Victor G. Laties

Behavior is an important component of many regulatory processes. Seeking shelter from the cold, for example, is an instance of behavioral thermoregulation. This last process has been studied quantitatively by exposing rats to cold and giving them access to a lever that turns on a heat lamp. Rats will keep warm by pressing the lever (Weiss and Laties, 1961).

Both metabolic and thermal variables govern the frequency with which rats turn on the lamp. One important metabolic variable is thyroid state. Thyroidectomy increases the frequency of responding while the administration of triiodothyronine decreases it (Laties and Weiss, 1959). One important thermal variable is the output of the heat lamp. If the output is low, the frequency of responding is high, and if the output is high, the frequency is low (Weiss and Laties, 1960). When the temperature under the skin is measured with a thermocouple probe, it can be demonstrated that the rat so varies the frequency with which it turns on the lamp that it maintains a relatively constant peripheral temperature (Weiss and Laties, 1961).

Our aim in the present experiments was to determine the effects upon thermoregulatory behavior of three widely studied drugs; amphetamine, chlorpromazine, and pentobarbital. Since most of the behavioral studies with these drugs have used food or water deprivation as motivating variables, we thought it possible that another type of situation—access to heat in a cold environment—would be affected by these agents in a unique manner. We had two reasons for this belief. The first was that in the heat reinforcement situation the animal does not have to make another type of response to obtain the reinforcement; he does not, as with food, have to find it, seize it, and swallow it. Nor can the reinforcement be avoided; the burst of heat warms the skin immediately, no matter what the rat does. These features of the situation avert the problem that has at times arisen with amphetamine, namely, that animals fail to eat food reinforcements (Weissman, 1959; Segal, 1962). The second was that, in contrast with the long chain of physiological and biochemical processes that intervene between the

From *Journal of Pharmacology and Experimental Therapeutics,* 1963, **140**, 1–7. Copyright © 1963 by The Williams and Wilkins Co., Baltimore, Md.

[1] Supported by grant MY-3229 from the National Institute of Mental Health and grant B-865 from the National Institute of Neurological Diseases and Blindness, National Institutes of Health.

ingestion of food and its metabolic effects, a burst of heat produces an immediate shift in heat balance. This would lead one to expect more responsiveness to homeostatic variables with thermoregulatory behavior.

Four studies will be reported; three examined the effects of these drugs on behavior maintained by the delivery of heat while the fourth examined the effects of these drugs on temperature fall in the cold.

METHODS

Apparatus. Four Plexiglas heat reinforcement chambers (illustrated in Weiss and Laties, 1961) were located in a refrigerated room maintained within $\pm$ 1°C of the thermostat setting. Each of these cylindrical chambers measured 7 inches in diameter. An infrared heat lamp (red bulb) was mounted 10 inches above each floor; the floors were made of Plexiglas rods. A plastic lever extended into each chamber. When it was depressed with a force of 20 grams, the lever closed a circuit that turned on the heat lamp. For the present experiment the output of a 375-watt heat lamp was set at 250 watts by a variable transformer and the duration of each heat reinforcement was set at 2 seconds by a timer. A single reinforcement produced a transient rise of about 3°C at the skin surface and about 0.6°C subcutaneously (Weiss and Laties, 1960). Each depression of the lever made while the lamp was off turned it on. Presses made while the lamp was on had no effect. The automatic recording and programming equipment was located in an adjoining room.

Procedure. All the subjects were adult male albino rats from the Sprague-Dawley strain maintained by Carworth Farms. Original training for the behavioral experiments consisted of a 16-hour session at 2°C with the reinforcement parameters noted above. Each rat in the experiment obtained at least 1,000 reinforcements within the 16 hours. During the subsequent experimental sessions, drug data were secured only after the rat had been responding at a steady rate for at least 1 hour. This determination is easy to make because the change from a zero rate to a steady one almost always occurs abruptly (Weiss and Laties, 1961). To give the drug, the animal was lifted out of the chamber, injected, and immediately put back. Fur was removed with an electric clipper before the start of an experimental session.

In two of the behavioral experiments, we obtained simultaneous records of skin temperature and behavior. The skin temperatures were obtained by securing a copper-constantan thermocouple junction to the back of the rat with a strip of Velcro which engirdled the rat's chest. The thermocouple leads were connected to a Minneapolis-Honeywell temperature recorder in the adjoining room. The resulting records were scored by estimating, from the record, the mean temperature for each 5-minute period.

The rats used to study temperature fall in the cold were first shaved, then injected with doses of the drugs used in the behavioral experiments. Immediately afterward, they were put into wire mesh cages located in the cold room, which was maintained at a temperature of 2°C. Rectal temperatures were taken with a thermocouple probe connected to the temperature recorder directly before drug administration and at hourly intervals during the period that the rats remained in the cold. Twelve rats were exposed during a single session. Each rat served just once. All dose levels of all the drugs and three saline controls were run during a single session. This experiment is reported last although it was the second one performed.

Drugs. The following dose levels were administered. Experiments 1 and 4: amphetamine, 1, 2, and 4 mg/kg; chlorpromazine hydrochloride, 1, 2, and 4 mg/kg; sodium pentobarbital, 5, 10, and 20 mg/kg. Experiment 2: amphetamine sulfate, 2 mg/kg; chlorpromazine hydrochloride, 2 mg/kg. Experiment 3: amphetamine sulfate, 2 mg/kg. All drugs were administered intraperitoneally.

RESULTS

Experiment 1.   *Reinforcement rate after amphetamine, chlorpromazine, and pentobarbital.*   In the first experiment 24 trained rats were randomly divided into three equal groups, one group assigned to each drug. Each rat supplied data for saline control sessions and at three levels of one drug. The sequence of treatments was counterbalanced for order. An experimental session lasted 4 hours. Figure 1 shows the data of this experiment in terms of deviations from the reinforcement rate prevailing during the hour immediately before drug administration. The absolute values appear in the figure legend and are represented by zero on the ordinates. Separate analyses of variance were calculated for each drug for the following periods: 00–30, 30–60, 60–120, and 120–240 minutes. The F ratios from these analyses are given in Table 1, along with the corresponding P values. The degrees of freedom appear as subscripts in this and the following tables. The differences significant by two-tailed *t* tests are also listed.

Amphetamine.   During the first 30 minutes after the drug was given, a dose of 4 mg/kg produced a considerable and statistically significant decrease. Doses of 1 and 2 mg/kg had little effect. The significant F ratio for this period was mainly the contribution of the fall in rate after the 4-mg/kg dose. For the next 90 minutes, the curves stayed fairly close together; the initial depressive effects of the 4-mg/kg dose wore off, and the 1- and 2-mg/kg curves tended to remain slightly above the control curve. During the last 2 hours, amphetamine at all dose levels increased the frequency of reinforcement. The significant variance among dose levels during this period was almost wholly due to the difference between saline and the three

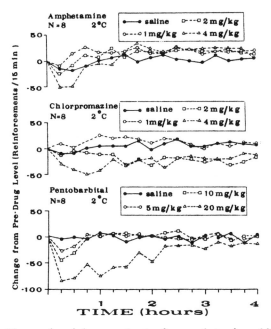

FIGURE 1.   Changes in reinforcement rate after amphetamine, chlorpromazine, and pentobarbital (Experiment 1). One hour pre-drug mean baseline values (reinf/15 min) were: amphetamine, 99.1; chlorpromazine, 92.9; pentobarbital, 92.9. These are the values represented by zero on the ordinates.

dose levels of amphetamine; these three doses did not differ significantly among themselves, but the rank order was in the expected direction.

Chlorpromazine.   In the first hour, 1 mg/kg produced a slight rise, while a dose of 2 mg/kg produced little change. The initial effect of 4 mg/kg, however, was a depression in reinforcement rate which became great enough between 30–60 minutes to produce a statistically significant F ratio. During the last 2 hours, however, the variance among treatments was not statistically significant. The lowered rate for the group as a whole at 4 mg/kg was mainly the contribution of three rats that did not respond at all after this dose.

Pentobarbital.   Pentobarbital depressed reinforcement rate in direct accordance with dose level for the first 30 minutes of the session. Although there was rapid recovery after 5 and 10 mg/kg, the curve for 20 mg/kg remained depressed for the next 90 minutes. There was no significant difference among dose levels during the last 2 hours. The slightly lower mean rate for the 20 mg/kg dose during this time was attributable to two rats that never responded at all at that dose level.

EXPERIMENT 2.   *Skin temperature and reinforcement rate after amphetamine and chlorpromazine.*   In order to determine whether the effects

TABLE 1.   Results of analyses of variance, Experiment 1.

	Minutes			
	0–30	30–60	60–120	120–240
Amphetamine				
$F_{3,21}$	4.79	0.96	0.83	4.12
P	<.05	N.S.	N.S.	<.05
t test P <.05	0–4[a]	—	—	0–1
				0–2
				0–4
CPZ				
$F_{3,21}$	1.90	5.87	2.72	1.48
P	N.S.	<.01	<.01	N.S.
t test P <.05	—	0–4	—	—
Pentobarbital				
$F_{3,21}$	14.06	12.64	6.66	0.51
P	<.001	<.001	<.01	N.S.
t test P <.05	0–10	0–20	0–20	—
	0–20			

[a] *i.e.*, only the difference between saline and 4 mg/kg was significant at the 0.05 level by two-tailed *t* test.

produced by amphetamine and chlorpromazine in the previous study were altering the temperature at which the rats maintained their skin, 9 trained animals were studied with doses of 2 mg/kg of amphetamine, 2 mg/kg of chlorpromazine, and saline. The sequences of treatments was counterbalanced for order. These dose levels were chosen on the basis of the results of Experiment 1 and Experiment 4.

The results of this experiment are given in Fig. 2 and Table 2, which are based on deviations from the pre-drug values. The absolute values, which are represented by the zero points on the ordinate, are given in the figure legends. Amphetamine produced a large rise and chlorpromazine a slight depression in reinforcement rate over the 3 hours that the animals were in the cold. By *t* test, the rises after amphetamine for 0–30, 30–60, and 60–120 minutes were significantly different from the control levels. Only at 60–120 minutes did the fall after chlorpromazine reach significance by *t* test, a result similar to Experiment 1 in that the depression produced by 2 mg/kg was slight but consistent.

Chlorpromazine led to a significant decrease in temperature while amphetamine produced hardly any effect. The lack of increase in skin temperature after amphetamine, despite the marked rise in reinforcement rate, was thought to be due to the possibility that at 2°C the rat loses heat

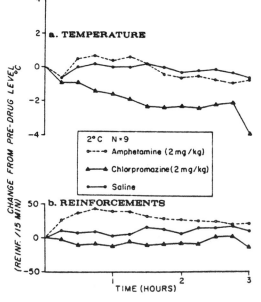

FIGURE 2.   Changes in skin temperature and reinforcement rate after amphetamine and chlorpromazine (Experiment 2). One hour pre-drug reinforcement baseline values (reinf/15 min) were: saline, 105.6; amphetamine, 100.3; chlorpromazine, 103.7. The corresponding pre-drug baseline temperatures were: 38.1°, 38.2°, and 38.3°C, respectively. These are the values represented by zero on the ordinates.

TABLE 2.   Results of analyses of variance, Experiment 2.

		Minutes		
	0–30	30–60	60–120	120–180
Temperature				
$F_{2,16}$	1.0	2.65	5.96	3.33
P	N.S.	N.S.	<.05	N.S. (0.10)
t test P <.05	—	—	0-CPZ	0-CPZ
Reinforcements				
$F_{2,16}$	4.75	11.73	8.87	2.82
P	<.05	<.01	<.01	N.S.
t test P <.05	0-Amphet.	0-Amphet.	0-Amphet. 0-CPZ	—

so rapidly that the effects of variations in reinforcement rate might be masked. The next experiment examined this notion.

EXPERIMENT 3.   *Skin temperature and reinforcement rate at 10°C after amphetamine.*   In this third experiment, a dose of 2 mg/kg of amphet-

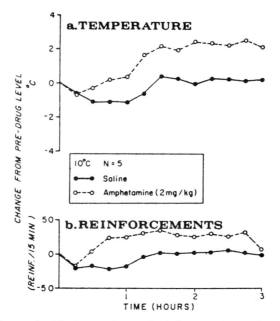

FIGURE 3.   Changes in skin temperature and reinforcement rate after amphetamine at 10°C (Experiment 3). One hour pre-drug reinforcement rates (reinf/15 min) were: saline, 60.4; amphetamine, 48.2. The corresponding pre-drug baseline temperatures were 37.4° and 35.6°C, respectively. These are the values represented by zero on the ordinates.

amine was again administered. Five trained animals were used. Each ran once under the drug and once under saline. The temperature of the cold room was maintained at 10°C. The data of this experiment are given in Fig. 3 and Table 3 as deviations from the pre-drug values. The absolute values appear in the figure legend. As can be seen there, amphetamine produced an increase in reinforcement rate considerably above that achieved with saline. Moreover, it produced a corresponding increase in the tempera-

TABLE 3.   Results of analyses of variance, Experiment 3.

	Minutes			
	0–30	30–60	60–120	120–180
Temperature				
$F_{1,4}$	0.20	1.09	6.47	15.40
P	N.S.	N.S.	$<.10$	$<.05$
Reinforcements				
$F_{1,4}$	0.59	4.76	19.58	6.72
P	N.S.	$<.10$	$<.05$	$<.10$

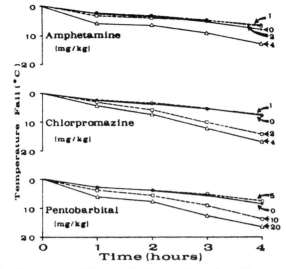

FIGURE 4.   Temperature fall at 2°C after amphetamine, chlorpromazine, and pentobarbital (Experiment 4). Pre-drug mean values were: amphetamine, 32.7°; chlorpromazine, 32.7°; pentobarbital, 32.5°C. These are the values represented by zero
on the ordinates.

ture maintained at the skin surface which was more marked this time than
previously, presumably because the higher ambient temperature did not
allow rapid dissipation of heat.

EXPERIMENT 4.   *Temperature fall at 2°C after amphetamine, chlorpromazine, and pentobarbital.*   The results of this experiment are shown in
Fig. 4 and Table 4. The actual pre-drug baseline temperatures are given
in the figure legend. Analyses of variance were calculated for each of the
4 hours after drug administration. All of these produced statistically significant F ratios.

The trends can be seen in Fig. 4. A dose of 4 mg/kg of amphetamine
produced a significantly faster drop in body temperature than the lower
doses. Both 2 and 4 mg/kg of chlorpromazine accelerated the fall in
temperature produced by cold exposure. Both 10 and 20 mg/kg of pentobarbital produced a significantly greater fall in temperature than saline as
determined by *t* test.

DISCUSSION

At appropriate dose levels, amphetamine and chlorpromazine can impair
behavioral thermoregulation. Amphetamine demonstrated such an effect
most clearly. In Experiments 1, 2, and 3, doses of 2 mg/kg of amphetamine

TABLE 4.   Results of analyses of variance, Experiment 4.

	Minutes			
	60	120	180	240
Amphetamine				
$F_{3.30}$	19.69	9.72	6.30	4.74
P	<.001	<.001	<.01	<.01
t test P <.05	0–2	0–4	0–4	0–4
	0–4			
CPZ				
$F_{3.30}$	9.58	6.42	7.51	8.46
P	<.001	<.01	<.001	<.001
t test P <.05	0–4	0–2	0–2	0–2
		0–4	0–4	0–4
Pentobarbital				
$F_{3\ 30}$	20.95	10.23	6.03	4.30
P	<.001	<.001	<.01	<.05
t test P <.05	0–10	0–10	0–10	0–20
	0–20	0–20	0–20	

caused the rats to increase the frequency with which they turned on the heat lamp. When the ambient temperature was high enough so that the added heat was not quickly dissipated (Experiment 3), skin temperature rose above its normal value. Experiment 4 demonstrated that this quantity of amphetamine did not affect the automatic mechanisms of temperature regulation enough to produce more than a transient change in the rate at which rectal temperature fell in the cold. We do not know, of course, the relative contribution of the various individual mechanisms such as metabolic rate, peripheral blood flow, spontaneous motor activity, *etc.* The end result, however, was a fall in temperature indistinguishable from that produced by saline. But whatever the mechanisms, the important fact is that after amphetamine, skin temperature was kept higher than normal, indicating deficient control of behavior by this physiological variable.

Chlorpromazine acted in a different way. Despite the fact that a dose of 2 mg/kg significantly enhanced the rate at which temperature fell in the cold (Experiments 2 and 4), there was no compensatory rise in the rate at which the rat turned on the heat lamp. In fact, there was a pronounced tendency, shown in both Experiments 1 and 2, for this rate to be maintained below its normal value. Experiment 4 confirms the data of other investigators on the acceleration of heat loss by chlorpromazine (for example, Forster *et al.,* 1956), a result arising from factors such as increased peripheral vasodilation (Chevillard and Giono, 1956), and sprawling (Le-

Blanc, 1958). Experiments 1 and 2 demonstrate impairment of the behavioral mechanisms as well. This disparity agrees with Schwartzbaum's finding (1955) that 10 mg/kg of chlorpromazine did not alter preferred environmental temperature in the rat but did interfere with a behavioral mechanism for regulating it, namely, nest building. A sharp contrast to this sort of disparity is offered by thyroid deficiency, which also impairs some of the reflex mechanisms but in which compensations are made by the behavioral ones (Laties and Weiss, 1959). The chlorpromazine data, however, are complicated by the possibility that the sedating properties of the drug may themselves be due in part to its propensity for lowering body temperature at environmental temperatures below that of the body (Lessin and Parkes, 1957).

Pentobarbital did not seem to impair behavioral thermoregulation despite its ability in higher doses to accelerate the decline in body temperature produced by exposing shaved rats to cold (Experiment 4). Dose levels that did not wholly immobilize the rat (less than 20 mg/kg) led to only a transient fall in the rate at which the heat lamp was turned on. Although this conclusion must be tempered by the lack of concurrent behavioral and temperature data for this drug, it appears reasonable because of the correlation between skin temperature and reinforcement rate in the cases of amphetamine and chlorpromazine.

The effects of a drug upon behavior are, in part, a function of the reinforcement schedule that maintains the behavior, that is, the program that states the relation between the behavior and the occurrence of reinforcements. The schedule used in the present experiments specified that each response made while the lamp was off turned it on. Such a program is called a continuous reinforcement schedule (CRF) and generally evokes a relatively low rate of responding compared to schedules of reinforcement on which only occasional responses are reinforced, for example, fixed ratio schedules which specify that a reinforcement will occur only every n responses. On a CRF schedule amphetamine tends to raise the frequency of responding. For example, increases in frequency of responding on CRF have been noted by Weissman (1959) after 1 mg/kg, by Stone *et al.* (1958) after 1.75 mg/kg, by Teitelbaum and Derks (1958) after 1 mg/kg. Amphetamine also increases the rate at which the lever is pressed to avoid electric shock (Verhave, 1958; Sidman, 1956) and to turn off a loud noise (Harrison and Abelson, 1959).

Chlorpromazine, in contrast, tends to reduce response frequency on a CRF schedule. Weissman (1959) noted such an effect after 5 mg/kg and Stone *et al.* (1958) after 1.5 mg/kg. The latter investigators also found that the main contribution to the decline in rate was the presence of rather long interresponse times, that is, long periods in which no responses occurred. In the cold, long interresponse times promote rapid heat loss and could account for the present observations. Doses in this range have also been observed to affect avoidance behavior (for example, Verhave *et al.,* 1958; Weissman, 1959). It must be stressed, however, as Dews and Morse (1961) have said, that such effects can be reversed by choosing another reinforcement schedule, and it is conceivable that this would be true of our situation as well. Indeed, we have presented elsewhere evidence of schedule effects in behavioral thermoregulation (Weiss and Laties, 1960).

As we said in the introduction, we expected that the drugs we used would affect thermoregulatory behavior differently from behavior maintained by food or water deprivation because the former is more responsive to homeostatic variables. One possible reason for not finding such differences is that both amphetamine and chlorpromazine can weaken the control that various stimuli exert over behavior. For example, amphetamine causes increased responding during extinction (periods when no reinforcement can be forthcoming) both in rats that are undergoing this procedure for the first time (Skinner and Heron, 1937) and in rats that have undergone training on reinforcement schedules on which extinction periods occasionally appear and are designated by an exteroceptive stimulus such as a light (Sidman, 1956; Weissman, 1959). Amphetamine also causes animals working on a schedule which specifies a minimum waiting period between successive responses to increase their response rate well above the optimum rate (Sidman, 1956; Segal, 1962). And, even more to the point from the standpoint of regulation, Teitelbaum and Derks (1958) have reported that amphetamine will also increase water lapping and consumption when such a response postpones shock, although amphetamine reduces drinking in the free situation. Thus, there is evidence that amphetamine reduces the ability of discriminative stimuli to control behavior. Chlorpromazine too impairs stimulus control; for example, chlorpromazine wipes out differences in performance elicited by two different components of a reinforcement schedule which are designated by exteroceptive stimuli both in pigeons (Dews, 1958) and in dogs (Waller, 1961). Chlorpromazine also reduces the ability of a conditioned stimulus to evoke an avoidance response to electric shock (Dews and Morse, 1961). If one looks upon thermoregulatory behavior as behavior controlled mainly by interoceptive stimuli (the skin or central temperature), then one could say that amphetamine and chlorpromazine weaken the control that these stimuli exert on behavior much as they weaken the control that exteroceptive stimuli exert.

Our data, then, in company with those of the investigators cited above, support the statement that the effects of these drugs on thermoregulatory behavior are similar to their effects on behavior maintained by food or water. That this occurred despite the atypical features of the heat reinforcement situation argues for the conclusion that the behavioral properties of these drugs are largely independent of the reinforcer that maintains the behavior or, put another way, of the motivational state that supports it.

SUMMARY

The effects of amphetamine, chlorpromazine, and pentobarbital were studied in rats trained to warm themselves in the cold by pressing a lever that turned on a heat lamp. Amphetamine, at a dose level that by itself did not increase the rate at which body temperature fell in the cold, increased the frequency with which the lamp was turned on even though the skin temperature was driven above normal. Chlorpromazine, at a dose level that accelerated heat loss in the cold, decreased the frequency with which the lamp was turned on. Pentobarbital produced only a transient depression directly correlated with dose level. Both amphetamine and chlorpromazine, therefore, impair behavioral regulation, the former by increasing and the latter by decreasing the optimal frequency of bursts of heat. These effects are similar to those observed by investigators who have used food or water to maintain behavior.

REFERENCES

Chevillard, L., and Giono, R.: *C.R. Soc. Biol.,* Paris 150:330, 1956.

Dews, P. B.: *Fed. Proc.* 17:1024, 1958.

Dews, P. B., and Morse, W. H.: *Annu. Rev. Pharmacol.* 1:145, 1961.

Forster, E., Kayser, C., Maier, A., and Schaff, G.: *Arch. Sci. physiol.* 10:363, 1956.

Harrison, J. M., and Abelson, R. M.: *J. exp. Anal. Behav.* 2:23, 1959.

Laties, V. G., and Weiss, B.: *Amer. J. Physiol.* 197:1028, 1959.

LeBlanc, J: *J. appl. Physiol.* 13:237, 1958.

Lessin, A. W., and Parkes, M. W.: *Brit. J. Pharmacol.* 12:245, 1957.

Schwartzbaum, J. S.: *Proc. Soc. exp. Biol.,* N.Y. 90:275, 1955.

Segal, E. F.: *J. exp. Anal. Behav.* 5:105, 1962.

Sidman, M.: *Ann. N.Y. Acad. Sci.* 65:282, 1956.

Skinner, B. F., and Heron, W. T.: *Psychol. Rec.* 1:340, 1937.

Stone, G. C., Calhoun, D. W., and Kloppenstein, M. H.: *J. comp. Physiol. Psychol.* 51:315, 1958.

Teitelbaum, P., and Derks, P.: *J. comp. Physiol. Psychol.* 51:801, 1958.

Verhave, T.: *J. exp. Anal. Behav.* 1:207, 1958.

Verhave, T., Owen, J. E., and Robbins, E. B.: *Arch. int. Pharmacodyn.* 116:45, 1958.

Waller, M. B.: *J. exp. Anal. Behav.* 4:351, 1961.

Weiss, B., and Laties, V. G.: *J. comp. Physiol. Psychol.* 53:603, 1960.

Weiss, B., and Laties, V. G.: *Science* 133:1338, 1961.

Weissman, A.: *J. exp. Anal. Behav.* 2:271, 1959.

30

Cocaine-reinforced behavior in rats: Effects of reinforcement magnitude and fixed-ratio size [1]

ROY PICKENS and TRAVIS THOMPSON

The reinforcing effects of drugs have been increasingly studied over the past ten years (Headlee *et al.*, 1955; Davis and Nichols, 1962). In these studies primary attention has been directed toward the reinforcing properties of opiates in animals previously made physically dependent on the drug. The effects of drug deprivation and nalorphine antagonism on morphine self-administration have been reported (Thompson and Schuster, 1964; Weeks, 1962). These investigations indicate that drug-deprivation conditions are an important factor controlling drug-reinforced behavior in physically dependent animals.

The self-administration of drugs which do not produce physical dependence (*e.g.*, cocaine) has also been reported (G. A. Deneau, personal communication). The extent to which drug deprivation alters the self-administration of these drugs is not known. The present study demonstrated that cocaine self-administration is a drug-reinforcement effect, and explored the effects of reinforcement magnitude (drug dose per infusion) and value of a fixed-ratio (FR) reinforcement schedule on this performance. In an FR schedule, reinforcement is presented following a fixed number of responses after the preceding reinforcement (Ferster and Skinner, 1957). These variables were selected for study since they are known to affect morphine-reinforced behavior in physically dependent animals (Weeks and Collins, 1964).

METHODS

EXPERIMENT 1. The self-administration of cocaine may be merely a reflection of the drug's non-instrumental or activity effects. Several control experiments were performed to establish that cocaine serves as a reinforcer for the behavior leading to drug injection.

Subjects. The subjects were two experimentally naive male Holtzman albino rats, about 150 days old. They were maintained on freely available food and water for the duration of the experiment.

From *Journal of Pharmacology and Experimental Therapeutics*, 1968, 161, 122–129. Copyright © 1968 by The Williams and Wilkins Co., Baltimore, Md.

[1] This research was supported in part by U.S. Public Health Service Research Grants MH-08565, MH-11135 and MH-14112 to the University of Minnesota.

298

Apparatus.   Each subject was equipped with a device that permitted the i.v. injection of drugs without interfering with the animal's normal movement. The device was similar to one described by Davis (1966), and consisted of a chronic jugular catheter which passed subcutaneously to an exit on the animal's back, where it connected to a length of needle tubing that passed through a hole in the top center of the cage. The needle tubing was attached at one end to the animal by a subcutaneously implanted shoulder harness and at the other end to a leakproof swivel, which was connected by rubber tubing to an infusion pump. Activation of the infusion pump was programmed to deliver a 50-sec infusion of 0.5 ml of drug solution,[2] which passed through the tubing and catheter and was injected into the animal's bloodstream in or near the heart.

The cages, measuring 10 by 10 by 9 inches, were equipped with single or double levers, food and water supplies and a stimulus light. Each cage was enclosed within a ventilated, sound-attenuating compartment. Programming and recording apparatus were located in a separate room.

Procedure.   Immediately after catheterization the subjects were placed in the injection cages where they lived for the duration of the experiment. The drug was available for infusion from about 9:00 A.M. until about 11:00 P.M. daily, during which time the animals were allowed to respond *ad libitum,* with each response delivering 0.5 mg/kg of cocaine hydrochloride in isotonic saline solution. All experimental manipulations were carried out when the mean number of reinforcements per hour was essentially constant, which occurred usually by the 3rd day after surgery.

Four response-infusion contingency manipulations were performed. These manipulations consisted of changing drug infusions from response-contingent to noncontingent, discontinuing drug infusion with and without stimuli normally correlated with infusion and requiring the animal to learn a new response to produce drug infusion. The effects of these manipulations on responding were recorded.

EXPERIMENT 2.   This experiment investigated the effect of reinforcement magnitude and the value of the FR schedule on cocaine-reinforced behavior.

Subjects and apparatus.   The subjects were three naive albino rats similar to those used in experiment 1, and the apparatus was the same.

Procedure.   The procedure for establishing cocaine self-administration was the same as in experiment 1, except that a stimulus light was always illuminated during drug infusion to facilitate conditioning.

The effect of magnitude of reinforcement (drug dose per infusion) on cocaine self-administration was determined with all three animals. By systematically varying the concentration of the drug solution the reinforce-

[2] The duration and volume of infusion were selected to avoid sudden changes in blood-fluid level at the heart, while maintaining accuracy of dose infusion.

ment dose was decreased, and then increased, until both upper and lower limits of magnitude of reinforcement effect were obtained. Each experimental condition was maintained for at least 6 hr, and was replicated twice for all animals. The effects of reinforcement magnitude were assessed on both frequency and temporal spacing of responses.

Several doses of cocaine were then used to study the effects of an FR schedule on response and reinforcement frequency. These effects were determined on two subjects; the third died after completion of the magnitude of reinforcement study. The effects of varying FR values from FR 5 through FR 80 were determined for doses of 0.25 to 3.0 mg/kg. For each dose, ratio value was increased until responding ceased altogether. Subjects were maintained at each condition for about 6 hr.

EXPERIMENT 3. In experiment 2, an inverse relationship was found between response rate and magnitude of reinforcement (infusion dose). However, in other studies using food and water as reinforcers, a direct relationship has been found between these variables (e.g., Shettleworth and Nevin, 1965). This difference may be due to the fact that in such studies food was available daily only for a relatively short period (usually 1 hr or less), whereas in our experiment cocaine was available for about 14 hr each day. The present experiment explores the effect of magnitude of reinforcement on rate of responding for food under conditions of increased availability, to account for apparent differences in the reinforcing effects of food and cocaine.

Subject. The subject was one naive albino rat, similar to those used in the previous experiments.

Apparatus. The apparatus was a standard operant-conditioning chamber with two levers, houselight, water bottle and food-delivery mechanism. The chamber was located in a sound-shielding cover box. All experimental events were controlled automatically.

Procedure. The subject lived in the conditioning chamber for the duration of the experiment. Each lever press by the subject was programmed to deliver 1, 5, 10 or 20 45-mg pellets of food, which were available 24 hr per day. Four days of responding were obtained at each reinforcement magnitude, and the procedure was then replicated three times, each time in a different order. A small stimulus light was illuminated during operation of the food-delivery mechanism. Responding was recorded in the same manner as that used with cocaine.

EXPERIMENT 4. In experiment 2, performance maintained by cocaine was characterized by unusually long post-reinforcement pauses, which were not seen with food reinforcement in experiment 3. While the long post-reinforcement pause obtained with cocaine may be interpreted as a drug-satiation effect, it may also reflect a disruption in performance produced by the drug and/or drug injection. The purpose of the present experiment, therefore, was to determine the effect of i.v. administered cocaine on performance maintained by another reinforcer.

Subject.   The subject was one naive albino rat similar to that used in the previous experiment, except that it was maintained at 80% of normal body weight.

Apparatus.   The apparatus was similar to that used in the previous experiment, but had been modified to incorporate the infusion device described previously. The infusion pump was shock-mounted outside the sound-shielding enclosure.

Procedure.   The subject was pretrained for 45 days to respond on an FR 10 schedule for a single pellet of food. Training sessions were conducted daily from Monday through Friday, and each session ended when 300 reinforcements had occurred. On the morning of the 46th training day the subject was prepared with an intravenous catheter and returned to the home cage. Infusions of 1.0 mg/kg of cocaine were administered automatically each hour until the start of the afternoon's training session 5 hr later, and 5 hr before the start of the training session on the following 2 days. The animal received hourly infusions of saline overnight.

During the training session on the days after surgery the animal was trained as usual, except that after a base-line interval of FR responding the infusion pump was activated, delivering either saline or a 0.5-, 1.0- or 1.5-mg/kg infusion of cocaine. Each dose was administered at least twice. Effects of the infusions on food-reinforced responding were recorded.

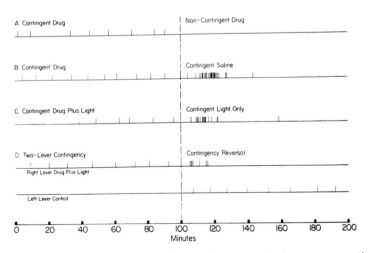

FIGURE 1.   Effects of response-infusion contingency variations on responding for 0.5-mg/kg cocaine infusion. Responding is shown as vertical deflections on event records. Contingency changes were made at the dashed vertical line 100 min into each session.

RESULTS

EXPERIMENT 1.   Figure 1 shows the effect of manipulations designed to demonstrate the reinforcing properties of cocaine. Such an effect would be indicated by the dependence of the behavior upon the contiguity between the response and its consequence. The data shown are for one animal, although similar results were also obtained with the second animal.

Figure 1A shows the effect of switching from response-contingent infusion of 0.5 mg/kg of cocaine to the same number of infusions per hour presented automatically, but not contingent on lever pressing. As can be seen, responding ceased altogether, indicating that drug-induced increases in activity or other noninstrumental effects were not maintaining responding.

If cocaine is serving as a reinforcer, discontinuation of the consequence of responding would eliminate the behavior through extinction. Figure 1B shows the effect upon response rate when saline was substituted for the drug. An initial rate increase characteristic of extinction was followed by cessation of responding. In Fig. 1C, cocaine infusion was discontinued, but the light which had been paired with infusion was continued. A pattern of responding similar to that seen with saline alone ensued, i.e., an initial rate increase followed by cessation of responding, indicating the light itself was not a reinforcer. Finally, in a two-lever cage, responses on one lever were followed by cocaine infusion and light while responses on the second lever had no consequence. As shown in figure 1D, regularly spaced responding occurred on the infusion lever, with no responding on the other lever. When the lever contingencies were reversed, there was an initial rate increase on the lever previously delivering infusion, followed by a rapid diminution of responding on that lever and a rather abrupt increase in rate on the second lever. The data in Fig. 1 clearly indicate that cocaine infusion is acting as a reinforcer, since cocaine self-administration was dependent on the contiguous relationship between the response and its consequence.

EXPERIMENT 2.   The effects of magnitude of reinforcement (drug dose per infusion) on drug-reinforced responding are shown in Fig. 2. In all cases, original effect and replication yielded essentially the same results, and for that reason were combined in the figure. The bar graphs illustrate frequency of self-infusion for each subject as a function of drug dose, and the event records show the temporal distribution of infusions. The 40-min event records presented were taken randomly during much longer infusion sessions. Doses high and lower than those shown for each animal did not maintain responding, but produced instead erratic performance leading to a cessation of responding at the low doses and abrupt cessation of respond-

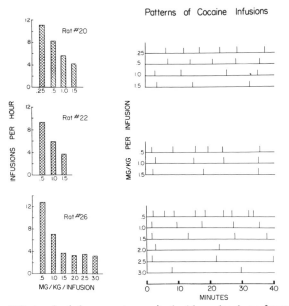

FIGURE 2.   Effects of reinforcement magnitude (drug dose) on frequency and temporal distribution of cocaine reinforcement. Data shown are for all doses that maintained responding.

ing at the high doses. As can be seen, increases in cocaine dose are associated with decreased frequency of reinforcement. This inverse relationship between dose and frequency of reinforcement approached linearity at the low and moderate doses of the drug. As is shown in the data for rat 26, increases in the higher doses of the drug did not produce corresponding decreases in frequency of reinforcement. There is, in fact, little difference between the self-administration of 2.0 and 3.0 mg/kg of the drug. The mean intakes of cocaine at all self-administered doses for the three animals were 5.3, 5.7 and 7.3 mg/kg/hr, and the mean intake of all animals at all doses was 6.1 mg/kg/hr.

The effects of varying the value of an FR schedule of reinforcement on response frequency and number of drug reinforcements are shown for a 1.0-mg/kg dose of cocaine in Fig. 3. All ratios found to maintain responding are presented. When the number of responses necessary for drug reinforcement was increased, proportionate increases in frequency of responding were found, with the result that about the same amount of drug was taken under each ratio value. The mean drug intake across all FR values at 1.0 mg/kg was 6.8 mg/kg/hr.

Figure 4 presents representative cumulative records of FR performance of one animal (rat 22) at all ratio values and reinforcement magnitudes which maintained responding. Responding was not sustained at ratios

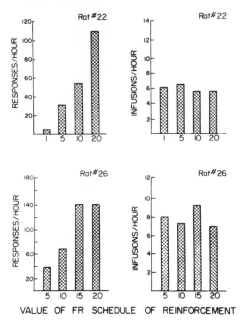

VALUE OF FR SCHEDULE OF REINFORCEMENT

FIGURE 3. Effects of value of FR reinforcement schedule on reinforcement frequency for 1.0 mg/kg of cocaine. Data shown are for all ratio values that maintained responding.

greater than FR 1 with reinforcement magnitudes below 0.5 mg/kg/infusion, and the largest reinforcement magnitude which would maintain performance was 1.5 mg/kg/infusion. Below 0.5 mg/kg infusion (0.25 mg/kg/infusion), performance became consistently ragged with long pauses, leading in some cases to cessation of responding. At drug doses greater than 1.5 mg/kg/infusion (2.0 and 2.5 mg/kg/infusion), two or three infusions would be taken and then responding would cease entirely. At these doses there was no progressive disruption or other changes characteristic of either extinction or satiation (Ferster and Skinner, 1957). Within the defined reinforcement-magnitude range, responding was maintained over a wide variety of FR values and magnitudes of reinforcement. For this animal, ratio performance was regular, with relatively long but constant interratio interval (post-reinforcement pause) and constant running rate up to FR 20 at 0.5 mg/kg/infusion, FR 60 at 1.0 mg/kg/infusion and FR 80 as 1.5 mg/kg/infusion. Increasing the ratio size above these values for a given reinforcement magnitude led to marked interruptions in responding, and finally to cessation of responding.

For rat 26, responding was sustained over a wider range of reinforcement magnitudes (0.5–3.0 mg/kg/infusion) but at lower ratio values, up to

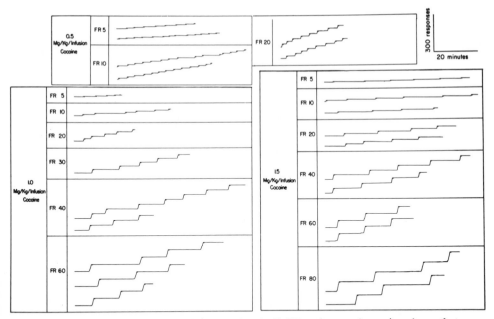

FIGURE 4. Sample cumulative records of all FR values and cocaine doses that maintained responding for rat 22. For each FR value and dose condition, upper record represents initial effect and lower record represents replication when given.

FR 15 (with 1.0–3.0 mg/kg/infusion) and up to FR 20 (with 1.0 mg/kg/ infusion). Only FR 10 performance was maintained by a 0.5-mg/kg infusion.

EXPERIMENT 3.   Responding for food reinforcement under conditions of unrestricted availability yielded an inverse relationship between response rate and reinforcement magnitude, similar to that observed with cocaine under conditions of availability for 14 hr daily. However, no regularly spaced pauses after reinforcement were evident with food, as had been found with cocaine. Figure 5 presents the effects of magnitude of food reinforcement on response rate. As shown in the figure, under these conditions increases in the number of food pellets per reinforcement were associated with decreases in response rate, and about the same number of pellets per day were taken at each reinforcement value. The mean number of responses per day was 19.8, 3.9, 1.9 and 1.1, and the number of pellets received per day was 19.8, 19.5, 19.0 and 22.0, for 1, 5, 10 and 20 food pellets per reinforcement, respectively, Thus, the apparent difference between magnitude of reinforcement effect obtained with food and that obtained with cocaine appears to be related to the conditions under which

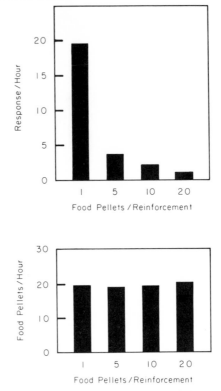

FIGURE 5. Effects of different magnitudes of food reinforcement on response frequency and total number of food pellets taken each day.

each was studied, and not entirely to differences in the reinforcers themselves.

EXPERIMENT 4.   Cocaine administered i.v. to an animal responding on an FR 10 schedule of food reinforcement produced a complete disruption of performance. These results are shown in Fig. 6, which presents representative cumulative records of the effects of saline and cocaine on FR performance. As can be seen, saline had little or no effect, whereas all doses of cocaine produced a complete cessation of responding. The lengths of the drug-induced paused were dose-dependent, with the mean pause interval (time between last food reinforcement before pause and first reinforcement after pause) of about 8 min for 0.5, 11 min for 1.0 and 15 min for 1.5 mg/kg of cocaine. After the pause, responding returned at about the same rate as that observed before drug injection.

The similarity of the length of the pauses produced by cocaine in FR food-reinforced responding and the length of cocaine post-reinforcement

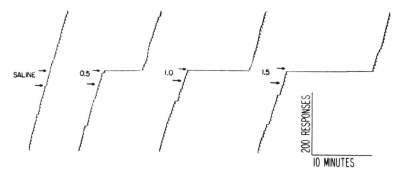

FIGURE 6.   Effects of i.v. infusion of saline and three doses of cocaine on FR 10 food performance. Lower arrow shows onset and upper arrow termination of infusion.

pauses (*e.g.,* Fig. 4) suggests that factors other than drug satiation alone may be operating to determine the latter.

DISCUSSION

The data from experiment 1 establish that the infusion of cocaine contingent on occurrence of an operant response serves as a reinforcer for the response. Stimulant effects or other indirect effects of cocaine could not account for the extinction effects, the discontinuation of responding when the same dose was given noncontingently or the differential responding in a two-lever cage on the lever which produced drug infusion. Thus, it seems clear that cocaine acts as an unconditioned reinforcer.

These data indicate that the reinforcement magnitude and value of an FR reinforcement schedule are important variables influencing cocaine-reinforced behavior. Direct comparisons with the data of Weeks and Collins (1964) on ratio size and dose of morphine per infusion are not possible, since their dependent variable was total drug intake per 24 hr. However, to the extent that total daily intake varied both with ratio size and dose of morphine per infusion, the findings of the present study on hourly cocaine intake appear to be similar.

The regularity in spacing of cocaine-reinforced responding is to be contrasted with Deneau's (personal communication) observation that no consistent pattern of cocaine self-administration by monkeys could be found. Deneau also reported observing an array of toxic signs in animals self-administering cocaine, including weight loss, tremors, ataxia and convulsions, which were observed infrequently and only at high drug doses in our animals. This suggests that the dose range used by him (0.25–1.0 mg/kg/infusion) may have exceeded the maximal effective reinforcing dose for the monkeys.

The mean hourly intake of cocaine was found to be relatively constant across all reinforcement magnitudes (6.1 mg/kg/hr) and ratio values (6.8 mg/kg/hr). When the reinforcement magnitude exceeded approximately one-fourth to one-half of the mean hourly intake (*i.e.,* 1.5 mg/kg/infusion for rat 22 and 3.0 mg/kg/infusion for rat 26) the drug no longer acted as a reinforcer. In one of the two animals studied across a range of doses and ratio values (rat 26), the cocaine-reinforced behavior reflected an interaction between reinforcement magnitude and value of the ratio schedule. When the reinforcement magnitude was relatively low (0.5 mg/kg and below) changes in performance characteristic of insufficient reinforcement with other reinforcers appeared, *e.g.,* intermediate rates and relatively long pausing (Ferster and Skinner, 1957). However, increasing the cocaine reinforcement magnitude above a certain maximal level produced an abrupt cessation of responding, which is rarely seen with food or water reinforcement. This effect is similar to the decreased rate of responding produced by intracranial reinforcement (Olds, 1958) and heat reinforcement (Weiss and Laties, 1960) when the magnitude of reinforcement is increased above an optimal level. Although pausing was relatively longer, increases in ratio size produced changes in performance similar to those commonly obtained with other reinforcers (Morse, 1966). However, rather than obtaining a gradual, overall negatively accelerated curve, animals tend to emit several ratio runs followed by long pauses. If the increased ratio has exceeded a critical value, responding ceases altogether.

SUMMARY

Cocaine was shown to serve as a reinforcer for the rat. The effects of different infusion doses and fixed-ratio schedules on cocaine self-administration were studied. Within the range of doses that maintained responding, the response rate was found to vary inversely as a function of drug dose per infusion (reinforcement magnitude) and directly as a function of size of the fixed ratio. Outside this range, low doses produced ragged performance and high doses caused responding to cease entirely. In general, ratio performance was somewhat dependent on reinforcement magnitude, with higher ratios being achieved by intermediate and higher drug doses. Food reinforcement under conditions resembling those used with cocaine also yielded an inverse relationship between reinforcement magnitude and response rate, reconciling what appeared to be a major difference between the reinforcers. The most striking characteristic of cocaine-reinforced behavior was long but regularly spaced pauses after reinforcement. Comparable pauses were obtained in food-reinforced fixed-ratio performance after cocaine infusion, suggesting the effect may be due at least in part to performance disruption produced by the drug.

REFERENCES

Davis, J. D.: A method for chronic intravenous infusion in freely moving rats. *J. Exp. Anal. Behav.* 9:385–387, 1966.

Davis, W. M., and Nichols, J. R.: Physical dependence and substained opiate-directed behavior in the rat. A preliminary report. *Psychopharmacology* 3:139–145, 1962.

Ferster, C. B., and Skinner, B. F.: *Schedules of reinforcement,* Appleton-Century-Crofts, New York, 1957.

Headlee, C. P., Coppock, H. W., and Nichols, J. R.: Apparatus and technique involved in a laboratory method of detecting the addictiveness of drugs. *J. Amer. Pharm. Ass.* 44:229–231, 1955.

Morse, W. H.: Intermittent reinforcement. In *Operant behavior: Areas of research and application,* ed. by W. H. Honig, pp. 52–108, Appleton-Century-Crofts, New York, 1966.

Olds, J.: Self-stimulation of the brain. *Science* (Wash.) 127:315–324, 1958.

Shettleworth, S., and Nevin, J. A.: Relative rate of response and relative magnitude of reinforcement in multiple schedules. *J. Exp. Anal. Behav.* 8:199–202, 1965.

Thompson, T., and Schuster, C. R.: Morphine self-administration, food-reinforced and avoidance behaviors in rhesus monkeys. *Psychopharmacologia* 5:87–94, 1964.

Weeks, J. R.: Experimental morphine addiction: Method for automatic intravenous injections in unrestrained rats. *Science* (Wash.) 138:143–144, 1962.

Weeks, J. R., and Collins, R. J.: Factors affecting voluntary morphine intake in self-maintained addicted rats. *Psychopharmacologia* 6:267–279, 1964.

Weiss, B., and Laties, V. G.: Magnitude of reinforcement as a variable in thermoregulatory behavior. *J. Comp. Physiol. Psychol.* 53:603–608, 1960.

31

Effects of intravenous injections of epinephrine and norepinephrine in a choice situation [1]

SETH K. SHARPLESS

Demonstrations that the autonomic nervous system is not essential for emotional behavior (Cannon, 1929; Sherrington, 1947) have never seemed altogether convincing to experimental psychologists. There has been a recurring suspicion that complex, learned responses motivated by fear may be mediated in some way by feedback stimulation from the peripheral autonomic system. The strongest theoretical formulation came from Mowrer (1947), who argued that the state of fear which motivates avoidance behavior consists precisely in the internal disequilibrium produced by a conditioned autonomic reaction. An attempt to subject this proposition to an experimental test was undertaken by Wynne and Solomon (1955). They found that once an avoidance response had been learned, it was completely unaffected by suppression of autonomic function. However, if autonomic function had been impaired prior to the initial learning, by sympathectomy or parasympathetic blockade or both, more trials were often required to learn the response and it was less resistant to extinction than in normal animals. These findings suggested that although autonomic reactions had no important role in the performance of avoidance responses already in the animal's repertoire, they might have a significant role in the initial learning of such responses.

There are several ways in which nervous or humoral feedback stimulation from autonomic reactions might conceivably play a role in the initial learning of emotional behavior. In the first place, feedback from autonomic reactions presumably contributes to the pool of afferent impulses maintaining activity in the reticular activating system and helps to sustain alertness. It is known, for example, that epinephrine in small quantities may act on the medial brain stem to produce EEG activation (Bonvallet, Dell, and Hiebel, 1954; Rothballer, 1956). In this way, autonomic reactions might contribute in a nonspecific way to any kind of learning—by maintaining an adequate degree of vigilance.

Secondly, feedback from autonomic reactions might function as a negative drive, in the sense that an animal will learn responses that lead to the

From *Journal of Comparative and Physiological Psychology*, 1961, **54**, 103–108. Copyright 1961 by the American Psychological Association, Washington, D.C.

[1] This investigation was supported by National Science Foundation Grant G-4459. The author gratefully acknowledges the help of Peter Ramos.

cessation or diminution of feedback stimulation from autonomic reactions. Thus, Solomon and Brush (1956) suggest that "the stimulus pattern from the viscera serves as an important aversive stimulus pattern (drive) in its own right" (p. 286).

Thirdly, feedback stimulation from autonomic reactions may be capable of acting as negative reinforcement, functioning as a kind of internal surrogate for punishment. It is known, for example, that epinephrine may inhibit learned responses, apparently by a direct action on the central nervous system, although the dose required (when administered intravenously) would seem to exceed physiological levels (Sharpless, 1959). Feedback from the baroreceptor elements also seems to exert generalized inhibitory effects on central nervous functions (Bonvallet *et al.,* 1954; Dell, Bonvallet, and Hugelin, 1954). It is therefore possible that the suppression of a learned response by punishment ("conditioned emotional response," Hunt and Brady, 1951) is mediated in the initial stages of learning by nervous or humoral feedback from autonomic reactions. Later, by a short-circuiting principle, the environmental stimulus might come to activate the inhibitory mechanism directly, and the autonomic reactions would become unnecessary.

The present study is concerned with the third alternative—the possibility that feedback from autonomic reactions has negative reinforcing value. It is possible to reproduce most of the effects of sympathoadrenal discharge by intravenous injections of small quantities of sympathomimetic drugs—epinephrine and norepinephrine. In this experiment, an attempt has been made to "punish" animals for making incorrect responses by injecting the drugs directly into the superior *vena cava* through implanted catheters at appropriate times during the animal's performance in a test situation. It was expected that if the pattern of interoceptive stimulation produced by sympathoadrenal discharge has significant negative reinforcing value, this would be revealed by changes in subsequent behavior.

METHOD. *Subjects.* The Ss were 45 male rats of the Sprague–Dawley strain, 10 to 15 weeks old at the beginning of the experiment. They were received in four separate lots, which were run at different times. The animals were divided into experimental groups in such a way that every group was drawn from several lots.

Apparatus and procedure. A T maze was used with 8-in. by 16-in. alleys. A swinging door at the choice point could be used to close off either side alley. Both side alleys contained food and functioned as goal compartments during the experiment. Two brass "shock" plates were attached to the floor of each side alley in such a way that the animal could not reach the food cup without running across both plates. During shock trials, the plates in one alley were charged with 700 v. through 750 k ohms.

The rats were maintained on a 23-hr. feeding schedule. Each animal received eight trials per day. It was placed in the starting alley with its back toward the choice point. When it entered a goal compartment, the door was closed, and the animal was locked in the goal compartment for 2 min. during which time it was free to eat or explore. At the end of 2 min., it was replaced in a "waiting compartment" adjacent to the starting alley and allowed to remain there for 3 min. before starting the next trial. Choice of goal compartment and running time were recorded.

The rats were trained in the maze for three days prior to the experiment. Polyvinyl catheters were then implanted in the superior *vena cava* (through the external jugular vein), and the animals were allowed to rest for one day. Chronic intravenous catheters and method of implantation have been described elsewhere for cats (Sharpless, 1959). The same method has been used in the present experiment with rats. On the first day of the experiment proper, the animals were run as usual, and the results were used to determine "preferences." On Days 2 to 6, a coiled, springlike polyethylene lead was attached to the animal's catheter and suspended above the maze in such a way that the rat was allowed unrestricted movement in the maze. An injection was then administered through the polyethylene lead each time the rat entered the goal compartment *for which it had exhibited a preference on the first day.* The injection was begun immediately after the rat entered the goal compartment, and required about 5 sec. Approximately 0.1 to 0.2 ml. of fluid was delivered in this time, dependent on the animal's weight. No injection was given if the animal entered the opposite (previously nonfavored) goal compartment.

At the end of the experiment, and occasionally at the end of one of the daily sessions, succinylcholine (0.15 mg/kg) was injected through the catheter to test its patency. If the rat showed muscular weakness immediately following the injection, the catheter was presumed to be intact and in the vein; otherwise, larger doses of succinylcholine were given, and if these also failed to produce the expected effect, the animal was discarded.

The rats were divided into five groups of 8 to 12 members each, receiving different treatment as follows: E: 9 rats, 5 μg/kg epinephrine (crystalline; Mann); NE: 8 rats, 5 μg/kg norepinephrine (as the bitartrate; Levophed, Winthrop Stearns); D: 12 rats, 5% dextrose in physiological saline; H: 8 rats, 8.75 mg/kg histamine (as the phosphate; Fisher); Sh: 8 rats, electric shock. (Doses are given as the weight of the base.) Epinephrine and norepinephrine were given in a solution of 5% dextrose in saline to delay oxidation. The total amount of dextrose administered during a single experimental session was negligible (40 to 80 mg. in 45 min.). The electric shock was not a severe punishment since it was easily escaped by simply running to either end of the goal compartment. However, all the shocked rats showed signs of emotional involvement: defecation, urination, vocalization, and refusal to eat while confined in the goal compartment.

The importance of dosage is discussed below. It should be pointed out here that the doses of epinephrine and norepinephrine were intended to be sufficient to produce a sympathomimetic reaction at least as great as the reflex response to a painful sensory stimulus. The doses were selected partly on the basis of pilot experiments on six rats in which blood pressure and heart rate were recorded. In general, the doses used were sufficient to produce sizable, but not maximal, responses. The heart rate in unanesthetized, unrestrained rats usually decreased following intravenous injections of catecholamines, due presumably to buffer reflexes mediated by baroreceptors. Thus, 5 μg/kg norepinephrine commonly produced cardiac slowing from 350 to 400 beats/min to something less than 200 beats/min, gradually returning to normal in 2 to 3 min.

Histamine was used as a control. It was chosen as a humor-like substance having a relatively brief action of a noxious character, which could be administered to rats in enormous doses without fatal consequences (Bovet and Bovet-Nitti, 1948, p. 718). The dose far exceeded anything that might have physiological significance; indeed, the amount given in a single injection was almost as great as that contained in the entire body of the rat (as judged from the data on the histamine content of various tissues provided by Bovet and Bovet-Nitti, 1948, p. 716). It was hoped that in large doses, the noxious effects of the substance would produce negative reinforcement, showing that the failure of the catecholamines to produce negative reinforcement could not be attributed to the timing of the injections or to other physical characteristics of the experiment. There was some basis in pilot experiments for believing that histamine would have such an effect.

RESULTS.   Aversive properties of the treatment might be revealed in one of the following ways: (*a*) The rats might show a change in preference, avoiding the side of the injection and running more and more frequently to the opposite side. (*b*) After a few initial injections (or shocks), a generalized fear of the apparatus might be established, so that the animal would hesitate to leave the starting box. (*c*) After several days' training, aversive properties of the treatment might be revealed by a difference in the mean running time to the two sides, i.e., the animal might be a little more hesitant in entering the side of injection than in entering the safe side.

The number of runs to the side of treatment on successive days is shown in Fig. 1. Injections were begun on Day 2. For purposes of analysis, each animal received as a score the total number of injections or shocks that it had received on Days 2 to 6. Duncan's multiple range test for heteroscedastic means (1957) was applied to the results. The mean numbers of approaches to the side of injection on Days 2 to 6 for the groups receiving epinephrine, norepinephrine, and dextrose were 21.0, 22.9, and 22, respectively (out of 40 trials). These means did not differ significantly from one another (at the .05 level). On the other hand, both the histamine and shock

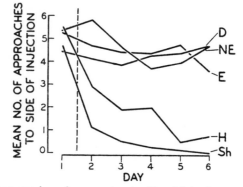

FIGURE 1.   Mean number of approaches to side of injection on successive days for dextrose, norepinephrine, epinephrine, histamine, and shock groups.

groups (an average of 8.1 and 2 approaches, respectively) differed from the other groups at the .01 level.

The question of whether the injection procedure itself produced any effect cannot be answered, since there was no noninjected control group. In Fig. 1, there appears to be a slight shift of preference away from the side of injection in the dextrose, epinephrine, and norepinephrine groups. It should be pointed out that if some of the animals had no real preference but vacillated in a random way from one day to the next, then one would expect a drop in the number of runs to the side of injection simply as a result of a systematic error in selecting the "preferred" side. In any case, a one-tailed t test failed to reveal significant changes of preference from Day 1 to Days 5 and 6 in the groups receiving dextrose, epinephrine, or norepinephrine.

Changes in mean log running time on successive days are shown in Fig. 2. It is especially interesting that both the histamine and shock groups increased in running time in the initial stages of the experiment (from Day 1 to Day 2), indicating that the anxiety associated with the treatment generalized at first to the whole situation. With further training, the running time of the histamine and shock groups gradually decreased until it matched that

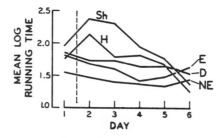

FIGURE 2.   Mean log running time to either side of T maze on successive days.

of the control group. The groups receiving epinephrine and norepinephrine, on the other hand, showed no initial increase in running time, but rather a slight decrease from day to day, as would have been expected as a result of practice in the absence of injections. Scores were assigned to animals on the basis of the changes in mean log running time from the first to the second day. The size of these changes was significant only in the case of the histamine group ($p < .01$), although the change in the shock group fell just short of significance (two-tailed t test). Application of Duncan's multiple range test showed that only the histamine and shock groups differed significantly from the others at the .05 level with respect to changes in running time. The dextrose, epinephrine, and norepinephrine groups did not differ significantly from one another.

The running time to the two sides on the last two days of the experiment were compared. The mean log running times to the injection side with 10% fiducial limits for the epinephrine and norepinephrine groups were 1.57 ± .25 and 1.49 ± .39, respectively, and to the safe side, 1.63 ± .35 and 1.41 ± 19, respectively. It is evident that there is no significant difference in the running time to the two sides. After five days of injections, the rats receiving epinephrine and norepinephrine ran to the side of injection as rapidly as to safe side.

In this experiment, the drugs were given on the side of the T maze that was preferred initially. However, in most cases, the initial "preference" was weak; all animals tended to alternate. Thus, a *positive* reinforcing effect should also have been revealed. No such effect was observed.

DISCUSSION.   These experiments were undertaken to test the hypothesis that nervous or humoral feedback from sympathoadrenal reactions may function in learning as a negative reinforcing agent. This hypothesis was suggested by the fact that blockade of the peripheral autonomic nervous system may retard the initial learning of an emotional response, although it has no effect on responses already in the animal's repertoire (Arbit, 1958; Cannon, 1929; Sherrington, 1947; Wynne and Solomon, 1955).

Experiments which have used autonomic blockade during tests of acquisition are open to the criticism that depression of the autonomic system may have unspecific effects. Thus, feedback afferent stimulation by way of both visceral and somatic nerves may contribute to reticular activation, and epinephrine released from the adrenal medulla into the systemic circulation may excite the reticular system (Bonvallet *et al.,* 1954; Dell and Olson, 1951; Rothballer, 1956, 1959). Blockade of the autonomic system might therefore lead to decreased input to the reticular system and hence, a diminished vigilance and alertness, with possible impairment of learning. Furthermore, autonomic blocking agents often have side effects, which may affect central nervous functioning directly, and surgical interference with the autonomic system may result in impaired homeostatic mechanisms which are revealed when the animal is required to learn something under stress.

In the present experiment, instead of trying to block autonomic reactions, an effort was made to elicit visceral reactions of the type believed to accompany fear and pain by intravenous injections of sympathomimetic drugs. There was no indication that the animals had the slightest aversion to a situation in which sympathomimetic drugs were injected, although controls indicated that the design of the experiments, the timing of the injections, etc. were such that negative reinforcing value, if present, should have been disclosed.

It is evident that dosage is important in the interpretation of these results. It is probable that by increasing the doses of epinephrine and norepinephrine to toxic levels, one could produce negative reinforcement similar to that which occurred with large doses of histamine in the present experiment. Intravenous injections of sympathomimetic drugs in toxic doses may cause ventricular fibrillation, pulmonary edema, and cerebral hemorrhage, and in man, overdoses have produced violent headaches, stabbing retrosternal and pharyngeal pain, vomiting, and other unpleasant symptoms (Goodman and Gilman, 1955). However, the demonstration that toxic doses can be used as negative reinforcement would be of little interest. The maximum dose used in the present experiments (5 μg/kg i.v. in rats) is the lower limit of the toxic dose range for epinephrine in rats, according to the data compiled by Bovet and Bovet-Nitti (1948). (This estimate may be somewhat conservative. Certainly no toxic effects were observed with the doses used in the present experiments.)

The injected amounts probably exceed the maximum capacity of the adrenal medulla when excited reflexly by sensory stimulation, although the doses may be within the capacity of the gland if excited directly by pharmacological agents such as nicotine, potassium, etc. (Bovet and Bovet-Nitti, 1948; Outschoorn, 1952, Satake, 1954; von Euler, 1956). The purpose of the injections, however, was not merely to match the effects of endogenous medullary secretions, but to mimic the sympathoadrenal reaction to a painful stimulus, including the effects mediated by sympathetic nerve fibers. As far as can be judged from what is known of sensitivities of various organs to catecholamines (von Euler, 1956), and the results of pilot experiments in which cardiovascular reactions were measured, the injections were adequate to produce very sizable, but not maximal, reactions. Nevertheless, it is difficult to determine whether the reactions to the injected drugs were sufficient to micmic the sympathetic reactions to painful stimuli, since autonomic reactions to peripheral stimuli tend to be quite variable in unanesthetized animals.

The possible importance of the *pattern* of autonomic activity is also difficult to assess. The classic investigations of Cannon (1929) showed that sympathoadrenal discharge characterizes fear, pain, rage, and allied emotions, and that most of the effects of this discharge can be reproduced by injected epinephrine. Many of the minor discrepancies observed by Cannon and his collaborators were later accounted for by the observation that norepinephrine rather than epinephrine is the predominant chemical mediator at the sympathetic neuroeffector junction. Norepinephrine also lacked negative reinforcing value in the present experiments. There are some features of sympathetic discharge that cannot be mimicked by exogenous catecholamines, including the activity of cholinergic sweat glands and certain kinds of sympathetic vasodilatation (Goodman and Gilman, 1955). It seems unlikely that these differences could be the essential factors converting the otherwise neutral feedback stimulation from a global sympathoadrenal discharge into a form of punishment.

In this experiment, an unsuccessful attempt was made to use the onset of a sympathomimetic reaction as negative reinforcement. It remains possible that the *termination* of such a reaction could serve as *positive* reinforcement —that a response leading to the diminution of sympathoadrenal discharge would be strengthened. This is the implication of the theory that feedback from sympathoadrenal discharge functions as an aversive drive stimulus in learning (Solomon and Brush, 1956). It should be pointed out in this connection that the effects of an injection of epinephrine or norepinephrine persist for several minutes. It is therefore unlikely that the termination of an intravenous injection of exogenous sympathomimetic amines would have reinforcing value, since the effects of the injection would persist for minutes after the injection itself had been stopped. Furthermore, human subjects receiving injections of epinephrine or norepinephrine do not usually comment on the aversive effects of the stimulus, although they occasionally recognize the subjective sensations as those which accompany emotional reactions ("cold emotions," see review by Rothballer, 1959).

SUMMARY.   An attempt was made to test the hypothesis that nervous or humoral feedback from sympathoadrenal discharge may function as a negative reinforcing agent in the acquisition of emotional behavior. The injection of sympatholmimetic drugs through permanently implanted intravenous catheters was substituted for electric shock as punishment in a maze situation. There was no evidence that the reactions to the injections had negative reinforcing value, although controls indicated that the design of the experiments, the timing of the injections, etc. were such that negative reinforcing value, if present, should have been revealed.

REFERENCES

Arbit, J. Shock motivated serial discrimination learning and the chemical block of autonomic impulses. *J. comp. physiol. Psychol.*, 1958, **51**, 199–201.

Bonvallet, M., Dell, P., and Hiebel, G. Tonus sympathique et activité électrique corticale. *EEG clin. Neurophysiol.*, 1954, 6, 119–144.

Bovet, D., and Bovet-Nitti, F. *Structure et activité pharmacodynamique des médicaments du système nerveux végétatif.* New York: Karger Bale, 1948.

Cannon W. B. *Bodily changes in pain, hunger, fear and rage.* (2nd ed.) Boston: Branford, 1929.

Dell, P., Bonvallet, M., & Hugelin, A. Tonus sympathique adrénaline et contrôle réticulaire de la motricité spinal. *EEG clin. Neurophysiol.* 1954, 6, 599–618.

Dell, P., and Olson, R. Projections secondaires mésencéphaliques, diencéphaliques et amygdaliennes des afferences viscérales vagales. *CR Soc. Biol., Paris,* 1951, 145, 1088–1091.

Duncan, D. B. Multiple range tests for correlated and heteroscedastic means. *Biometrics,* 1957, 13, 164–176.

Goodman, L. S., and Gilman, A. *The pharmacological basis of therapeutics.* (2nd ed.) New York: Macmillan, 1955.

Hunt, H. F., and Brady, J. V. Some effects of electroconvulsive shock on a conditioned emotional response ("anxiety"). *J. comp. physiol. Psychol.,* 1951, 44, 88–98.

Mowrer, O. H. On the dual nature of learning: A reinterpretation of "conditioning" and "problem-solving." *Harvard educ. Rev.,* 1947, 17, 102–148.

Outschoorn, A. S. The hormones of the adrenal medulla and their release. *Brit. J. Pharmacol.* 1952, 7, 605–615.

Rothballer, A. B. Studies on the adrenaline-sensitive component of the reticular activating system. *EEG clin. Neurophysiol.,* 1956, 8, 603–621.

Rothballer, A. B. The effects of catecholamines on the central nervous system. *Pharmacol. Rev.,* 1959, 11, 494–547.

Satake, Y. Secretion of adrenaline and sympathins. *Tohoku J. exp. Med.,* 1954, 60, Suppl. 2.

Sharpless, S. K. The effects of intravenous epinephrine and norepinephrine on a conditioned response in the cat. *Psychopharmacologia,* 1959, 1, 140–149.

Sherrington, G. *The integrative action of the nervous system.* Cambridge Univer. Press, 1947.

Solomon, R. L., and Brush, E. S. Experimentally derived conceptions of anxiety and aversion. In M. Jones (Ed.), *Nebraska symposium on motivation, 1956.* Lincoln: Univer. Nebraska Press, 1956. Pp. 212–305.

von Euler, U. S. *Noradrenaline.* Springfield, Ill.: Charles C Thomas, 1956.

Wynne, L. C., and Solomon, R. L. Traumatic avoidance learning: Acquisition and extinction in dogs deprived of normal peripheral autonomic functioning. *Genet. psychol. Monogr.,* 1955, 52, 241–284.

32

Morphine self-administration, food-reinforced, and avoidance behaviors in rhesus monkeys *

TRAVIS THOMPSON and CHARLES R. SCHUSTER

Research techniques based upon the behavioral principles of operant conditioning have provided a complementary approach to the standard pharmacologic analysis of physical dependence upon opiates (Seevers 1936, 1958). With these techniques, a simple arbitrary response is conditioned by following it with a reinforcement. For example, a food deprived rhesus monkey learns to press a lever because pressing a lever leads to a pellet of food. By the same token, if a lever pressing response is followed by the injection of an opiate to a physically dependent animal, that response will be learned.

Using the general principle outlined above, several investigators have recently demonstrated that it is possible to condition physically dependent rats to emit operant responses for morphine reinforcement. Nichols and co-workers (1956, 1959), have shown that dependent rats will learn to drink water containing morphine rather than the initially preferred morphine-free tap water. Weeks (1960, 1962) has recently shown that unrestrained rats can be conditioned to emit a lever-pressing response to receive intravenously infused morphine on a fixed ratio reinforcement schedule. In addition, he has shown that pretreatment with nalorphine produces an increase in rate of responding for the drug, presumably produced by the induced abstinence syndrome.

GENERAL PROCEDURE. The experimental approach we have used is an extension of the lines of investigation based upon the principle of reinforcement of behavior by opiate administration, to permit an analysis of the interaction of pharmacological and behavioral variables in opiate dependence (Schuster and Thompson, 1962). Rhesus monkeys seated in restraining chairs obtain all of their food and avoid painful electric shocks by pressing levers under specific visual or auditory stimulus conditions. When a yellow light is present, pressing the lever leads to food. When a clicker is presented, pressing the lever postpones an electric shock. The ani-

From *Psychopharmacologia* (Berl.), 1964, **5**, 87–94. Copyright 1964 by Springer-Verlag, Heidelberg, Germany.

* This research was supported by research grant MY-1604 from the National Institute of Mental Health and grant NsG 189-61 from the National Aeronautics and Space Administration, to the University of Maryland.

mals are in the experiment for 24 hours a day, so that large and continuous samples of the animal's behavior can be brought under experimental control. Interspersed with periods when the animal is working for food or avoiding shock, occasions are provided when a response will lead to the infusion of morphine sulphate through a chronically indwelling jugular catheter. Since the various stimuli associated with food, shock and drug periods, as well as the drug administration and data recording are all controlled electronically by devices located in an adjacent control room, it is not necessary to distrub the animal for the measurement of drug-effects or to administer the opiate. Because of this degree of experimental control, it is possible to obtain highly reliable measures of behavioral output from day to day over a period of 6 months. Thus, the experimenter has at his disposal a double bladed instrument for the analysis of drug-behavior interaction. It is possible to measure the effects of conditions of the opiate administration on food and shock-avoidance behaviors, and at the same time to measure the animal's disposition to administer the drug to himself.

Experiment 1. In this preliminary study, the feasibility of conditioning monkeys to work for a morphine reinforcement was established. These experiments employed 3 adult male rhesus monkeys weighing approximately 3.5 kg. Following surgical implantation of the jugular catheter (Niemann, Schuster and Thompson 1962), the animals were infused 4 times daily with 7 mg of morphine sulphate in isotonic saline, for a period of 30 days. Food and water were available at all times. Following this period during which physical dependence was developed, the monkeys were conditioned to emit a specific behavioral sequence in order to obtain subsequent intravenous infusions of morphine. The final series of behaviors required is called a fixed interval-fixed ratio chain (FI-FR chain). The fixed interval component is indicated by the onset of a tone. The first occurrence of a response after two minutes in the presence of the tone turned on a white light signaling a change to a fixed ratio schedule. A fixed ratio of 25 responses in the presence of the white light produced the infusion of 7 mg of morphine over a period of 60 seconds. During the infusion of morphine a red light was presented. Thus, in order to obtain the drug, the animal must first complete the two-minute fixed interval giving it the opportunity to emit 25 more responses to be followed by morphine infusion. Each 24 hour experimental session was divided into 4 cycles of 6 hours duration. In each cycle the subjects had the opportunity of self-administer ¼ of its total daily morphine intake of 28 mgs or 8.0 mg/kg.

Following stabilization of the FI-FR behavior sequence, the infusion and stimulus presentation apparatus was turned off for 24 hours. The following day the 6 hour FI-FR schedule was reinstated and changes in behavior as a function of the increased deprivation condition were observed. Figure 1 presents cumulative response records for the session following 24 hours deprivation of morphine. The number of responses in the fixed interval are

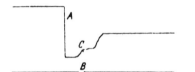

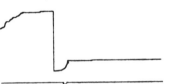

Last FI-FR prior to nalorphine pretreatment

Last FI-FR prior to morphine deprivation

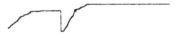

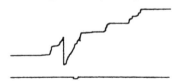

1.0 mg nalorphine 45 minutes pretreatment

First FI-FR following 24 hours morphine
deprivation

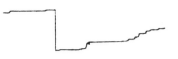

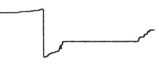

6 hours 45 minutes following nalorphine
pretreatment

Second FI-FR following 24 hours morphine
deprivation

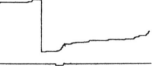

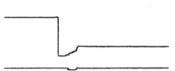

12 hours 45 minutes following nalorphine
pretreatment

Third FI-FR following 24 hours morphine
deprivation

FIGURE 1.   Representative cumulative response records of fixed interval-fixed ratio performance following 24 hours of morphine deprivation compared FI-FR performance 45 minutes after the administration of 1.0 mg nalorphine, i.v.

A Reset of response pen indicating the onset of 2 minute FI with accompanying tone.
B Deflection of event marker indicating the FR period with accompanying white light.
C Brief deflection of response pen indicates infusion of morphine and presentation of a red light.

dramatically increased as compared with the baseline condition. It can also be seen that the latency to completion of the 25 responses in the FR is reduced. After the FI-FR behavior had reached the pre-deprivation baseline, 1.0 mg of nalorphine was administered I.V. 45 minutes prior to the scheduled FI-FR period. As can be seen in Fig. 1, the number of responses in the fixed interval is markedly increased. In addition, the time taken to completion of the ratio is much shorter than any of the baseline periods. Subsequent stabilization of the FI-FR chain was followed by a series of sessions on which the animals were pretreated with 7.0, 14.0 or 21.0 mg of morphine 45 minutes before a FI-FR period. The effect of morphine pretreatment is illustrated in Fig. 2. As can be seen, there is a progressive disruption in the tendency to work for the drug as an increasing

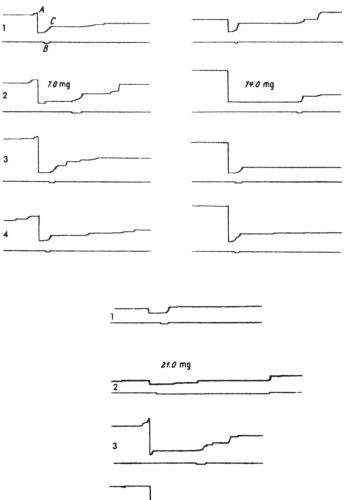

FIGURE 2.   Representative cumulative response records of fixed interval-fixed ratio performance following 45 minutes pretreatment with 7.0, 14.0, and 21.0 mg of morphine, i.v.

1 Last FI-FR prior to morphine pretreatment.   *2* 45 minutes pretreatment with 7.0, 14.0 and 21.0 mg morphine.   *3* 6 hours 45 minutes following morphine pretreatment. *4* 12 hours 45 minutes following morphine pretreatment.

A Reset of response pen indicating the onset of 2 minute FI with accompanying tone. *B* Deflection of event marker indicating the FR period with accompanying white light. *C* Brief deflection of response pen indicates infusion of morphine and presentation of a red light.

function of dose. These effects have been replicated on three different animals.

Experiment 2.   Subsequent experiments have interspersed food and shock-avoidance periods between the four drug-reinforced behavior periods. Each six hour cycle consisted of 4 shock avoidance periods, 4 food periods and 1 drug reinforced FI-FR period.

The presentation sequence of these periods was as follows: Food, Shock, Food, Shock, FI-FR drug period, Shock, Food, Shock, Food. A minimum of 8 and maximum of 32 minutes separated the presentation of the various periods.

The food period consisted of five successive fixed ratios of thirty-five responses. If the animal failed to complete the five ratios the food period was automatically terminated after 8 minutes.

The shock avoidance periods were presented for a maximum of 8 minutes or until the animal received 5 shocks. The shock schedule consisted of a 10 second warning clicker presented on a variable time schedule with an average interval of 60 seconds. Responses between the warning stimulus presentations had no consequence. Responses in the warning stimulus terminated the clicker and avoided the 0.5 second electric shock. The 1.5 ma electric shock was delivered to the subject through eight stainless electrodes mounted on the inside of a leather waist belt.

Figure 3 shows baseline performance over a period of 30 days, for food reinforced responses, shock avoidance responses, responses in the fixed interval leading to the opportunity to work for morphine, and the length of time to complete a ratio of 25 responses to be infused with morphine.

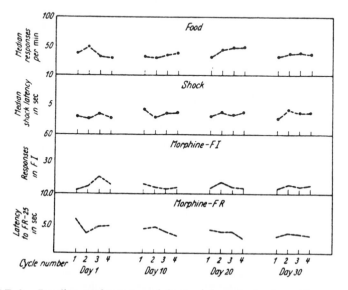

FIGURE 3.   Baseline performance of food-reinforced, shock avoidance, and fixed interval-fixed ratio drug-reinforced behaviors, over a period of 30 days.

The effects of abstinence from the drug (by not providing the opportunity to work for the drug) on food-reinforced and shock-avoidance behaviors were superimposed upon this stable baseline performance. Figure 4 presents the changes in the food reinforced and shock-avoidance behaviors during 48 hours of abstinence. As can be seen, there is a progressive reduction in tendency to work for food, and the shock-avoidance latencies increase. Following the first drug infusion after 48 hours of abstinence, the food reinforced behavior returns immediately, and the shock-avoidance latencies begin decreasing toward the pre-abstinence baseline. This effect has been replicated on three animals over a period of 4 months, with consistently the same result. A placebo effect was demonstrated for the infusion process by substitution of saline for morphine during the 60 second red light on the first self-administration opportunity after 48 hours abstinence. This effect is illustrated in the lower half of Fig. 4. The animals began working again immediately after the saline infusion. However, their food and shock performance showed progressive disruption as time without the drug increased.

The subjects' FI-FR performance in these 4 periods in which saline was

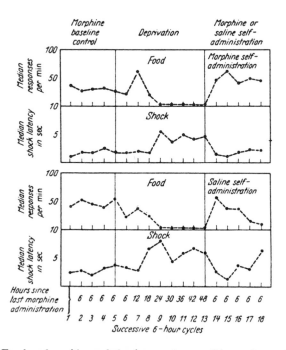

FIGURE 4.   Food and avoidance behaviors under conditions of morphine baseline control, 48 hours without the opportunity to self-administer morphine, followed by (upper graph) return to morphine baseline control procedure, or (lower graph) return to baseline condition with saline substituted for morphine self-administration.

substituted for morphine showed no progressive changes indicative of extinction.

DISCUSSION. The reinforcing effects of morphine to physically dependent animals has been well established. The present investigation has examined the properties of a more complex sequence of behaviors maintained by morphine administration, in relation to other aspects of the organism's behavior.

A two-member behavioral chain leading to the intravenous infusion of morphine was maintained with great reliability for 6 months. The FI-FR chain proved to be a reliable and sensitive index of the morphine deprivation conditions. The similarity of the effects of deprivation from morphine and pretreatment with the morphine antagonist, nalorphine, on the FI-FR chain, demonstrates the value of this procedure for the assessment of both environmental and pharmacological variables. Morphine pretreatment further illustrates the sensitivity of the chain to deprivation conditions. The functional relationship between the morphine pretreatment dosage and the characteristics of the subsequent FI-FR behavior provides a direct statement of the relationship between the degree of motivation and the animal's propensity to work for the drug.

Abstinence was found to produce changes not only in the morphine reinforced behavior, but also other behaviors essential to the animal's maintenance. Profound disruption of food and shock avoidance behaviors was produced by 48 hours deprivation, with an immediate return to baseline conditions following a single morphine self-administration. The same immediate return to baseline behavioral levels was observed when saline was substituted for morphine in the first red light infusion period following 48 hours of deprivation. This placebo effect was transitory as indicated by the fact that succeeding self-administered saline infusions were seen to be associated with progressive disruption of the food and avoidance behaviors. The fact that the saline infusion, in conjunction with the red light, maintained the FI-FR sequence for four periods suggests the conditioned reinforcing properties of stimuli previously associated with the morphine infusion reinforcement. Thus, the degree to which the physically dependent animal effectively deals with its environment is controlled, not only by the drug but also by the stimulus conditions associated with the prior self-administration of the drug.

SUMMARY. 1. A fixed interval-fixed ratio chain of behavior was maintained for periods as long as 6 months by intravenously administered morphine.

2. The morphine reinforced FI-FR chain was found to be a sensitive and reliable index of motivational changes induced by drug deprivation, nalorphine antagonism and pretreatment with morphine.

3. Profound behavioral disruption occurred in both shock avoidance and food reinforced ratio behavior under conditions of drug deprivation.

4. The behavioral disruption of the food reinforced and shock avoidance behaviors was ameliorated by a single self-administration of morphine. Substitution of saline for the morphine solution produced a transitory placebo effect characterized by an immediate return of the food and avoidance behaviors to their pre-deprivation baseline conditions, but followed by progressive disruption as time without the drug increased.

REFERENCES

Davis, W. M., and Nichols, J. R.: Physical dependence and sustained opiate-directed behavior in the rat. *Psychopharmacologia* (Berl.) 3, 139 (1962).

Nichols, J. R., and Davis, W. M.: Drug addiction II. Variation of addiction. *J. Amer. pharm. Ass.* 48, 259 (1959).

Nichols, J. R., Headlee, C. P., and Coppock, H. W.: Drug addiction 1. Addiction by escape training. *J. Amer. pharm. Ass.* 45, 788 (1956).

Niemann, W. H., Schuster, C. R., and Thompson, T.: A surgical preparation for chronic intravenous infusion in rhesus monkeys. University of Maryland, Laboratory of Psychopharmacology Technical Report No. 62–39, September, 1962.

Schuster, C. R., and Thompson, T.: Self-administration of morphine in physically dependent monkeys. University of Maryland, Laboratory of Psychopharmacology Technical Report No. 62–29, July, 1962.

Seevers, M. H.: Opiate addiction in monkeys; methods of study. *J. Pharmacol. exp. Ther.* 56, 147 (1936).

Seevers, M. H.: Ch 19 in *Pharmacology in medicine* (V. A. Drill, ed.). New York: McGraw-Hill Book Co. 1958.

Weeks, J. R.: Self-maintained morphine "addiction": A method for chronic programmed intravenous injection in unrestrained rats. *Fed. Proc.* 20, 397 (1961) (abst).

Weeks, J. R.: Experimental morphine addiction: Method for automatic intravenous injections in unrestrained rats. *Science* 138, 143 (1962).

33

Experimental morphine addiction: Method for automatic intravenous injections in unrestrained rats

James R. Weeks

Operant conditioning has been applied in recent years to the study of the effect of drugs on animal behavior. This report describes a method for using drug administration as a positive reinforcer of a lever-press response in rats. It was presumed that such operant behavioral studies would require relatively unrestrained animals and intravenous injections to minimize the time between lever press and drug effects. Many animal studies have demonstrated that repeated administration of opiates can lead to tolerance and physical dependence, as evidenced by an abstinence syndrome and a desire to continue opiate administration (1).

With the method I used, rats could move freely about their cages, carrying a lightweight saddle strapped behind the forelegs. The saddle was connected by a sprocket chain to a small swivel and stuffing box to permit injection of drugs. Intravenous injections were made through a polyethylene cannula passed down the jugular vein into the right heart. Cannulae could be expected to remain functional for at least several weeks (five of ten lasted 9 months), and differed from other rat heart canulae (2) in two important details: the intravenous portion was drawn down to 0.2 to 0.4 mm outside diameter, and the exit through the skin was reinforced (3). Injections were by automatic syringe drivers or burettes whose output was programmed on film. Rats were albino females weighing 200 to 250 g.

Two series of experiments were conducted. In the first, physical dependence upon morphine sulfate was established by hourly doses increased in a 2.5-percent geometric progression from 2 to 40 mg/kg of base (122 doses), the last dose being repeated for 1 to 2 days. Next, a lever was put into the cage, which, when pressed, caused injection of 10 mg/kg of morphine as the sulfate. After experiencing drug effects a few times by chance lever pressing, rats responded regularly. After 2 days the dose was reduced to 3.2 mg/kg, whereupon the response rate promptly increased. Abrupt withdrawal by disconnecting the syringe led to a prompt increase in response rate (sevenfold average) which lessened gradually after the first 3 hours (Table 1). Response rate increased before overt signs of abstinence appeared. Overnight withdrawal caused an abstinence syndrome of weight loss (about 20 percent), tremor, hypersensitivity, agitation, soft stools, and increased respiration, but the rats remained gentle.

From *Science*, 1962, **138**, 143–144. Copyright 1962 by the American Association for the Advancement of Science, Washington, D.C.

TABLE 1. Responses per hour for self-administered morphine by addict rats on continuous (1:1) reinforcement.

Condition		Responses per hour						Daily intake (mg/kg)
Reinforce-ment ratio	Dose (mg/kg)	Rat 95	Rat 224	Rat 255	Rat 261	Rat 402	Av.	
1:1	10	2.4	2.0	1.3	0.9	1.2	1.6	384
1:1	3.2	5.5	3.1	2.9	2.5	2.1	3.2	240
Withdrawal*		33	11	21	27	17	22	

* Calculations on first 3 hours only.

In the second series, reinforcement ratio (responses per injection) was also varied. Physical dependence was established as before, except that the dose was increased to a maximum of only 20 mg/kg (94 doses). For the first 12 to 24 hours, each response injected 3.2 mg/kg; then for periods of 23 to 34 hours each the program was 5 : 1 at 3.2 mg/kg, next, 10 : 1 at 3.2 mg/kg, and finally 10 : 1 at 10 mg/kg. The change from continuous reinforcement to 5 : 1 decreased net morphine intake. Presumably, the delay enforced by extra responses allowed full effects of a dose to be felt before a second was taken. When the ratio was increased from 5 : 1 to 10 : 1, response rate about doubled; when the dose was then increased to 10 mg/kg, the response rate decreased (Table 1). Performance of one rat is shown in Fig. 1.

Nalorphine, a morphine antagonist, temporarily induces an acute abstinence syndrome (4). These same four rats, when on a 10 : 1 ratio at 10 mg/kg, were given 4 mg/kg of nalorphine hydrochloride intraperitoneally. Within the next hour, three responded 50 times each, and the fourth, 20 times.

The most interesting aspect of ratio reinforcement was the response pattern after about 2 days on the same ratio and dose. Prolonged periods of no responding alternated with brief periods at a high rate terminated by an injection (Fig. 1D). This evidence indicates that the drug was a reinforcer that produced almost immediate satiation.

TABLE 2. Responses per hour for self-administered morphine by addict rats on fixed-ratio reinforcement.

Condition		Responses per hour					Daily intake (mg/kg)
Reinforce-ment ratio	Dose (mg/kg)	Rat 470*	Rat 483	Rat 485	Rat 490	Av.	
1:1	3.2	1.8	1.1	1.9	3.5†	2.6	160
5:1	3.2	7.4	4.4	7.1	5.2	6.0	91
10:1	3.2	13	7.6	12	12	11	84
10:1	10	5.4	4.7	5.2	4.7	5.0	120

* Illustrated in Fig. 1.   † Records of only last 7½ hours of 24-hour period available.

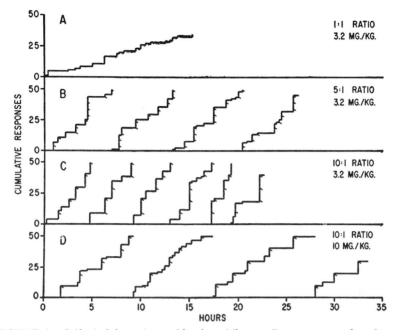

FIGURE 1.   Self-administered morphine by addict rat. Responses are plotted to the nearest 15 minutes, performance continuous. In *A*, there was one injection for each response. In *B*, *C*, and *D*, injections were at diagonal marks. For the last 15 hours in *D*, responses, in groups of 7 to 10, were terminated by an injection.

SUMMARY.   An operant behavioral study on morphine addiction utilized a self-injection technique for giving intravenous injections to relatively unrestrained rats. The rate of self-injection varied inversely with the dose. Morphine was a reinforcer that produced almost immediate satiation.

REFERENCES AND NOTES

1. H. Krueger *et al.*, *Public Health Repts. (U.S.) Suppl.* **165**, 1 (1941); M. H. Seevers, *Ann. N.Y. Acad. Sci.* **51**, 98 (1948); S. D. S. Spragg, *Comp. Psychol. Mongr.* **15**, 1 (1940); J. R. Nichols *et al., J. Pharm. Sci.* **45**, 788 (1956); J. R. Nichols and W. M. Davis, *ibid.* **48**, 259 (1959); H. D. Beach, *Can J. Psychol.* **11**, 104 (1957); A. Wikler *et al., Federation Proc.* **19**, 22 (1960).
2. V. Popovic and P. Popovic, *J. Appl. Physiol.* **15**, 727 (1960); M. A. Slusher and B. Browning, *Am. J. Physiol.* **200**, 1032 (1961).
3. Details of fabrication and the use of cannula, saddle, and swivel have been deposited as Document No. 7304 with the ADI Auxiliary Publications Project, Photoduplication Service, Library of Congress, Washington 25, D.C.
4. L. A. Woods, *Pharmacol. Rev.* **8**, 175 (1956).

34

Comparison of drug effects on approach, avoidance, and escape motivation [1]

HERBERT BARRY III and NEAL E. MILLER

Effects of drugs on different motives have sometimes been compared by means of the conflict test (Barry and Miller, 1962; Barry, Wagner, and Miller, 1963), in which approach to a desired goal (such as food for a hungry animal) is pitted against avoidance (threat of shock at the goal). By comparing the opposing tendencies, the conflict test balances out any effects, such as ataxia or general depression, which can be assumed to act equally on both. However, this technique has the disadvantage of permitting each motive to be measured only in relation to a contrary one. The same response cannot be used for comparing the different motives, because opposing motives require opposite directions of response.

In some experiments the same response (pressing a bar in an operant-conditioning situation) has been studied under different motives by means of a "multiple schedule" which presents signals for different motivational conditions (Boren, 1961; Ray, 1963; Weissman, 1959). The same animals are tested under all the conditions, so that the problem of discriminating the signals becomes a complicating factor in the situation; furthermore, becoming associated with one motivational condition is likely to influence performance under different motivational conditions. It is highly desirable to use the same response but different groups of animals when comparing the effects of a drug on different motives.

Several studies, reviewed by Dews and Morse (1961), have compared the effects of drugs on two similar aversive motives: avoidance motivated by fear of electric shock and escape from the shock itself. In most of these studies, a drug dosage which had little or no effect on escape produced a great decrement in avoidance performance. However, fear of shock is an anticipatory motive which tends to be weaker than the pain of the shock itself; and the avoidance tends to be performed more slowly and less reliably than the escape. Therefore, a reasonable explanation of the differential

From *Journal of Comparative and Physiological Psychology,* 1965, 59, 18–24. Copyright 1965 by the American Psychological Association, Washington, D.C.

[1] This experiment was supported by Grant MY-2949 from the National Institute of Mental Health, United States Public Health Service; preparation of the article was supported by Grant MH-07824 from the same source. Roberta Pritzker conducted the experimental testing. The statistical analysis was done in part at the University of Pittsburgh Computation and Data Processing Center, supported by National Science Foundation Grant G-11309.

drug effect is that the drug may have had a greater detrimental effect on the weaker motive, which in this case happened to be the avoidance. It is obvious that for comparison of the effects of drugs on different motives, the strength of the different motives under the nondrug condition should be equalized.

In the present experiment an identical response in the same apparatus was measured under three motivational conditions: food-approach, shock-avoidance, and shock-escape. Separate groups of animals, equalized in non-drug performance, were used for testing each of these motivations. Thus the motivational conditions were highly comparable (same response, equalized performance) yet independent of each other (separate groups).

METHOD.   *Subjects.*   The *S*s were 24 male albino rats of Sprague-Dawley strain, housed in individual cages. They were 100–120 days old at the beginning of the experiment and had been received from the Holtz-man Company, Madison, Wisconsin at 90 days of age.

Apparatus.   A straight alley 5 in. high, with a hinged Plexiglas lid, comprised a start box 7 in. long, a runway 26 in. long, and a goal box 6 in. long. The start box and runway were 6 in. wide, with white wooden walls; the floor consisted of steel bars $\frac{1}{16}$ in. in diameter, spaced $\frac{3}{8}$ in. apart, mounted into the side walls. The runway was separated from the start box by an aluminum guillotine door. The goal box was 4 in. wide, with black wooden walls, and with a black cardboard floor $\frac{1}{8}$ in. higher than the floor of the runway and start box. There was no barrier separating the goal box from the runway.

Starting time was measured, to the nearest .01 sec., by an electric timer which started automatically when the start-box door was opened and stopped when *S* reached a photocell 2 in. beyond the start box. A similar timer recorded the running time for the 24-in. distance between this photo-cell and another photocell at the entrance to the goal box. A 60-cycle ac electric shock, with the voltage selected by *E*, could be delivered through a 100,000-ohm resistance to the steel bars comprising the floor of the start box and runway. Alternate bars were wired to the two sides of the shock output; the floor of the goal box was insulated from the shock.

Test procedures.   The *S*s were divided randomly into groups of eight, one group assigned to each motivational condition: Approach, Avoidance, and Escape. Each trial began when *E* placed *S* in the start box and released a counterweight which raised the start-box door. The *S* was removed from the apparatus 2 sec. after entering the goal box, or after 30 sec. if it did not go to the goal box. Six trials were given per day, with a 30-sec. wait in a nearby cage before each trial. For the Approach group, four food pellets (.045 gm. each, from the P. J. Noyes Company, Lancaster, New Hamp-shire), were available in a small cup mounted on the back wall of the goal box. The cup was not present for the other two groups. For the Escape group a shock of 80 v. was delivered continuously to the steel floor bars, beginning automatically when the start-box door was raised. For the Avoidance group the shock was 150 v., beginning at variable intervals of time after the start-box door was raised (1, 2, or 4 sec.). In all drug and placebo tests, the shock was omitted on three of the six trials per day (the first two and either the fourth or fifth) in order to provide an avoidance situation without any need to escape.

All Ss were maintained on the same food-deprivation schedule, with 12-gm. Purina lab chow checkers given each day, 1 hr. after testing. Every 2 weeks the Avoidance and Escape groups were given the same quantity of reward pellets in their cages as the Approach group had received in the test apparatus. Water was available ad lib in the cages.

Test of drug effects.   Drug tests were begun on the sixth day of the test procedures. Most of the drugs were tested with three dosages plus a placebo test. Drugs and placebo were injected intraperitoneally, in a solution of isotonic saline. The drugs, with dosages, concentrations (mg/ml), and time intervals between injection and testing, were as follows:

Methamphetamine hydrochloride: ½, 1, 2 mg/kg; 1 mg/ml; 40 min.
Amobarbital sodium: 10, 20, 30 mg/kg; 10 mg/ml; 15 min.
Ethyl alcohol: 600, 1200, 1800 mg/kg; 80 mg/ml; 15 min.
Chlordiazepoxide hydrochloride: 5, 10, 15 mg/kg; 5 mg/ml; 15 min.
Morphine sulfate: 3 mg/kg; 3 mg/ml; 40 min.
Chlorpromazine hydrochloride: 1, 2, 4 mg/kg; 2 mg/ml; 40 min.
Morphine sulfate: 3, 6, 9 mg/kg; 3 mg/ml; 40 min.
Caffeine with sodium benzoate: 10, 20, 40 mg/kg; 20 mg/ml; 15 min.
Amobarbital sodium: 10, 20, 30 mg/kg; 10 mg/ml; 15 min.
Methamphetamine hydrochloride: ½, 1 mg/kg; 1 mg/ml; 40 min.

Different time intervals between injection and testing were used for different drugs in order to give the tests during the approximate peak action of each drug. Each S was tested under each dosage of each drug, with only a few exceptions.[2] The different drugs were given in the sequence shown above; as may be seen, some drugs given near the beginning of the series were repeated near the end. Any daily fluctuations were controlled by testing equal numbers of animals under the different dosages and placebo on each day.

The weekly schedule consisted of three drug tests and one placebo test (Tuesday–Friday), plus a nondrug test on Monday in order to provide a

[2] One S, in the Escape group, died after the chlorpromazine tests. The missing data were filled in by the same S's prior scores, where possible, or by the average of the other 7 Escape Ss. For analysis of variance tests, the missing scores are subtracted from the degrees of freedom. The caffeine dosages were incomplete, because an error in the schedule caused each S to receive only two of the three scheduled dosages, with different Ss having a different one of the dosages omitted.

warm-up after the weekend interruption. Most of the drugs used in this experiment are short-acting and would be expected to be almost completely detoxified within the 24-hr. minimum interval between tests. The possibility of the drug effects persisting for longer durations does exist, especially in the case of chlorpromazine and morphine, but any persisting effects of a particular drug dosage were counterbalanced by giving drugs with different sequences of dosages, including the zero (placebo) dosage, to different Ss. During tests under the same placebo or drug condition, animals given different dosage sequences seldom showed any differences in performance attributable to differences in their placebo or drug condition on the preceding day.

RESULTS.   Each time score was converted into its reciprocal to obtain a measure of speed. Figure 1 compares the three groups in running speed during each of the 10 placebo tests. The data shown are for the first two trials per day, because these were the only trials in which the shock was always omitted for the Avoidance group during the placebo and drug tests. The first of these placebo tests was given after 6 days (33 trials) of preliminary training. It is evident that performance was reasonably stable during the placebo tests, despite the brevity of prior training and the 10-week time span, filled with 27 drug tests, which intervened between the first and last of the placebo tests. Differences among the 10 tests were not statistically significant, as estimated by analysis of variance ($F = 1.95$, $df = \frac{9}{185}$). Furthermore, the three groups were reasonably similar in performance throughout the tests; there were no significant differences among the groups with the 10 tests averaged together ($F = 0.90$, $df = \frac{2}{21}$), and no significant interaction between groups and tests ($F = 1.60$, $df = \frac{18}{185}$).

Whereas Fig. 1 compares the three groups during nondrug tests, Fig. 2 compares the three groups in drug effects, showing running speed in the

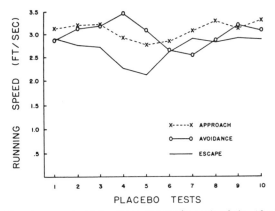

FIGURE 1.   Running speeds of the three groups in each of the 10 placebo tests.

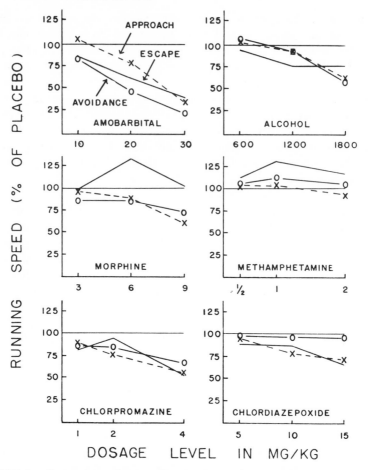

FIGURE 2. Comparison of drug with placebo performance for each of the three groups, showing three dosages of each of six drugs.

first two trials per day under each drug condition as a percentage of the placebo performance. Since there were no significant differences in performance among the placebo tests, each of the drug tests was compared with the average of the 10 placebo tests. A percentage score was calculated separately for each S, and these percentage scores were used for the averages in Fig. 2 and for the tests of statistical significance of the results. For amobarbital, methamphetamine, and morphine, the two series of tests, given at different times, yielded similar results and are averaged together.

Pooling the three groups and comparing the dosages, significant differences among the three dosages were found for amobarbital ($F = 65.00$, $df = \frac{2}{42}$, $p < .01$), alcohol ($F = 18.74$, $df = \frac{2}{42}$, $p < .01$), morphine

($F = 6.52$, $df = \frac{2}{40}$, $p < .01$), chlorpromazine ($F = 6.46$, $df = \frac{2}{42}$, $p < .01$), and chlordiazepoxide ($F = 4.36$, $df = \frac{2}{42}$, $p < .05$). For all of these five drugs except morphine, progressive increases in dosage resulted in progressively slower running speeds. The drug dosages were compared with each other and not with placebo performance. Two stimulant drugs (methamphetamine and caffeine) showed no significant differences among dosage levels, but when the three dosages were pooled for a comparison with the average of the placebo tests, running speed was found to be significantly increased by methamphetamine ($F = 15.45$, $df = \frac{1}{21}$, $p < .01$) and by caffeine ($F = 26.48$, $df = \frac{1}{20}$, $p < .01$).

Since the scores in Fig. 2 are measures of drug effects, any significant difference among the three groups under the same drug, pooling the three dosage levels, would indicate that the drug had a differential effect on the Approach, Avoidance, and Escape groups. The groups differed significantly in the effects produced by amobarbital ($F = 9.81$, $df = \frac{2}{21}$, $p < .01$), apparently because this drug caused the Approach group to be highest and the Avoidance group lowest, relative to placebo performance. Significant differences among the groups were also found in the effects of morphine ($F = 5.37$, $df = \frac{2}{20}$, $p < .01$), with the Escape group being conspicuously above the other two. The groups did not differ significantly in the effects produced by any of the other four drugs shown in Fig. 2. However, certain trends may be noteworthy. Under methamphetamine the Escape group was the highest and the Approach group was the lowest; under chlorpromazine the Approach group tended to be lowest and under chlordiazepoxide the Avoidance group was highest; contrary to the effects of amobarbital; under the lower dosages of alcohol the Escape group was lowest, contrary to the effects of morphine and methamphetamine. Caffeine, which is not included in Fig. 2 because the dosage administration was incomplete, showed no evidence of differential effects among the three groups.

Whereas the three groups during placebo tests were very similar in running speed, they differed considerably in starting speed. The average speed in ft/sec for the first two trials of the day in the 10 placebo tests was 0.62 for the Approach group, 0.26 for the Avoidance group, and 0.31 for the Escape group. The corresponding reciprocal scores, showing the time required to traverse the 2-in. distance into the alley, were 0.27, 0.63, and 0.53 sec. The differences among groups in starting speed were highly significant ($F = 46.03$, $df = \frac{2}{21}$, $p < .01$). It is paradoxical that the fastest starters were the Approach animals, whose motivation for running might seem to have been least urgent. Presumably the shock (for the Escape group) and the threat of shock (for the Avoidance group) produced a crouching or withdrawal reaction which interfered with a fast start. During placebo tests the starting speeds were less stable than were the running speeds. The two measures of performance showed generally similar drug effects, but one difference seems worth noting, specially because Posluns (1962) has reported that in an avoidance situation, chlorpromazine decreased starting more than running performance. In the present experiment, chlorpromazine produced a much larger percentage reduction in starting speed than in running speed for the Escape group; there was a small difference between the two measures in the same direction for the Avoidance group and in the opposite direction for the Approach group. The three groups differed significantly with respect to the relative effects of chlorpromazine on the two measures of performance ($F = 14.04$, $df = \frac{2}{14}, p < .01$).

The data we have reported on running and starting speeds are for the first two trials per day. Performance varied only slightly during the six daily trials in placebo tests and under most of the drugs. The time span of less than 3 min., between the first and sixth trial, was insufficient for any sizable changes in the physiological effects of the drugs. However, certain changes in running speed on successive trials did occur, as shown in Fig. 3. For this portrayal the drug dosages are averaged together. Under amobarbital the running speed of the Avoidance group increased greatly on successive trials. In all of the conditions shown in Fig. 3 (placebo, amobarbital, and chlorpromazine), shock was omitted for the Avoidance group on the first, second, and fifth trials. Comparison among these three

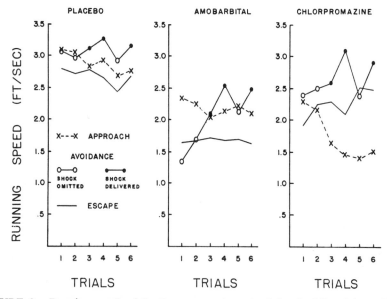

FIGURE 3.   Running speeds of the three groups in each of the six daily trials, under amobarbital and chlorpromazine and in the corresponding placebo tests.

nonshock trials shows that the Avoidance group ran progressively faster under amobarbital ($F = 14.23$, $df = \frac{2}{14}$, $p < .01$ for the difference among these three trials) but not in the placebo tests or under chlorpromazine. Shock was delivered to the Avoidance group 4 sec. after the start-box door was opened on the third trial and 1 or 2 sec. after the door was opened on the fourth and sixth trials. The Avoidance group tended to run faster on the trials when shock was delivered than on the trials when it was omitted. The Ss usually were not able to reach the goal box before the shock was delivered on trials with the 1-sec. delay, but they successfully avoided the shock in most of the trials with the longer delays, at least during placebo tests.

Under chlorpromazine the running speed of the Approach group decreased drastically in the later trials of the day to a level markedly below the other two groups, as shown by a significant difference among the three groups on the fifth trial ($F = 4.48$, $df = \frac{2}{21}$, $p < .05$), whereas the groups did not differ significantly from each other in the first two trials. The Approach group showed a progressive decrease in the placebo tests also, and was significantly slower in the last two trials of the day than in the first two trials ($F = 17.43$, $df = \frac{1}{7}$, $p < .01$), but in the placebo tests this change was relatively small and the Approach group never sank below both of the other groups.

DISCUSSION.   Running speed was decreased by four depressant drugs (amobarbital, alcohol, chlorpromazine, and chlordiazepoxide) and increased by two stimulants (methamphetamine and caffeine). The effects of all six drugs were significant, five of them beyond the .01 level. For each of the four depressant drugs a clear dose-response relationship was demonstrated in a comparison among the three dosages, without regard to the placebo condition. Therefore, the present technique clearly provided a sensitive measure of the overall drug effects.

The effects of these drugs were very similar for groups with Approach, Avoidance, and Escape motivation. There was no consistently greater decrement in Avoidance than in Escape performance under the depressant drugs and no confirmation at all of prior findings reviewed by Dews and Morse (1961) that chlorpromazine has a much greater detrimental effect on avoidance than on escape. This discrepancy is probably due to the fact that in prior studies on effects of chlorpromazine, avoidance was a weaker motivation than was escape from the same shock. In the present experiment, the strength of the two motivations was equated by comparing avoidance of a severe shock with escape from a milder shock. This technique for equating avoidance with escape has been used previously (Miller and Murray, 1952) but not for tests of drug effects.

A complete absence of significant differences in drug effect among the experimental groups might signify that the present technique was a satisfactory measure only of the overall drug effects, such as ataxia produced by depressants, while failing to differentiate among the conditions represented by the three groups. Contrary to such a supposition are the significant differences among the groups in the effect of amobarbital. Previous experiments have given evidence that amobarbital reduces the shock-avoidance component of a conflict more than the food-approach component (Miller, 1961, 1964). The present study compared these motivations with separate groups of animals, each performing the same simple, literally straight-forward response. The present findings, shown in Fig. 2, give important confirmation of the evidence from conflict tests that the drug reduces avoidance more than approach. The intermediate position of the Escape group, in the present experiment, is consistent with the previous finding (Barry and Miller, 1962) that the avoidance-reducing effect of amobarbital in a series of conflict tests was diminished when shocks at the goal were delivered instead of omitted.

Further evidence that pain and stress may counteract the sedative effect of amobarbital is found in successive trials of the same day, shown in Fig. 3. Presentation of shocks on Trials 3, 4, and 6, which slightly increased speed of the Avoidance group in the placebo tests, had an exaggerated effect under amobarbital. Even in the three nonshock trials, the repeated exposures to the stress situation progressively increased Avoidance speed under amobarbital. These data for individual trials demonstrate that apparently small variations in the situation can greatly alter drug effects. Under amobarbital, the Avoidance group was markedly below the other two groups in the first trial of the day but above them in two of the last three trials.

Different conclusions would also be made about the effects of chlorpromazine, depending on whether one looked at the first two trials or the last four trials of the day. The conspicuous decrease in Approach speed on successive trials under chlorpromazine was an accentuation of a trend also found in the placebo tests. The low Approach performance in the later trials under chlorpromazine, agrees with prior findings that the drug decreased approach more than avoidance (Ferster and Skinner, 1957; Geller, Kulak, and Seifter, 1962) but is contrary to a finding by Weissman (1959). In our laboratory, chlorpromazine decreased approach less than avoidance in a lever-pressing situation (Barry et al., 1963; Grossman, 1961) but not in a straight alley (Barry and Miller, 1962). Therefore, the relative effect of this drug on different motives is evidently determined in large part by certain features of the situation.

Morphine has a mixture of stimulant and depressant effects at all levels of the central nervous system (Goodman and Gilman, 1955). In view of the well-known analgesic effects of morphine, it is surprising that the stimulating effect of the drug apparently predominated in the Escape group. Presumably the mild but consistent pain experienced by the Escape animals either diminished the depressant effect or enhanced the stimulant effect of the drug. The differential effects for the three groups in the present experiment agree well with a prior report (Edwards, 1961) that a much higher dosage of morphine was required to produce a decrement in a pain-escape response than in a food-approach response, with an intermediate dosage being required to produce a decrement in shock-avoidance. Edwards used very diverse test situations for the three types of motivation. The important situational determinants of drug effects, some of which are demonstrated in our present findings, indicate the value of our use of similar apparatus, procedures, and level of nondrug performance when comparing effects of drugs on different motives.

The foregoing analyses of differential drug effects on the three groups should not obscure the overall finding of the present experiment that performance of all the groups was very similarly affected by most of the drugs. Previous experimental findings would lead us to expect alcohol to decrease Avoidance more than Approach performance (Barry and Miller, 1962) and methamphetamine to decrease Approach while increasing Avoidance and Escape performance (Poschel, 1963). Any such differential effects were slight and not statistically significant in the present experiment. The similarity of the three groups in apparatus, procedures, and nondrug performance may have enhanced the similarity of the groups in drug effects.

SUMMARY.   Three groups of 8 albino rats were trained to run down the same straight alley at approximately the same speed during placebo tests, with 1 group approaching food, the 2nd avoiding a strong shock, and the 3rd escaping a weaker shock. Running speed was decreased by 4 depressants (chlorpromazine, amobarbital, alcohol, and chlordiazepoxide) and increased by 2 stimulants (methamphetamine and caffeine), with tests under 3 dosages of each drug. Under amobarbital, the Avoidance group decreased most and the Approach group decreased least in speed; under morphine, the Escape group was above the 2 others. During 6 massed trials per day, the Avoidance group when under amobarbital greatly increased and the Approach group when under chlorpromazine greatly decreased in speed.

REFERENCES

Barry, H., III, and Miller, N. E. Effects of drugs on approach-avoidance conflict tested repeatedly by means of a "telescope alley." *J. comp. physiol. Psychol.,* 1962, **55,** 201–210.

Barry, H., III, Wagner, S. A., and Miller, N. E. Effects of several drugs on performance in an approach-avoidance conflict. *Psychol. Rep.,* 1963, **12,** 215–221.

Boren, J. J. Some effects of adephine, benactyzine, and chlorpromazine upon several operant behaviors. *Psychopharmacologia,* 1961, **2**, 416–424.

Dews, P. B., and Morse, W. H. Behavioral pharmacology. *Ann. Rev. Pharmacol.,* 1961, **1**, 145–177.

Edwards, R. E. Methods of detecting behavioral effects of morphine in rats. *Federat. Proc.,* 1961, **20**, 397. (Abstract)

Ferster, C. B., and Skinner, B. F. *Schedules of reinforcement.* New York: Appleton-Century-Crofts, 1957.

Geller, I., Kulak, J. T., Jr., and Seifter, J. The effects of chlordiazepoxide and chlorpromazine on a punishment discrimination. *Psychopharmacologia,* 1962, **3**, 374–385.

Goodman, L. S., and Gilman, A. *The pharmacological basis of therapeutics.* (2nd ed.) New York: Macmillan, 1955.

Grossman, S. P. Effects of chlorpromazine and perphenazine on bar-pressing performance in an approach-avoidance conflict. *J. comp. physiol. Psychol.,* 1961, **54**, 517–521.

Miller, N. E. Some recent studies of conflict behavior and drugs. *Amer. Psychologist,* 1961, **16**, 12–24.

Miller, N. E. The analysis of motivational effects illustrated by experiments on amylobarbitone. In H. Steinberg, A. V. S. de Reuck, and J. Knight (Eds.), *Ciba Foundation symposium, jointly with the co-ordinating committee for symposia on drug action, on animal behavior and drug action.* London: Churchill, 1964. Pp. 1–18.

Miller, N. E., and Murray, E. J. Displacement and conflict: Learnable drive as a basis for the steeper gradient of avoidance than of approach. *J. exp. Psychol.,* 1952, **43**, 227–231.

Poschel, B. P. H. Effects of methamphetamine on hunger and thirst motivated variable-interval performance. *J. comp. physiol. Psychol.,* 1963, **56**, 968–973.

Polsuns, D. An analysis of chlorpromazine-induced suppression of the avoidance response. *Psychopharmacologia,* 1962, **3**, 361–373.

Ray, O. S. The effects of tranquilizers on positively and negatively motivated behavior in rats. *Psychopharmacologia,* 1963, **4**, 326–342.

Weissman, A. Differential drug effects upon a three-ply multiple schedule of reinforcement. *J. exp. Anal. Behav.,* 1959, **4**, 271–299.

35

Effects of chlorpromazine on appetitive and aversive components of a multiple schedule [1]

Marcus B. Waller and Patricia F. Waller

Many investigators have been particularly interested in comparing the effects of drugs on behavior maintained by positive reinforcement with their effects on behavior maintained by negative reinforcement. Much of this interest has resulted from the clinical use of drugs and the interpretations of their clinically observed effects. The purpose of the present experiment was to investigate the effects of chlorpromazine (CPZ) on a multiple schedule having both appetitive and avoidance components.

Research comparing drug effects on schedules of positive and negative reinforcement has yielded ambiguous results. Weissman (1959), using a multiple-schedule procedure with rats, found that CPZ had a more depressing effect on avoidance than on food-maintained behavior. On the other hand, Olds (1959), using rats and a brain-stimulation technique, found that CPZ inhibited responding to positive stimulation (approach), but failed to do so to negative stimulation (escape).

A similar state of affairs exists over the behavioral effects of reserpine. For example, Wenzel (1959) has reported that reserpine tends to increase response latencies to a greater extent and for a longer period of time on an avoidance schedule than on a food-reinforced schedule. Other reports fail to support Wenzel's result (Miller, 1956; Weiskrantz and Wilson, 1955). Furthermore, Dews and Morse (1960) have questioned Wenzel's results on methodological grounds. More data would seem desirable because of these ambiguous results.

The method used by Weissman (1959) and Wenzel (1959) offers several advantages over other methods. Because it is a special case of a multiple schedule having both appetitive and avoidance components (Herrnstein and Brady, 1958; Herrnstein, 1958; Brady, 1959), drug effects can be observed on both positively and negatively reinforced behavior in the

From *Journal of the Experimental Analysis of Behavior,* 1962, **5,** 259–264. Copyright 1962 by the Society for the Experimental Analysis of Behavior, Inc., Bloomington, Ind.

[1] This research was supported by Grant MY 1775 from the National Institute of Mental Health of the U.S.P.H.S. The authors wish to thank Doctors John L. Fuller, Arlo K. Meyers, and William H. Morse for their careful reading of the manuscript and helpful suggestions; and Mr. Jack Kirshenbaum for assistance in collecting and tabulating the data. The chlorpromazine used in this research was donated by Smith Kline & French Laboratories.

same subject almost simultaneously. The food-reinforced component in Weissman's schedule has several limitations, however. For example, the CRF schedule used placed a very low upper limit on response-output measures, *i.e.,* number and rate. A less constrained schedule would seem more appropriate.

METHOD. *Subjects.* The subjects were two male beagle dogs approximately 2 years old at the start of the experiment. They were maintained throughout the experiment on 300 g of Big Red dog chow per day plus a vitamin-mineral supplement once a week. This regime kept the animals at approximately 80% of their free-feeding weights.

Apparatus. The apparatus consisted of a cubical with a specially constructed grid floor and a nose manipulandum (Waller, 1960). Discriminative stimuli were presented by a 100-watt bulb in a flush-mounted ceiling fixture which directed the light on the manipulandum. Food was presented through a tube connected with a Gerbrands universal feeder. Each reinforcer consisted of two pellets of Big Red dog chow having a combined weight of approximately 5 g. The electric shock, administered through the grid floor and programmed through a grid scrambler had an intensity of 2.5 ma and a duration of 1 sec.

Procedure. Subjects were deprived of food and shaped *via* CRF to a VI 1 min schedule for food reinforcement. The program was then altered to a mult VI 1 min S^Δ 25 min. Continuous light was the stimulus condition correlated with the VI 1-min component, and the no-light condition was correlated with the S^Δ 25 min. After a stable performance developed, the schedule was altered to mult VI 1 min S^Δ 25 min avoid RS 20 sec SS 20 sec S^Δ 25 min. A flashing light (on 0.5 sec, off 0.5 sec) was correlated with the avoidance component. Both Ss were then shaped to the avoidance component in a single 9-hr session in which the avoidance component was introduced as a single 6-hr block. In the following sessions, components were of variable duration, *i.e.,* either 10, 20, 30, or 40 min. Under these conditions, Ss were run daily in 5-hr sessions until performance on all components was stable (approximately 400 hr), at which point the first drug procedure was carried out.

The initial drug procedure consisted of administering either 30, 75, 105, 180, or 225 mg of CPZ in "Spansule" form (sustained release capsules) 2 hr before a session. Subjects were run 7 days a week, with drug administered on alternate days. Four observations were taken for each drug dosage. The order of dosage was counterbalanced within these limitations. After approximately 10 months, during which time various changes had been made in the schedule, the schedule was returned to mult VI 1 min S^Δ 25 min avoid SS 20 sec RS 20 sec S^Δ 25 min for a second drug analysis.

In the second drug experiment, CPZ was used in soluble form ("thorazine" pills) at four dose levels: 25, 50, 100, and 150 mg. Subjects were run 5 days each week, and the drug was administered on Friday 2 hr before the session began. These sessions were 4 hr long. Each dose of the drug was administered twice for each *S*.

RESULTS.   The data reported in all figures are based upon performance during the fifth and sixth hours after drug administration, which were the third and fourth hours after the session began. This particular selection was based on the repeated observation that drug effects were maximal and stable during this period. The numbers reported in Fig. 1 were obtained by measuring the cumulative records.

Figure 1A shows the results of the first drug analysis, in which "Spansule" CPZ and a somewhat chronic drugging procedure were used. This procedure restricts the interpretation of these data, since the data cannot be interpreted as a dose-response function. No systematic change indicating drug tolerance was observed. The *S*s are presented separately.

By plotting output ratio, *i.e.,*

$$\frac{\text{mean drug rate of response}}{\text{mean control rate of response}}$$

on the ordinate, relative changes in response output for both the variable-interval and the avoidance components can be compared directly. Each point represents the mean of four drug observations. Thus, the change with

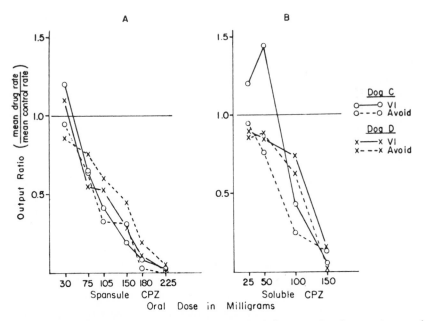

FIGURE 1. Output ratios based upon responses/minute under drug and control conditions. Figure 1A shows means of four replications with "Spansule" CPZ. Figure 1B shows means of two replications with soluble CPZ in oral doses.

increasing amounts of drug is comparable in most respects for the two components. For both subjects, however, the rate on the food-reinforced component tended to increase at the lowest dose, whereas a small decrease was observed on the avoidance component. Both components show decreases after greater doses which are progressive to the maximum dose given. Performance in the S^Δ components is not shown because response output was minimal under all conditions.

Figure 1B shows the results of the later drug experiment. In this figure, each point represents the mean of two drug observations. Only a single valid observation was obtained for Dog D at the 150-mg dose. A second observation of this dose was grossly deviant: Both components showed virtually no drug effect, indicating that the animal vomited following the oral administration. Evidence of nausea following large oral doses of CPZ was not uncommon. The similarity of the drug effects on the two components is striking for Dog D. Dog C showed an increase in rate on the VI 1-min component at low doses of chlorpromazine. Further, for Dog C, CPZ may have a greater depressing effect on avoidance responding. The first obvious depression of responding in both subjects followed the 100-mg dose.

Figure 2 shows segments of the cumulative records for both subjects. Because neither time nor the response count is directly comparable from segment to segment, records must be compared as to slope. Figure 2A shows segments of the cumulative records for Dog C taken from the "Spansule" procedure. These segments were from the records approximately 4–6 hr after drug administration. Note the comparability of the drug effect on the variable-interval component and on the avoidance component. Figure 2B shows comparable segments of the cumulative records for Dog D taken from the records for the later drug analysis in which soluble CPZ was used in oral doses. Again, a similar effect is observed on both the food and shock-avoidance components. The S^Δ components are not shown because virtually no responding was evident in S^Δ under any condition.

DISCUSSION. The results of these experiments suggest that over a considerable dose range, chlorpromazine has a similar effect on both food- and avoidance-maintained behavior. At very low doses the rate of food-reinforced responding tended to increase when compared with control performance, whereas a slight decrease in rate occurred in avoidance-maintained responding. At higher dose levels, both food and avoidance responding were generally depressed to a comparable degree. If by sensitivity we mean any deviation from control performance, the results suggest that food-maintained behavior is more sensitive to the effects of CPZ than is avoidance responding. Although low doses of CPZ tended to increase re-

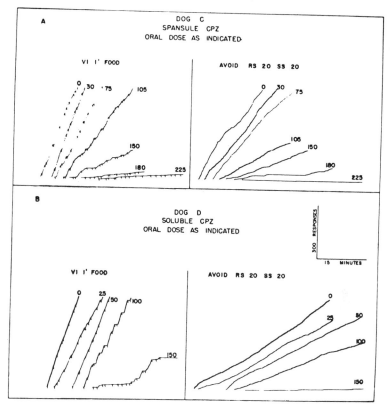

FIGURE 2. Portions of the cumulative records obtained during the 5th and 6th hours after the drug administrations indicated. Figure 2A shows the performance of Dog C following "Spansule" CPZ administration, and Fig. 2B shows Dog D after oral dosage with soluble CPZ.

sponse output in the food-reinforced component, the same doses had little or no effect on the avoidance component.

A second observation is of some interest. The drugging operation was somewhat different in the two drug procedures. In the first series, chlorpromazine was administered every other day and in "Spansule" form—a relatively chronic procedure; but in the second procedure, the regular oral form of chlorpromazine was administered once a week. The similarity of the two dose-response functions indicates that for gross approximations the chronic procedure is probably an adequate method for establishing the shape of the dose-response function for chlorpromazine.

The failure to find a gross difference in the effects of CPZ on food-reinforced and avoidance-maintained responding raises several questions which should be discussed at length. The first concerns the logic underlying cross-schedule comparisons, in general, and positively versus negatively reinforced schedules, in particular. The second question deals with cross-schedule versus cross-drug interaction, *i.e.,* when several drugs are compared on the basis of their cross-schedule effects. Although drugs will be used as a variable to develop both arguments, the analysis is more general and is applicable to other variables as well.

Schedule of reinforcement is not a unitary variable. A logical analysis will reveal that "schedule" encompasses a number of variables, two of which are rather obvious. Schedule specifies "contingency of reinforcement," *i.e.,* fixed ratio, fixed interval, DRL, or variable ratio. Furthermore, within broad limits, contingency of reinforcement can be manipulated independently of parameter value or "density of reinforcement." Experimental evidence supports this logical analysis. In a series of recent experiments, Dews (1958, 1960) has demonstrated unequivocally that parameter value or "density of reinforcement" is a variable of importance in the analysis of drug effects where contingency of reinforcement is held constant. There is no unequivocal evidence that contingency of reinforcement is a variable determining drug effects, but there is considerable evidence that contingency of reinforcement has an effect on behavior (Ferster and Skinner, 1957; Hearst, 1958).

If both density of reinforcement and contingency of reinforcement are variables determining drug effect, cross-schedule comparisons that do not consider both variables are obviously confounded. In fact, because schedule is not a unitary variable, comparisons across schedules are necessarily second-order comparisons, *i.e.,* comparisons of the interactive function of two variables. Although such comparisons are legitimate both logically and empirically, the interactive function must be specified.

Comparison of positively and negatively reinforced behavior, particularly where schedules are involved, is somewhat more complex. Parameter value or density of reinforcement and contingency of reinforcement seem rather inappropriate as variables specifying schedules of negative reinforcement. Even if shock-shock intervals and response-shock intervals could be translated into variables having scale properties similar to density and contingency of reinforcement (and this may well be experimentally feasible), other variables present equally difficult problems of experimental analysis. One of these is equivalence of magnitude of reinforcement. Obviously, shock, the avoidance of shock, the reduction of anxiety, or whatever serves as the negative reinforcer, is scaled on a different continuum than is food of water. Logically, a quantitative comparison of positive versus negative reinforcement requires that the magnitudes of reinforcement can be equated. Empirically, a quantitative comparison of positive and negative reinforcement demands that the magnitudes of reinforcement be scalable and that these scales be known.

The comparability of dependent variables should also be considered. There is reason to believe that an avoidance response is not directly comparable with a food-reinforced response (Sidman, 1958). However, there is little reason to believe that other indices of responding are any better. Certainly, the practice (Herrnstein, 1958; Weissman, 1959) of comparing number of shocks taken on the avoidance schedule with rate of response on the food schedule only complicates matters further.

There is no easy way out of the problems of cross-schedule comparisons. The problem is not unlike that of comparisons across species in comparative psychology. Only a careful experimental analysis will yield the functional relations which are necessary for such comparisons. Although the "double dissociation" experimental design described by Weiskrantz (1959, pp. 53–56) represents a logical improvement over simpler designs, it does not and, as currently used, cannot generate the basic functional relations required for cross-schedule comparisons. In fact, the addition of a cross-drug dimension to cross-schedule experiments leads to further difficulties in experimental analysis in that the new dimension generates other requirements.

SUMMARY. A multiple schedule having both an appetitive and an avoidance component was maintained in two dogs to create a complex behavioral base line for observing the effects of chlorpromazine. Both soluble and "Spansule" chlorpromazine generated similar functions relating drug dose to measures of behavioral output. Although the dose ranges and the drugging procedures differed markedly for the different preparations of CPZ, the functions generated were comparable. There was no evidence that chlorpromazine had a differential depressing effect as a function of type of reinforcement. At low doses, rates of responding on the food-reinforced components increased slightly, whereas rates on the avoidance components remained relatively unchanged. At higher doses, both components showed an approximately equal depression of responding. These results are discussed with reference to some of the logical and experimental difficulties inherent in making comparisons across components of a multiple schedule and across schedules in general.

REFERENCES

Brady, J. V. Animal experimental evaluation of drug effects upon behavior. In: Braceland, P. J. (Ed.), *The effects of pharmacologic agents on the nervous system.* Baltimore, Md.: Williams & Wilkins Co., 1959. Pp. 104–125.

Dews, P. B. Studies on behavior. IV. Stimulant actions of methamphetamine. *J. Pharmacol. & exp. Therap.,* 1958, **122**, 137–147.

Dews, P. B. Free-operant behavior under conditions of delayed reinforcement. I. CRF-type schedules. *J. exp. Anal. Behav.,* 1960, 3, 221–234.

Dews, P. B., and Morse, W. H. Behavioral pharmacology. *Ann. Rev. Pharmacol.*, 1961, 1, 145–174.

Ferster, C. B., and Skinner, B. F. *Schedules of reinforcement.* New York: Appleton-Century-Crofts, 1957.

Hearst, E. Multiple schedules of time-correlated reinforcement. *J. exp. Anal. Behav.*, 1960, 3, 49–62.

Herrnstein, R. J. Effects of scopolamine on a multiple schedule. *J. exp. Anal. Behav.*, 1958, 1, 351–358.

Herrnstein, R. J., and Brady, J. V. Interaction among components of a multiple schedule. *J. exp. Anal. Behav.*, 1958, 1, 293–300.

Miller, N. E. Effects of drugs on motivation: The value of using a variety of measures. *Ann. N.Y. Acad. Sci.*, 1956–57, 65, 318–333.

Olds, J. Studies of neuropharmacologicals by electrical and chemical manipulation of the brain in animals with chronically implanted electrodes. In Bradley, P. D., Deniker, P., and Radouco-Thomas, C. (Eds.), *Neuro-psychopharmacology,* Princeton, N.J.: Elsevier Publishing Co., 1959. Pp. 20–32.

Sidman, M. Some notes on "bursts" in free-operant avoidance experiments. *J. exp. Anal. Behav.*, 1958, 1, 167–172.

Waller, M. B. A manipulandum for use with dogs. *J. exp. Anal. Behav.*, 1960, 3, 311–312.

Weiskrantz, L. In Bradley, P. B., Deniker, P., and Radouco-Thomas, C. (Eds.), *Neuro-psychopharmacology,* Princeton, N.J.: Elsevier Publishing Co., 1959. Pp. 53–56.

Weiskrantz, L., and Wilson, W. A. The effects of reserpine on emotional behavior of normal and brain operated monkeys. *Ann. N.Y. Acad. Sci.*, 1955, 61, 36–55.

Weissman, A. Differential drug effects upon a three-ply multiple schedule of reinforcement. *J. exp. Anal. Behav.*, 1959, 2, 271–287.

Wenzel, Bernice. Relative resistance to reserpine of responses based on positive as compared with negative reinforcement. *J. comp. physiol. Psychol.*, 1959, 52, 673–681.

36

An analysis of chlorpromazine-induced suppression of the avoidance response *

DONALD POSLUNS

Chlorpromazine, one of the phenothiazine derivatives, suppresses the avoidance response at doses which neither produce ataxia nor impair the performance of an escape response (Cook *et al.;* Miller *et al.,* 1957a; Maffii). The avoidance response suppression is a property of most, if not all, phenothiazine derivatives (Fellows and Cook; Irvin; Stone; Cook and Kelleher), and can be manifested during acquisition and extinction (Ader and Clink; Miller *et al.,* 1957a, 1957b), as well as maintenance, of the response (Cook and Weidley; Verhave *et al.*). The avoidance-suppressing property of the phenothiazine derivatives may be related to the drugs' action in relieving psychotic disorders, because a rank order relation has been demonstrated between the dose at which any one phenothiazine derivative suppresses the avoidance response and its relative potency in psychotic relief (Cook and Kelleher). However, some nonataractic compounds, including morphine and belladonna alkaloids such as atropine and scopolamine, also specifically suppress the avoidance response (Mikhelson *et al.* cited by Berger; Maffii; Paskal and Vanderwolf). A more detailed discussion can be found in Herz's review of drug-induced avoidance response suppression.

The three experiments reported here form part of a systematic search for the factors underlying the specific suppression of the avoidance response by chlorpromazine. Two separate conclusions have been reached to explain chlorpromazine-induced avoidance response suppression. Some investigators (e.g., Ader and Clink; Miller *et al.,* 1957a; Torres) have suggested that chlorpromazine reduces "fear" or "anxiety" the presence of which is believed necessary for the reinforcement of the avoidance response. The "fear reduction" suggestion has an intuitive plausibility to it because of the drug's therapeutic effect, but other investigators (e.g., Killam and Killam; Bradley; Key) have concluded that chlorpromazine produces an impairment of "sensory-arousal" functions, an impairment which could suppress the avoidance response by inhibiting cue functions or arousal functions or

From *Psychopharmacologia* (Berl.), 1962, 3, 361–373. Copyright 1962 by Springer-Verlag, Heidelberg, Germany.

* This research was supported by Grant No. APT-36 from the National Research Council of Canada to Dr. D. Bindra. Chlorpromazine was supplied free of charge, as *Largactil,* by Poulenc Ltd., Montreal. While conducting the experiments, the author held a Bursary from the National Research Council of Canada.

both. From an examination of the results of the present and previous experiments, an alternative conclusion is reached here.

In Experiment 1, an attempt was made to partially overcome chlorpromazine's decremental effect on the avoidance response by manipulating selected parameters of the avoidance situation. Partly because increasing the preshock interval was the only manipulation which improved avoidance response performance under the drug, it was suggested that chlorpromazine induced a locomotor deficit. In order to see whether the locomotor deficit was one of motor performance (as opposed to one attributable to fear reduction), Experiment 2 was planned to investigate chlorpromazine's effect on avoidance learning as measured by later, undrugged, performance. In Experiment 3, the relations between avoidance response suppression and chlorpromazine's effect on selected component acts of the avoidance response were investigated.

METHODS AND RESULTS

Subjects. Fifty-seven naive male hooded rats of the Long-Evans strain, obtained from the Royal Victoria Hospital colony, served as subjects. At the start of the experiments, the animals were about 110 days old. During the experiments, they were housed two to a cage in which food and water were continuously available.

Apparatus and materials. The avoidance apparatus used in all experiments was a wooden box, 106.7 cm long, 14.6 cm wide and 50.8 cm deep. The walls of one half of the box were painted black and the walls of the other half white; the color of the walls divided the box into two equal-sized compartments with no structural separation between them. The floor of the apparatus was a grid of 0.16 cm steel rods set about 1.25 cm apart. The grid floor of the black compartment could be electrically charged with a shock "scrambled" through 15 separate output leads; the nonelectrified white compartment was the goal compartment.

The compounds used in the experiments were chlorpromazine hydrochloride B.P. and a 0.9% solution of sodium chloride. The fluid contents of commercial vials of the chlorpromazine (5 mg drug/ml water) were mixed with sufficient additional distilled water to attain a concentration (in mg/ml) which was numerically equal to the dose used (in mg/kg). The use of such concentrations kept the volumes of both the drug and the isotonic saline constant at 1 ml/kg. The drug was freshly mixed for each experiment. Administration in all cases was by intraperitoneal injection.

General procedure. The avoidance response in the present experiments required locomotion from a starting point at the end of the black compartment into the white compartment. Under "standard conditions," there were no specific warning signals and a 1.2 mA electric shock was administered after a 5 sec preshock interval. In all experiments, the intertrial interval was 30 sec, during which the animal remained in the white compartment. After the intertrial interval, the animal was manually replaced at the starting point and another trial administered. Trials were administered in each session until an animal had performed 9 successful avoidance responses in 10 consecutive trials, with a maximum of 30 trials. The attainment of the 90% criterion or the 30-trial maximum defines a session for all experiments. Avoidance response performance was measured by the total number of shocks received (that is, escape responses) in reaching the 90% criterion or 30-trial maximum. The compounds were injected 30 min. before the start of the appropriate session. "Standard conditions" were used in all training sessions.

EXPERIMENT 1.   In this experiment, an attempt was made to increase the number of avoidance responses made under the influence of chlorpromazine by increasing, in turn, one of 3 parameters. The 3 manipulated parameters were the magnitude of warning signals, the intensity of electric shock, and the length of the preshock interval.

Procedure.   Twenty-six rats were first given 4 sessions of avoidance training, using the "standard conditions" (no specific warning signals, a 1.2 mA shock, and a 5 sec preshock interval). After training, there were 3 Test Phases. No drug was administered during training; 3.0 mg/kg chlorpromazine were injected prior to each Test Phase.

In each Test Phase, the essential plan was to compare the drugged animals' avoidance performance during a session in which the "standard conditions" were used (Standard Session) with the same animals' performance during a session in which the value of one of the 3 parameters was increased (Experimental Session). To this end, the animals used in each Test Phase were assigned to two equal groups which were tested in a counterbalanced order. One group was tested first in an Experimental Session, and then, immediately afterwards, was tested in a Standard Session. The reverse order of Standard and Experimental Sessions was used with the other group. All 26 rats were used in the first Test Phase; 14 of the 26 were selected for the second and third Test Phases. In each Test Phase, one parametric value was increased and all other conditions were held constant.

In the first Test Phase, the magnitude of the warning signals was manipulated (Warning Signals Phase). In the Experimental Session, the warning signals were used; in the Standard Session, no specific warning signals were used. The warning signals comprised a 100 watt bulb and a 5000 cps. tone of about 70 db., both of which were simultaneously applied when the animal was placed at the starting point, and terminated when the animal entered the white goal compartment. Twelve rats (6 tested first in the Experimental Session and then in the Standard Session, and 6 tested in the reverse order) were tested with the warning signals positioned directly over the entrance to the goal compartment. For the remaining 14 (7 from each of the counter-balanced orders), the warning signals were positioned over the starting point.

In the second Test Phase, the intensity of electric shock was manipulated (Shock Intensity Phase). In the Experimental Session, a 2.8 mA shock was used; in the Standard Session, a 1.2 mA. shock was used.

In the third Test Phase, the length of the preshock interval was manipulated (Preshock Interval Phase). In the Experimental Session, a 15 sec preshock interval was used; in the Standard Session, a 5 sec preshock interval was used.

Results. When the Experimental and the Standard Sessions were pooled, and the differences between first and second sessions only were examined, there were no significant differences between the first and second sessions in either the Warning Signals Phase or the Preshock Interval Phase. In the Shock Intensity Phase, however, the number of shocks received decreased by a mean value of 2.7 from the first session to the second ($p < .05$; Wilcoxon matched-pairs, signed-ranks test, two-tailed).

Comparisons between the Standard and Experimental Sessions for all 3 Test Phases are shown in Table 1. Of the 3 manipulated variables, lengthening the preshock interval was the only manipulation which increased the number of avoidance responses performed under the influence of chlorpromazine ($p < .01$; Wilcoxon matched-pairs, signed-ranks test, two-tailed).

The results from the Warning Signals Phase were also analyzed for the effects of the position of the signals. These results are shown in Table 2. Disregarding the order of presentation of Experimental and Standard Sessions, the warning signals had a tendency to improve avoidance performance when they were positioned over the starting point, but a tendency to decrease performance when they were positioned over the goal entrance (for both, $p < .05$; Wilcoxon matched-pairs, signed-ranks test, two-tailed).

The behavior of the animals in this experiment was observed closely, and a specific pattern of responding could be observed when an animal made an avoidance response during the 15 sec preshock interval. During

TABLE 1.   Changes between the Standard and Experimental Sessions in the three Test Phases, in mean number of shocks received.

Phase	Changes between sessions		
	Standard session	Experimental session	Change
Warning signals	14.38	13.35	− 1.03
Shock intensity	19.28	19.00	− 0.28
Preshock interval	19.50	11.21	8.29*

* $p < .01$; Wilcoxon matched-pairs, signed-ranks test, two-tailed.

TABLE 2.   Changes between the Standard and Experimental Sessions of the Warning Signals Phase, in relation to the position of the warning signals. Scores represent mean number of shocks received.

Position of warning signals	Changes between sessions		
	Standard session	Experimental session	Change
Goal entrance	6.83	10.08	3.25*
Starting point	20.71	16.14	−4.57*

* $p < .05$;   Wilcoxon   matched-pairs,   signed-ranks test, two-tailed.

the total avoidance response, 3 or 4 separate behavioral "units" or "component acts" could be isolated by pauses between them. First, the animal typically executed an orienting movement, turning its head to one side or, often, turning completely around to face the white compartment. Orienting tended to occur rapidly. Second, there was a considerable pause, following which the animal quickly moved towards the white compartment. Third, some animals paused just before entering the white compartment, frequently sustaining a shock during the pause. Fourth, many animals also paused just after entering the white compartment, after which they would typically continue to the far end of the compartment. For purposes of convenient description, I have used the term *segmentation* to describe this pattern of motion and pauses because the total response appears segmented into various bits or component acts. Complete segmentation, that is, all 3 pauses in the same trial, was seen only about a dozen times, but each pause was observed at least twice in all animals which made any response. The first pause, between orienting and the initial locomotion, was by far the most frequent; this pause occurred on almost every trial.

EXPERIMENT 2.   Rats were first given two sessions of avoidance training while under the influence of chlorpromazine. Then, in a third session, they were tested, undrugged, in order to see if the avoidance response had been acquired.

Procedure.   Twenty-two rats were first randomly assigned to either a Chlorpromazine Group ($n = 12$) or a Saline Group ($n = 10$). Then all animals received 3 sessions of avoidance training in all of which the "standard conditions" were used. The Saline Group received isotonic saline prior to all 3 sessions. The Chlorpromazine Group received injections of 2.5 mg/kg chlorpromazine prior to the first two sessions; for the third session, this group also received injections of isotonic saline.

Results.   The results of the experiment are shown in Table 3. In the first two sessions, the Chlorpromazine Group received more shocks than the Saline Group ($p < .002$; Mann-Whitney U test, two-tailed). In the third session, however, when only saline was administered to both groups, all

TABLE 3. Mean number of shocks received by the Saline and Chlorpromazine Groups in learning the avoidance response. In the 3rd session, both groups received only saline.

Session	Group	
	Saline	Chlorpromazine
1st	7.4	16.5*
2nd	1.6	13.1*
3rd	0.8	1.3**

* Greater than the Saline Group in the same session ($p < .002$; Mann-Whitney U test, two-tailed).

** Less than the Saline Group in the 1st session ($p < .002$; Mann-Whitney U test, two-tailed).

animals received about the same number of shocks. The mean improvement in performance from the first to the second session was about the same for both groups. The performance of the Chlorpromazine Group in the third session was superior to the performance of the Saline Group in the first session ($p < .002$; Mann-Whitney U test, two-tailed).

EXPERIMENT 3.   This experiment represents an attempt to specify more precisely the effect of chlorpromazine on the avoidance response by differentiating the drug's effect upon locomotor initiation and upon the running time after initiation. An attempt was also made to relate the severity of segmentation to the degree of avoidance response suppression induced by the drug.

Procedure.   Nine rats were first given 3 sessions of avoidance training, using "standard conditions," followed by two Test Phases. Prior to the first Test Phase, each animal received isotonic saline (Control Phase). Prior to the second Phase, each animal received 2.5 mg/kg chlorpromazine (Chlorpromazine Phase). In all other respects the two Test Phases were identical.

Paired comparisons on each animal were made between the two Test Phases. First, in both Test Phases, a regular session of trials was administered (that is, with the 90% criterion and 30-trial maximum), using the "standard conditions." During the regular session, the total number of *shocks received* was noted for each animal.

Then, immediately following the regular session, the shock was discontinued and 10 additional trials were administered. On the odd-numbered nonshock trials, the time between placing the animal at the starting point and its subsequent initiation of locomotion was recorded; this was called the *locomotor initiation latency*. If an animal did not move within 30 sec, it was manually placed in the white compartment and assigned a latency of 30 sec for that trial. On the even-numbered nonshock trials, the time be-

TABLE 4. Comparisons of mean group scores between the Control Phase and the Chlorpromazine Phase.

Measure		Test phase	
		Control	Chlorpromazine
Regular session	Number of shocks received	1.55	5.66*
Nonshock trials	Locomotor initiation latency (in sec)	0.68	3.32*
	Running time (in sec)	0.85	0.82

* Greater than the same measure in the Control Phase ($p < .01$; Wilcoxon matched-pairs, signed-ranks test, two-tailed).

tween the locomotor initiation and the subsequent entry into the goal compartment was recorded; this was called the *running time*. If an animal initiated locomotion, but paused before entering the goal compartment, the trial was discounted and another was immediately administered in its place. Both the locomotor initiation latency and the running time were measured with a manually operated stopwatch.

Results. Means of the 5 locomotor initiation latencies and of the 5 running times were computed for each animal, for both Test Phases. Table 4 shows group means for all 3 measures in both Test Phases. Under the influence of chlorpromazine, the animals received more shocks and had longer locomotor initiation latencies than without the drug (for both, $p < .01$; Wilcoxon matched-pairs, signed-ranks test, two-tailed). However, the drug did not alter the running time.

Using the results of the Chlorpromazine Phase only, product-moment correlation coefficients were computed among the 3 measures. The coefficients are shown in Table 5. The locomotor initiation latency under chlorpromazine was highly and positively correlated with the number of shocks received under the drug ($p < .01$, two-tailed). The running time was negatively correlated with the number of shocks received ($p = .02$, two-tailed) to about the same degree and in the same direction that the running time was correlated with the locomotor initiation latency ($p < .05$, two-tailed).

In this experiment, another phenomenon was observed, which had been

TABLE 5. Product-movement correlation coefficients among the three measures, during the Chlorpromazine Phase.

	Number of shocks received	Running time
Locomotor initiation · latency	0.94***	−0.65*
Running time	−0.69**	—

* $p < .05$, two-tailed test. ** $p = .02$, two-tailed test. *** $p < .01$, two-tailed test.

noted but disregarding previously. In the Chlorpromazine Phase, four rats had a tendency to shriek while sitting on the grid, when no shock was being applied. This conditioned vocalization (Vanderwolf) was not the squealing associated with placing an animal at the starting point nor picking up the animal from the grid. For the four animals, conditioned vocalization occurred on 10% to 75% of the trials in the Chlorpromazine Phase, primarily during the nonshock trials. The animals which showed conditioned vocalization made fewer avoidance responses than the other animals, but within the group of four conditioned vocalizers there did not seem to be a rank order relation between the number of shocks received and the number of conditioned vocalizations.

DISCUSSION

The results of Experiment 1 suggested that chlorpromazine induced a locomotor deficit in suppressing the avoidance response. The locomotor deficit was specifically suggested by the finding that lengthening the pre-shock interval from 5 to 15 sec increased the number of avoidance responses made under chlorpromazine. It appeared that the drugged rats could make the avoidance response, but merely required more time. The failure of both introducing warning signals and increasing the shock intensity to increase the number of avoidance responses suggested that the locomotor deficit could not be attributed to sensory deficits.

Although the warning signals were ineffective in improving the avoidance response performance under chlorpromazine (Table 1), the same signals acted as aversive stimuli, directing the drugged animals away from the source of stimulation (Table 2). It is clear, from the escape responses to the warning signals, that the drugged animals sensed and attended to the stimuli, and were aroused by them. Therefore, if chlorpromazine had induced a sensory deficit sufficient to suppress the avoidance response, the introduction of the warning signals should have improved the avoidance response performance, because the signals clearly were perceived.

Similarly, if chlorpromazine decreased sensitivity to electric shock, the increase in shock intensity from 1.2 mA to 2.8 mA should have improved avoidance response performance under the drug. Undrugged rats reach an asymptotic minimum in the avoidance response latency at about 1 mA (Kimble; Black et al.). If chlorpromazine had decreased the sensitivity to electric shock, the avoidance response latency would not yet have reached its minimum at the lower intensity, and the increase to 2.8 mA would shorten the response latency. For that reason the increased locomotor latency induced by chlorpromazine cannot be attributed to a decreased sensitivity to electric shock.

Although the results of Experiment 1 suggested a locomotor deficit without accompanying sensory impairments, chlorpromazine might have reduced the "fear" or "anxiety" the presence of which is believed necessary for the reinforcement of the avoidance response. The results of Experiment 2, however, demonstrated that the chlorpromazine drugged rats learned the avoidance response as well as the saline control groups, as shown by the performance in the third session (Table 3); apparently the drug prevented the performance of the response in the first two sessions. It is difficult to understand how the avoidance response could be acquired under the influence of chlorpromazine if the drug reduced the efficacy of the reinforcer during training to the point where the performance of the response was suppressed. Avoidance training under chlorpromazine results in more rapid extinction than training without drug (Ader and Clink; Miller *et al.,* 1957b) and also blocks mediated acquisition of the avoidance response (Davis *et al.*). However, the maintenance of the electric shock in the present Experiment 2 demonstrates rapid avoidance response acquisition under chlorpromazine, even though the ease with which the acquisition can be shown varies with different procedures.

It has thus been concluded that chlorpromazine induces a locomotor deficit without impairing the pertinent sensory or motivational processes. The results of Experiment 3 specify the locomotor deficit more precisely as a deficit in initiation; chlorpromazine delays locomotor initiation without affecting the speed of locomotion after initiation. Applying a variance interpretation (Ferguson, p. 107) to the correlation coefficient between the length of the locomotor initiation delay and the number of shocks received (Table 5), it can be estimated that over 85% of the avoidance response suppression is attributable to the delay in locomotor initiation. The failure of chlorpromazine to affect the running time supports the conclusion of Miller *et al.* (1957a) that the drug does not suppress the avoidance response by producing peripheral muscular inabilities. The negative correlation between the number of shocks received and the running time can be interpreted as further evidence that chlorpromazine does not alter the efficacy of shock and shock termination, that is, the rats which have been shocked more often tend to run faster. Results similar to those obtained in Experiment 3 were also found in an unreported experiment in which the avoidance response required jumping rather than running to the goal.

If chlorpromazine suppresses the avoidance response by delaying the initiation of locomotion, the first segmentation pause (Experiment 1) is understandable. However, the pauses just before and just after entering the goal compartment are not easily understood unless entering the goal and moving to its far end constitute separate locomotor acts the initiation of which chlorpromazine also delays. While training 18 naive undrugged rats in the same apparatus, for another experiment, it was noted that 14 of the animals made pauses during the first training session just like the pauses made by chlorpromazine-drugged rats in the present experiments. Both normal naive rats, during the initial training trials, and chlorpromazine-drugged rats, in later as well as the initial trials, paused between orienting and running, just before entering the goal compartment, and just after the entrance. The rank order frequency of the pauses is the same for both normal naive and chlorpromazine-drugged rats. It thus appears that orienting, approaching the goal, entering the goal, and moving to its far end all constitute separate component acts in the avoidance response. Under normal conditions, continued practice decreases the initiation latencies of the components acts until they become integrated into one smooth response. Chlorpromazine, by delaying the initiation of locomotor acts, reinstates the segmentation (as opposed to integration) observed during normal training, leaving the latency of the nonlocomotor orienting act and the running speed relatively intact.

Some other experimental results are also pertinent to the conclusions drawn here. Chlorpromazine depresses locomotion in both open field and activity wheel situations (Boyd and Miller; Jasmin and Bois; Janssen *et al.*), and the amount of locomotor decrement, like the degree of avoidance suppression, is directly related to the dose level (Fellows and Cook; Miller *et al.*, 1957a). Fellows and Cook, as well as Irvin, also found that, within a group of phenothiazine derivatives, the dose at which any one of the compounds suppressed the avoidance response was related to the dose required to depress locomotor activity. Using a time-sample method in which locomotor acts were included, Bindra and Baran found that chlorpromazine decreased the number of activity *changes,* that is, the number of initiations of new acts.

If chlorpromazine delays locomotor initiation, it follows that the drug should not affect the acquisition or maintenance of a response which requires no locomotion. In keeping with this conclusion, Hunt demonstrated that a high dose of chlorpromazine impaired neither the acquisition nor the maintenance of a conditioned emotional response, as measured by the suppression of bar pressing and by defecation. The observation of conditioned vocalization in Experiment 3 seems similar to Hunt's findings, and has similar implications. Moreover, Blough found that chlorpromazine actually facilitated the acquisition and maintenance of a response which required pigeons to stand still for food reinforcement.

In delaying locomotor initiation, chlorpromazine must selectively affect only certain kinds of locomotor acts, for both escape response initiation and the reactin time to unconditioned stimulation seem unimpaired by the drug. As the evidence suggests a direct motor deficit, the selective action of the drug must be attributed to differences in the locomotor initiation mechanisms among the responses. Assuming a continuum from completely stimulus-bound to completely voluntary responses, chlorpromazine may selectively suppress the initiation of the more voluntary responses, that is, of responses the initiation of which is more dependent upon mediating processes (Hebb, p. 48). The avoidance response is often regarded as a kind of escape response to which classical conditioning has been added, but the implication of a mediating process in the avoidance response requires a more complex mechanism. The more complex mechanism is required, in part, by the evidence that chlorpromazine suppresses the avoidance response while disrupting neither the classical conditioned response (Hunt), nor the escape response (Maffii), nor the instrumental response (Aceto *et al.;* Blough).

CONCLUSION.   Chlorpromazine suppresses the avoidance response by delaying the initiation of the more voluntary locomotor acts, and when a number of such acts are components of some integrated response, the initiation of each component act is delayed. The locomotor initiation delay is a motor performance deficit induced through the inhibition of some central nervous system function.

SUMMARY

Three experiments were reported, as part of a search for the factors underlying chlorpromazine-induced suppression of the avoidance response. The avoidance response required moving from the end of one compartment in a two-compartment box into the other compartment. The experiments were conducted upon the hooded rat.

The results of the experiments may be summarized as follows.

1. Lengthening the preshock interval increased the number of avoidance responses made under the influence of chlorpromazine by rats which had been previously trained without drug. Neither intensifying the electric shock nor introducing warning signals affected the number of responses made under the drug. It was concluded that chlorpromazine induces a locomotor deficit which is not attributable to sensory deficits.

2. Chlorpromazine did not impair avoidance response acquisition when the drug was injected just prior to two training sessions and omitted for the third, the test, session. It was concluded that the drug did not alter the efficacy of the avoidance response reinforcer.

3. Chlorpromazine induced a delay in the initiation of locomotion without affecting the running time. The length of the locomotor initiation delay correlated highly with an independent measure of avoidance response suppression. It was concluded that the avoidance suppression was attributable to the inability to initiate locomotion under chlorpromazine, and that the inability resulted from the drug's action upon some central motor function.

REFERENCES

Aceto, M. D., Lynch, V. D., and Thoms, R. K.: Effects of drugs on conditioning in the rat. II. Synthesis of a centrally active drug and the effects of nine drugs on operant conditioning and extinction. *J. pharm. Sci.* **50**, 823–827 (1961).

Ader, R., and Clink, D. W.: Effects of chlorpromazine on the acquisition and extinction of an avoidance response in the rat. *J. Pharmacol. exp. Ther.* **131**, 144–148 (1957).

Berger, F. M.: The chemistry and mode of action of tranquilizing drugs. *Ann. N.Y. Acad. Sci.* **67**(10), 685–700 (1957).

Bindra, D., and Baran, D.: Effect of methylphenidylacetate and chlorpromazine on certain components of general activity. *J. exp. Anal. Behav.* **2**, 343–350 (1959).

Black, R., Adamson, R., and Bevan, W.: Runway behavior as a function of apparent intensity of shock. *J. comp. physiol. Psychol.* **54**, 270–274 (1961).

Blough, D. S.: New test for tranquilizers. *Science* **127**, 586–587 (1958).

Boyd, E. M., and Miller, J. K.: Inhibition of locomotor activity by chlorpromazine hydrochloride. *Fed. Proc.* **13**, 338 (1954).

Bradley, P. B.: The central action of certain drugs in relation to the reticular formation of the brain. In H. H. Jasper, L. D. Proctor, R. S. Knighton, W. D. Noshay, and R. T. Costello (eds.), *Reticular formation of the brain.* Boston: Little, Brown & Co. 1958.

Cook, L., and Kelleher, R. T.: Drug effects on the behavior of animals. *Ann. N.Y. Acad. Sci.* **96**(1), 315–335 (1962).

Cook, L., and Weidley, E.: Behavioral effects of some psychopharmacological agents. *Ann. N.Y. Acad. Sci.* **66**(3), 740–752 (1957).

Cook, L., Weidley, E., Morris, R., and Mattis, P.: Neuropharmacological and behavioral effects of chlorpromazine. *J. Pharmacol. exp. Ther.* **113**, 1–11 (1955).

Davis, W. M., Capehart, J., and Llewellin, W. L.: Mediated acquisition of a fear-motivated response and inhibitory effects of chlorpromazine. *Psychopharmacologia* (Berl.) **2**, 268–276 (1961).

Fellows, E. J., and Cook, L.: The comparative pharmacology of a number of phenothiazine derivatives. In S. Garattini and V. Ghetti (eds.), *Psychotropic drugs.* Amsterdam: Elsevier Publ. Co. 1957.

Ferguson, G. A.: *Statistical analysis in psychology and education.* New York: McGraw-Hill 1959.

Hebb, D. O.: *A textbook of psychology.* Philadelphia: W. B. Saunders Co. 1958.

Herz, A.: Drugs and the conditioned avoidance response. *Int. Rev. Neurobiol.* **2**, 229–227 (1960).

Hunt, H. F.: Some effects of drugs on classical (type S) conditioning. *Ann. N.Y. Acad. Sci.* **65**(4), 258–267 (1956).

Irvin, S.: Comparative potency of phenothiazine tranquilizers in suppressing avoidance and locomotor behavior: its implications. *Pharmacologist* **1**, 51 (1959).

Janssen, P. A. J., Jageneau, A. H. M., and Schellekens, K. H. L.: Chemistry and pharmacology of compounds related to 4-(4-hydroxy-4-phenyl-piperidino)-butyrophene. IV. Influence of haloperidol (R 1625) and of chlorpromazine on the behavior of rats in an unfamiliar "open field" situation. *Psychopharmacologia* (Berl.) **1**, 389–392 (1960).

Jasmin, G., and Bois, P.: Effects of centrally-acting drugs on muscular exercise in rats. *Canad. J. Biochem.* **37**, 417–423 (1959).

Key, B. J.: The effect of drugs on discrimination and sensory generalization of auditory stimuli in cats. *Psychopharmacologia* (Berl.) **2**, 352–363 (1961).

Killam, K. F., and Killam, E. K.: Drug action on pathways involving the reticular formation. In H. H. Jasper, L. D. Proctor, R. S. Knighton, W. C. Noshay, and R. T. Costello (eds.), *Reticular formation of the brain*. Boston: Little, Brown & Co. 1958.

Kimble, G. A.: Shock intensity and avoidance learning. *J. comp. physiol. Psychol.* **48**, 281–284 (1955).

Maffii, G.: The secondary conditioned response of rats and the effects of some psychopharmacological agents. *J. Pharm. Pharmacol.* **11**, 129–139 (1959).

Mikhelson, M. I. A., Rozhkova, E. K., and Savateev, I. A.: Antagonistic action of cholinolytic and anticholinesterase substances on the higher nervous functions in man and animals. *Biul. eksp. Biol. Med.* **37**, 7–12 (1954).

Miller, R. E., Murphy J. V., and Mirsky, I. A.: The effect of chlorpromazine on fear-motivated behavior in rats. *J. Pharmacol. exp. Ther.* **120**, 379–387 (1957a).

Miller, R. E., Murphy, J. V., and Mirsky, I. A.: Presistent effects of chlorpromazine on extinction of an avoidance response. *Arch. Neurol. Psychiat.* (Chic.) **78**, 526–530 (1957b).

Paskal, V., and Vanderwolf, C. H.: Some effects of atropine sulfate on learning in the rat. Paper read at Canadian Psychological Association, Hamilton, Ont., June, 1962.

Stone, G. C.: Effects of some centrally acting drugs upon learning of escape and avoidance habits. *J. comp. physiol. Psychol.* **53**, 33–37 (1960).

Torres, A. A.: Anxiety versus escape conditioning and tranquilizing action. *J. comp. physiol. Psychol.* **54**, 349–353 (1961).

Vanderwolf, C. V.: Medial thalamic functions in voluntary behavior. *Canad. J. Psychol.* **16**, 318–330 (1962).

Verhave, T., Owen, J. E., and Robbins, E. B.: Effects of chlorpromazine and secobarbital on avoidance and escape behavior. *Arch. int. Pharmacodyn.* **116**, 45–53 (1958).

37

Brain stimulation reward "thresholds" self-determined in rat

LARRY STEIN and OAKLEY S. RAY

Behavioral training procedures that permit an animal to stimulate his brain electrically through permanently implanted electrodes can provide unique information about central nervous system processes (Olds, Brady). These self-stimulation procedures may be extended quantitatively by allowing the magnitude as well as the rate of the stimulation to be manipulated by the animal; in this way, information about stimulation preferences and thresholds may be obtained and stable baselines established for the study of variables. In a recent paper (Stein and Ray), we reported a technique for determining the preferred (selected as optimal by the animal) current intensity for stimulating positively reinforcing brain sites. In this report, we describe a related method which gives a continuous assay of the smallest current levels that will stimulate positive cell groups sufficiently to produce a rewarding effect.

METHODS.   The animals were trained in a small sound-resistant box with two levers in one wall. Responses at one lever (stimulation lever) delivered a brief train of positively reinforcing brain stimulation. Each succeeding response at the stimulation lever produced brain-shock rewards that decreased stepwise in intensity. In the present experiments, there were 15 equal current steps between a moderately reinforcing, but a clearly suprathreshold, top value (generally less than 10 ma) and zero ma. The current steps were programmed with a stepping switch, activated by operations of the stimulation lever, which introduced graded resistances into the stimulating circuit.

The second lever (reset lever) could be operated at any time to reset the current to the top step. The reset lever never gave brain shocks. Ideally, the method has the animal work the stimulation lever repetitively for the brain-shock rewards until the current intensity is driven down below a maintaining or reinforcing level, respond once at the reset lever to reset the current to the top step, and then return to the stimulation lever and start the next cycle. This procedure may be recognized as an adaptation for animal subjects of the classical psychophysical method of minimal changes (Guilford) with an operant response (reset) substituted for a verbal judgment.

From *Psychopharmacologia* (Berl.), 1960, 1, 251–256. Copyright 1960 by Springer-Verlag, Heidelberg, Germany.

Continuous records of the current step at which resets occurred were drawn by a recording potentiometer whose input voltage, controlled by the stepping switch through an auxiliary bank of resistances, was always proportional to the stimulating current. A cumulative response recorder and impulse counters simultaneously provided records of the self-stimulation rate.

The stimulation waveform was supplied from a Lilly-type pulse-pair generator and is described in more detail elsewhere (Lilly *et al.*, Stein and Ray). The paired pulses were opposite in sign, each 50 μsec in duration, and separated by 200 μsec. A brain-shock reward in the experiments reported here consisted of a 0.25 sec current train at 50 pulse pairs sec.

Six male albino rats with bipolar electrodes (0.01 inch platinum wires, twisted together and insulated except at the tips) permanently implanted in posterior hypothalamic and midbrain tegmentum sites have been studied. In preliminary training the animals learned to obtain fixed, moderately reinforcing (approximately 5 ma) brain shocks by operating first either lever and then only the stimulation lever. After the self-stimulation rates had stabilized, threshold-determination training was begun.

With assistance from the experimenter, the rats could frequently be trained in the essentials of this procedure in less than 20 minutes. This aid consisted mainly in resetting the current to the top step when it was driven to zero or near-zero levels by the animal. Training was greatly facilitated by "shaping" the reset response; this was accomplished by resetting the current at first only when the animal oriented toward the reset lever, and then later requiring approaching and investigating responses at this lever before resetting.

RESULTS. After a few two or three hour sessions, stable cycles of self-stimulation and resetting as described above were obtained with most animals. Current resetting was quite precise; even with small intensity steps (roughly, 1–2 per cent of the total range that gives reinforcement), a good animal would reset at the same step 50–60% of the time, and place 90–95% of the resets within one step above and below the modal step. Typically, the threshold would increase during the first 10–20 minutes of an experimental session; then it leveled off and was stable for hours, although variability increased somewhat as the session progressed. With rest periods of 2–3 days between experimental sessions, performance has been found, at least for the two animals most extensively studied, to be stable for more than three months.

A representative record of threshold-determining behavior obtained from a well-trained animal with an electrode in the midbrain tegmentum is shown in the right-hand portion of Fig. 1. The recording pen moves downward one step (0.42 ma) with each successive response at the stimulation lever, and returns to the top (6.4 ma) with every response at the reset lever; hence, the jagged edge of the curve indicates the current intensities

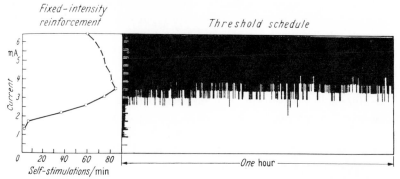

FIGURE 1. Comparison of two indices of the threshold for brain-stimulation re-ward: (left) self-stimulation rate obtained with fixed-intensity reinforcement vs. (right) current intensity at reset in threshold schedule. The horizontal markings to the left of the threshold record indicate the 16 current levels (15 steps) available from 6.4 ma to zero ma. In the one-hour period shown, the animal gave himself 4,247 brain shocks and reset the current 558 times.

at which resets occurred. On the left, plotted against the same current scale, are the self-stimulation rates obtained when the current steps were presented singly, each for several minutes, as fixed-intensity reinforcements for lever-pressing. In this manner, estimations of the "reinforcement thresh-old" given by the present technique may be directly compared with the minimum current level required to maintain self-stimulation in the fixed-intensity situation.

Figure 1 shows that resetting tended to center about an intensity level (3.4 ma) that maintained a high self-stimulation rate, but below which performance dropped off sharply.[1] Similar findings were obtained from a second tegmental animal and an animal with an electrode in posterior hypothalamus. The new procedure thus seems to give, at least for these electrode placements, an estimate of the reward threshold that is slightly higher than the minimum maintaining level for self-stimulation under fixed-intensity reinforcement.[2]

The effect of manipulating the frequency (repetition-rate) of the stimulating waveform is depicted in Fig. 2. Two similar experiments are shown,

[1] Studies of intensity preference indicate that the fall-off in self-stimulation rate with intensities higher than 3.4 ma should not be attributed to a decline in reinforcing value. For the preparation shown in Fig. 1, the preferred intensity is about 25 ma, and occasionally, after long periods of stimulation, values as high as 50 ma may be selected. Possibly, this decline in rate reflects longer lasting after effects of higher intensity brain shocks: put loosely, the rate declines because the animal does not "need" the next stimulation as soon.

[2] It will be recalled that the range of current intensities used for the threshold determination occupies only a small segment of the low end of the total range giving reinforcement (footnote 1). The discrepancy, then, between the estimates of the "reinforcement threshold" given by the two procedures, although reliable, is relatively minor.

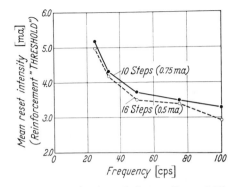

FIGURE 2. Rat H-38 posterior hypothalamus. Reward "threshold" (mean intensity at reset) as a function of the repetition-rate of the stimulating waveform. Each point is the average current intersity of approximately 75 resets obtained in 10-min test periods.

one involving relatively coarse intensity steps (0.75 ma) and the other finer steps (0.5 ma). In both experiments the animal was exposed to five repetition-rates, each for 15 minutes, presented in an ascending series. Each point is the mean intensity at which resets occurred during the last 10 minutes that any repetition-rate was in force. The experiments, in good agreement, gave negatively accelerated, decreasing curves relating the reinforcement threshold and frequency. That the technique discriminates so clearly a shift from 25 to 33 cps testifies to its sensitivity.

Some sample drug actions are shown in Fig. 3. Clorpromazine hydrochloride at 1.5 mg/kg raised the threshold for reinforcement (resets at higher intensities) with the onset of action occurring about 15 minutes after the intraperitoneal injection. In contrast, *dl*-amphetamine sulphate (0.75 mg/kg) lowered the threshold (resets at smaller intensities) with the first indications of activity at about 5 minutes.[3] A more complete report describing the actions of other centrally-acting drugs [e.g., reserpine, phenethylamine, sodium pentobarbital, serotonin, LSD-25, phenylisopropylhydrazine (JB-516)] is in preparation.

COMMENT. The method has considerable promise as a tool for the investigation of the central nervous system actions of drugs. The use of discrete stimulation to specific brain structures gives some information about sites of action. Because the determination is continuous, the time course of drug action is directly charted. Finally, the use of the threshold intensities

[3] The rate of self-stimulation was increased by this dose of chlorpromazine and decreased by amphetamine. These effects on rate may appear at first to conflict with the threshold data, but, following the reasoning in footnote 1, these actions may be reconciled by assuming that chlorpromazine shortens and amphetamine prolongs the aftereffects of a brain shock.

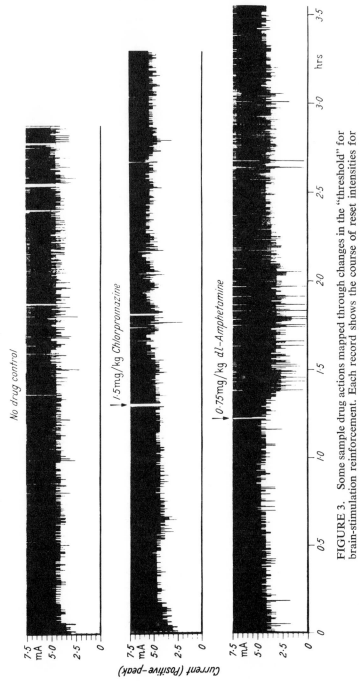

FIGURE 3. Some sample drug actions mapped through changes in the "threshold" for brain-stimulation reinforcement. Each record shows the course of reset intensities for an entire daily session. The ordinal markings indicate the 10 current levels that were available. Rat H38 posterior hypothalamus.

366

for stimulation may be expected to lend considerably to the sensitivity of the method.

SUMMARY.   The self-stimulation technique of Olds is modified to permit a continuous determination of the smallest current levels that will produce a rewarding effect by stimulating positive brain sites. The animal receives brief brain shocks that decrease in intensity in small steps by operating one lever, and indicates which current step stimulated insufficiently by resetting the current at a second lever. Preliminary data suggest that the technique will provide a valuable tool for the investigation of the central nervous system actions of drugs.

REFERENCES

Brady, J. V.: Temporal and emotional effects related to intracranial electrical self-stimulation. In Henry Ford Hospital Internat. Symposium: *The reticular formation of the brain*. Boston: Little, Brown & Co. 1958.

Guilford, J. P.: *Psychometric methods,* New York: McGraw-Hill 1936.

Lilly, J. C., Hughes, J. R., Alvord, E. C., Jr., and Galkin, T. W.: Brief non-injurious electric waveform for stimulation of the brain. *Science* 121, 468–469 (1955).

Olds, J.: Self-stimulation of the brain. *Science* 127, 315–324 (1958).

Stein, L., and Ray, O. S.: Self-regulation of brain-stimulating current intensity in rat. *Science* 130, 510–512 (1959).

38

Changes in pain tolerance and other behavior produced by salicylates [1]

BERNARD WEISS and VICTOR G. LATIES

Pharmacologists have developed many methods for evaluating analgesics in animals. While some of these methods reflect the clinical potency of the narcotic analgesics fairly well they tend to be insensitive to the milder agents such as salicylates (Beecher, 1957). Those that are sensitive to the salicylates, such as the "writing syndrome" (Siegmund et al., 1957), respond to other classes of drugs besides analgesics (Koster et al., 1959; Hendershot and Forsaith, 1959). Perhaps one reason for the lack of correlation with clinical data is that while the current animal methods rely mainly on simple unlearned responses, the response to a painful stimulus in humans is a complex learned one. It therefore seemed worthwhile to study the action of salicylates on more complex animal behavior than has typically been used. Hill et al. (1957) have demonstrated how behavioral techniques could be useful in studying certain aspects of the action of morphine.

The technique used in the present studies to measure analgesia is called a titration schedule (Weiss and Laties, 1958, 1959). Animals are trained to depress a lever to reduce the intensity of an electric shock applied through the floor of the experimental chamber. The intensity of the shock is programmed to undergo periodic rises. By recording the intensity of the shock, we can determine the level of shock great enough to produce lever pressing; or, more loosely, the amount of "pain" tolerated by the subject. We reasoned that an effective analgesic should raise the shock level at which responding is maintained.

The experiments are divided into four sections. Section 1 consists of four experiments using the titration schedule. In the first, we studied the effect of parenteral sodium salicylate on shock level as a function of how rapidly the shock increased in intensity. We suspected an interaction with drugs because we found earlier that the more rapid the rate of rise, the higher the level at which the rat keeps the shock (Weiss and Laties, 1959). Morphine

From *Journal of Pharmacology and Experimental Therapeutics*, 1961, 131, 120–129. Copyright © 1961 by The Williams and Wilkins Co., Baltimore, Md.

[1] This work was supported in part by grants from the Institute for the Study of Analgesic and Sedative Drugs, and from the National Institute of Neurological Diseases and Blindness, National Institutes of Health (Grant B-865). The authors wish to thank Mrs. Catharine Nass for helping to conduct the experiments and Mr. Arthur Oleinick for advice on some of the statistical problems that arose.

was included in this experiment to get a notion of how a narcotic analgesic affects this behavior. The second experiment examined the relation between the level at which the shock was kept and dose of parenteral sodium salicylate. The third experiment examined the relation between the level at which the rat kept the shock and dose of oral aspirin. The fourth experiment assessed the effect of pentobarbital on shock level. It was an attempt to observe the effect of an agent with marked depressive action and very slight analgesic potency. It represented, therefore, a control for general behavioral impairment.

Section 2 consists of two experiments on escape performance in which we measured the latency of escape from an electric shock. One experiment studied the effect of sodium salicylate, the other the effect of aspirin. We sought in these two experiments to obtain a measure of the amount of motor impairment (the ability to press the lever) produced by dose levels of sodium salicylate and aspirin that produced significant effects on titration performance.

Sections 3 and 4 studied the effects on positively reinforced behavior of sodium salicylate and aspirin. These were attempts to assess other behavioral effects of the salicylates produced by doses which charged the shock level maintained on the titration schedule. We studied timing behavior in section 3 and variable-interval schedule performance in section 4, using a water reinforcement each time. Section 4 also included a control experiment on the effects of pentobarbital.

METHODS

TITRATION SCHEDULE. The subjects in studies A, B, C and D were tested in an experimental chamber [2] that measured 25 × 26.5 × 30 cm. It possessed aluminum sides, a glass top, and a floor of stainless steel rods spaced 2 cm apart. To reduce distracting stimuli the chamber was enclosed in a housing whose walls were packed with fiberglass. Two levers connected to microswitches projected into the chamber. They were 5 cm long and 1.3 cm in diameter.

The electric shock stimulus came from a constant-current stimulator. It was continuously delivered to the experimental chamber *via* a scrambling device that kept switching the relative polarities of the floor rods. The walls and lever were also included in this circuit. The output of the stimulator (half-wave 60 cycle) varied from a minimum of 0.07 to a maximum of 0.65 mA (average value of the wave) in 25 discrete and nearly equal steps. Pulses to an add-subtract stepping switch changed the intensity of the shock stimulus in the following way. Periodic pulses from a timer, by driving the stepping switch in one direction, raised the intensity by one step for each

[2] Manufactured by Foringer and Co., Rockville, Md.

pulse. Whenever the rat in the chamber pressed either one of the levers with a force of 16 grams or more, a pulse was delivered to the stepping switch which drove it in the opposite direction and lowered the output of the stimulator by one step. A brief tone sounded in the chamber each time one of the levers was pressed.

Programming and recording were automatic. The equipment used for this purpose was in an adjoining room. Recordings were made of stimulator output, responses, and the amount of time spent at each of the 25 steps from the minimum to the maximum values of the shock.

The rats used in this series of experiments were trained until their performance was stable both within sessions and from session to session.

All of the rats used throughout the paper were adult male albinos from Wistar and Holtzman stock.

ESCAPE PERFORMANCE. In studies E and F the subjects performed in an experimental chamber similar to the one used in the experiments on titration schedules except that it contained only one lever. The rats were run on an escape program with the following features. Every 30 seconds an electric shock came on. The shock intensity was 0.64 mA (60 cycle a.c.) delivered through a series resistance of 0.25 megohms and *via* a scrambler to the floor and walls of the chamber. The first depression of the lever after the shock came on turned it off. The total amount of time that the shock was on during the 2-hour period (240 trials) was recorded on a running time meter. Each rat received 2 hours of training on this program before starting on the study.

TIMING BEHAVIOR. The subjects in studies G and H were first trained to press the lever for water. Each reinforcement consisted of a dipper of water containing 0.05 ml that remained accessible to the rat for 3 seconds. The subjects were then put on a reinforcement schedule that reinforced only those responses made at least 20 seconds after the previous response. Each response, whether it was reinforced or not, reset a timer to zero and another 20 seconds had to pass before a reinforcement could be obtained. This schedule has been named a DRL schedule because of its *D*ifferential *R*einforcement of *L*ow rates (Ferster and Skinner, 1957).

After considerable practice, the frequency distribution of inter-response times showed a pronounced peaking, with the mode occurring close to 20 seconds. Each of the rats used in Study G had received, before the study began, about 60 hours of training on this schedule. By the end of this time they were peaking consistently from session to session. Each time a session was run in Study G, the rat had been without water for about 48 hours.

The distribution of inter-response times was recorded on counters in ten 4-second blocks, plus an eleventh counter which recorded the number of responses occurring more than 40 seconds after the last response. A running time meter recorded the total amount of time that successive responses were separated by more than 40 seconds.

Variable interval performance. The subjects in experiments I, J and K worked on a reinforcement schedule which occasionally reinforced a lever press with a dipper of water. The intervals between such occasions varied from 5 to 237 seconds, with a mean interval of 120 seconds. The actual distribution of intervals was the one used by Clark (1958). Such a schedule typically leads to a fairly steady rate of lever-pressing.

Six rats were trained until their performance was fairly consistent from session to session as judged by the cumulative records and the total number of responses per session. They performed under a 24-hour water deprivation with 30 minutes of access to water after each session.

RESULTS

TITRATION SCHEDULES. *Study A. The effects of sodium salicylate on median shock level under two different rates of rise in shock intensity.* Study A examined the effects on shock level of 250 mg/kg of sodium salicylate. Saline and morphine sulfate (2.5 mg/kg) served as control agents. These dosages were selected on the basis of preliminary experiments with other rats. The interval between shock increments (i–i) was also varied by using two such intervals: 2 seconds and 10 seconds. With i–i = 2 seconds the shock level rose by one step every 2 seconds. With i–i = 10 seconds the shock level rose by one step every 10 seconds. Six animals were run under all drug conditions at both i–i intervals. The sequence of drugs for a particular rat within each interval was randomly chosen.

The drugs were given in the following concentrations: morphine sulfate, 2.5 mg/ml; sodium salicylate, 25 mg/ml, a nearly isotonic solution (used because of indications from earlier experiments that hypertonic solutions caused irritation). On half the occasions when placebo was scheduled the subjects received a volume of isotonic saline equal to 10 ml/kg. The other times they received a volume of saline equal to 1 ml/kg. This was done to match the respective volumes of sodium salicylate and morphine sulfate used. (No differences due to volume were found and so the results for both control treatments were combined.) All drugs were administered intraperitoneally.

Immediately after injection, the rat was placed in the chamber and run for 100 minutes, only the last 90 of which were used to obtain the distributions of time over shock levels; that is, the amount of time spent at each of the 25 steps from the minimum to the maximum shock intensity. The first 10 minutes served as a warm-up period. The animals were usually more variable at this time than during the rest of the session and we did not wish to incorporate this extraneous variability into the results.

The results of Study A are given in Fig. 1 as the median shock level for each treatment condition. The median shock level is the point above which (and below which) the shock intensity was kept half the time during the session. The medians were calculated by considering step 1 of the 25 steps from the minimum to the maximum shock level to extend from 1.00 to 1.99, step 2 from 2.00 to 2.99, and so on.

Note, first of all, the higher median shock level at i–i = 2 seconds than i–i = 10 seconds. This confirms our earlier finding (Weiss and Laties, 1959). Also, note that the differences among drug treatments are much greater at i–i = 2 seconds than at i–i = 10 seconds. To determine the statistical significance of the drug differences at i–i = 2 seconds we performed

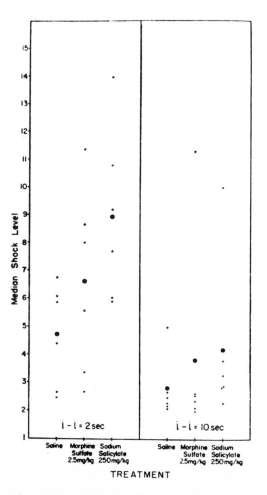

FIGURE 1. Median shock levels with saline, 2.5 mg/kg morphine sulfate, and 250 mg/kg sodium salicylate at i–i = 10 sec and i–i = 2 sec. The large dots show the means of the medians. The individual subjects are shown by the small dots.

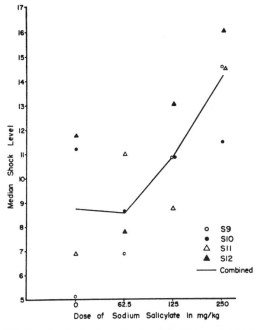

FIGURE 2. Median shock levels with 0, 62.5, 125, and 250 mg/kg sodium sali-cylate. The line represents the mean of the medians.

an analysis of variance (McNemar, 1955, p. 284 ff.). Drug differences were statistically significant: $P < 0.05$. Drug differences at i–i $= 10$ seconds were not significant.

We estimated the 95% confidence limits of the differences between the means of the three treatments by the Scheffé method (Scheffé, 1953).[3] This method gives a more conservative estimate of the reliability of the differences than the t test. Only the 95% limits for the difference between placebo and 250 mg/kg of sodium salicylate did not include zero, indicating that the significant variance among treatments was due mostly to this difference.

Study B. The effects of sodium salicylate on shock level. Study B com-pared doses of sodium salicylate of 0, 62.5, 125 and 250 mg/kg. All doses were given intraperitoneally as an isotonic solution in a volume of 10 ml/kg with isotonic saline added to obtain the matched volumes. Each of four subjects ran once under each of the four conditions in a balanced Latin square design. Immediately after injection, the subject was placed in the chamber and run for 100 minutes, only the last 90 of which were used to obtain the distribution of time over shock levels. The i–i interval was 2 seconds.

Figure 2 shows the results of Study B. Rats maintained a higher shock

[3] Whenever Scheffé tests are discussed in this paper, we refer to the 95% confidence limits.

level with the two higher doses of sodium salicylate (125 and 250 mg/kg) than with the doses of 0 and 62.5 mg/kg. The analysis of variance (performed as in Study A) gave a P-value for differences among doses of less than 0.01. Scheffé estimates gave bounds that did not include zero only for the difference between the two lowest doses (0 and 62.5 mg/kg) and the highest dose (250 mg/kg). However, since the linear response component (Goulden, 1952, chap. 10) accounts for 85% of the treatment variance ($P < 0.001$), we can conclude that the dose-response relation is significant and linear.

Study C. The effects of aspirin on shock level. Study C compared the following doses of oral aspirin: 0, 125, and 250 mg/kg. The aspirin was delivered as a suspension *via* stomach tube. The suspension was made up by first dissolving the dose of aspirin assigned for the session in 2 ml of polyethylene glycol (Carbowax 300) and then suspending this soluition in 8 ml of a 0.5% solution of carboxymethylcellulose to give a final volume of 10 ml. The volume administered was equal to 10 ml/kg.

The subject ran for 130 minutes, starting 60 minutes after the drug was administered. Only the last 120 minutes contributed to the results.

Ten rats took part in the experiment. The sequence of doses was randomly determined for each animal. The i–i interval was 2 seconds.

Figure 3 shows the results of Study C. The higher the dose of oral aspirin, the higher the median shock level. Differences among dose levels

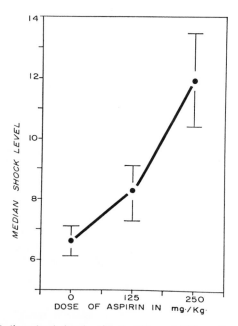

FIGURE 3. Median shock levels with 0, 125, and 250 mg/kg aspirin based on the mean of 10 animals. The standard errors for each dose are also drawn.

were tested by an analysis of variance. The F for treatments was significant: $P < 0.05$. Scheffé estimates indicated that only the difference between 0 and 250 mg/kg was significant. The linear response component, however, accounts for 94% of the treatment variance and is statistically significant.

Study D. The effects of pentobarbital on shock level.   Study D evaluated the effects of placebo and 10 mg/kg of sodium pentobarbital (i.p.). This dose of pentobarbital produces a severe depression of response rate on a schedule in which occasional lever presses are reinforced by access to water (Study K); in many animals, it also produces clearly observable ataxia.

The subject was put into the chamber directly after injection and run for 130 minutes. Only the last 120 minutes were used to obtain the distribution of time over shock level. The subjects were nine of the rats that had served in Study C. The order of treatments was randomly determined.

The mean of the median shock levels was 6.59 for placebo (almost exactly the value obtained with these same rats for placebo in Study C) and 9.43 for pentobarbital, giving a difference of 2.84. Four of the subjects gave a higher shock level with placebo while five gave a higher level with the pentobarbital. The standard error of the difference was 1.87, giving a t of 1.52. A t of 2.31 would be necessary to attain significance at the 0.05 level. It should be noted that most of the difference between treatments was contributed by one animal that became so severely ataxic that it could not press the lever for most of the session. Without its data, the mean for placebo becomes 6.11 and that for pentobarbital 7.44.

ESCAPE PERFORMANCE.   *Study E. The effects of sodium salicylate on escape behavior.*   Eight rats served in this study. Each was run twice with an intraperitoneal dose of 250 mg/kg sodium salicylate (administered in the concentration and volume used in Studies A and B) and twice with a matched volume of physiological saline. Thirty minutes after drug administration, the subject was placed in the experimental chamber and run for 2 hours on an escape program.

Sodium salicylate did not change the latency of the escape response. The mean length of time that the shock was on (for a total of 480 trials) came to 3.16 minutes for saline and 3.31 minutes for 250 mg/kg sodium salicylate. This difference was not significant: $\text{S.E.}_{\text{diff.}} = 0.296$.

Study F. The effects of aspirin on escape behavior.   Seven of the eight rats that served in Study E were used in Study F. Each rat was run twice with an oral dose of aspirin equal to 250 mg/kg and twice with placebo. These were administered as in Study C. One hour after drug administration the subject was placed in the chamber and run for 2 hours under the conditions described for Study E. Oral aspirin did not change the latency of the escape response. The mean length of time that the shock was on (for a total of 480 trials) came to 3.50 minutes for saline and 3.09 minutes for 250 mg/kg oral aspirin. This difference was not significant: $\text{S.E.}_{\text{diff.}} = 0.252$.

TIMING BEHAVIOR.   *Study G. The effects of sodium salicylate on timing behavior.*   Three highly trained rats were used in this study. Each animal ran four times on the following four conditions: "low" placebo, "high" placebo, 125 mg/kg sodium salicylate, 250 mg/kg sodium salicylate. The sodium salicylate was given intraperitoneally in a concentration of 25 mg/ml. The "low" and "high" placebo represented two different volumes of saline corresponding to the low and high doses of sodium salicylate. We wished to see whether volume alone had any effect. The injections were given 30 minutes before the start of a 2-hour experimental session. Each rat received the four treatments in a different order. The results of Study G are summarized in Table 1. The subjects made fewer total responses after the drug than after saline. An analysis of variance of the total response data (McNemar, 1955, p. 281 ff.) gave an F for treatments significant at the 0.01 level. Scheffé estimates showed that neither the difference between the two control levels nor the difference between the two drug levels was significant. But both levels of the drug were significantly different from their respective controls.

The distribution of inter-response times—a measure of the acuity of the temporal discrimination—is shown for the grouped data in Fig. 4. These data can be described in various ways. The differences among treatments in the number of extremely long inter-response times (greater than 40 seconds) were examined both by counting the number of responses in this category and by recording the amount of time cumulated on the clock that ran only after 40 seconds had passed since the last response. Both indices show a significant effect of sodium salicylate. Scheffé tests made after significant F's were obtained by analyses of variance indicate that both drug levels increased the number of long responses while only the high dose (probably because of the small number of subjects) significantly increased the amount of time over 40 seconds.

The median inter-response time reflects the distribution without unduly weighting the extremes. This measure (see Table 1) shows that while the two control doses and the lower dose of sodium salicylate did not differ

TABLE 1.   Effects of sodium salicylate on timing behavior (means based on $N = 3$).

	Placebo Low	Placebo High	125 mg/kg	250 mg/kg	P*
Total responses	359.3	322.7	230.0	205.3	<0.01
Total inter-response time over 40 seconds in minutes	0.05	1.55	22.65	22.59	<0.05
Total responses over 40 seconds	1.00	2.67	23.67	33.67	<0.01
Median inter-response time in seconds	18.43	19.61	20.93	23.75	<0.001
Total reinforcements	96.3	144.7	127.7	148.0	>0.10

* These values refer to the overall F's from the analyses of variance.

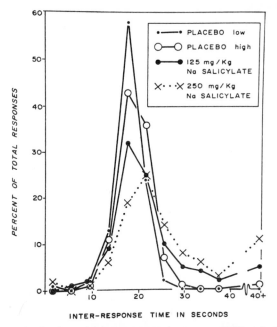

FIGURE 4.   Distribution of inter-response times on a DRL schedule with 125 and 250 mg/kg sodium salicylate and matched volumes of saline. (Mean of three rats.)

significantly, the higher dose of the drug did increase the median inter-response time significantly ($P < 0.01$). The total number of reinforcements did not differ as a function of treatment.

Study H. The effects of aspirin on timing behavior.   Study H examined the effects of 0, 125, and 250 mg/kg oral aspirin on DRL 20 performance, the same schedule used in Study G. The drugs were administered as in Study C. The same three rats used in Study G were used here, too. Each rat ran three times under each of the three treatments, with order of administration being randomized within each replication. Each session followed a 48-hour period of water deprivation. A single session lasted 2 hours and started 1 hour after the drug had been given. In both Study G and Study H, successive sessions were spaced about a week apart.

Oral aspirin had a smaller effect than parenteral sodium salicylate (Study F) on the performance of rats working for water on a DRL schedule of reinforcement. The data are summarized in Table 2 and Fig. 5. Only the total number of responses was affected to a statistically significant extent, with Scheffé tests showing the differences between control and 250 mg/kg and between 125 and 250 mg/kg to be significant. The dose-response relation was significantly linear ($P < 0.01$) and this linear component accounted for 95% of the treatment sum of squares.

TABLE 2.   Effects of aspirin on timing behavior (means based on $N = 3$).

	0	125 mg/kg	250 mg/kg	P*
Total responses	350.3	321.0	254.9	<0.05
Total inter-response time over 40 seconds in minutes	3.29	5.50	18.09	>0.10
Total responses over 40 seconds	4.0	6.2	18.2	>0.10
Median inter-re-sponse time in sec-onds	19.21	19.75	20.65	>0.10
Total reinforcements	125.0	141.4	128.8	>0.10

* These values refer to the overall F's from the analyses of variance.

VARIABLE INTERVAL PERFORMANCE.   *Study I. Effects of sodium salicy-late on variable interval performance.*   Each of the 6 rats ran at two drug levels, 125 and 250 mg/kg sodium salicylate, and two placebo levels, each matching one drug level, in the manner of Study G. The drug was given intraperitoneally 30 minutes before the start of a 60-minute session. The four treatments were given to each subject in a random order within each of two replications.

The rate at which rats pressed a lever to obtain water decreased after i.p. doses of sodium salicylate. The mean response rates (in responses per min-ute) were: control (low volume), 6.0; control (high volume), 5.9; 125 mg/kg, 3.9; 250 mg/kg, 2.2. The analysis of variance of these data give a significant F ($P < 0.001$). Scheffé tests showed that neither the difference between high and low control volumes nor the difference between the drug doses was significant. Each dose differed significantly from its appropriate control.

Study J. Effects of aspirin on variable interval performance.   The same 6 rats used in Study I were given oral administrations of 0, 125, and 250 mg/kg of aspirin. Order of treatment was again randomized within each of two replications. The treatments were given 1 hour before the start of a 2-hour session under the same conditions outlined in Study I.

Oral aspirin decreased response rate on a variable interval reinforcement schedule. The mean response rates (in responses per minute) were: con-trol, 4.1; 125 mg/kg, 2.9; 250 mg/kg, 2.2. The analysis of variance showed that the differences among treatments were significant at the 0.01 level. Scheffé tests showed that only the difference between the control and 250 mg/kg treatments was significant. But the linear component of the treat-

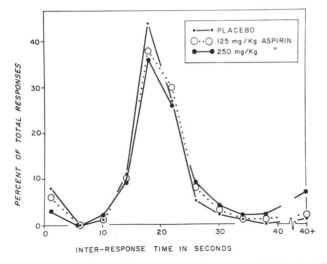

FIGURE 5. Distribution of inter-response times on a DRL schedule with 0, 125, and 250 mg/kg aspirin. (Mean of three rats.)

ment variance is significant $(P < 0.01)$ and accounts for 98% of the treatment sum of squares.

Study K. Effects of sodium pentobarbital on variable interval performance. The same dose of pentobarbital used in Study D was evaluated in variable interval performance with the same 6 rats that had served in Studies I and J. Each rat ran twice, once after an injection of saline and once after an injection of 10 mg/kg sodium pentobarbital (i.p.) Order of treatment was random. An experimental session lasted 2 hours and started immediately after injection. The conditions of the experiment were otherwise the same as in the two previous variable interval experiments.

The mean response rate decreased from 3.38 per minute after injections of saline to 1.03 after pentobarbital. This drop was significant at the 0.01 level.

DISCUSSION

Table 3 summarizes the results of the 11 experiments reported in this paper. The experiments on titration behavior demonstrate that parenteral sodium salicylate and oral aspirin raise the level at which rats will keep the intensity of an electric shock. Is this a true analgesic effect or does the increase in shock level merely reflect a general impairment of behavior? The collateral studies performed offer some evidence on this point. Doses of drugs that altered titration performance produced significant changes in certain features of DRL performance and in response rate on the variable-

TABLE 3.   Summary of the results.

Study	Type of Behavior	No. of Subjects	Drug	Dose Levels	Effect
				mg/kg	
A	Titration (i–i = 2 and i–i = 10 sec)	6	Na salic. and morphine	0, 250 Na salic., 2.5 morphine (i.p.)	Increase in median shock level with both drugs, but more pronounced for Na salic., at i–i = 2. No effect at i–i = 10.
B	Titration (i–i = 2 sec)	4	Na salic.	0, 62.5, 125, 250 (i.p.)	Increase in median shock level with 2 highest doses. Significant linear dose-response relation.
C	Titration (i–i = 2 sec)	10	Aspirin	0, 125, 250 (p.o.)	Increase in median shock level. Significant linear dose-response relation.
D	Titration (i–i = 2 sec)	9	Na pentobarbital	0, 10 (i.p.)	Nonsignificant increase in median shock level despite observable ataxia.
E	Escape	8	Na salic.	0, 250 (i.p.)	No effect.
F	Escape	7	Aspirin	0, 250 (p.o.)	No effect.
G	DRL (timing)	3	Na salic.	0, 125, 250 (i.p.)	Significant decrease in total responses and significant effect on inter-response time distribution (median IRT increased).
H	DRL (timing)	3	Aspirin	0, 125, 250 (p.o.)	Decrease in total responses. No effect on inter-response time distribution.
I	Variable interval	6	Na salic.	0, 125, 250 (i.p.)	Both Na salic. doses decreased response rate compared to control.
J	Variable interval	6	Aspirin	0, 125, 250 (p.o.)	Significant linear relation in depression of response rate.
K	Variable interval	6	Na pentobarbital	0, 10 (i.p.)	Significant depression of response rate.

interval schedule. Since part of the rise in median shock level due to drug treatment comes from some rats allowing the shock intensity to reach the maximum value for certain periods of time—and these are periods during which they press at a very low rate—the possibility that it reflects a general impairment cannot be discounted.

However, other collateral experiments contradict the thesis that a general malaise is the major contributor to the rise in tolerated shock level with salicylates. First, salicylates produced no impairment in how promptly rats turned off a shock whose intensity corresponded to the top level of the titration schedule. Also, we found that pentobarbital sodium in a dose (10 mg/kg) that produced a striking and significant depression of variable interval performance did not have a significant effect on median shock level. An even smaller dose than this (8 mg/kg) completely disrupts timing behavior (Sidman, 1956). We also observed that 10 mg/kg of pentobarbi-

tal produced ataxia, a phenomenon we never saw after salicylate administration.

But, without a clear dissociation between the effects of salicylates on
titration performance, which we explored as a device for measuring analgesia, and behavior under the control of positive reinforcement, the results
are equivocal. It is not possible to state at this time whether performance
on a titration schedule measures analgesia, general CNS depression, both,
or something wholly extraneous such as nausea. One main difficulty is the
remarkable pharmacological versatility of the salicylates. Because of their
widespread effects it is virtually certain that any attempt to measure analgesia
in animals completely unconfounded with any other effect will fail.

This sort of ambiguity or incomplete dissociation of effect is not uncommon. Take, for example, morphine. Morphine is a potent analgesic in man.
Yet, in doses that produce satisfactory analgesia, we find complaints of diz-
ziness, nausea, itchiness, headache, warmth, lethargy, *etc.* (Smith and
Beecher, 1959). And in rats, the degree to which a dose of morphine attenuates a conditioned emotional response is closely related to how much
it depresses responding for food (Hill *et al.,* 1957).

Perhaps the problem is, by its very nature, insoluble. As Sidman says,
"It is clear that the relations between drugs and behavior are a function not
only of the drug but also of the conditions under which the behavior is generated. The evidence also suggests that while drugs and behavior interact
differentially, it will be difficult if not impossible to find a drug whose effects are confined to one specific behavior-environment contingency" (Sidman, 1956, p. 301).

At least, however, the study of complex behavior offers some possibility
of reaching a conclusion. Most of the other techniques in widespread use
not only have failed to include measures of the behavioral specificity of the
technique but also have been unsuccessful in detecting salicylate effects except with dose levels higher than those used in the present series of experiments. For example, Hart (1947), using a modification of the radiant heat
method, obtained an AD50 of 350 mg/kg with oral aspirin. Gibson *et al.*
(1955), using the squeak response to electrical stimulation, obtained a
minimum effective dose of 450 mg/kg of oral aspirin. And Cunningham *et
al.* (1957) found no effect of 1000 mg/kg of oral aspirin on the skin temperature that provoked a withdrawal response in the rat. The possible confounding of side effects with analgesia at their higher doses offers even more
of a problem.

SUMMARY

Parenteral sodium salicylate and oral aspirin raise the level at which rats
keep the intensity of an electric shock that periodically rises in intensity
while lever presses by the rats reduce this intensity. The rise in shock level

is proportional to drug dose. The same doses of sodium salicylate and aspirin that produce changes in tolerated shock level also produce changes in two kinds of positively reinforced responding: timing behavior and variable-interval schedule performance. Ordinary escape performance was not affected at these doses. Sodium pentobarbital has little effect on shock level but depresses positively reinforced behavior. It is not now possible to state whether the effect on shock level is an analgesic one, the result of general CNS depression, or both.

REFERENCES

Beecher, H. K.: *Pharmacol. Rev.* **9**:59, 1957.

Clark, F. C.: *J. exp. Anal. Behav.* **1**:221, 1958.

Cunningham, D. J., Benson, W. M., and Hardy, J. D.: *J. appl. Physiol.* **11**:459, 1957.

Ferster, C. B., and Skinner, B. F.: *Schedules of reinforcement,* Appleton-Century-Crofts, New York, 1957.

Gibson, R. D., Miya, T. S., and Edwards, L. D.: *J. Amer. pharm. Ass., Sci. Ed.* **64**:605, 1955.

Goulden, C. H.: *Methods of statistical analysis,* 2nd ed., John Wiley & Sons, New York, 1952.

Hart, E. R.: *J. Pharm. exp. Ther.* **89**:205, 1947.

Hendershot, L. C., and Forsaith, J.: *J. Pharm. exp. Ther.* **125**:237, 1959.

Hill, H. E., Pescor, F. T., Belleville, R. E., and Wikler, A.: *J. Pharm. exp. Ther.* **120**:388, 1957.

Koster, R., Anderson, M., and deBeer, E. J.: *Fed. Proc.* **18**:412, 1959.

McNemar, Q.: *Psychological statistics,* 2nd ed., John Wiley & Sons, New York, 1955.

Scheffé, H.: *Biometrika* **40**:87, 1953.

Sidman, M.: *Ann. N.Y. Acad. Sci.* **65**:282, 1956.

Siegmund, E., Cadmus, R., and Lu, G.: *Proc. Soc. exp. Biol., N.Y.* **95**:729, 1957.

Smith, G. M., and Beecher, H. K.: *J. Pharm. exp. Ther.* **126**:50, 1959.

Weiss, B., and Laties, V. G.: *Science* **128**:1575, 1958.

Weiss, B., and Laties, V. G.: *J. exp. Anal. Behav.* **2**:227, 1959.

39

The effect of drugs on a fixed-ratio performance suppressed by a pre-time-out stimulus [1,2]

Charles B. Ferster, James B. Appel, and
Richard A. Hiss

Under several conditions, the stimulus preceding a time out from positive reinforcement may suppress responding on the base-line schedule as it does when a stimulus precedes an electric shock (Estes and Skinner, 1942). Herrnstein (1955) and Ferster (1958, 1960) have described the procedures. In all of the earlier experiments studying the effect of a pre-time-out stimulus, the base line was a variable-interval schedule of positive reinforcement. Furthermore, the procedure had little effect on responding elsewhere than in the pre-time-out stimulus, except, perhaps, for some frequent pausing (Ferster, 1958). The pausing was difficult to interpret because such a deviation may be a result of other conditions. However, in this experiment, the pre-time-out stimulus was imposed on a fixed-ratio base line; and the procedure was similar to one used earlier by Ferster (1958), in which no time out occurred in the absence of responding in the critical part of the pre-time-out stimulus. A fixed-ratio (FR) schedule was used for several reasons. First, because rate changes are easier to identify in a fixed-ratio rather than a variable-interval (VI) schedule, any disruptions in the base line produced by the pre-time-out stimulus would be much easier to detect. Second, in an FR, changes in the rate of responding alter the frequency of reinforcement, so that any variable that increases pausing or lowers the rate of responding can be used to produce low frequencies of reinforcement. In contrast, in VI, the frequency of reinforcement can be altered significantly at only extreme rate changes. Third, in an FR, the probability of a response being reinforced does not increase during a pause. Consequently, if pausing should emerge in the presence of a pre-time-out stimulus, the pause would not be counteracted by the increased probability of reinforcement resulting from the interval basis of the schedule. Finally, reinforcement under FR ratio schedules more frequently occurs while the rate of responding is high. Because the increase in the number of

From *Journal of the Experimental Analysis of Behavior,* 1962, **5**, 73–88. Copyright 1962 by the Society for the Experimental Analysis of Behavior, Inc., Bloomington, Ind.

[1] This research was carried out with the support of a grant from the National Science Foundation (G-7617).

[2] Experiment I was carried out by C. B. Ferster with the technical assistance of R. Hiss. Experiment II was carried out by all three authors.

responses emitted may function as a conditioned reinforcement, at any point in a fixed ratio the conditioned reinforcement provides a basis for the reinforcement of high rates. The final factor would impede the development of pausing during the pre-time-out stimulus to the extent that the FR schedule generates sustained rates of responding under normal conditions. Usually, once the ratio has begun, it is completed. On the other hand, because reinforcement always occurs at high rates, any pausing once begun might be maintained.

PROCEDURE

The experiments were carried out in a standard experimental space with one key which would be illuminated red or green. The subjects were two White Carneaux cock pigeons.

GENERAL PROCEDURE.   The pre-time-out stimulus, a red light, occurred after a response in the fixed ratio; for example, the red light might come on after the fifth response following reinforcement. Responses during the first part of the warning stimulus continued to advance the fixed ratio, and were not followed by a time out. However, responses during the final part of the pre-time-out stimulus were followed by a time out. If the bird did not respond in the last part of the pre-time-out stimulus, the pre-time-out stimulus terminated and the FR requirement for the food-magazine operation could be completed. Thus, no food reinforcement was possible unless the bird allowed the pre-time-out stimulus to terminate without a response.

VARIATIONS IN PROCEDURE.   In the first exposure to the time-out contingencies, both animals had already achieved a stable FR 85 performance. The pre-time-out stimulus occurred after the 50th response after reinforcement in every third FR segment. The maximum duration of the pre-time-out stimulus was 3 sec $(2 + 1)$, but only responses in the final second produced a 20-min time out. Because the two birds' performances differed under the time-out procedure, all of the major variables in the procedure were adjusted to make the deviant bird conform.

Schedule of occurrence of the pre-time-out stimulus.   In the early stages of the experiment, the pre-time-out stimulus was made to occur more and more frequently. First, it occurred in each fixed-ratio segment. Then, the fixed ratio was reset following each time out. Finally, every time a response in the pre-time-out stimulus was followed by a time out, the very next response the animal made reintroduced the time out, and the fixed ratio could not be completed until the bird ceased responding during the pre-time-out stimulus.

The time out.   Whenever the frequency of time outs was very high, particularly with Bird 4Y, the duration of the time out was reduced so that a sufficient number of reinforcements could occur for the bird to be exposed to the contingencies. As the pre-time-out procedure produced suppression during the pre-time-out stimulus, the duration of the time out was increased to the values noted below.

Duration of the pre-time-out stimulus. The duration of the pre-time-out stimulus was kept very small until it suppressed responding, at which point it was gradually increased. This procedure was used on the assumption that a gradual increase in the duration of the pre-time-out stimulus is a condition which will produce suppression, whereas as sudden exposure to a long duration of the pre-time-out stimulus will not.

The size of the fixed ratio. Particularly with Bird 4Y, the size of the fixed ratio was increased in order to produce suppression in the pre-time-out stimulus. As the results indicated, suppression with Bird 4Y was easier to achieve at large fixed ratios.

FINAL PROCEDURE AFTER THE PRE-TIME-OUT STIMULUS SUPPRESSED THE BASE-LINE PERFORMANCE IN BOTH BIRDS. The main data to be reported is the final effect of the procedures rather than the transitory states and the effects of the intermediate procedures. We did not study these intermediate states thoroughly enough so we could be sure which of the early procedures were essential for the final state.

Bird 3Y. In the first part of the experiment, the maximum duration of the pre-time-out stimulus was 3 sec, and responses in the first two sessions advanced the fixed ratio but had no effect on the time out. Responses in the final 1 sec produced a 20-min time out, and the pre-time-out stimulus occurred following the first response in the fixed ratio. When the position of the pre-time-out stimulus in the fixed ratio was varied, the maximum duration of the pre-time-out stimulus was increased to 9.5 sec, and only responses in the final 2 sec produced a 10-min time out. During the intermediate stages of the experiment, the size of the fixed ratio was varied between 60 and 210. However, in the final procedure, in which the position of the pre-time-out stimulus was varied, the fixed ratio remained at 100.

Bird 4Y. The size of the fixed ratio varied from 100 to 250. The maximum duration of the pre-time-out stimulus was 4 sec, and a 3-min time out followed only those responses in the final 2 sec.

RESULTS

Figure 1 illustrates the main difference between the two birds, whose performances were recorded after considerable exposure to the pre-time-out stimulus. The data here include only the procedure in which the pre-time-out stimulus followed the first response in the fixed ratio and reappeared

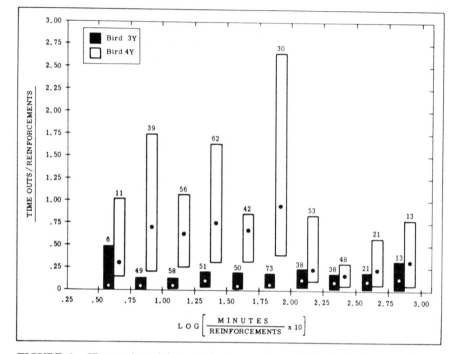

FIGURE 1.   The number of time outs in the pre-time-out stimulus is given as a function of the amount of strain in the fixed ratio (time per reinforcement). Each point is the median time-out level of experimental sessions falling in a given class interval of fixed-ratio pausing. The bar gives the interquartile range, and the number over each bar gives the number of sessions falling into each class interval.

after each time out. The graph shows the number of time outs (expressed as time outs per reinforcement) occurring as a function of the amount of fixed-ratio straining. Each point gives the median of the session; the bar gives the interquartile range; and the number over each bar is the number of experimental sessions falling in the indicated class interval. This figure shows that Bird 3Y's tendency to respond in the pre-time-out stimulus was much lower than that of Bird 4Y. The median number of time outs per reinforcement never exceeds 0.1 time out per reinforcement. Also, the degree of suppression by the pre-time-out stimulus does not appear to depend upon the amount of fixed-ratio straining, except, perhaps, that the pre-time-out responding has some slight tendency to increase at extreme degrees of fixed-ratio strain. However, Bird 4Y showed suppression only when the base-line, fixed-ratio, performance showed considerable strain. Time outs occurred in less than 50% of the pre-time-out stimuli only when the mean time per reinforcement exceeded 10 min. Nevertheless, the data in the first bar are an exception. This was the only phase of the experiment in which the pre-time-out stimulus suppressed responding even though the bird was responding at a high rate. This level of suppression occurred at an early phase of the experiment, when the size of the fixed ratio varied between 120 and 140 and the performance was very well sustained. Thereafter, the size of the ratio was reduced to FR 50, and the amount of pre-time-out stimulus responding increased greatly. After the exposure to FR 50 and the loss of suppression, the pre-time-out stimulus suppressed responding only when the size of the fixed ratio and other conditions of the experiment were such as to produce considerable straining in the base-line performance. Even after this bird developed suppression in the pre-time-out stimulus with large fixed ratios, decreasing the size of the fixed ratio again increased the number of times out.

THE EFFECT OF THE PRE-TIME-OUT STIMULUS ON THE FR PERFORMANCE.   *Bird 3Y*.   The predominant effect of the pre-time-out stimulus on the fixed-ratio performance was an increase in pausing after reinforcement, scalloping rather than the usual "square" FR performance, and variability in the terminal rate of responding. Figure 2 contains all of the segments from an experimental session. These segments are arranged in order of length of pause, and the numbers on each give the actual order of occurrences. The schedule of food reinforcement was FR 210, and the pre-time-out stimulus occurred after the first response for 4 sec. Only responses in the first 2 sec produced time outs; and after a time out, the pre-time-out stimulus reappeared with the next response. Segment 7 (high) and Segment 8 (low) illustrate the large variability in the terminal rate of responding in the FR. Scattered responding occurred throughout many of the strained ratios, as, for example, in Segments 15 and 19 at the top of the figure. The shift to the terminal rate of responding was sometimes abrupt, as in Segment 17; but frequently it was gradual, as in Segment 12, where the performance is similar to that under an FI schedule.

Even after the size of the fixed ratio was reduced to 90, the extreme pausing, curvature, and intermediate rates of responding continued. Figure 3 shows a performance when the schedule of reinforcement had been FR 90 for 7 sessions following 63 sessions of continuously downward adjustment of the fixed ratio. The pre-time-out stimulus still occurred after the first response in the fixed ratio for a maximum duration of 4 sec. The entire experimental session is again presented, with each FR segment arranged in order of the length of time required to complete the fixed ratio. There was still considerable pausing (15 min in the top two curves), and the terminal rate of responding doesn't exceed 2 responses per sec except at the very end of the FR segment. Frequently, the rate did not exceed 1 response per sec (Segment 48). In general, the over-all rate of responding was high at the start of the session but fell during the session, as often happens with strained fixed ratios. Most of the segments show curvature

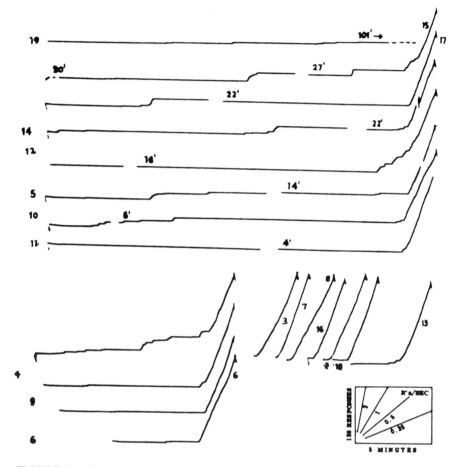

FIGURE 2.   Final performance on FR 210 showing extreme pausing after reinforcement and a wide range of terminal rates of responding. The pre-time-out stimulus (TO 20) occurred after the first response in the FR for a maximum of 4 sec. Time outs followed only responses in the last 2 sec of the 4-sec pre-time-out stimulus.

and scalloping more nearly resembling a fixed-interval performance than that of a fixed ratio.

At one stage of the experiment, this bird stopped responding during the pre-time-out stimulus without extreme curvature or intermediate rates of responding. Figure 4 shows such a performance for Bird 3Y when the fixed ratio was 100 and the pre-time-out stimulus was 4 sec. Long pauses followed reinforcement, without disruption of the normal fixed-ratio pattern of responding. Only one time out (at the arrow) occurred during the session. The pause after reinforcement frequently lasted up to 20 min; but once responding began, the bird frequently reached the terminal rate of

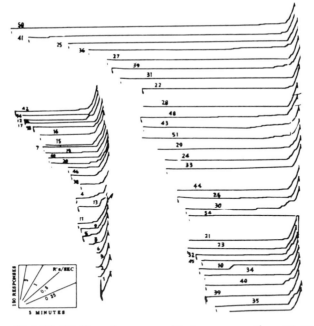

FIGURE 3.   Bird 3Y. FR 90 performance, with the same pre-time-out procedure as in Fig. 2, showing extreme curvature. The segments are arranged in order of length of time, and the actual order of occurrence is given by the number above each segment.

responding immediately. Occasional curvature did occur, however, as in the fifth segment from the end of the session.

Bird 4Y.   Figure 5 shows two consecutive sessions of Bird 4Y's performance on FR 140. The pre-time-out stimulus occurred after the first response in the FR for a maximum duration of 4 sec, and time outs occurred during the final 2 sec. The pre-time-out stimulus reappeared on the first response following a time out (TO 3). Bird 4Y sustained respond-

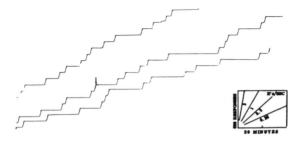

FIGURE 4.   Bird 3Y. Performance on FR 100 with a 3-sec pre-time-out stimulus (TO 20) showing considerable pausing but minimal curvature. The pre-time-out stimulus occurred after the second response in the fixed ratio.

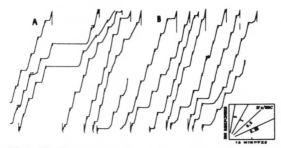

FIGURE 5. Bird 4Y. Two consecutive daily sessions on FR 140 illustrating the early development of suppression of responding by the warning stimulus. The pre-time-out stimulus followed the first response in the fixed ratio for a maximum duration of 4 sec. Only responses in the final 2 sec were followed by a time out (3 min).

ing throughout the experiment at high fixed ratios better than Bird 3Y. The performance recorded in Fig. 5 occurred just after responding in the pre-time-out stimulus fell to the point where time outs occurred only occasionally. During the next 15 sessions, the median number of time outs per reinforcement was 0.30; $Q_1 - Q_3$ was 0.10 to 0.91; and the range was 0.0 to 10.40. Records A and B are two consecutive daily sessions illustrating the range of performances during this phase of the experiment. Record A shows 16 time outs (at the arrows) compared with 4 in Record B. Although the curvature was much less than with Bird 3Y, variations in the magnitude of the running rate were extreme, as in the last three reinforcements of the third segment of Record A, for example. In spite of the high overall rate of responding, most of the pre-time-out stimuli occurred without time outs.

Figure 6 illustrates the extreme of the effect of the pre-time-out stimulus on the fixed-ratio performance, 17 sessions after Fig. 5 when the size of the fixed ratio had reached 230 and when responding had virtually ceased during the critical part of the pre-time-out stimulus. There were no time outs during the session, although 21 responses occurred during the first 2

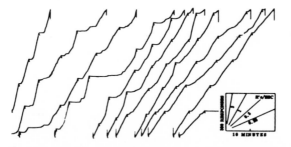

FIGURE 6. Bird 4Y. An FR 230 performance showing a predominance of intermediate rates of responding. The pre-time-out stimulus procedure was the same as in Fig. 5.

sec of the 4-sec, pre-time-out stimulus. Occasional instances of extreme curvature appeared; however, the main effect of the pre-time-out stimulus on the fixed-ratio responding was sustained responding at intermediate rates that is more characteristic of interval than ratio schedules. Occasional instances of high rates of responding immediately preceding the reinforcement still occurred, as well as typical "normal" fixed-ratio segments. An example is in the fourth recorder excursion.

REMOVAL OF THE PRE-TIME-OUT STIMULUS FOR BIRD 3Y.   Early in the experiment, when the pre-time-out stimulus was suppressing responding on FR 60 and also producing considerable strain and curvature in the base-line FR performance, the pre-time-out stimulus was removed for 13 sessions. During this period, there was no indication that the base-line performance was returning to normal, and the pre-time-out procedures were again resumed. Once more, we attempted to recover a normal fixed-ratio performance by discontinuing the pre-time-out procedure after the drug experiments reported in Experiment II. But the curvature did not disappear until this bird had prolonged exposure (151 sessions) to very small fixed ratios. During 25 sessions on FR 100, we gave five consecutive injections of chlorpromazine to see whether the increased rates of responding under the drug (Experiment II) would continue after drug administrations were discontinued. The injections produced normal FR rates of responding, but the base line returned to its previously strained condition when the drug was discontinued. For the next 35 sessions, the size of the fixed ratio was progressively increased from FR 40 to FR 130. After these procedures did not change the bird's performance, the fixed ratio was again decreased to FR 30, and the program of increasing the size of the FR to FR 100 was made even more gradual (over 90 sessions). Reinforcement was maintained at each value of the fixed ratio until it was sustained normally, and then it was increased. Any time rate changes atypical of a normal FR schedule occurred, the fixed ratio was kept at that value or decreased. And the curvature and intermediate rates of responding disappeared only toward the end of this 90-session period.

POSITION OF PRE-TIME-OUT STIMULUS IN THE FIXED RATIO.   While Bird 4Y's procedures were being adjusted to produce suppression during the pre-time-out stimulus, the position of the pre-time-out stimulus in the FR 100 food schedule was varied for Bird 3Y.

Figures 7 and 8 summarize the over-all rate of responding and frequency of time outs, respectively, as the position of the pre-time-out stimulus was varied. The maximum duration of the pre-time-out stimulus was 9.5 sec (7.5 + 2) to 10. The first determination was made with the pre-time-out stimulus after the first response in the fixed ratio. After the performance stabilized at this value, the procedure was altered to produce the pre-time-out stimulus after the 5th response in the fixed ratio; then, the

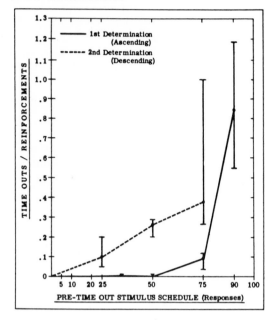

FIGURE 7.   Bird 3Y. FR 100, 4-sec pre-time-out stimulus, TO 20. The frequency of
time outs was a function of the position of the pre-time-out stimulus in the fixed ratio.
The determinations were made in order, first ascending then descending. The median
and interquartile range are given for the last five sessions on each value of the independent variable.

10th, 20th, 35th, 50th, 75th, and 90th response (10 responses before the
reinforcement). Some of the original values were then recovered in a descending series as given in the graphs. The pre-time-out stimulus suppressed responding more when it occurred early in the fixed ratio. When
the pre-time-out stimulus occurred after the 75th response, responding in
the pre-time-out stimulus increased. After the 90th response, responding
in the pre-time-out stimulus increased to produce the highest level of time
out that this bird had shown since the control by the pre-time-out stimulus
was first established. The increased pre-time-out responding continued
even when the pre-time-out stimulus was moved to a position earlier in the
fixed ratio during the descending series of measurements. However, suppression finally became complete when the pre-time-out stimulus occurred
again after the first response.

Moving the position of the pre-time-out stimulus toward the end of the
fixed ratio did not decrease the over-all rate of responding until it occurred after the 75th response in the fixed ratio in the descending series.
The over-all rate fell, probably as a cumulative result of the exposure to
FR 90 and FR 75; but, thereafter, it reached essentially the base-line values
at FR 50, 25, and 1. The reliability of the measurements is sufficiently

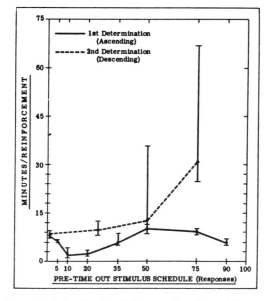

FIGURE 8.   Amount of fixed-ratio strain as a function of the position of the pre-time-out stimulus in the fixed ratio. The determinations were made in order, first ascending then descending. The median and interquartile range are given for the last five sessions on each value of the independent variable.

good that the decrease in rate of responding on FR 5 and 10 is significant. Possibly, there is an optimal point for interrupting the fixed ratio with minimum disruption of the FR performance: It is early enough in the fixed ratio so that the tendency to respond is not so high as to make it virtually impossible to stop responding in the pre-time-out stimulus; yet, it is far enough into the fixed ratio so that the disposition to respond is enough for the performance to be sustained.

EXPERIMENT I

DISCUSSION.   These experiments confirm the observation that when the pigeon can avoid a time out if it stops responding in the warning signal, the pre-time-out stimulus controls a lower rate of responding. Control by the pre-time-out stimulus was generally easier to establish with large fixed ratios; but once the warning stimulus suppressed the bird's responding, it continued to do so even after the size of the fixed ratio was reduced, particularly for Bird 3Y. The two birds differed markedly in the conditions under which the early control of the pre-time-out stimulus developed. The control developed readily in Bird 3Y and remained intact, regardless of the size of the fixed ratio. But for Bird 4Y, which had generally higher rates of responding, the pre-time-out stimulus suppressed responding only after the performance was weakened following the increase in the fixed ratio to values producing extreme amounts of pausing.

Even when the pre-time-out stimulus occurred only after the first response in the fixed ratio, the normal FR performance was grossly disrupted for the remainder of the fixed ratio. With both birds, a typically long pause occurred after reinforcement, as well as extended curvature more typical of fixed-interval than of fixed-ratio schedules. The order of magnitude of disruption of the FR pattern of responding recorded in this experiment does not occur under simple FR schedules of reinforcement, except perhaps as a transitory condition. Prolonged curvature was recorded, for example, under a tandem fixed-ratio, fixed-interval schedule (Ferster and Skinner, 1957) preliminary to almost complete cessation of responding. Equally significant are the large order-of-magnitude declines in the terminal rate of responding for Bird 4Y, which would suddenly respond evenly at only I response per sec throughout the ratio. This gross disruption of the base-line performance is further evidence of the aversiveness of the pre-time-out stimulus, and confirms the previous findings that time out from even relatively unfavorable (low frequency of reinforcement) schedules of reinforcement continues to suppress responding (Ferster, 1960). For Bird 3Y, the suppression by the pre-time-out stimulus disappeared when this stimulus occurred toward the end of the fixed ratio. This bird received many time outs because it responded during the warning stimulus. In general, the closer the warning stimulus was to the end of the ratio, the more difficult it was for the bird to stop responding.

Even under those conditions in which the bird showed a very low disposition to peck (*e.g.,* in an 8-hr experimental session when only two or three fixed reinforcements might occur), the normal FR responding ceased whenever the pre-time-out stimulus occurred. Thus, the pre-time-out stimulus apparently will more easily suppress responding when the disposition to respond generated by the base-line schedule of positive reinforcement is low.

When the base-line schedule of reinforcement is variable-interval, the small size of the pre-time-out stimulus might frequently fall within normal inter-response times. Hence, the frequency of responding in the pre-time-out stimulus might fall solely because of the decreased rate of responding. In ratio schedules, however, regardless of how low the over-all rate of responding may be, local rates of responding remain high. Therefore, the fact that the pre-time-out stimulus was response-contingent guaranteed that it would be programmed regularly whenever there was some substantial disposition to respond. Thus, the low rate of responding in the pre-time-out stimulus in the FR schedule is a suppression of the bird's performance at a time when it has a substantial frequency of responding. If the pre-time-out stimulus were programmed on a time rather than a fixed-ratio basis, it would occur most frequently during the long pauses of the strained fixed ratio. Thus, it would not be possible to know if the low rate is due to the pause generated by the base-line schedule of positive reinforcement or the suppression by the time-out procedure, if the pre-time-out stimulus were programmed as a temporal basis.

Because the probability of a response being reinforced does not increase with passage of time in fixed-ratio schedules, long pauses are not followed by reinforced responses as they are in variable-interval schedules. Under interval schedules of reinforcement, the probability that the next response will be reinforced increases in a pause and might lead to an increase in the rate of responding in the warning stimulus in spite of the ensuing time-out (Ferster, 1958, 1960). A similar factor, counteracting the possible aversive effects of the time out, might also operate in ratio base lines, even though the probability of reinforcement does not increase with pauses. In the FR schedule, the very high rate of responding and strong over-all disposition to peck generated by the conditioned reinforcement of increased number of responses probably counteracts the zero probability of food reinforcement in the pre-time-out stimulus.

The occurrence of time outs because of responding during the pre-time-out stimulus is related to the general topic of self-control (Skinner, 1957), in which a response is reinforced positively but also has aversive consequences, which may be avoided if the positively reinforced response is withheld. The FR schedule generates a strong disposition to respond that must be reduced during the pre-time-out stimulus. The bird must temporarily cease strong, positively reinforced behavior, especially, for example, when the pre-time-out stimulus appears toward the end of the fixed ratio. Responding during the pre-time-out stimulus seemed to depend on both the over-all disposition to respond as a result of the schedule of positive reinforcement and the aversive consequence of responding in the pre-time-out stimulus.

EXPERIMENT II

INCREASED RESPONDING AFTER INJECTION OF AMOBARBITAL, PENTOBARBITAL, CHLORPROMAZINE, AND, d-AMPHETAMINE.   Many behavioral experiments with compounds classified pharmacologically as sedatives show both increases and decreases in rate of responding, depending upon both the dose and the nature of the performance (Dews, 1955, 1956, 1958; Morse and Herrnstein, 1956; Verhave, 1959; Boren, 1959; Kelleher and Cook, 1959). Increased rates of responding predominately occur at low doses or when the major effect of the drug is passed and the normal base line is returning. Furthermore, these increased rates of responding are observed in both interval and ratio schedules; however, the effect is usually more pronounced in fixed-interval schedules, since the fixed-ratio performances which were measured were already near maximum rates because of the small size of the ratios. This experiment demonstrates similar increased rates of responding when a low over-all rate of responding on a fixed-ratio schedule is produced by the time-out procedures of Experiment I. We explored a range of doses of amobarbital, and repeated the experiment with pentobarbital, chlorpromazine, and d-amphetamine in order to determine what were the characteristics of the behavioral effects with these compounds. Sodium pentobarbital, sodium amobarbital, chlorpromazine, and d-amphetamine all produced essentially the same behavioral effects. At larger doses, the behavioral effects of the injection had two phases. First, the pause following the injection reached 120 min after the largest doses. Second, this pause was followed by a period when the extreme pausing (badly strained ratio) yielded to a more typical fixed-ratio performance, with the sustained responding almost immediately after reinforcement continuing until the next reinforcement. Because of the biphasic drug action, the average rate of responding would give a misleading picture of the effect of the drug. The dose-response curve was therefore reported as a median number of seconds required to complete a fixed ratio in the session. Thus, the median and interquartile range of this measurement described the predominant effects of the drug. The remaining aspect of the drug's action can be described by the time following the injection to the time when the bird resumes responding. Drugs dissolved in isotonic saline solution were injected intramuscularly in the breast muscle, and approximately 15 sec elapsed between this injection and the actual start of the session.

Figure 9 gives dose-response curves with sodium amobarbital and pentobarbital for both birds. Each point is the median time per reinforcement for a single experimental session, and the bracket gives the interquartile range. The left panel for Bird 3Y shows dose-response curves for pentobarbital and amobarbital which are similar. The open and closed circles at the left part of the graph give the median number of seconds per reinforcement for each of the experimental sessions preceding the drug injections. The control values are typically variable, ranging from 180 to 1313 sec. The median time for reinforcement decreased to minimum values at the 5-mg dose of the injection drug. Even though the injections disrupted responding completely for as long as 1 or 2 hr at the 7- and 8-mg doses, once the bird began responding the predominant effect of the drug was to increase the rate of responding. As given by the interquartile range around each point, the marked decrease in variability occurred because the birds responded at near the maximum rate. The effect of the pentobarbital injections for Bird 4Y, shown in the right-hand panel of Fig. 9, depends upon the base-line performance. The pentobarbital injections represented by the bottom curve were given early in the experiment, when the schedule of reinforcement was FR 125 and the pre-time-out stimulus had not yet sup-

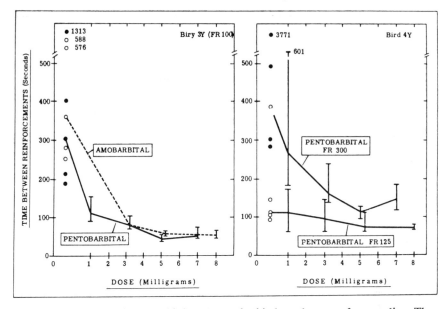

FIGURE 9.   Effect of amobarbital and pentobarbital on the rate of responding. The ordinate gives the number of seconds taken to complete a single fixed ratio, and the abscissa gives the amount of drug injected. The bird's performance is expressed as the median and interquartile range of the number of seconds required to complete each fixed ratio. The open and closed circles at the extreme left of each panel give the median values for control sessions in which a drug was injected. The curves begin at the median values of the control sessions. The pre-time-out stimulus occurred after the first response in the fixed ratio (7.5 + 2) TO 10 for Bird 3Y and (1 ± 1) TO 3 for Bird 4Y.

pressed the bird's performance. Rates of responding increased slightly, particularly in the interquartile range or the 8-mg doses; but the order of magnitude of the effect of the drug injection was not nearly so large as with Bird 3Y, because the over-all rates of responding were already near maximum. One control point, representing a session when the rate of responding was atypically low, falls in the range of the control points recorded at FR 100. Later, when the size of the fixed ratio was increased to 300, the baseline performance became considerably more strained, as the filled circles at the left show. These circles indicate the control values at this time. The pentobarbital injections given on this base line produced the same results as with Bird 3Y: an increase in rates of responding to near-maximum values. When the base-line schedule was FR 300, Bird 4Y confirmed the reversal of the curve at 7 mg.

Bird 3Y, whose responding ceased almost completely during the pre-time-out stimulus, did not show any increase in pre-time-out responding despite the very large increase in its over-all rate of responding. On the other hand, for Bird 4Y, which responded in the pre-time-out stimulus more than Bird 3Y, the number of time outs under drug also remained approximately the same as during control sessions.

Bird 3Y's data with pentobarbital is shown in more detail in Fig. 10, which contains frequency distributions, at each dose, of the number of seconds required to complete each of the 55 reinforcements received during the respective experimental sessions. The midpoints of the class intervals (20 sec) of the distribution are indicated on a log scale because of the wide range of the measurements from control to experimental sessions. Except for the 7-mg dose, the curves have peaks which shift to the left end of the distribution as the dose is increased. The 7-mg curve reflects the slight upward bend in the dose-response curve of Fig. 9, and indicates a reversal in the direction of the effect of the drug at the higher doses.

With Bird 3Y, injections of chlorpromazine produced some of the rate increases evident in Fig. 9 with pentobarbital and amobarbital; but the performances recorded with chlorpromazine differed in several important

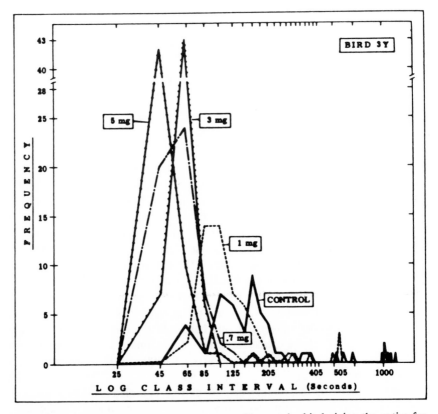

FIGURE 10. Bird 3Y. Dose-response curve with pentobarbital giving the entire frequency distribution of inter-reinforcement times for each amount of drug which was administered.

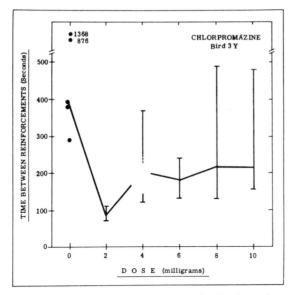

FIGURE 11.   The effect of chlorpromazine on the fixed-ratio performance. The conditions of the experiment are the same as those described in the legend of Fig. 9.

details. Figure 11 shows that at doses larger than 2 mg, periods of no effect were intermixed with periods when the rate of responding was normal. An example is the large increase in the 75th percentile, which indicates that more and more fixed-ratio segments are being emitted with pausing comparable with control values. The cumulative curves (Fig. 16) show the effect in more detail. However, the lower part of the range shows that many of the fixed ratios continued to be emitted much more rapidly than control values. Additional injections of amobarbital, pentobarbital, and chlorpromazine confirmed the results reported here.

The results with pentobarbital were compared with those for *d*-amphetamine for Bird 4Y. The general result, shown in Fig. 12, is similar: The responding increased at smaller doses and through the middle range, but fell off at the larger doses. However, the median time between reinforcements did not reach values so low as those with pentobarbital, for which the median values varied between approximately 130 and 160 compared with almost 300 sec for *d*-amphetamine injections.

With several injections of pentobarbital, amobarbital, and *d*-amphetamine, the pre-time-out procedure was discontinued for Bird 4Y during the session of the drug administration in order to show the drug effects without the interruptions in the performance during the time outs. The typical results was still obtained. It was also clear in the control experiments described in Experiment I, in which the pre-time-out stimulus procedure was discontinued in an attempt to recover the normal FR performance. The

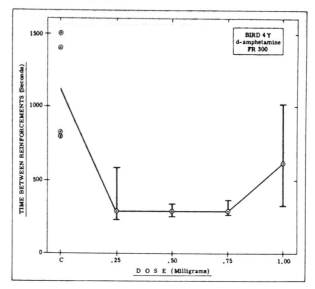

FIGURE 12.   Bird 4Y. The effect of *d*-amphetamine on the performance at FR 300. The conditions of the experiment are the same as those described in the legend of Fig. 9.

over-all rate of responding increased only after prolonged reinforcement on FR alone. The brief exposure to the FR without the time-out procedure during drug sessions could not have contributed to any rate increases.

Figure 13 shows representative daily sessions at the pentobarbital doses reported in the dose-response curve of Fig. 9 for Bird 3Y. The figure shows the over-all rate changes during the session by giving complete sessions in reduced form. The control performance was a low, over-all rate of responding that was roughly constant except for a brief period around the first six reinforcements. After the 1-mg injection, the initial rate of responding was sustained for slightly over an hour before it returned to the base line. After 3 mg, the over-all rate of responding increased further, and was sustained for approximately 100 min. After 5 mg, the over-all rate increased even further, and was sustained to the end of the session, when 55 reinforcements were delivered. A pause occurred only after the 8-mg injection; but the disruption was brief, and the remaining responding in the session occurred at the highest rate yet recorded. The panel in the upper part of the figure shows two enlarged segments from each of the experimental sessions represented in the figure. Besides reducing the pause after reinforcement, the drug injections increased the local rate of responding and changed the form of the curve from curvature to the typical "square pattern" of pause and shift to a terminal rate of responding characteristic of the normal FR schedule.

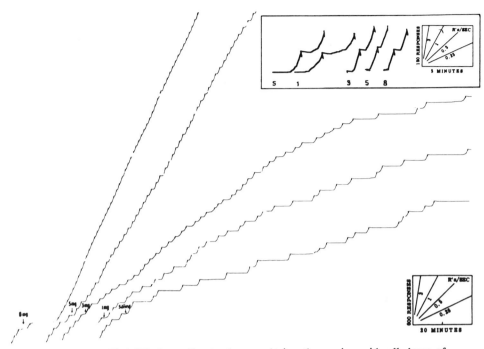

FIGURE 13.   Bird 3Y. Over-all rate changes during the session with all doses of pentobarbital. The data and the conditions of the experiment have already been presented in the legend of Fig. 9.

Figure 14 shows the typical drug effect in more detail for Bird 4Y at a 5-mg dose of pentobarbital. The top part of the figure shows the entire session preceding the drug injection. The arrows indicate pre-time-out stimuli which were followed by time outs; and the numbers above the breaks in the curve indicate pauses, in min, which were deleted from the graphic record. Pausing was extreme, and the over-all rate of responding was very low. The result shown in the bottom part of the figure was a 5-mg injection of pentobarbital at the start of the experimental session. The injection stopped the responding within several minutes, and the first reinforcement did not occur until approximately 40 min later. After another pause of about 10 min, the performance was thereafter sustained until the end of the experimental session, no pause exceeding 2.5 min. The increased rate of responding was caused not only by the reduction in the pause, but also by the substantial increase in the terminal rate of responding in the fixed ratio.

After larger injections of pentobarbital, rates of responding remained high for several sessions, and performances were similar to those just after drug injections. Figure 15 shows the effect on Bird 3Y of a 7-mg injection of pentobarbital. The increased rates persisted for 5 days following the

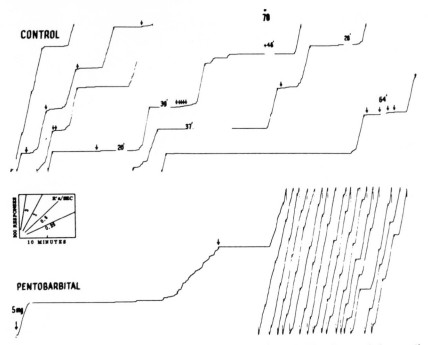

FIGURE 14.   Detail of effect of pentobarbital for Bird 4Y. The data and the conditions of the experiment have already been presented in the legend of Fig. 9.

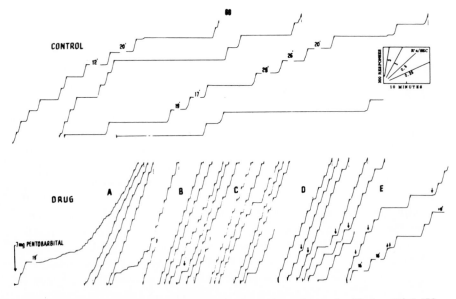

FIGURE 15.   Illustration of the effect of a large dose of pentobarbital on Bird 3Y, and the continued effect over several sessions. The conditions of the experiment were the same as those described in the legend of Fig. 9.

injection. The control performance in the upper curve shows the typical strained, FR performance, with very marked pausing and curvature generally increasing toward the end of the experimental session. At the start of the experimental session in Record A, the 7-mg injection of pentobarbital produced the characteristic effect after some initial pausing. However, in Records B and C, the next two experimental sessions, the rate of responding remained substantial; and only in the final part of Record D, the fourth session following injection, and Record E, the fifth session, did the rate of responding begin to fall to values approaching that of the control session shown in the top part of the figure.

Figure 16 shows two complete experimental sessions illustrating the effect of chlorpromazine in detail. The control session in the top part of the figure shows the normal, strained, control performance. The 6-mg chlorpromazine injection at the start of the session in the bottom part of the figure had an almost immediate effect in reducing the amount of pausing. However, the over-2-hr pause after the 7th reinforcement far exceeded pauses observed during control sessions. Subsequently, the over-all rate of responding remained substantial, although 5- to 30-min pauses still occurred frequently. The results here differed from the effects of pentobarbital largely in the frequent continuation of pausing and curvature

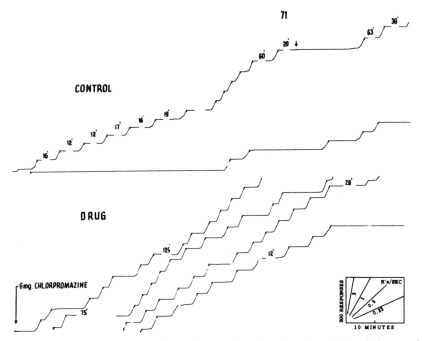

FIGURE 16. Bird 3Y. Complete daily sessions showing the effect of 6 mg of chlorpromazine and the preceding control session.

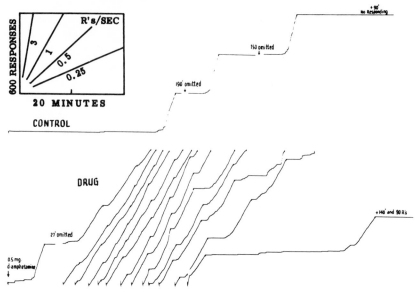

FIGURE 17.   Bird 4Y. FR 300. The effect of 0.5 mg of *d*-amphetamine. The upper curve is the entire experimental session preceding the injection. The pre-time-out procedures were discontinued during the drug session.

intermixed with sustained responding. The terminal rates of responding in the fixed-ratio segments did not increase over control rates, as they did with pentobarbital.

Figure 17 shows a detailed effect of the 0.5-mg injection of *d*-amphetamine, when the base-line performance was very badly strained. As the upper part of the figure shows, only three reinforcements occurred during the entire experimental session preceding the injection. Although a 27-min pause followed this injection, the performance thereafter was sustained until after 42 reinforcements, when the prolonged pausing again reappeared.[3] The effect of *d*-amphetamine on the local rate of responding was different from that of pentobarbital, amobarbital, or chlorpromazine. Here, the actual terminal running rate of responding in the fixed ratio during the drug sessions was considerably less than the control rates, as other investigators have reported (Morse and Herrnstein, 1956; Kelleher *et al,* 1959a, 1959b; Owen, 1960). The increase in the over-all rate of responding was almost entirely due to reduction in the amount of pausing after reinforcement.

DISCUSSION.   These experiments confirm the results of previous investigators who have shown increases in rate of responding under fixed-ratio

[3] The time-out procedure was discontinued during the session in which the drug was administered.

schedules of reinforcement with barbiturates and amphetamines (Ferster and Skinner, 1957; Dews, 1958; Kelleher *et al,* 1959a, 1959b, 1960; Morse and Herrnstein, 1956). In the experiments reported here, however, the low rate of responding in the FR schedule was produced by a pre-time-out stimulus rather than by the size of the fixed ratio. In addition to increasing the over-all rate responding, the drugs injected in this experiment also altered the very major deviations from a normal FR performance. Desultory responding at the start of the fixed interval, curvature during the early parts of the fixed-ratio segment, and gross variations from segment-to-segment in the terminal rate of responding disappeared whenever the drugs were injected. Dews (1958) has shown that pentobarbital had very little effect on very large fixed ratios (FR 900). The discrepancy between Dews' findings at FR 900 and the other conditions under which pentobarbital does increase rates of responding suggests that the drug is not creating new behavior, but is making it available by altering some of the relevant variables. In our experiment, the increases in over-all rate of responding under drugs may have been due to a disruption of the control of the FR performance by the pre-time-out stimulus, whereas at FR 900 no set of conditions might exist (other than variables such as increased amounts of reinforcement) that might increase the rate of responding. Similarly, the increases in rate observed with more medium-range FR's may be due to a disruption of the factors which produce pausing in spite of the relatively high frequency of reinforcement, as, for example, the number of responses in the FR as a discriminative stimulus. The effect of a drug injection on a medium-size FR might be analogous to a transition from an FR to a VR with mean value equal to the FR. Performances are sustained under VR at substantially higher over-all rates than those occurring on the FR, probably because the number of responses emitted between reinforcements does not control the organism's behavior.

We have confirmed the main findings of this experiment using a fixed-ratio schedule without a pre-time-out stimulus. The increases in rate of responding recorded on a simple FR schedule under the same conditions and with the same doses of drug as in this experiment suggest that the drug effects reported here do not depend upon the pre-time-out procedure. Rather, the pre-time-out procedure probably represents a procedure which produces grosser disturbances from a normal FR pattern which can then be "normalized" by the drug injections.

Increases in rates of responding under the pre-time-out stimulus procedure occurred at doses considerably higher than those reported with pentobarbital in other base lines in previous experiments except for the effects of chlorpromazine on observing responses (Kelleher *et al,* 1960). Typically, the range of doses producing increased rates of responding on fixed-interval performances is 0.5-2.0 mg with the pigeon. Some increases in rate of responding on interval schedules have been reported after recovery from large doses (Verhave, 1959); however, the number of observations is small, and our experience in this laboratory has been that such effects tend to be transitory. The increased rates over a wide dose range under the FR schedule suppressed by the time-out procedure may be due to the relatively favorable frequency of reinforcement in terms of responses per reinforcement. The drug might act by giving the bird behavior it has potentially available by disrupting the control by the pre-time-out stimulus. The rates of responding potentially available are those normally produced by the FR schedule undisturbed by the time-out procedure.

SUMMARY

Pecking was reinforced by a fixed-ratio schedule with food, and responses during a red light produced a time out. If the bird did not respond during the red light, the light terminated and the bird could complete the FR schedule of positive reinforcement uninterrupted. The bird stopped responding during the red light sufficiently to avoid most of the possible time outs. In general, the pre-time-out stimulus suppressed responding more when the FR schedule was large than when it was small. The occurrence of the pre-time-out stimulus in the fixed ratio produced FR strain and extreme curvature atypical of normal fixed ratios of this size. Amobarbital, pentobarbital, chlorpromazine, and d-amphetamine injected when the FR performance was strained by the pre-time-out procedure produced marked increases in responding. The drug administration lowered the rate of responding only at larger doses; and then this occurred predominantly just after the injection.

REFERENCES

Boren, J. J., and Navarro, A. P. The action of atropine, benactyzine, and scopolamine upon fixed-interval and fixed-ratio behavior. *J. exp. Anal. Behav.*, 1959, **2**, 107–115.

Brady, J. V. Assessment of drug effects on emotional behavior. *Science* 1956, **123**, 1033–1034.

Dews, P. B. Studies on behavior. I. Differential sensitivity to pentobarbital of pecking performance in pigeons depending on the schedule of reward. *J. Pharmacol & exp. Therap.*, 1955, **113**, 9.

Dews, P. B. Modification by drugs of performances on simple schedules of positive reinforcement (Techniques for the study of behavioral effects of drugs). *Ann. N.Y. Acad. Sci.*, 1956, **65**, 268–281.

Dews, P. B. Studies on behavior. IV. Stimulant actions of methamphetamine. *J. Pharmacol. & exp. Therap.*, 1958, **122**, 137–147.

Dews, P. B. Effects of chlorpromazine and promazine on performance on a mixed schedule. *J. exp. Anal. Behav.,* 1958, 1, 73–82.

Ferster, C. B. Control of behavior in chimpanzees and pigeons by time out from positive reinforcement. *Psychol. Monogr.,* 1958, 72, No. 14 (Whole No. 461).

Ferster, C. B. Suppression of a performance under differential reinforcement of low rates by a pre-time-out stimulus. *J. exp. Anal. Behav.,* 1960, 3, 143–153.

Ferster, C. B., and Skinner, B. F. *Schedules of reinforcement.* New York: Appleton-Century-Crofts, 1957.

Herrnstein, R. J. Behavioral consequence of removal of a discriminative stimulus associated with variable-interval reinforcement. Unpublished doctoral dissertation, Harvard Univer., 1955.

Kelleher, R. T., and Cook, L. Effects of chlorpromazine, meprobamate, *d*-amphetamine, mephenesin, or phenobarbital on time discrimination in rats. *The Pharmacol.* (2) 1959, 51.

Kelleher, R. T., and Cook, L. Effects of *d*-amphetamine, meprobamate, phenobarbital, mephenesin, or chlorpromazine on DRL and FR schedules of reinforcement with rats. *J. exp. Anal. Behav.,* 1959, 2, 267. (Abstract)

Kelleher, R. T., Riddle, W. C., and Cook, L. A behavioral analysis of qualitative differences among phenothiazines. *Federation Proc.,* 1960, 19, 22.

Morse, W. H., and Herrnstein, R. J. Effects of drugs on characteristics of behavior maintained by complex schedules of intermittent positive reinforcement (Techniques for the study of behavioral effects of drugs). *Ann. N.Y. Acad. Sci.,* 1956, 65, 303–317.

Owen, J. E., Jr. The influence of *dl-, d-* or *l*-amphetamine and *d*-methamphetamine on a fixed-ratio schedule. *J. exp. Anal. Behav.,* 1960, 3, 293–310.

Skinner, B. F. *Science and human behavior.* New York: Macmillan, 1958.

Verhave, T. The effect of secobarbital on a multiple schedule in the monkey. *J. exp. Anal. Behav.,* 1959, 2, 117–120.

40

Effect of amobarbital and chlorpromazine on punished behavior in the pigeon *

WILLIAM H. MORSE

Punishment is defined as a procedure in which an aversive stimulus follows a response. The usual effect of punishment is to suppress rate of responding. Over the past few years evidence has been accumulating which suggests that chlorpormazine and related phenothiazines differ from meprobamate, chlordiazepoxide, and barbiturates in their effects on punished behavior (see Cook and Kelleher 1963). These latter drugs appear to attenuate the suppression produced by punishment with electric shock in a wide variety of situations, whereas drugs such as chlorpromazine have no appreciable tendency to restore behavior suppressed by punishment with electric shock. For example, Naess and Rasmussen (1958) found that amobarbital and meprobamate, but not chlorpromazine, increased drinking in water-deprived rats that were punished with electric shock for each drinking response. Geller and Seifter (1960) and Geller et al. (1962) found that meprobamate, pentobarbital, phenobarbital, and chlordiazepoxide, but not chlorpromazine, promazine, or trifluoperazine attenuated the suppression of lever-pressing responses that produced both food and electric shock.

Although distinctions can be made among drugs on the basis of their effects on punished responding, the proper interpretation of these results is uncertain. Since they have been obtain in situations in which behavior is punished, the tendency is to accept uncritically the hypothesis that the drug effects are specifically related to the effects of punishment. Both Naess and Rasmussen (1958) and Geller and Seifter (1960) describe their results in terms of conflict, but Geller and Seifter also point out that it is not yet possible to isolate the factors that produce these effects.

A possible explanation of these effects of drugs on punished behavior is that they simply reflect the general tendency for these drugs to enhance or diminish the level of responding. The effects of drugs on punished responding have been studied mainly in the rat. In this species moderate doses of meprobamate and barbiturates have a tendency to enhance responding,

From *Psychopharmacologia* (Berl.), 1964, 6, 286–294. Copyright 1964 by Springer-Verlag, Heidelberg, Germany.

* This work was supported by grants MH 02904 and MH 07658 from the U.S. Public Health Service and by a research career program award 5-K3-GM-15, 530 from the Institute of Mental Health. The author wishes to thank Mrs. Catherine Jackson for her assistance with the experiments.

while chlorpromazine decreases responding in situations not involving punishment (Kelleher et al. 1961). There are species, however, in which chlorpromazine can cause an appreciable enhancement in responding. Waller (1961) found that low doses of chlorpromazine increased responding maintained by food in the dog, and in many situations chlorpromazine can enhance performance in the pigeon (Dews 1958a, b; Ferster et al. 1962; Kelleher et al. 1962). Because chlorpromazine has graded effects on the behavior of the pigeon over a 100-fold range of doses (Dews 1958a), it is of interest to investigate the effects of chlorpromazine on punished responding in this species. Since the rate-decreasing effects of chlorpromazine on the pigeon's responding appear to be less in situations involving changing stimuli (Dews 1958b), the punishment was introduced as a component of a multiple schedule. In different pigeons, different degrees of suppression were studied. The drug experiments confirmed the findings of Geller and Seifter (1960), and Geller et al. (1962) that barbiturates increase the rate of responding suppressed by punishment, but chlorpromazine does not.

METHOD. *Subjects and procedure.* Behavioral studies were made on three pigeons, designated 21, 22, and 180, each maintained at a body weight of about 80% of its weight when given free access to food. Prior to this experiment all the birds have been conditioned with food to peck a transilluminated response key (Ferster and Skinner 1957), and their performance on a variety of schedules of reinforcement had been studied. In the present experiment 3-minute variable-interval reinforcement (VI) was used as the maintenance schedule. This schedule specifies that the first response after a predetermined, but variable, time period will be reinforced. At the beginning of the session the key was transilluminated with a blue light. After four minutes the key color changed to white and thereafter the color of the key alternated every four minutes for a total of 16 4-minute periods. Identical, but independent punched tapes programmed the 3-minute VI schedules during the blue and the white stimulus periods (Mult VI VI).

Prior to the first delivery of punishment, each subject was exposed for about 10 hours to the Mult VI VI schedule. Next, punishment was introduced by having each response in the presence of the white light produce a 25 msec electric shock, 60 cycles AC. The current was held constant for the individual bird but was different for each bird. The shocking circuit consisted of a variable voltage in series with a 10,000 ohm resistor in series with the bird's resistance. The current was 2 mA for Bird 22, 6 mA for Bird 21, and 8 mA for Bird 180. The electric shocks were delivered according to the method described by Azrin (1959, 1960). Gold wire electrodes were implanted around bone in the tail region and attached to a leather harness that the subject wore at all times. During experimental sessions a jack was attached to a plug in the harness; the wires leading from the jack were attached to a swivel mounted at the roof of the experimental chamber. This arrangement insured reliable delivery of shocks while permitting the bird to move freely about the chamber. The electrical resistance of each bird was determined at the time of implantation and checked frequently during the course of the experiment. The measurements were made by nulling the current flow in a bridge circuit delivering a maximum current of 0.6 mA through the bird. The impedances of the birds varied from 1000 to 1200 ohms initially and remained unchanged throughout the experiment.

The birds were maintained for about 50 sessions on the Mult VI VI+ punishment schedule comprising a nonpunishment (blue stimulus) and a punishment (white stimulus) component. Sessions were conducted daily from Monday to Friday. The control observations reported are the means and standard deviations of 10 control sessions selected randomly from control sessions immediately preceding drug sessions. A session was used as a control day only if the bird's performance appeared consistent with its stable performance in previous sessions without drug.

Drugs. Chlorpromazine hydrochloride [1] and amobarbital sodium [2] were dissolved in saline and injected intramuscularly. Chlorpromazine was given 50 min and amobarbital was given 15 min before the session. Doses were given in terms of salts and duplicate observations were made at each dose. Some observations were made on Bird 21 with imipramine hydrochloride,[3] given 50 min before the session. At the end of the experiment the schedule was changed for Bird 21 so that only the punishment component appeared, and additional observations were made with amobarbital.

RESULTS.   Figure 1 shows the stable nonpunished and punished performances for the three birds. Punishing each response in the presence of the white stimulus resulted in a reduction in the rate of responding during the punishment component relative to the nonpunishment component. The suppression was only slight (about 10%) for Bird 22, shocked with 2 mA; the suppression was more pronounced (about 40%) for Bird 180, shocked with 8 mA; and the suppression was almost complete (97%) for Bird 21, shocked with 6 mA. That the 6 mA shock produced greater suppression than the 8 mA shock is consistent with Azrin's (1960) report of differences between pigeons in susceptibilities to punishment by electric shock.

The results from the drug experiments are shown in the Table. Increasing doses of chlorpromazine decreased responding on both the nonpunishment and punishment components of the schedule (excepting that these doses did not further reduce the already low level of responding of Bird 21 during the punishment component). There is some suggestion that on both

[1] Kindly supplied by Smith Kline & French Laboratories.
[2] Kindly supplied by Eli Lilly and Company.
[3] Kindly supplied by Geigy Pharmaceuticals.

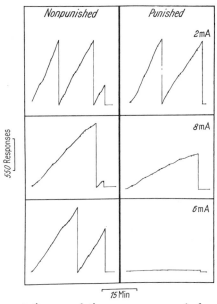

FIGURE 1.   Representative cumulative response records for daily sessions on Mult VI VI+ punishment. The nonpunishment and punishment components of the schedule alternated every 4 min. The nonpunishment periods are shown on the left, the punishment periods on the right. The top record is for Bird 22, the middle record is for Bird 180, and the bottom record is for Bird 21. The diagonal marks on the records show food deliveries. Each response during the punishment periods produces a 25 msec electric shock of the indicated current. The suppression during the punishment components is slight for Bird 22, moderate for Bird 180, and virtually complete for Bird 21.

components the decrease is greater when the control rate is high than when it is low.

In contrast to chlorpromazine, amobarbital had biphasic effects, both increasing and decreasing responding relative to appropriate control levels in all three birds. The lowest dose studied for each bird increased responding on both components, with the proportional increase above the control level being greater for the punishment component than for the nonpunishment component. Relative to control levels, higher doses of amobarbital decreased nonpunished responding to a greater extent than punished responding; in fact, after certain doses for Birds 21 and 180, nonpunished responding was decreased while punished responding was increased.

The dose-effect curve for amobarbital on punished responding seems to be steepest for Bird 22 (the least suppressed subject), and less steep for Birds 21 and 180 (Fig. 2). All of the doses increased punished responding markedly for Bird 21. Unlike amobarbital, chlorpromazine did not increase punished responding significantly in any of the birds, although again it ap-

TABLE. Effects of drugs on nonpunished and punished variable-interval performance in the pigeon.

The drug observations for each bird are means of the total number of responses per session during two drug sessions. The control means and standard deviations are based on 10 representative daily sessions preceding drug injections

Drug and Dose (mg)	Bird 22		Bird 180		Bird 21	
	Non-punished	Punished (2 mA)	Non-punished	Punished (8 mA)	Non-punished	Punished (6 mA)
Control	2368±217	2090±130	1016±122	621±77.5	1512±168	44±11
CPZ						
0.1			1024	644		
0.3	2165	1910	765	560	1450	41
1	1463	1243	656	377	1100	48
3	1040	888	647	283	909	59
10	755	717	547	134	917	32
17			608	55		
Amobarbital						
3			1180	869		
5.6	2637	2430	925	755	1660	502
10	1680	1570	611	465	1093	533
13.3	715	756			613	327
Imipramine						
0.3					1389	16
[1					1459	26
3					937	1
10					0	0

pears that the slope of the dose-effect function is steepest for Bird 22 (the least suppressed) the least steep for Bird 21 (the most suppressed) (Fig. 3).

Figure 4 shows a cumulative record for Bird 21 for the nonpunished and

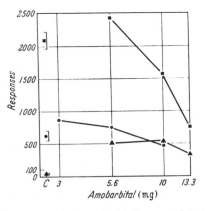

FIGURE 2. Dose-effect curve for amobarbital on punished responding for three pigeons. Squares: Bird 22; circles: Bird 180; triangles: Bird 21.

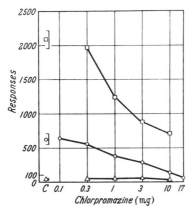

FIGURE 3.   Dose-effect curve for chlorpromazine on punished responding for three pigeons. Squares: Bird 22; circles: Bird 180; triangles: Bird 21.

punished components on a control day and on a day following 10 mg amobarbital. The effect of amobarbital on the punished component is to increase the number of responses emitted and its effect on the nonpunished component is to decrease the number of responses emitted. This opposition in the effect on the two components occurred on all of the four occasions when Bird 21 received 10 or 13.3 mg amobarbital and on both occasions when Bird 180 received 5.6 mg amobarbital.

At the end of the experiment Bird 21 was studied on the punishment

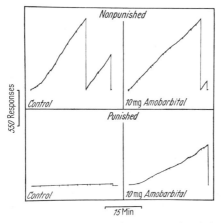

FIGURE 4.   Cumulative response records for a control and drug session on Mult VI VI+ punishment for Bird 21. The control records are shown on the left, the drug records for the following day are on the right. The shock current during the punished components was 6 mA which greatly suppressed the level of responding. After 10 mg amobarbital the level of nonpunished responding is somewhat decreased (top right), while the level of punished responding is greatly increased (bottom right).

component alone. The control performance was approximately the same as before, and amobarbital still reliably increased the rate of punished responding. Responses per half-session following single doses of 5.6, 10, and 13.3 mg were 89, 372, and 232, respectively. This represents a several-fold increase in punished responding, but it is less than that shown in the Table.

DISCUSSION.   The findings of Geller and Seifter (1960) and Geller *et al.* (1962) that barbiturates, but not chlorpromazine, attenuate the suppression of responding by punishment with electric shock were confirmed in these experiments on the pigeon. The results offer no support for the view that these drug effects on punished responding simply reflect a non-specific enhancement or diminution in level of responding. Chlorpromazine does not have a pronounced tendency to decrease responding in the pigeon; in fact, under certain circumstances it greatly increases rate of responding (Dews 1958a, b; Kelleher *et al.* 1962). In the present experiments an appreciable level of responding was maintained over a 30-fold dose range of chlorpromazine, but no increases occurred in the rate of responding suppressed by punishment. Likewise, imipramine is a drug which can have a pronounced tendency to enhance responding in the pigeon under certain circumstances (Dews 1962), but it failed to increase the level of responding suppressed by punishment (see the Table).

Opposition in the direction of drug effects during punishment and nonpunishment components provides still stronger evidence that increases in rate of responding during punishment components are not simply nonspecific enhancements of responding. In the present experiments, increases in punished responding were obtained with doses of amobarbital that greatly decreased nonpunished responding. Similarly, Geller and Seifter (1960) report many instances in which meprobamate, phenobarbital, and pentobarbital increased responding during the punishment component and decreased responding during the nonpunishment component of a multiple schedule. They also report instances in which *d*-amphetamine increased the rate of nonpunished responding and decreased the rate of punished responding.

Chlorpromazine and barbiturates differ in their effects on punished responding, but it has not been established that these effects are specific to the behavioral processes of punishment. The effectiveness of barbiturates in increasing the rate of punished responding under many different punishment procedures is suggestive evidence favoring an explanation of this drug effect in terms of the dynamics of punishment, but other explanations cannot be excluded. The tendency of barbiturates to enhance the rate of occurrence of a response depends upon the control level of responding (Morse 1962; Waller and Morse 1963; Dews 1964). In the present experiments increases in punished responding produced by amobarbital were greatest for the subject with the lowest control rates and least for the subject with the highest control rates. Rather than representing any specific effect upon punished responding *per se,* the effect of barbiturates on the punishment procedure may arise because punishment lowers the control rate of responding. Further quantitative experiments are needed, i. e., comparisons between the effects of barbiturates and the control level of punished responding, as well as comparisons between different procedures, including punishment, which produce gradations in rate of responding.

That this effect of amobarbital on punished responding is due simply to a change in the control exerted by the stimuli correlated with the two components of the schedule may be excluded, since in the final experiment, amobarbital attenuated punished responding even when the nonpunished component was eliminated. It is unlikely that this effect of amobarbital on punished responding is due to an analgesic property of the drug reducing the effectiveness of the shock itself. In the first place, amobarbital is not considered to have strong analgesic properties (Eddy 1928). Secondly, in the experiments of Geller *et al.* (1963), barbiturates, meprobamate, and chlordiazeproxide were effective in increasing the level of punished responding, but morphine was not. Thirdly, Azrin (1960) reported that a reduction in the intensity of shock did not lead to an immediate dramatic increase in the rate of a punished response comparable to that obtained when shock is eliminated completely.

Whether or not it is reasonable to describe the effect of amobarbital in this experiment as a specific effect on punished behavior, the fact remains that amobarbital and chlorpromazine differed greatly in their effects on this procedure. The results offer no support for the widespread belief that chlorpromazine has specific effects to attenuate suppression of responding by punishment (see Dews and Morse 1961; Cook and Kelleher 1963). One should not assume that any procedure which involves the presentation of an aversive stimulus to a subject will necessarily be affected by drugs of the tranquilizer class.

SUMMARY. The effects of amobarbital and chlorpromazine were studied on punished behavior in the pigeon. Key-pecking responses, maintained by a variable-interval schedule of food reinforcement, were punished by brief electric shocks. Under this simultaneous food and punishment schedule, responding is suppressed and occurs at a fairly uniform rate that is inversely related to the punishment intensity. Amobarbital partially restores responding suppressed by punishment, but chlorpromazine has no tendency to attenuate suppression by punishment.

REFERENCES

Azrin, N. H.: A technique for delivering shock to pigeons. *J. exp. Anal. Behav.* **2**, 161–163 (1959).

Azrin, N. H.: Effects of punishment intensity during variable-interval reinforcement. *J. exp. Anal. Behav.* **3**, 123–142 (1960).

Cook, L., and Kelleher, R. T.: Effects of drugs on behavior. *Ann. Rev. Pharmacol.* **3**, 205–222 (1963).

Dews, P. B.: Effects of chlorpromazine and promazine on performance on a mixed schedule of reinforcement. *J. exp. Behav.* **1**, 73–82 (1958a).

Dews, P. B.: Analysis of effects of psychopharmacological agents in behavioral terms. *Fed. Proc.* **17**, 1024–1030 (1958b).

Dews, P. B.: A behavioral output enhancing effect of imipramine in pigeons. *Int. J. Neuropharmacol.* **1**, 265–272 (1962).

Dews, P. B., A behavioral effect of amobarbital. *Naunyn-Schmiedebergs Arch. exp. Path. Pharmak.* **248**: 296–307 (1964).

Dews, P. B., and Morse, W. H.: Behavioral pharmacology. *Ann. Rev. Pharmacol.* **1**, 145–174 (1961).

Eddy, N. B.: Studies on hypnotics of the barbituric acid series. *J. Pharmacol. exp. Ther.* **33**, 43–68 (1928).

Ferster, C. B., Appel, J. B., and Hiss, R. A.: The effect of drugs on a fixed-ratio performance suppressed by a pre-time-out stimulus. *J. exp. Anal. Behav.* **5**, 73–88 (1962).

Ferster, C. B., and Skinner, B. F.: *Schedules of reinforcement.* New York: Appleton-Century-Crofts 1957.

Geller, I., Bachman, E., and Seifter, J.: Effects of reserpine and morphine on behavior suppressed by punishment. *Life Sci.* **4**, 226–231 (1963).

Geller, I., Kulak, J. T., and Seifter, J.: The effects of chlordiazepoxide and chlorpromazine on a punishment discrimination. *Psychopharmacologia* (Berl.) **3**, 374–385 (1962).

Geller, I., and Seifter, J.: The effects of meprobamate, barbiturates, *d*-amphetamine and promazine on experimentally induced conflict in the rat. *Psychopharmacologia* (Berl.) **1**, 482–492 (1960).

Kelleher, R. T., Fry, W., Deegan, J., and Cook, L.: Effects of meprobamate on operant behavior in rats. *J. Pharmacol. exp. Ther.* **133**, 271–280 (1961).

Kelleher, R. T., Riddle, W. C., and Cook, L.: Observing responses in pigeons. *J. exp. Anal. Behav.* **5**, 3–13 (1962).

Morse, W. H.: Use of operant conditioning techniques for evaluating the effects of barbiturates on behavior. In *First Hahnemann Symposium on Psychosomatic Medicine.* J. H. Nodine and J. H. Moyer (Eds.). Philadelphia: Lea & Febiger 1962.

Naess, K., and Rasmussen, E. W.: Approach-withdrawal responses and other specific behaviour reactions as screening test for tranquillizers. *Acta pharmacol.* (Kbh.) **15**, 99–114 (1958).

Waller, M.: Effects of chronically administered chlorpromazine in multiple-schedule performance. *J. exp. Anal. Behav.* **4**, 351–360 (1961).

Waller, M., and Morse, W. H.: Effects of pentobarbital on fixed-ratio reinforcement. *J. exp. Anal. Behav.* **6**, 125–130 (1963).

41

Observing responses in pigeons

Roger T. Kelleher, William C. Riddle, and
Leonard Cook

In visual-discrimination experiments, different exteroceptive stimuli are correlated with different conditions of reinforcement. For example, pressing a lever (response A) will be reinforced in the presence of a green light (positive stimulus) but not in the presence of a red light (negative stimulus). We will refer to response A as the food-producing response. When the organism develops a visual discrimination, food-producing responses occur in the presence of the positive stimulus but not in the presence of the negative stimulus. However, the development of a visual discrimination implies the concurrent development of observing responses which enable the organism to perceive the positive and negative stimuli. For example, the organism may have to move its eyes or its head to see the stimulus. For the experimental analysis of observing responses, Wyckoff (1952) and Kelleher (1958) required subjects to make a clearly specified response, such as pressing a second lever (response B), in order to produce the appearance of the positive and negative stimuli. We will refer to response B as the observing response. The experiments of Wyckoff (1952) and Kelleher (1958) demonstrated that observing responses ceased when they did not produce the positive and negative stimuli or when the stimuli were not correlated with reinforcement conditions. These results indicate that the appearance of the positive and negative stimuli reinforced observing responses.

The present experiments investigated observing-response rates and observing-response patterns as a function of: (1) varying the number of observing responses required to produce the positive and negative stimuli; (2) giving prolonged exposure to a given observing-response requirement; and (3) administering chlorpromazine.

METHOD. *Subjects.* The seven subjects were adult male pigeons (White Carneaux) maintained at 75% of their free-feeding weights. Four birds (P2, P4, P7, and P15) had no experimental history and three birds (P1, P9, P10) had had previous experience on various schedules of reinforcement.

Apparatus. Two experimental chambers were used, each containing

From *Journal of the Experimental Analysis of Behavior,* 1962, **5**, 3–13. Copyright 1962 by the Society for the Experimental Analysis of Behavior, Inc., Bloomington, Ind.

two Plexiglas response keys mounted 4 in. apart in one wall. A food magazine located below and between the response keys occasionally permitted a 4-sec access to grain. Each chamber was in a ventilated picnic icebox; the two iceboxes, which we will identify as A and B, were enclosed in a larger, sound-resistant, ventilated chamber. The programming and recording equipment has been generally described (Ferster and Skinner, 1957).

General procedure. Birds P2, P4, and P7 were trained in box A. Following magazine training, these birds were conditioned to peck each response key. They received 10 sessions on a 1-min, variable-interval schedule, which alternated unpredictably between the two response keys. This procedure established approximately equal response rates on both keys. Following this variable-interval training, these birds were subjects in a long series of observing-response experiments. We studied P2 and P7 for 3 years and P4 for 2.5 years, before P4 died from an overdose of a drug. Bird P15 replaced P4 for the remainder of the study; it was magazine trained and then conditioned to peck each key. After this brief training, P15 was shifted directly to the observing-response procedure.

Experiments in box B were conducted during the third year of experiments in box A, with Birds P1, P9, and P10. Because of their experimental histories, these birds were started on observing-response experiments without any special training.

The basic experimental procedure was similar to that reported by Kelleher (1958). Pecks on the left key were designated *food-producing responses,* and pecks on the right key, *observing responses.* Periods when food-producing responses were reinforced by food on a 100-response, variable-ratio (VR 100) schedule alternated with periods of extinction (EXT); the duration of each type of period varied from 10 sec to 10 min, averaging 5 min. A white light (mixed stimulus) illuminated the chamber unless observing responses occurred. Observing responses produced 30 sec of either a red light (negative stimulus) correlated with EXT, or a green light (positive stimulus) correlated with VR 100. If the periods alternated during the 30 sec, the stimulus changed accordingly. Each daily session ended when 50 reinforcements had been delivered or 4 hr had elapsed.

Preliminary training. All birds started on a procedure in which each observing response produced the positive or negative stimulus. Figure 1 shows stable performances of three birds on this procedure. The cumulative-response records in the upper part of each frame show food-producing responses. All birds developed high food-producing response rates in the positive stimulus (indicating VR 100) and extremely low response rates in the negative stimulus (indicating EXT). Birds P2 and P4 developed observing-response rates that were high enough to keep the positive and negative stimuli on for almost the entire session. However, P7 developed relatively low observing-response rates, and the mixed stimulus was on for more than half of each session. In the presence of the mixed stimulus, P7

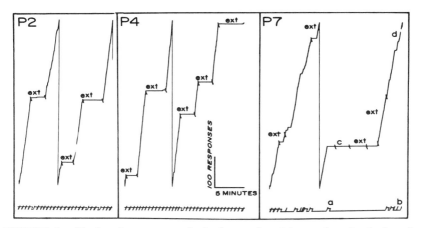

FIGURE 1.   Final performances on the basic experimental procedure (each observing response producing the discriminative stimulus). Cumulative records of food-producing responses are shown in the upper part of each frame. Food deliveries are not indicated. Pips indicate alternations between EXT and VR 100 periods; EXT periods are labelled. The lower record is displaced upward to show 30-sec intervals when the positive or negative stimulus is on (as at *a*). Brief upward displacements (as at *b*) indicate reinforcements occurring while the white stimulus is on. Both recorders stopped only during reinforcement cycles.

either paused (as at *c*) or responded at a high rate on the food-producing key (as at *d*). Birds P1, P9, and P15 developed performances comparable with those shown for P2 and P4; the performance of P10 was comparable with that shown for P7.

EXPERIMENT I: INCREASING THE OBSERVING-RESPONSE REQUIREMENT. *Procedure.*   A specified number of observing responses was required to produce the positive or negative stimulus; that is, observing responses produced the positive or negative stimulus according to a fixed-ratio (FR) schedule. The FR value was increased until observing responses ceased. Then, the FR value was decreased to FR 1 and increased again. Four pigeons (P2, P4, P7, and P15) were used.

Results.   Figure 2A shows the performance of P2 on an FR 10 schedule of observing. Food-producing responses (upper records) and observing responses (lower records) were simultaneously recorded on separate cumulative-response recorders. When the white stimulus was on, observing responses occurred at a high rate until the FR was completed. During the 30-sec intervals in which the red or green stimulus was on, no observing responses occurred. This response pattern on the FR schedule of observing is similar to response patterns on FR schedules of food reinforcement. The vertical lines at *a* and *b* indicate simultaneously recorded segments in which the bird paused briefly on the food-producing key while completing the FR on the observing key. Frames B and C of Fig. 2 show the first two ses-

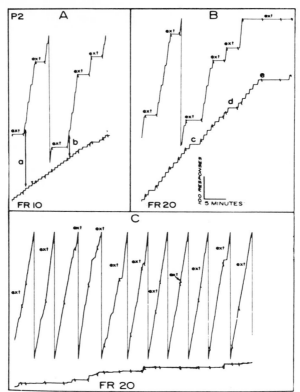

FIGURE 2. Effects of increasing the observing-response requirement to FR 10 and FR 20 with P2. Food-producing responses (upper records in each frame) and observing responses (lower records) were simultaneously recorded on two cumulative-response recorders. Both recorders stopped only during reinforcement cycles.

sions on an FR 20 schedule of observing. Although the observing-response pattern was maintained for most of the first session on FR 20 (frame B), some pauses occurred (as at *c, d,* and *e*). In the second session on FR 20 (frame C), observing-response rates decreased markedly and high food-producing response rates were maintained throughout most of the session. Following this session, the response requirement was decreased to FR 1 and then increased again.

Figure 3 shows the performance of P2 at FR 15 and FR 20 as the observing-response requirement was increased for the second time. The distribution of food-producing and observing responses changed. High food-producing response rates were maintained throughout most of each session. The bird occasionally paused on the food-producing key in order to respond on the observing key. If observing responses produced the positive stimulus, the bird immediately returned to responding at a high rate on the food-producing key (as at *a*). However, if observing responses produced

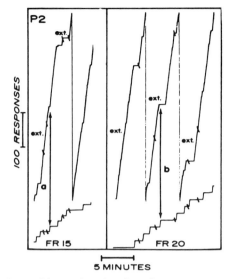

FIGURE 3.   Effects of increasing the observing-response requirement for the second time with P2.

the negative stimulus, the bird paused until the red stimulus went off and then returned to responding on the food-producing key (as at *b*).

Figure 4 shows the performance of P4 as the observing-response requirement was increased for the first time. Although observing-response performances of P4 could be maintained at relatively high FR values, the results are qualitatively similar to those of P2. Pauses on the observing key increased at the FR was increased, but stable observing-response performances were maintained at FR 30 (frame A) and FR 60 (frame B). High observing-response rates were also maintained during the first session on FR 90 (frame C). During the second session on FR 90 (frame D), however, observing-response rates fell to zero, and the bird responded at a continuous high rate on the food-producing key.

Figure 5 shows the performance of P4 at FR 25 and FR 30 as the observing-response requirement was increased for the second time. The results for P15 were comparable with those for P4.

Bird P7 developed low observing-response rates on FR 1 (Fig. 1). When the observing-response requirement was increased to FR 5, observing-response rates fell to very low values, and the bird responded almost continuously on the food-producing key. When the observing-response requirement was gradually increased to FR 20 over 20 experimental sessions, Bird P7 did maintain low observing-response rates on FR 20. From the start of the experiment, the performance of P7 was similar to that for the other birds when the FR was increased for the second time.

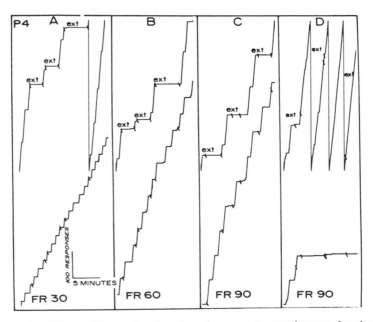

FIGURE 4.   Effects of increasing the observing-response requirement for the first time with P4.

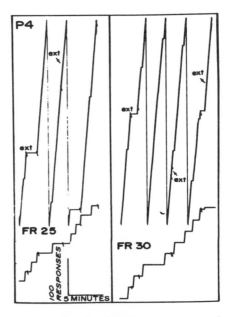

FIGURE 5.   Effects of increasing the observing-response requirement for the second time with P4.

EXPERIMENT II: PROLONGED EXPOSURE TO AN FR 20 SCHEDULE OF OB-
SERVING. *Procedure.* Following the study of the effects of increasing the
observing-response requirement, Birds P2, P4, and P7 were shifted to an
FR 20 schedule of observing. For P1, P9, P10, and P15, the observing-
response requirement was gradually increased to FR 20 following preliminary training. The duration of exposure to this procedure ranged from 5
months for P15 to more than 2 years for P2 and P7. All birds were frequently used in drug experiments during this time; base-line performance
was always recovered following drug administration.

Results. All birds developed similar response patterns. When observing
responses produced the negative stimulus, the bird paused on both keys.
When the negative stimulus went off, the bird responded on the observing
key until the negative or positive stimulus appeared. If the positive stimulus
appeared, the bird responded at a high rate on the food-producing key.
When the positive stimulus went off, the bird continued to respond on the
food-producing key in the mixed stimulus until several hundred responses
occurred without reinforcement. Because of this pattern, observing-response
rates were higher in EXT than in VR 100.

To show the difference between observing-response rates VR 100 and
EXT, observing responses were recorded on two cumulative-response recorders. One recorder ran only during EXT, and the other only during VR
100; both recorders stopped when the positive or negative stimulus was on.
Figure 6 shows observing-response records for P2, P4, and P7 after they
had been on FR 20 for about 6 months. Although observing-response rates
differed among birds, the results show that each bird maintained higher observing-response rates during EXT than during VR 100.

Figure 7 shows representative performances of the other birds after
about 5 months on FR 20. Observing responses here were cumulated on
one recorder. Again, the cumulative-response records show that these
pigeons produced the negative stimulus (correlated with EXT) more frequently than they produced the positive stimulus (correlated with VR
100).

Occasionally, we tested the effects of observing-response extinction, that
is, when observing responses did not produce the positive or negative
stimulus. Figure 8 shows the effects of observing-response extinction upon
the performance of P7. Frame A shows food-producing responses and
frame B, observing responses. For the first 10 min, the bird alternated responses between the two keys. For the next 50 min, the bird responded almost continuously on the observing key; then, after the first hour, the bird
responded almost continuously on the food-producing key. Observing-
response rates remained near zero for the rest of the session.

EXPERIMENT III: EFFECTS OF CHLORPROMAZINE ON OBSERVING RE-
SPONSES. *Procedure.* In this experiment, we studied the effects of

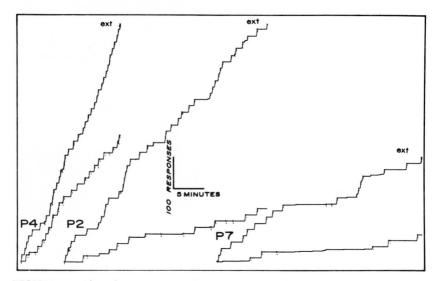

FIGURE 6.   Observing-response performance after prolonged exposure to an FR 20 schedule of observing. The upper records show observing responses in EXT periods; the lower records show observing responses in VR 100 periods. The recorders did not run during 30-sec intervals in which the positive or negative stimulus was on. When observing responses produced either stimulus, both recorders show a pip.

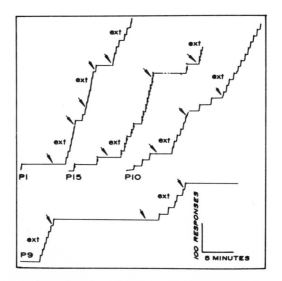

FIGURE 7.   Observing-response performance after prolonged exposure to an FR 20 schedule of observing. The cumulative records show only observing responses. Small arrows indicate alternations between VR 100 and EXT periods; EXT periods are labelled. The recorder did not run during the 30-sec intervals in which the red or green light was on.

chlorpromazine hydrochloride on performance on the FR 20 schedule of observing. The drug was administered orally 1 hr before the start of the session. The volume of solution administered never exceeded 1 ml, and all doses are in terms of the salt. The effects of doses ranging from 2.5 to 30 mg/kg were determined for P2, P4, and P7, and the effects of doses of 5 or 10 mg/kg were determined for P1, P9, P10, and P15.

Results. Figure 9 shows the effects of 10 mg/kg of chlorpromazine on the observing-response performances of P2, P4, and P7. The upper frames show representative control performances for each bird; pauses of variable duration alternate with bursts of responses in which the observing-response requirement is completed. These records do not show the 30-sec periods in which either the red or green stimulus was on. The records show that this dose of chlorpromazine markedly increased observing-response rates by decreasing or eliminating periods of pausing; and these effects were confirmed with P1, P9, P10, and P15.

Figure 10 shows the effects of the full range of doses upon the observing-response performance of P2. Doses of 5, 20, or 30 mg/kg produced extremely high observing-response rates.

For further analysis of dose-effect relationships, we computed a ratio for each control and drug session. The number of food-producing responses in VR 100 in the presence of the green stimulus was divided by the total number of food-producing responses in VR 100. We will refer to this ratio as

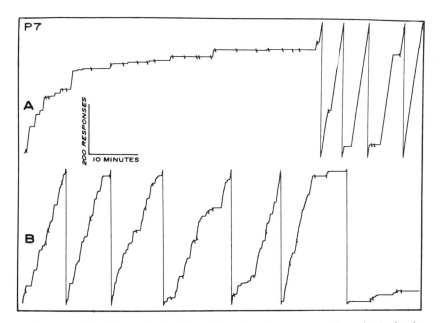

FIGURE 8.   The effects of extinction of the observing response. The mixed stimulus appeared throughout the entire session.

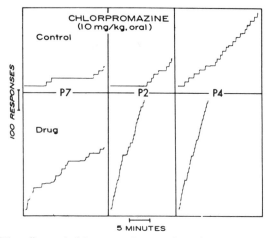

FIGURE 9.   The effects of chlorpromazine on observing-response performance. The cumulative records show only observing responses. The recorder did not run during the 30-sec intervals in which the red or green light was on.

the *observing* ratio. If no observing responses occurred in a session, the green stimulus would not appear and the observing ratio would be zero. If many observing responses occurred in a session, the green stimulus would appear frequently and the observing ratio would approach 1.00 (as-

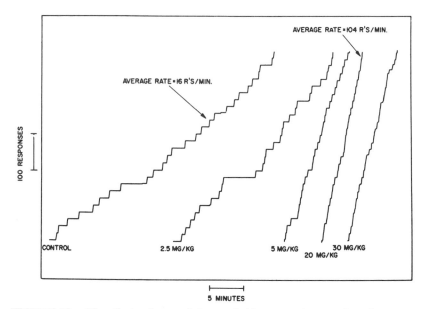

FIGURE 10.   The effects of several doses of chlorpromazine on observing-response performance. The cumulative records show only observing responses. The recorder did not run during the 30-sec intervals in which the red or green light was on.

suming that the bird responded on the food-producing key in the presence of the green stimulus). Also, we computed *total response rate* for each control and drug session. The total response rate is the total number of responses, observing and food-producing, occurring in each session divided by time in the session.

Figure 11 shows observing ratios and total response rates for P2, P4, and P7 as a function of doses of chlorpromazine. The medians and ranges from control sessions are shown at the left of each graph. The solid lines and dashed lines indicate the first and second determinations, respectively, of the effects of chlorpromazine; and a single point indicates the effects of a third dose of 10 mg/kg for P7. The experiments in the first and second determinations were separated by about 1 year. The results show that the observing ratio is increased by doses ranging from 5 to 30 mg/kg. Except possibly for P7, the dose-effect relationship is almost flat between these doses. The total response rate was inversely related to the dose of chlorpromazine. At all doses tested, the discrimination between the positive and negative stimuli was intact. In summary, as the dose of chlorpromazine was increased, the total response rate decreased accordingly; however, over this same range of doses, observing-response rates increased markedly and remained high.

In another experiment, we studied the effects of chlorpromazine on per-

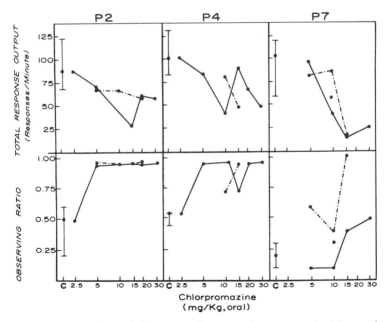

FIGURE 11.   The effects of chlorpromazine on total response output (upper frames) and observing ratios (lower frames). The medians and ranges from control sessions (C) are shown at the left of each frame. The abscissa is a logarithmic scale.

formance during the extinction of observing responses. Figure 12 shows representative effects with two pigeons. Birds P2 and P4 had three successive sessions of observing-response extinction. Chlorpromazine (10 mg/kg) was administered to P2 before the second session of observing-response extinction, and to P4 before the third session of observing-response extinction. Chlorpromazine did not retard or reverse the effects of extinction on observing-response rates.

In a subsequent experiment in which the positive and negative stimuli appeared throughout each session independently of observing responses, observing-response rates were near zero. Chlorpromazine (10 mg/kg) did not increase observing-response rates under these conditions.

DISCUSSION.   These observing-response experiments are similar to schedule-preference experiments (Ferster and Skinner, 1957). If observing responses do not occur, a mixed VR 100 EXT schedule is in effect on the food-producing key; that is, the same exteroceptive stimulus is correlated with both VR 100 and EXT. If observing responses do occur, a multiple

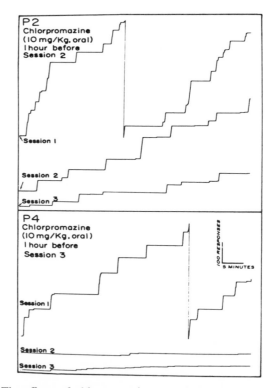

FIGURE 12.   The effects of chlorpromazine on extinction of observing responses. The mixed stimulus appeared throughout all three sessions.

VR 100 EXT schedule is in effect for 30 sec; that is, different exteroceptive stimuli are correlated with VR 100 and EXT. The results for the preliminary training procedure (see Fig. 1), in which the observing-response schedule was FR 1, indicate that the birds kept the multiple schedule in effect for most of each session. The results also suggest that the net conditioned reinforcing effect of the positive and negative stimuli correlated with 0.01 and zero probabilities of food reinforcement, respectively, is greater than the conditioned reinforcing effect of the mixed stimulus correlated with an intermediate probability of reinforcement. Using a delay of reinforcement procedure with rats in a T-maze, Prokasy (1956) obtained similar results. These findings support the notion that as the probability or frequency of reinforcement correlated with a stimulus increases, the conditioned reinforcing effect of the stimulus increases in a positively accelerated fashion (cf. Wyckoff, 1959). On FR schedules of observing, observing responses occurred in a regular biphasic pattern. In the mixed stimulus, the birds either paused on the observing key (initial pause) or responded at a high rate (the terminal rate) that was maintained until the positive or negative stimulus appeared. This pattern of responding is similar to that which would occur on an FR schedule of food reinforcement. As the FR schedule of observing was increased, the durations of the initial pauses increased, but terminal response rates were maintained until a maximum FR value was reached. Beyond this maximum FR, which differed for individual birds, the birds responded only on the food-producing key. In general, the present results confirm the results of previous observing-response experiments with chimpanzees (Kelleher, 1958).

For some of the birds, relatively high observing-response rates were maintained when the FR schedule of observing was increased for the first time. These high response rates probably were maintained because the birds had not had sufficient exposure to the mixed schedule. Pauses on the observing key in the mixed stimulus were accompanied by pauses on the food-producing key; that is, these birds did not respond on the mixed schedule. When the FR schedule was increased for the second time, or when the birds had prolonged exposure to an FR schedule, all birds developed high food-producing response rates in the mixed stimulus; and the observing-response patterns of the different birds became more comparable. If the birds had been exposed to both multiple and mixed schedules before the preliminary training procedure, the individual differences in observing-response patterns that occurred when the FR was increased for the first time could probably have been minimized.

Kelleher (1958) reported that average observing-response rates of chimpanzees were higher in VR periods than in EXT. Two reasons may explain our opposite results in this study with pigeons. First, the chimpanzees did not have the prolonged training on a single FR schedule of observing that the pigeons did. Second, the chimpanzees made observing responses and food-producing responses at the same time by using both hands; for the pigeons, observing responses and food-producing responses were mutually exclusive.

Perhaps because the two responses were mutually exclusive, the pigeons made a complex adjustment to schedule contingencies on the FR 20 schedule of observing. In the presence of the positive stimulus, the birds responded at a high rate on the food-producing key. In the presence of the negative stimulus, the birds did not respond on either key. In the presence of the mixed stimulus, the disposition to respond on the observing key was in competition with the disposition to respond on the food-producing key. The actual response dispositions at any moment appeared to be a function of preceding stimulus conditions. When the mixed stimulus followed the positive stimulus, the VR 100 period was probably still in effect; thus, the disposition to respond on the food-producing key was prepotent over the disposition to respond on the observing key. As time passed in the presence of the mixed stimulus, it became less probable that the VR 100 period was still in effect; and the disposition to respond on the observing key increased until it became prepotent. When the mixed stimulus followed the negative stimulus, the EXT period was probably still in effect; thus, the disposition to respond on the observing key was prepotent over the disposition to respond on the food-producing key. This interpretation is consistent with the finding that observing-response rates were higher during EXT than during VR 100.

The striking effects of chlorpromazine on behavior on the observing-response schedule deserve careful consideration. The increase in observing-response rates after chlorpromazine is not part of a generalized increase in responding. Indeed, the total response output decreases as the dose of chlorpromazine increases; this finding is consistent with almost all reports of the effects of chlorpromazine on response output in animals. Chlorpromazine did not increase observing-response rates when observing responses were undergoing extinction or when the discriminative stimuli were on throughout the session. The effect of chlorpromazine on observing responses is apparently specific to the particular contingencies in effect on the FR schedule of observing.

After receiving chlorpromazine, the birds remained on the multiple schedule for most of the session. Dews has suggested that "discriminatory behavior not based on exteroceptive stimuli is more readily disrupted by drugs than discriminatory behavior based on explicit environmental stimuli" (Dews, 1958, p. 80). As we noted above, the patterns of responding on the FR 20 schedule of observing appear to be based upon a complex adjustment to the schedule contingencies, including a discrimination between mixed-following-negative and mixed-following-positive. If chlorpromazine disrupted this complex discrimination, it would increase the disposition to respond on the observing key. This interpretation of the effects of chlorpromazine must remain speculative until further experiments are conducted with modifications of the observing-response procedure.

SUMMARY.   Pigeons were trained on an observing-response procedure in which periods of VR 100 and EXT alternated unpredictably during a white light (mixed stimulus). During VR 100, responses on a food-producing key (the first key) were intermittently reinforced. Responses on the observing key (the second key) produced a green light (positive stimulus) when VR 100 was in effect, and a red light (negative stimulus) for EXT. The birds did not respond on either key during the negative stimulus, but they responded on the food-producing key when the positive stimulus appeared. When observing responses produced the positive or negative stimulus on FR, observing responses were maintained until the FR reached a maximum; beyond this, only food-producing responses occurred. When observing responses did not produce either stimulus, the observing-response rates fell to zero. With prolonged exposure to an FR 20 schedule of observing, observing-response rates during EXT were higher than during VR 100. Chlorpromazine hydrochloride decreased the total response output but markedly increased observing-response rates except when it was administered before sessions of observing response extinction.

REFERENCES

Dews, P. B. Effects of chlorpromazine and promazine on performance on a mixed schedule of reinforcement. *J. exp. Anal. Behav.,* 1958, **1,** 73–82.

Ferster, C. B., and Skinner, B. F. *Schedules of reinforcement.* New York: Appleton-Century-Crofts, 1957.

Kelleher, R. T. Stimulus-producing responses in chimpanzees. *J. exp. Anal. Behav.,* 1958, **1,** 87–102.

Prokasy, W. F. The acquisition of observing responses in the absence of differential external reinforcement. *J. comp. physiol. Psychol.,* 1956, **49,** 131–134.

Wyckoff, L. B., Jr. The role of observing responses in discrimination learning: Part I. *Psychol. Rev.,* 1952, **59,** 431–442.

Wyckoff, L. B., Jr. Toward a quantitative theory of secondary reinforcement. *Psychol. Rev.,* 1959, **66,** 68–78.

42

Differential effects of two phenothiazines on chain and tandem schedule performance [1]

JOHN R. THOMAS

Several experiments concerned with the performances of pigeons on schedules of positive reinforcement (Ferster and Skinner, 1957) have suggested that one of the effects of chlorpromazine and other compounds is to attenuate the discriminative control which some exteroceptive and interoceptive environmental stimuli have over the occurrence of behavior (Blough, 1957; Dews, 1958a,b; Dews and Morse, 1961; Ferster and Appel, 1963; Ferster et al., 1962). Precise analysis of stimulus control of behavior may be investigated with sequences of behavior provided by chained schedules of reinforcement (Ferster and Skinner, 1957; Kelleher and Gollub, 1962). In a chained schedule, responding in the presence of one exteroceptive stimulus produces a second exteroceptive stimulus; responding in the presence of the second stimulus produces a third stimulus, and so forth. A primary reinforcer usually terminates the chain. Each exteroceptive stimulus, including the primary reinforcer, defines a component of the chained schedule. A specific rate and pattern of responding in one chain component may be reinforced and maintained by the production of the stimulus associated with the following component. Stimuli in a chain also serve as discriminative stimuli controlling a given rate and pattern of responding in their presence.

In the sequence of behavior in a tandem schedule of reinforcement, changes from one component to the next are contingent upon responding, as in chained schedules; however, the same exteroceptive stimulus appears in all components (Ferster and Skinner, 1957; Kelleher and Gollub, 1962). A tandem schedule can have the identical response requirements in each component as a chained schedule and can be used as a control procedure for the reinforcing and discriminative aspects of the stimuli in a chained schedule. Both chain and tandem schedules may be programmed in a single experimental session by a multiple base-line procedure with the same subject. The multiple base-line procedure allows the effects of stimu-

From *Journal of Pharmacology and Experimental Therapeutics,* 1966, **152,** 354–361. Copyright © 1966 by The Williams & Wilkins Co., Baltimore, Md.

[1] This investigation was conducted at the Laboratory of Psychopharmacology, University of Maryland, and was supported by U.S. Public Health Service Research Grant MH-01604 from the National Institute of Mental Health. The chlorpromazine hydrochloride and the trifluoperazine dihydrochloride were kindly provided by Dr. L. Cook of the Smith, Kline and French Laboratories, Philadelphia, Pa.

lus control in the components of a chained schedule to be compared directly with the components of a tandem schedule (Thomas, 1964).

The present study investigated the effects of chlorpromazine and trifluoperazine upon the behavior of pigeons trained to respond on a multiple chain-tandem base line.

METHODS. *Subjects.* The subjects were three White Carneaux pigeons (T4, T7 and T9) weighing between 488 and 546 g when allowed free access to grain and water. The subjects were maintained at about 80% of their free-feeding weight during the study.

Apparatus. The experimental chamber was a picnic icebox similar in design to that described by Ferster and Skinner (1957). The pigeons' compartment was 13 by 13 by 14 inches, and was illuminated by a 115 V a.c., 7-w house light. The chamber contained a single plastic response key on one wall which the subjects were trained to peck for food reinforcements. The response key could be illuminated by any one of several different colored 115 V a.c., 7-w key lights located behind it. Directly below the response key, a 2- by 2-inch opening allowed access to a food magazine, which could be raised into place for 4 sec to provide access to the grain reinforcer. The key light and the house light went off simultaneously with the operation and illumination of the food magazine. A cup containing fresh water was mounted on the side wall of the chamber. The chamber contained a centrifugal blower for ventilation purposes, and a masking noise was continuously provided by a white-noise generator. Programming was accomplished by a system of switching relays and timers. Data were recorded automatically on counters and a cumulative recorder.

Procedure. Experimental sessions were run daily except on days when apparatus failures occurred. Each session lasted for 40 reinforcement or for 2½ hr, whichever occurred first. The experimental base line was a multiple (fixed ratio chain) (fixed ratio tandem) procedure. Some properties of the multiple (FR chain) (FR tandem) base line have been described previously (Thomas, 1964). In brief, the procedure was the following. The subjects obtained a food reinforcement upon emitting 180 responses (FR 180). The FR requirement was programmed under two different stimulus conditions. In one condition, the response requirement was broken into three blocks of 60 responses, each block having its own exteroceptive stimulus. Responses 1 to 60 were emitted in the presence of a red key light, and the 60th response produced a white key light. Responses 61 to 120 were emitted in the presence of the white key light, and the 120th response produced a green key light. The 121st to 180th responses were emitted in the presence of the green key light, and the 180th response produced the food reinforcement. The above procedure is technically a three-component chain, in which the requirement in each component is FR 60.

The second stimulus condition also consisted of three component blocks of 60 responses, and changes from one component to the next were contingent on every 60th response; however, the same exteroceptive stimulus (a yellow key light) appeared in all components. Each component followed the other in tandem without correlated stimuli. The second stimulus condition is technically a three-component tandem schedule, in which the requirement in each component is FR 60, although the schedule may be viewed as a simple FR 180. During an experimental session, the chain and tandem schedules alternated in an irregular order.

The effects of doses of chlorpromazine hydrochloride ranging from 2.5 to 30 mg/kg and trifluoperazine dihydrochloride ranging from 0.25 to 2.5 mg/kg were determined for the three subjects. All injections were made intramuscularly 30 min before the start of a session in volumes of 0.1 ml/100 g b.wt. from an appropriate solution in 0.9% NaCl. At least two determinations were made for each dose. A session in which saline was administered always preceded a drug session, and served as a control for the drug effects. Saline was occasionally administered also during control sessions that did not precede a drug session. There were at least 4 sessions between successive drug administrations.

RESULTS.   *Multiple chain-tandem performance.*   Presented in Fig. 1A is a cumulative response record for one subject which shows control performance on the multiple chain-tandem base line. For all three subjects, response rates (responses/min) in the first chain component were lower than rates in the first tandem component. The mean response rate in the first chain component, based on the last 5 control sessions, for T4 was 9.4 ± 3.8 responses/min. The rate for T7 was 12.4 ± 0.8 and for T9, 40.2 ± 0.6. The mean rate in the first tandem component for T4 was 25.2 ± 3.1 responses/min. The rate in the first tandem component for T7 was 52.1 ± 3.5, and for T9 was 66.3 ± 3.4. Long pauses before responding began usually occurred in the first chain component (Fig. 1A). The second chain components also had lower response rates than those of the second tandem components. Response rates in the second chain components were 129.8 ± 2.1 for T4, 127.8 ± 2.8 for T7 and 143.3 ± 2.0 for T9. Response rates in the second tandem component were 134.0 ± 1.9 for T4, 236.5 ± 4.4 for T7 and 176.9 ± 3.3 for T9. Brief pauses often occurred at the start of the second chain component. Mean response rates in the third chain components were 155.1 ± 4.0, 271.7 ± 7.4 and 221.8 ± 3.0; response rates in the third tandem component were 138.2 ± 3.8, 304.1 ± 5.5 and 210.0 ± 2.6 for T4, T7 and T9 respectively. Performances in the present study were similar to performances on multiple (FR chain) (FR tandem) base lines observed previously (Thomas, 1964).

Effects of chlorpromazine on multiple chain-tandem performance.   The effects of chlorpromazine were evaluated in terms of the ratio of response rates in each chain component to the response rates that occurred in each

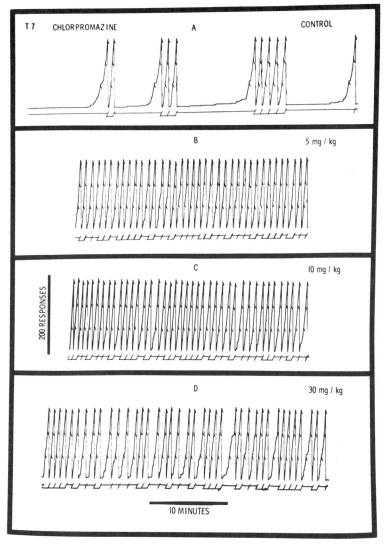

FIGURE 1. Cumulative response records of performances on multiple chain/ tandem base line for control and for several doses of chlorpromazine. Ordinate, cumulated responses; abscissa, time in minutes. Excursions of the recording pen during which the bottom pen is up indicate chain schedules; excursions with the bottom pen down are tandem schedules. Each pip during an excursion of the recording pen indicates the completion of each fixed ratio-60 component and the pen resets each time food reinforcement occurs.

comparable tandem component. Chlorpromazine increased the chain/tandem ratio of all three subjects above control values in all three components, followed by a decline in the ratio, as a function of dose (Fig. 2). The rela-

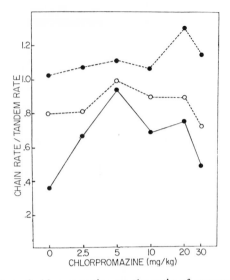

FIGURE 2. Effect of chlorpromazine on the ratio of response rates in each chain component to the response rates that occurred in each comparable tandem component. Ordinate, chain/tandem ratio; abscissa, dose plotted on a log scale. Black circles, solid line: chain/tandem ratio of first components; white circles, dashed line: ratio of second component; black circles, dashed line: ratio of third components. Each point represents the mean of at least two determinations for each of three subjects. The points plotted at zero dose are control values.

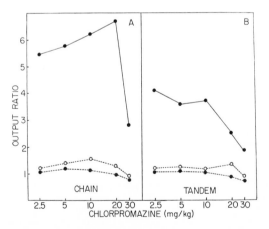

FIGURE 3. Effect of chlorpromazine on the ratio of response rate during a drug session to response rate during the preceding control session (output ratio) for the chain (A) and the tandem (B) schedules. Ordinate, output ratio; abscissa, dose and log scale. Black circles, solid line: output ratios in first components; white circles, dashed line: output ratios for second components; black circles, dashed line: output ratios in third components. Each point represents the mean of at least two determinations for each of three subjects.

tionship shown in Fig. 2 is representative of each of the subjects. There was a larger increase in the chain/tandem ratio in the first component than in the second and third components.

Figure 3 presents an account of the behavioral changes producing the increases in the chain/tandem ratios as a function of dose of chlorpromazine. Behavioral changes are expressed as the ratio of response rates during a drug session to response rates during the preceding saline control session (output ratio). In Fig. 3, it may be seen that the increase in the chain/tandem ratio in the first component, and to some extent in the second component, was due to a relatively larger increase in the behavior output in the chain schedule (Fig. 3A) than in the tandem schedule (Fig. 3B). The increase in the chain/tandem ratio for the third component at higher doses of chlorpromazine was due to a slightly larger decrease in the behavioral output for the tandem schedule than for the chain schedule. Cumulative response records showing chain and tandem performances for several doses of chlorpromazine are presented in Fig. 1B to D.

Effects of trifluoperazine on multiple chain-tandem performance. The effects of trifluoperazine on the chain/tandem ratio are presented in Fig. 4. The 0.25 mg/kg dose of trifluoperazine increased the chain/tandem ratio of the first component above control values. The three higher doses of

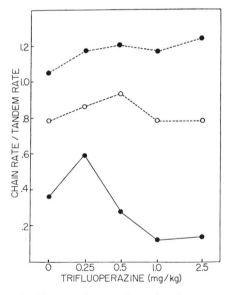

FIGURE 4. Effect of trifluoperazine on the ratio of response rates in each chain component to the response rates which occurred in each comparable tandem component. Ordinate, chain/tandem ratio; abscissa, dose, plotted on a log scale. Black circles, solid line: chain/tandem ratio of first components; white circles, dashed line: ratio of second components; black circles, dashed line: ratio of third components. Each point represents the mean of at least two determinations for each of three subjects. The points plotted for zero dose are control values.

trifluoperazine decreased the chain/tandem ratio of the first component below control values. The chain/tandem ratio of the second component first increased and then returned to control values as a function of dose. The chain/tandem ratio of the third component generally increased as a function of dose. The changes in the chain/tandem ratio of the first component as a function of trifluoperazine were similar for all three subjects. There was more variability among the subjects in the changes in the chain/tandem ratio of the second and third components. The change in the chain/tandem ratio of the second and third components was not too different from that produced by chlorpromazine.

Figure 5 presents the output ratio for the chain and tandem schedules as a function of dose of trifluoperazine. The decrease in the chain/tandem ratio in the first component was produced by a relatively larger decrease in the behavioral output of the first chain component (Fig. 5A) as compared to the first tandem component (Fig. 5B). The increase in the chain/tandem ratio of the terminal member was produced by a larger decrease in the behavioral output of the third tandem component than of the third chain component. At higher doses, the effects of trifluoperazine on the terminal members were similar to the effects of chlorpromazine on the terminal members. Trifluoperazine produced a larger decrease in the behavioral out-

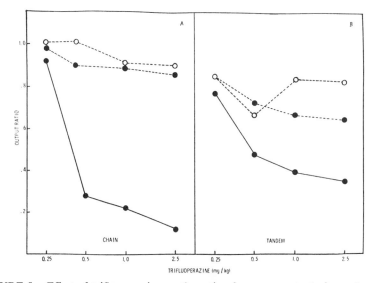

FIGURE 5. Effect of trifluoperazine on the ratio of response rate during a drug session to response rate during the preceding control session (output ratio) for the chain (A) and tandem (B) schedules. Ordinate, output ratio; abscissa, dose, plotted on a log scale. Black circles, solid line: output ratios in first components; white circles, dashed line: output ratios for second components; black circles, dashed line: output ratios for third components. Each point represents the mean of at least two determinations for each of three subjects.

put of the second tandem component than for the second chain component, although the effects were not systematically related to dose. Cumulative response records showing chain and tandem performances for several doses of trifluoperazine are presented in Fig. 6A to C.

DISCUSSION.   In the present study, the behavioral effects differentiating chlorpromazine and trifluoperazine appeared most clearly in the first components of the schedules, although differential drug effects were also observed in the second and third components. Chlorpromazine, particularly in the first component of the chain and tandem schedules, reduced the difference between performances in the presence of the chain and tandem stimuli. The reduction in the difference between performances under differential stimulus control by chlorpromazine has been reported previously (Dews, 1958a). One interpretation of the present results might be that chlorpromazine attentuates the environmental stimulus control over the occurrence of behavior.

Trifluoperazine increased the difference between performances in the chain and tandem schedules, especially in the first components. Chlorpromazine and trifluoperazine have been behaviorally differentiated with a procedure that differs from the present study, but which also involves exteroceptive stimulus control of behavior (Cook and Kelleher, 1962; Kelleher et al., 1960, 1962). Pigeons were trained on an observing response procedure in which positive periods of intermittent food reinforcement and negative periods of extinction alternated unsystematically during the presence of a single exteroceptive stimulus. Responses on an observing key intermittently produced a brief exposure of one of two stimuli that was correlated either with the positive or the negative periods. Chlorpromazine increased the stimulus-producing or observing responses markedly, while it reduced food-producing responses. Trifluoperazine was found to decrease the observing responses as well as the food-producing responses.

An alternative interpretation of the results of the present study and of the observing response procedure to the attenuation of stimulus control involves the conditioned reinforcing properties of a stimulus. Each component stimulus in a chained schedule may function as a conditioned reinforcer for responding in the component which precedes it (Ferster and Skinner, 1957; Kelleher and Gollub, 1962). The relatively larger increase in rate of responding in the first and second chain components, compared to tandem controls, as a function of chlorpromazine, could be accounted for by an increase in the reinforcing effectiveness of the stimuli associated with the following component. The observing response experiments reported above have also been interpreted as involving conditioned reinforcement (Kelleher and Gollub, 1962). The two exteroceptive stimuli associated with the positive and negative periods function as the conditioned reinforcement maintaining the observing behavior. As chlorpromazine selectively increased responses which produced the conditioned reinforcing stimuli and decreased concurrent food-producing responses, the results may also be interpreted as the effects of chlorpromazine upon the conditioned reinforcing effectiveness of the stimuli. Chlorpromazine did not increase observing response rates when the two stimuli were on throughout a session or when observing responses were undergoing extinction (Kelleher *et al.,* 1962). Since trifluoperazine decreased response rates on the chain relatively more than the tandem control and decreased observing responses, the results may be interpreted as a reduction of the reinforcing aspects of the conditioned reinforcing stimuli.

In an experiment in which pigeons were required to perform an avoidance response to avoid the withdrawal of a conditioned reinforcer (a discriminative stimulus associated with an intermittently reinforced food schedule), chlorpromazine was found to increase selectively the output of the avoidance behavior while it decrease concurrent performances (Thomas,

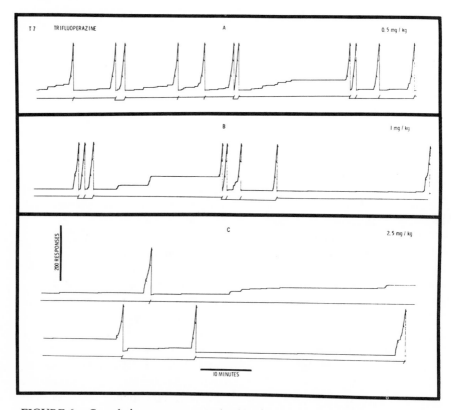

FIGURE 6. Cumulative response records of performances on multiple chain/tandem base line for three doses of trifluoperazine. Ordinate, cumulated responses; abscissa, time in minutes. Excursions of the recording pen during which the bottom pen is up indicate chain schedules. Each pip indicates the completion of each fixed ratio-60 component and the pen resets each time a food reinforcement occurs.

1965), again suggesting that chlorpromazine increased the effectiveness of the conditioned reinforcing stimulus.

SUMMARY.   The effects of chlorpromazine and trifluoperazine on the behavior of pigeons trained to respond on a multiple (fixed ratio chain) (fixed ratio tandem) schedule of reinforcement were studied. The behavioral effects differentiating the two drugs occurred most clearly in the first component of the chained schedule. Differentiation of drug effects was not as clear for the other components. Chlorpromazine increased response rate in the first chain component relatively more than it increased the rate in the first tandem component. Trifluoperazine decreased response rate in the first chain component relatively more than it decreased the rate in the first tandem component.

REFERENCES

Blough, D. S.: Some effects of drugs on visual discrimination in the pigeon. *Ann. N.Y. Acad. Sci.* 66:733–739, 1957.

Cook, L., and Kelleher, R. T.: Drug effects on the behavior of animals. *Ann. N.Y. Acad. Sci.* 96:315–335, 1962.

Dews, P. B.: Analysis of effects of psychopharmacological agents in behavior terms. *Fed. Proc.* 17:1024–1030, 1958a.

Dews, P. B.: Effect of chlorpromazine and promazine on performance on a mixed schedule of reinforcement. *J. exp. Anal. Behav.* 1:73–82, 1958b.

Dews, P. B., and Morse, W. H.: Behavioral pharmacology. *Ann. Rev. Pharmacol.* 1:145–174, 1961.

Ferster, C. B., and Appel, J. B.: Interpreting drug-behavior effects with a functional analysis of behavior. In *Psychopharmacological methods,* ed. by Z. Votava, pp. 170–181, Pergamon Press, New York, 1963.

Ferster, C. B., Appel, J. B., and Hiss, R. A.: The suppression of a fixed-ratio performance by a pre-time-out stimulus. *J. exp. Anal. Behav.* 5:73–88, 1962.

Ferster, C. B., and Skinner, B. F.: *Schedules of reinforcement,* Appleton-Century-Crofts, New York, 1957.

Kelleher, R. T., and Gollub, L. R.: A review of positive conditioned reinforcement. *J. exp. Anal. Behav.* 5:543–597, 1962.

Kelleher, R. T., Riddle, W. C., and Cook, L.: A behavioral analysis of qualitative differences among phenothiazines. *Fed. Proc.* 19:22, 1960.

Kelleher, R. T., Riddle, W. C., and Cook, L.: Observing responses in pigeons. *J. exp. Anal. Behav.* 5:3–13, 1962.

Thomas, J. R.: Multiple baseline investigation of stimulus functions in an FR chained schedule. *J. exp. Anal. Behav.* 7:241–245, 1964.

Thomas, J. R.: Discriminated time-out avoidance in pigeons. *J. exp. Anal. Behav.* 8:329–338, 1965.

Section **F**   CONSEQUENCE VARIABLES:
                    SCHEDULES OF REINFORCEMENT

The importance of reinforcement schedules in determining the behavioral actions of drugs has generally been underestimated. Inasmuch as the contingencies for reinforcement are perhaps the single most important determinant of the rate and pattern of responding, it should not come as a surprise that drugs affect behavior maintained by different schedules differentially. A schedule in which a single contingency exists between responding and reinforcement (e.g., an amount of elapsed time, a number of responses) is called a *simple schedule*. Non-intermittent simple schedules are distinguished by the fact that the consequence of every response is the same: e.g., every response is reinforced, or every response goes unreinforced. Article 43 illustrates effects of two phenothiazines and a barbiturate on such non-intermittent simple schedules. Simple schedules may also be reinforced intermittently (e.g., every 10 responses or every five minutes). Response rate under some intermittent schedules may be markedly increased by a given dose of a drug, but behavior maintained by other schedules is relatively unaffected by the same dose of the same drug (Articles 44 and 45). Within a given type of schedule, the value of the

443

schedule may also be an important determinant of whether the drug diminishes responding and the exact way in which overall rate is changed (Article 46). Distinctions based on presumed underlying process can be misleading. For example, the assumption that two schedules both involve a "temporal discrimination" can be deceiving, when the contingencies are in fact quite different. It should not be surprising that drugs differentially affect behaviors as a function of the contingencies rather than a presumed underlying process (Article 47). Behaviors controlled by certain temporal contingencies (e.g., DRL schedules and time-correlated schedules) have proved sensitive to drug manipulations. The influence of schedule parameters in such cases has been significant, as illustrated by Articles 48 and 49.

Compound reinforcement schedules involve two or more contingencies in effect either sequentially or concurrently. Article 50 illustrates the use of a *multiple* reinforcement schedule in which simple fixed-interval and fixed-ratio schedules, each with a distinctive stimulus, are programmed sequentially, each maintained by food reinforcement. In another study (Article 51), similar contingencies were in effect sequentially; however, no discriminative stimuli indicated which schedule was in effect. Such a *mixed* schedule can be used to assess the degree to which the behavior is under schedule control. Another multiple schedule was used to illustrate that the development of behavioral tolerance is dependent on the reinforcement contingencies (Article 52).

Parallel arrangements of operants in *concurrent schedules* have been used to illustrate differences in the way schedules control behavior under the influence of drugs. One such schedule has been a concurrent VI DRL schedule following *dl*-amphetamine administration (Article 53).

Complex reinforcement schedules are distinguished by the presence of two or more contingencies which either change systematically over time or as a function of some property of the subject's preceding behavior. Article 54, using human subjects, illustrates the interaction between methamphetamine and complex schedule requirements involving both numbers of responses (ratio) and elapsed time (DRL) contingencies. The efficiency under the influence of the drug was found to be dependent on parameter values of the schedules. While this experiment involved complex reinforcement scheduling, it was not aimed at systematically examining reinforcement contingencies. Article 55 is explicitly concerned with the role of schedule parameters in controlling the effects of drugs on *adjusting avoidance*. In this schedule the number of responses necessary to avoid a forthcoming shock varies as a function of the pause following the last ratio. The effects of drugs on behavior maintained by an *interlocking* schedule of reinforcement are illustrated in Article 56. On such a schedule, the magnitude of one schedule value changes as a function of the characteristics of responding on the other schedule.

The importance of schedule variables in determining the behavioral actions of drugs is only minimally represented by these studies. The fact that drug-behavior interactions (Article 57) are a major concern has been known since the mid-1950's; however, the general significance of this observation has not been widely appreciated. In a particulary eloquent series of experiments, Article 58 deals with the general problem of schedule-drug interactions with specific reference to punished and escape behavior. These investigations clearly indicate that reinforcement schedules can more profoundly alter the behavioral actions of drugs than any other variable. It is essential, therefore, that research designed to assess the role of any other variable (reinforcement magnitude, kind of reinforcement, etc.) take into consideration any possible differences in schedule or schedule parameters.

43

The effect of two phenothiazines and a barbiturate on extinction-induced rate increase of a free operant [1]

Travis Thompson

An earlier paper introduced a method of analysis of the change in frequency of emission of a lever pressing response induced by the onset of extinction (Thompson, 1961). In that study rats trained to obtain water on a regular reinforcement schedule (CRF) were given a test trial in which 6 min. of CRF was followed by a 3-min. extinction period. The increased frequency of emission of the response was expressed as an extinction inflection ratio (EIR) of a pre- and postextinction-onset lever presses.[2]

In the study cited above the effects of a 1.5 mg/kg ip. dose of chlorpromazine on the EIR were examined in comparison with the EIR of controls receiving isotonic saline. It was found that while the overall rate of lever pressing was significantly depressed in the chlorpromazine animals, they exhibited a relatively greater increase in rate of pressing following extinction onset.

The purpose of the present study was to determine the extent to which the foregoing effects of chlorpromazine are reducible to motor retardation and generalized sedation, and to explore the relationship of drug dose to the EIR. This was accomplished by comparing the effects of three doses of chlorpromazine with those of thioridazine, another phenothiazine derivative similar in behavioral action (Heistad and Torres, 1959; Taeschler and Cerletti, 1958; Torres, 1961) and phenobarbital, used as a motor-retarding control.

EXPERIMENT 1: EFFECTS ON RATE OF LEVER PRESSING

The purpose of Experiment 1 is to determine dose-response-rate curves for the three drugs, and to select three doses of the three drugs producing

From *Journal of Comparative and Physiological Psychology*, 1962, **55**, 714–718. Copyright 1962 by the American Psychological Association, Washington, D.C.

[1] This research was supported in part by Research Grant MY-2273 from the National Institute of Mental Health under the direction of Gordon T. Heistad.

[2] The increased frequency of responding following extinction-onset is one readily measurable aspect of that class of behaviors frequently described as "aggressive" (Lawson and Marx, 1958). It was this relationship to a supposed emotional state that suggested the exploration of the effect of tranquilizing drugs.

comparable effects on the rate of lever pressing to be used in Experiment 2.

METHOD. *Subjects.* Nine experimentally naive male albino, Sprague-Dawley rats, 120 days old at the beginning of the experiment, served as Ss.

Apparatus. Three standard Foringer-type, two-lever Skinner boxes with accompanying automatic control devices served as the experimental apparatus.

Procedure. After arriving in the laboratory, the animals were maintained on a 23½-hr. water-deprivation schedule for 4 weeks, receiving 30 min. of water per day with food constantly available. The animal quarters were maintained at a mean temperature of 72° F. with a range of 6° F. and a 12-hr. light-dark cycle.

The following training schedule was used:

Day 1: The animals were placed in the boxes and received six gratis water reinforcements at 20-sec. intervals followed by 28 min. of CRF (regular) reinforcement.

Days 2–4: Each animal received 30 min. of CRF. On the basis of the number of presses in the third and fourth sessions, animals were rank ordered and one member of each successive triad was randomly assigned to each of the three drug groups (three animals per drug).

Days 5–6: No training; injection with the lowest dose of the appropriate drugs listed below.

Days 7–end: The dose was increased daily according to the following schedule: Phenobarbital: 30, 40, 50, 60, 70, 80, 90, 100, 110, 120 mg/kg ip. Chlorpromazine and thioridazine: 75, 1.50, 3.50, 5.50, 7.00, 9.00, 12.00, 15.00, 17.00, and 20.00 mg/kg ip. Training and drug administration were continued until the mean presses for each group fell below 10 presses in a given session.

All drugs were administered intraperitoneally 30 min. before placing the animals in the boxes.

RESULTS. Figure 1 graphically presents the reduction in lever pressing produced by successive increments of phenobarbital, chlorpromazine, and thioridazine. It will be noted that the doses of chlorpromazine and thioridazine are expressed on a scale from 1 to 19 mg/kg and the corresponding values of phenobarbital are these scale values multiplied by 6. An examination of the three curves suggests that administration of these three drugs in successive small increments leads to a less profound reduction in motor activity than would be expected from other data (e.g., Taeschler and Cerletti, 1958, found s.c. ED50's to be 1.9 for chlorpromazine and 7.2 mg/kg for thioridazine). This apparent tolerance effect was taken into account in selecting doses producing 15%, 25%, and 40% reduction in lever pressing as compared with the mean of the last 2 days before drug administration. The values and the curves presented in Fig. 1 were used in choosing the

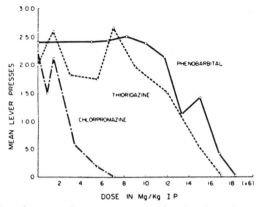

FIGURE 1. Dose by mean lever press curves for the three drug groups in Experiment 1.

doses for Experiment 2: phenobarbital: 30, 48, 64 mg/kg; chlorpromazine: .90, 1.83, 3.0 mg/kg; and thioridazine: 3.0, 6.7, 11.5 mg/kg ip.

EXPERIMENT 2: Effects on Extinction-Induced Rate Increase

METHOD.   *Subjects.*   The *S*s were 27 experimentally naive male albino, Sprague-Dawley rats 100 to 120 days old at the beginning of the experiment.

Apparatus.   The apparatus was the same as that used in Experiment 1.

Procedures.   The animals were maintained on a 23½-hr. water-deprivation schedule with ad libitum food for 2 weeks prior to the beginning of training. The following training schedule was used:

Day 1:   The animals were placed in the box and received six gratis water reinforcements at 20-sec. intervals followed by 28 min. of CRF.

Days 2–3:   Animals received 15 min. of CRF. On the basis of total number of presses on Days 2 and 3, the animals were rank ordered and one member of each successive triad randomly assigned to each of the three drug groups. Then within each drug group the nine animals were randomly assigned to three dosage levels. The resulting design is a 3 × 3 factorial, with triple replication per cell. After the training session each animal was given the appropriate dose of the assigned drug via intraperitoneal injection.

Days 4–5:   No training session; drug administration the same as Day 3.

Day 6:   Thirty minutes after ip. administration of drugs, each animal received a 10-min. CRF session, followed by 5 min. of extinction. All responses were recorded automatically on an Elmeg print-out counter. Immediately after the extinction period, each animal was tested for ataxia, using four independent measures. This procedure required about 5 min. per animal.

Unpublished research has indicated that the greatest increase in rate with extinction onset is obtained following 45 to 75 min. of CRF. Further, the magnitude of the EIR is a decreasing function of the time interval before and after extinction onset. As a consequence a total of 70 min. of CRF was selected to maximize the extinction effect and a 2-min. interval to measure most accurately the brief rate increase. However, instead of using the lever presses during the 2-min. period immediately preceding extinction onset as well as after, we have taken the mean of the 10-min. interval and multiplied it by 2 to give the pre-extinction measure and, therefore, more accurately reflect any change due to nonreinforcement. Thus, the final form of the extinction inflection ratio used here is: (presses 2 min. post-ext.) − (mean presses 10 min. pre-ext. × 2)/mean presses 10 min. pre-ext. × 2.

The percentage of the predrug presses emitted during the 10 min. prior to extinction onset was calculated to determine the relative motor-reducing effects. In addition a multiple ataxia scale was used to assess the degree of motor incoordination produced. The ratings on the following four ataxia scales were summed to yield a total ataxia score.

1. *Rearings:* 0, normal; 1, slight instability or staggering when rearing onto hind legs; 2, marked staggering, falling, or inability to rear.

2. *Inclined-plane behavior:* The animal was placed on a sheet of plate glass 18 in. square, with one end raised 4 in. off the horizontal plane. 0, animal walks off the glass without slipping or falling; 1, animal slips or crawls off cautiously; 2, animal falls, slips, is unable to move.

3. *Narrow-walkway behavior:* A strip of wood 36 in. long and 1½ in. wide was placed between two platforms, 24 in. off the floor. The animal was placed on the middle 12-in. portion of the board and was allowed 1 min. to walk to the platform on either end of the board. 0, crawls off successfully; 1, walks to either end-segment but not onto the platform; 2, falls off or has not moved off the middle segment at the end of 1 min.

4. *Walking in short alley:* An enclosed runway 6 in. wide by 6 in. high, and 24 in. long, with wire-mesh floor and top, was used to measure ability to walk or run in an alley situation. 0, normal ambulation; 1, slight incoordination of hind legs, weaving, or staggering; 2, marked staggering, falling, or dragging of hind legs.

RESULTS.   The effects of high, medium, and low doses of the three drugs on the extinction inflection ratio (EIR) is expressed in Fig. 2. An overall analysis of variance of these data yielded an F ratio which was statistically significant, and which, when further analyzed into components, was found to be attributable to a significant dose effect ($F = 10.279$,

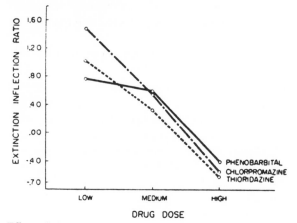

FIGURE 2.   Effect of three dosages of phenobarbital, chlorpromazine, and thtorida-
zine on the EIR.

$p < .01$), with drug and interaction effects failing to reach significance. An
examination of the curves in Fig. 2 indicates that for all three drugs there is
an inverse relationship between dose and magnitude of the EIR.

In Fig. 3 are presented the percentages of the predrug presses on the last
day before drug administration, emitted during the 10-min. period before
extinction onset in the test session. Like the EIRs it is seen that there is an
inverse relationship between drug dose and the percentage of predrug rate.
The overall F ratio based on the 3×3 analysis of this variable was sufficiently large to be considered nonchance, leading to further analysis of the
constituents. It was found that there were significant dose ($F = 9.203$,

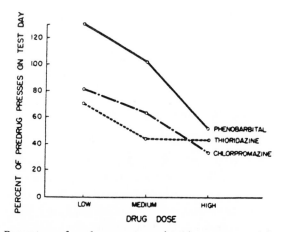

FIGURE 3.   Percentage of predrug presses emitted by groups receiving three doses of
phenobarbital, chlorpromazine, and thioridazine on the test day.

$p < .01$) and drug ($F = 7.328$, $p < .01$) effects, but no discernible interaction between the two variables. Since the dose effect was consistent with the EIR data and seemed to be a reasonable expectation, only the drug difference was further analyzed. Subcomparisons of the three drug groups lead to the conclusion that the differences between drugs can be attributed to the deviation of the phenobarbital group from the two phenothiazines ($F_{\text{phen} \times \text{chl}} = 8.968$, $p < .01$; $F_{\text{phen} \times \text{thio}} = 12.703$, $p < .01$) while there is no significant difference between the thioridazine and chlorpromazine groups.

The dose effects on total ataxia scores are presented in Fig. 4. The overall analysis of variance yielded a significant F ratio which was found to be due to significant dose ($F = 12.883$, $p < .01$) and drug ($F = 5.184$, $p < .05$) effects when further analyzed. Subcomparisons indicate that the difference in drug effects is a reflection of the deviation of the phenobarbital group ($F_{\text{phen} \times \text{chl}} = 8.723$, $p < .01$; $F_{\text{phen} \times \text{thio}} = 6.680$, $p < .01$), which is very clearly different from the relationship between drug dose and the ataxic effect for all drugs.

DISCUSSION

A comparison of the chlorpromazine data presented in Fig. 2 with the EIRs obtained in the previous study (Thompson, 1961) tends to corroborate the original finding that at a 1.5 mg/kg ip. dose, chlorpromazine animals exhibit a marked rise in EIR. At doses of .90 to 1.83 mg/kg ip., the mean EIRs for the chlorpromazine groups are +.55 and +1.48, as compared with a median EIR at +.38 at 1.5 mg/kg in the earlier report.

The results of the analysis of variance of the EIR data along with the graphic presentation in Fig. 2 clearly indicate that the three drugs had no

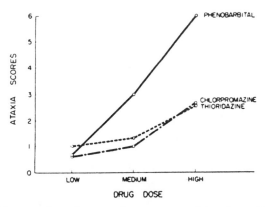

FIGURE 4.   Mean total ataxia scores for groups receiving three doses of phenobarbital, chlorpromazine, and thioridazine.

significantly different effect on the EIR; however, there was a very marked inverse relationship between the dose of the three drugs and the EIR. This suggests that there were no differences in "tranquilizing" action of the three drugs on this behavior despite the great pharmacological dissimilarity of the barbiturate and the phenothiazines. The obtained inverse relationship between dose and frequency of lever pressing as compared with predrug rate is consistent with other data on these drugs (Blough, 1956; Cook, Weidley, Morris, and Mattis, 1955; Dews, 1956).

While these data would appear to indicate no basic advantage in using the phenothiazines for the control of this class of behavior, an examination of the ataxia scores casts a different light on value of these compounds. The ataxia scores for the phenobarbital group were significantly higher than those obtained by the two phenothiazine, which did not differ significantly from one another. This markedly higher degree of incoordination and inability to carry out gross locomotor activities suggests that while phenobarbital is capable of altering extinction-induced rate increase, it also produces a high degree of undesirable ataxia.

It would certainly appear that the primary effect on the EIR for chlorpromazine, thioridazine, and phenobarbital is one of dose. The implication of these findings for our initial queston is that while the phenothiazine derivatives and barbiturates are known to differ in mode and sites of action (Berger, 1960; Killam, 1956), as far as their effects on this behavior is concerned, the drugs cannot be distinguished. However, an examination of the effects of the two phenothiazines and a barbiturate on the degree of ataxia indicates that there are differences which might have a great deal of importance in efforts to control one class of behavior without altering the other.

SUMMARY

The present study was carried out in two parts. Experiment 1 was designed to determine the effect of various doses of phenobarbital, thioridazine, and chlorpromazine on rate of lever pressing for water reinforcement on a CRF schedule. From the dose-lever press curves, high, medium, and low doses of the three drugs were selected which produced comparable degrees of reduction in pressing. Experiment 2 employed the three doses of the same three drugs to examine drug and dose effects on the extinction inflection ratio (EIR), on depression in lever pressing, and on degree of ataxia. The experimental design was a 3 × 3 factorial, with triple replication per cell. The findings were as follows: (a) There were no significant drug or interaction effects, only dosage differences on EIR. The EIR for all drugs bore an inverse relation to dose. (b) There were significant dose and drug differences in amount of reduction of lever pressing, but no interaction effect. The drug difference was contributed by the phenobarbital group, which deviated significantly from the two phenothiazines. Like the EIR, this variable was inversely related to dosage. (*c*) There were significant dose and drug effects but no interaction effect in the total ataxia scores. The drug effect was contributed solely by the phenobarbital group. The ataxia scores were directly related to dose.

The data were interpreted as indicating no basic difference in effect of the three drugs on the extinction-induced rate increase but a very significant difference in ataxic effect, which presumably has practical implications.

REFERENCES

Berger, F. M. Classification of psychoactive drugs according to their chemical structure and sites of action. In L. Uhr and J. G. Miller (Eds.), *Drugs and behavior*. New York: Wiley, 1960.

Blough, D. S. Technique for studying the effects of drugs on discrimination in the pigeon. *Ann N.Y. Acad. Sci.,* 1956, **65**, 334.

Cook, L., Weidley, E. F., Morris, R. W., and Mattis, P. A. Neuropharmacological and behavioral effects of chlorpromazine (Thorazine hydrochloride). *J. Pharmacol. exp. Ther.,* 1955, **113**, 11.

Dews, P. B. Modification by drugs of performance on simple schedules of positive reinforcement. *Ann. N.Y. Acad. Sci.,* 1956, **65**, 268.

Heistad, G. T., and Torres, A. A. A mechanism for the effect of a tranquilizing drug on learned emotional responses. *U. Minn. med. Bull.,* 1959, **30**, 518.

Killam, E. K., The pharmacological aspects of certain drugs useful in psychiatry. In J. O. Cole and R. W. Gerard (Eds.), *Psychopharmacology: Problems in evaluation*. Wash., D.C.: National Academy Sciences—National Research Council, 1956.

Lawson, R., and Marx, M. H. Frustration: Theory and experiment. *Genet. Psychol. Monog.* 1958, **57**, 393–464.

Taeschler, M., and Cerletti, A. The pharmacology of thioridazine hydrochloride, Mellaril. *Schweiz. med. Wschr.* 1958, **88**, 1216.

Thompson, T. Effects of chlorpromazine on "aggressive" responding in the rat. *J. comp. physiol. Psychol.,* 1961, **54**, 398–400.

Torres, A. A. Anxiety versus escape conditioning and tranquilizing action. *J. comp. physiol. Psychol.,* 1961, **54**, 349–353.

44

Differential sensitivity to pentobarbital of pecking performance in pigeons depending on the schedule of reward [1,2]

PETER B. DEWS

The use of experimental animals in the analysis of behavioral effects of drugs has been hampered by a paucity of objective, quantitative methods of study. However, the techniques developed by Skinner and his colleagues permit a strictly operational approach to these problems (Skinner, 1953; Ferster, 1953). The animal is confronted with a device which it can operate; the "response" of the animal is defined as such an operation. The animal is suitably rewarded for responding. Rewards can be made intermittent, i.e. not every response need be rewarded. The rate of response at different times depends upon the contingencies which determine which response will be rewarded (see below). These contingencies can be specified and responses are automatically recorded; so the methods are both objective and quantitative.

As long ago as 1937, Skinner and Heron studied the effects of caffeine and of amphetamine on the performance of rats working in a Skinner box. The following year, Wentink (1938) reported on the effects of a variety of other drugs. In spite of the interesting results obtained, the studies were not continued. Recently, Wikler (1954) has presented a preliminary communication on use of the Skinner box technique to study the effects of morphine on "behavior-disrupting anticipatory responses to painful stimuli" in rats.

In the present work, the experimental animals have been pigeons. The birds were confronted with a device (the key), which was operated by a peck. Reward was access to food; this was rewarding because the birds were maintained in a state of partial food deprivation.

To show promise of usefulness for the analysis of behavioral effects of

From *Journal of Pharmacology and Experimental Therapeutics*, 1955, 113, 393–401. Copyright © 1955 by The Williams & Wilkins Co., Baltimore, Md.

[1] This work was supported in part by funds received from the William F. Milton Fund of Harvard University, and in part by funds received from The Roche Anniversary Foundation of Hoffmann-LaRoche, Inc. The author wishes to express his indebtedness to Dr. Charles B. Ferster of the Psychological Laboratories of Harvard University for invaluable help in the initiation of these experiments. Thanks are also due to Mr. Brian Connor for conscientious assistance and to Abbott Laboratories who generously supplied the pentobarbital sodium.

[2] For a more detailed account of the principles involved in the design of the apparatus see Ferster (1953).

drugs a method should enable a behavioral effect to be detected and measured following doses insufficient to cause gross disturbance of the animal. The principal object of the present communication is to present the Skinner box technique as a method of potential usefulness to pharmacologists, and to give evidence that the above requirement for promise is met. The drug chosen was pentobarbital sodium because its duration of action was convenient.

MATERIALS AND METHODS. *Apparatus.*   In all the studies reported here, the same Skinner pigeon box has been used; its general arrangement is shown in Fig. 1 (not to scale). The pigeon is placed in a soundproofed ventilated box. The key is a recessed disc of light translucent plastic in one wall, at a convenient height for the pigeon to peck. When the pigeon pecks it, an electrical contact is broken. On release, a spring restores the key to its original position and so remakes the circuit. The maximum permitted excursion of the key is only a few millimeters, and the strength of the spring is such that the cycle of make and break of the key circuit can be repeated at least 10–15 times per second. Behind the key is a small (6W) electric bulb (the key light).

A tray of food can be lifted by an electromagnet so that it is accessible to the pigeon through an opening in the pigeon chamber below the key. At each reward, the food is made accessible, and brightly illuminated, for 4–5 seconds. The rest of the time, the food is out of reach of the pigeon.

The electrical connections from the box lead to an arrangement of simple switching, timing and counting devices which automatically program the schedules to be described.

Responses were recorded on a Gerbrands' cumulative recorder. Paper

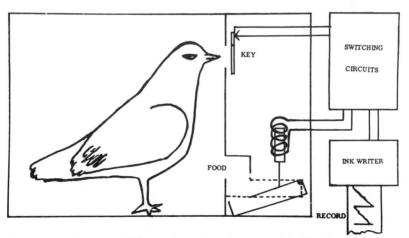

FIGURE 1.   Diagram of Skinner pigeon box (not to scale). For details see text.

feeds through the recorder at constant speed; each response moves an ink pen a constant distance at right angles to the direction of movement of the paper. After approximately 900 responses, the pen resets automatically. The records have thus time as abscissa and cumulative responses as ordinate; the slope of the curve gives the rate of response. Also, occurrence of rewards can be shown on the records. In addition, responses can be counted with digital counters.

SCHEDULES (see Fig. 2). 1. *Fixed ratio of responses to rewards.* The bird was put into the completely darkened box. Fifteen minutes later, the key light came on and remained on for five minutes. During this five minute period, every 50th response was rewarded. At its conclusion, the bird was removed from the box, the drug injected, and the bird returned to the box. Fifteen minutes later, the key light came on again, and remained on for fifteen minutes, during which time, again, every 50th response was rewarded. This schedule will be referred to as FR50. On this schedule, the higher the rate of response, the sooner a reward was obtained.

2. *Fifteen minute fixed interval.* The key light came on fifteen minutes after the bird was placed into the darkened box. The first response made after the key light had been on for fifteen minutes (the "fixed interval") was rewarded. Responses occurring before the end of the fixed interval were not rewarded; the key light remained on after the end of the fixed interval until the first response occurred. At the time of the reward, the key light went out and remained out for fifteen minutes; it then came on

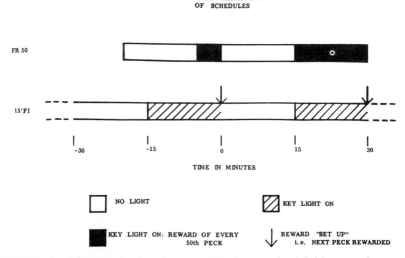

FIGURE 2. Diagram showing the sequence of events in definitive experiments on the two schedules. The drug injection was given at time 0. On the 15'FI several light on-light off cycles were run both before and after drug.

again and the whole cycle was repeated. After three or four repetitions, the drug was administered immediately following a reward. Hence, as on fixed ratio schedule, the key light came on fifteen minutes after drug administration, and so the subsequent fifteen minute sample of behavior was comparable in its time relations to drug administration to the fifteen minute post-drug period studied on FR50. Usually, the bird was allowed to remain in the box through several cycles following the drug. This schedule will be referred to as 15'FI. On this schedule, rate of response during the fixed interval had no effect on the time of reward.

Sources of error.   In the experiments on the ratio schedule, the pecks were counted with Veeder Root digital counters, which were able to follow considerably higher rates than the maximum pecking rate encountered in these experiments (2/sec) and are, therefore, virtually errorless. In the interval schedule experiments, the numbers of pecks were estimated by measurements on the ink record; the measurements were subject to an average error not exceeding 3 per cent. Periods of time on both schedules were timed with Eagle Signal Corporation Timoflex Timers and were subject to a random error not exceeding 1.5 per cent. Errors arising from these sources will be included in the empirical estimates of errors given in the results section. A systematic source of error not so included arose from the error of adjustment of the timers to the specified intervals; this did not exceed 10 seconds. The cumulative systematic error resulting from comparison of rates over periods timed by different timers (as in the ratio experiments) does not exceed 5 per cent.

Animals.   Male white pigeons, not less than two years old, and weighing between 400 and 500 grams have been used. Throughout the experiments each pigeon was kept close to a running weight, which was approximately 80 per cent of the weight it attained when given free access to food. At the same time each day, and after the experimental run, the bird was weighed, and fed a weight of grain equal to the difference between its running weight and the weight at the time of weighing.

Training.   The hungry bird was placed in the box and, without closing the top, the food tray was raised and kept up until the bird ate from it. After allowing the bird to eat for a few seconds the food tray was lowered and the procedure repeated 10–20 times at irregular intervals until the bird approached and started eating from the tray immediately after it was raised. The food tray was then automatically raised for the usual reward time (4–5 seconds) at irregular intervals of from a few seconds up to thirty minutes. This procedure was continued until the bird not only ate from the tray immediately after it was raised, but did not attempt to get at the food when the tray was lowered and not illuminated. At least 100 rewards were given in this way. Then a grain of wheat was stuck on the key under a small piece of transparent adhesive tape and the key transilluminated. The circuits were arranged so that each peck of the key caused the food tray to rise. Sooner or later, usually within a few minutes, the bird would peck at the grain of wheat, and so obtain a reward. After remarkably few repetitions—often as few as 2 or 3, rarely more than 5—the bird came to peck the key immediately after the food tray descended. The grain of wheat could be removed from the key at this stage. After about 100 individual pecks had been rewarded, training on the appropriate schedule was started. The above training procedure was conducted in a series of sessions, individual sessions often being separated by several days. During training on the schedules, and through the subsequent experimental period, the birds had a single daily session in the box, except, usually, on Sundays.

Procedure. Two pigeons were run on FR50 and two on 15′FI. Each bird was given, in random order, a series of graded doses of pentobarbital, each dose and saline alone being given once only. The schedules were then crossed over; the pigeons working on FR50 were put on 15′FI and *vice versa.* After the birds had worked for 1 to 2 weeks on the new schedule, the series of doses of pentobarbital was repeated. The basic information obtained is of the effect of 5 doses of pentobarbital and one of saline in each of 4 pigeons and on each of 2 schedules; 24 experiments in all.

Pentobarbital sodium was dissolved in 0.9 per cent sodium chloride solution and injected intramuscularly. Dosages are given in terms of the sodium salt and give the total dose administered.

Gross effects of the drug were studied by placing the pigeon after dosing in a large open glass jar, and observing throughout the time of drug effect.

RESULTS.   *Effect of schedule.*   As reported by Skinner and his colleagues (see e.g., Skinner, 1953), the response rates were markedly affected by the schedule of reward. A comparison of the average rate of pecking in the control (before drug) period of four birds, when they were working on FR50 and when they were working on 15′FI is shown in Table 1. Response rates were much higher on FR50. The lowest mean rate among the four birds when working on FR50 was more than twice as great as the highest mean rate when working on 15′FI.

The standard deviations give an estimate of the variation from day to day in the mean rates; 15′FI gave much less stable performance in this regard (mean coefficient of variation 37 per cent) that did FR50 (mean coefficient of variation 17 per cent).

Another difference between the performances on the two schedules is illustrated in Fig. 3. It shows typical records for each of two birds working successively on FR50 and 15′FI. On FR50 the rate of response was constant throughout the fifteen minute period of observation. In contrast, on 15′FI the rate of response showed a progressive increase through the

TABLE 1.   Mean response rates (pecks per minute) during the control period on six days.

Pigeon No.	Schedule			
	15'FI		FR50	
	Mean rate	S.D.	Mean rate	S.D.
1	27	8.2	130	7.2
2	14	3.8	90	14.5
3	23	9.4	86	19.8
4	31	15.9	111	24.9
Grand mean.....	24		104	

fifteen minute period, giving the records of each individual interval an upward concavity.

It should be emphasized that the only change in the apparatus made as between the two schedules was a change in the switching circuits determin-

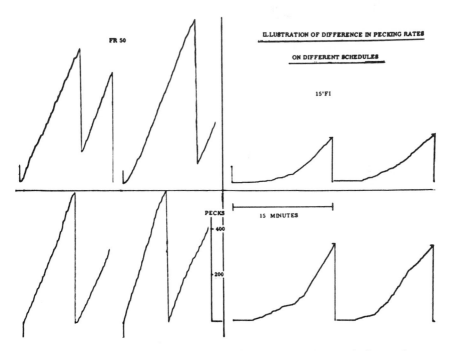

FIGURE 3.   Pecking rates of pigeons on different schedules. Typical records, two birds working on FR50 (on left) and on 15'FI (on right). For each schedule, two control periods of fifteen minutes are shown. On the 15'FI records the time of reward is shown by the short horizontal mark at the end of each period. Rewards are not shown on the FR50 records.

ing the schedule of reward. All features of the box proper, and so all constant features of the environment observable by the pigeon were identical on the two schedules. Hence, the difference between the high constant rate of response on FR50 and the generally lower, but accelerating, rate of response on 15'FI must be attributed to the difference in the schedule of reward.

Effects of pentobarbital.   The gross effects of various doses of pentobarbital sodium are summarized in Table 2; a dose of more than 2 mgm. was necessary to cause unequivocally observable effects.

The effects of pentobarbital sodium on performance in the Skinner box are summarized in Fig. 4. The drug effect (ordinate) was estimated as the ratio of the mean rate of response after the drug to the mean rate of response before the drug on the same day. These ratios were averaged over the four birds to give the points shown. This method of expressing the drug effect eliminates variability due to day to day changes in overall mean rate but includes that due to the difference between the birds in their sensitivity to pentobarbital.

The mean of the ratios of experiments in which no injection was given was 0.94 (S.E. 0.037) for FR50 and 0.92 (S.E. 0.110) for 15'FI. Each of these figures is based on 20 experiments. When saline alone was injected the mean ratios were 0.84 (S.E. 0.040) for FR50 and 0.57 (S.E. 0.065) for 15'FI. There is thus evidence that handling the birds and injecting saline has an appreciable effect on subsequent performance.

The much greater sensitivity to depression by pentobarbital of performance on 15'FI than that on FR50 is shown in Figs. 4 and 5. For example, compared to saline alone, 1 mgm. of pentobarbital caused a significant ("t" = 3.5, d.f.6, P < .02) decrease in the mean ratio of the birds when working on 15'FI but an increase in the mean ratio when the birds were working on FR50. The difference in the dosage of pentobarbital

TABLE 2.   Directly observable effects of pentobarbital sodium on pigeons.

Dose of Pentobarbital Sodium (i. m.)	Grossly Observable Effects
mgm.	
5.6	Loss of righting reflexes within 5 minutes of injection, but eyes remained open and pigeons appeared "aware" of surroundings. Apparent recovery in 20–30 minutes
4	Marked inco-ordination of movements and weakness within 10 minutes of injection. Apparent recovery in 20 minutes
2	No gross effects. Birds able to run without apparent inco-ordination. Suggestion of reduced "aggressiveness" in a bird well known to the observer, but effect not apparent to observer not familiar with bird
1	No effect apparent in any of the birds

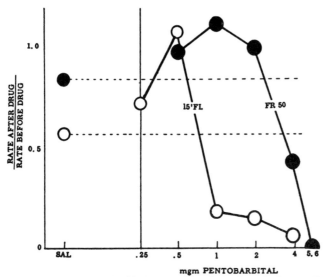

FIGURE 4. Effect of pentobarbital on pecking behavior of pigeons. Log dose-effect curves. Each point represents the arithmetic mean of the ratios for the same four birds at each dosage level on each schedule. Open circles: mean effects, birds working on 15'FI. Solid circles: birds working on FR50.

necessary to depress the response rate depending on the schedule of reward is shown again by the estimated ED50 values (Table 3). The ED50 was defined as the dosage of pentobarbital necessary to cause a reduction in mean response rate to 50 per cent of its value before the drug. It was estimated by linear interpolation on the log dose effect curve.

The individual interval records of birds working on 15'FI not under the influence of a drug, showed overall upward concavity with extreme regularity (Figs. 3 and 5). After small doses of pentobarbital, and during the recovery phase from larger doses, there was a marked tendency for the concavity to be lost; sometimes the records showed an upward convexity, an appearance never seen in the records of normal birds except in the initial stages of training.

TABLE 3. Differential sensitivity of response rates to depression by pentobarbital according to schedule.

Pigeon No.	E. D. 50 Pentobarbital (mgm.)	
	15'FI	FR50
1	0.78	3.3
2	0.68	4.0
3	0.85	4.9
4	0.50	3.0

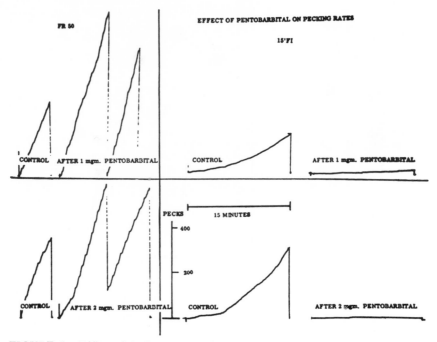

FIGURE 5.   Differential effect of pentobarbital on pecking performance depending on schedule of reward. On the left, records from two pigeons working on FR50 showing a five minute control run before drug and then a fifteen minute run starting fifteen minutes after drug administration. On the right, records from the same two birds working on 15′FI showing an interval record before the drug, and then the record of the interval which started fifteen minutes after drug administration.

DISCUSSION.   The pecking performance of pigeons working in a Skinner box on 15′FI schedule was significantly affected by a dose of 1 mgm. pentobarbital sodium. This dose caused no change in the behavior of the birds detectable by simple observation; even after twice the dose (2 mgm.) the directly observable effects were so slight as to be equivocal. Hence use of the Skinner box technique permits the effect of a drug on a behavioral activity of an animal to be detected and measured following a dose insufficient to cause gross disturbance of the animal.

Following doses of 1 or 2 mgm. to birds working on FR50 the rate of response was, on the average, higher than following saline alone. Clearly, these doses of pentobarbital do not interfere with the pigeon's physical ability to execute the response at a high rate. Yet these same doses caused marked reductions in response rates when the same pigeons were working on 15′FI. The use of the two schedules has thus permitted the effect in performance on 15′FI of doses of pentobarbital in the range 1 to 2 mgm. to be identified as an effect on the "higher" central nervous processes determining rate of response, and not as an effect on the physical capacity of the pigeon to peck the key rapidly such as would result, for example, from gross inco-ordination or weakness. When the pigeons were working on FR50 they maintained a constant rate of response throughout the period when the key light was on. On the other hand, on 15'FI the response rate progressively increased through the interval, although all environmental stimuli remained constant. Thus the response rate on 15'FI must be determined by factors additional to simple physical environmental stimuli. The greater sensitivity to modification of performance on 15'FI by small doses of pentobarbital suggests that it is the control of rate of response by these additional factors which is more easily disrupted by pentobarbital.

It is interesting to note that, for each schedule, a dosage of pentobarbital was found which led to an increase in average rate of response; this might properly be considered a behavioral stimulating effect.

SUMMARY.   Pigeons working in a Skinner box developed different rates of pecking depending on the schedule of reward.

When every 50th peck was rewarded (FR50) the rate of response was high and constant.

When the first peck after an interval of fifteen minutes was rewarded (15'FI) the average rate of pecking was low and there was a steady increase in rate through the interval.

Pecking of the birds on 15'FI was markedly reduced by doses of pentobarbital which had no effect, or caused an increase in rate of pecking of the same birds working on FR50. This differential sensitivity to depression by pentobarbital of performance on different schedules shows that by use of these techniques a behavioral effect of a drug can be detected and measured under circumstances when the drug does not affect the physical ability of the pigeon to execute a peck.

REFERENCES

Skinner, B. F.: *Am. Psychologist,* 8:69, 1953.
Ferster, C. B.: *Psychol. Bulletin,* 50:263, 1953.
Skinner, B. F., and Heron, W. T.: *Psychol. Record,* 1:340, 1937.
Wentink, E. A.: *J. Exper. Psychol.,* 22:150, 1938.
Wikler, A., Hill, H. E., and Belleville, R. E.: *Fed. Proc.,* 13:417, 1954.

45

Stimulant actions of methamphetamine [1]

PETER B. DEWS

Methamphetamine is generally regarded as a stimulant of behavior. However, it is almost a truism that, even in optimum dosage, it does not stimulate all behavior under all circumstances (see, for example, review by Ivy and Krasno, 1941). Except for the general statement that the stimulant effects tend to be greater in states of fatigue, there is little information on the factors determining the behavioral effects of methamphetamine. The present work was designed to provide some information of this kind.

Appropriate doses of methamphetamine cause an increase in "spontaneous" motor activity of small animals as measured either by the jiggle-cage technique (Novelli and Tainter, 1943) or by frequency of interruption of a light beam (Dews, 1953). The word "spontaneous" in this context means only that many of the important determinants of the behavior have not been identified. Very often, however, the frequency of occurrence of the behavior under study (the "response") can be shown to be determined by the consequences of the behavior in the past. Behavior of this type has been called "operant behavior" by Skinner (1938). When no physical constraint is imposed on when the response can be made, the term "free operant" is used. Increased output of responses by rats in a free operant situation following administration of *dl*-amphetamine was reported long ago by Skinner and Heron (1937) and by Wentink (1938) and following *d*-amphetamine by Sidman (1956) and Brady (1956). However, in an earlier study in this series using a free operant situation, it was found that methamphetamine caused only very slight increase in output of recorded pecking behavior of pigeons (Dews, 1955b). The absence of a substantial stimulant effect in that study might have been attributed to a species difference between pigeons and rats, or to a difference between amphetamine and methamphetamine. Neither of these possibilities appeared likely, and the difference was suggested to be due to the nature of the performance engendered by the schedule of reward used. If this is true, then stimulant actions of methamphetamine on free operant behavior in the pigeon should be demonstrable by use of other schedules of reward.

From *Journal of Pharmacology and Experimental Therapeutics,* 1958, **122**, 137–147. Copyright © 1958 by The Williams & Wilkins Co., Baltimore, Md.

[1] This work was supported by funds received from the U.S. Public Health Service (M-1226). The author wishes to thank Mrs. Pina von Henneberg for help with the experiments.

Therefore, the effects of methamphetamine on three other schedule-con-trolled performances in pigeons were compared with its effects on the per-formance engendered by the "1-minute variable interval schedule" (1' VI) used in the earlier investigation. It has been found that the output of peck-ing behavior in pigeons working on one of these other schedules was not appreciably increased by methamphetamine, while great increases were obtained with the other two schedules. On the basis of these differential effects, an attempt has been made to identify the characteristics of a per-formance that determine whether or not it will be susceptible to "stimula-tion" by methamphetamine.

MATERIALS AND METHODS.   The apparatus used was that previously described (Ferster, 1953; Dews, 1955a).

Subjects of the experiments were thirteen white male Carneaux pigeons. All had been trained as previously described (Dews, 1955a). They were maintained close to a constant weight which was about 80 per cent of their weight on *ad lib.* feeding and which varied from 400 to 450 gm. in this series of pigeons. The birds were subjected to a standard procedure daily five or six times per week on one or other of the schedules to be described. When no systematic change in the performance from day to day was tak-ing place, observations on drug effects were started.

Most of the birds had had extensive past experience on a variety of schedules prior to these studies. Care was taken to ensure that the individ-ual birds working on each schedule differed in their past history as much as did the birds on the different schedules. This deliberate mixing of his-tories leads presumably to an increase in the variations from bird to bird of performance on each schedule. However, it greatly reduces the likeli-hood that a consistent change in the performance following a drug could be related to a fortuitous circumstance in the previous history of the bird rather than to the designated schedule currently in operation.

Schedules.   The 1-minute variable interval schedule (1' VI) used has been previously described in detail (Dews, 1955b). Briefly, a single peck was reinforced when a predetermined time had elapsed following a previ-ously reinforced peck. The time that necessarily elapsed between consecu-tive reinforcements varied from 0 to 190 seconds with a mean of 62 seconds.[2]

FR 50 and 15' FI have also been described before (Dews, 1955a). When FR 50 was in operation, every 50th peck the pigeon made was reinforced. On 15' FI, the first response made after the elapse of 15 minutes was reinforced. Each reinforcement was followed by 15 minutes with no light behind the key.

[2] This is not strictly a 1-minute variable interval schedule since the mean interval is 62 seconds rather than 1 minute. For the purposes of this paper this difference is of no consequence, so the schedule will be referred to as 1' VI.

FR 900 was identical with FR 50 except that only every 900th peck was reinforced instead of every 50th.

Procedure.   Seven birds were studied on 1' VI. Periods of 5 minutes of operation of 1' VI were alternated with periods of 5 minutes of presentation of other stimuli during which no pecks were reinforced. The alternations were continued 30 minutes, giving a total of 15 minutes presentation of 1' VI.

The FR 50 procedure was studied in four birds. FR 50 presentations were continuous for 15 minutes. Three birds were studied on 15' FI; here the 15-minute period studied was a natural unit of the schedule.

Three birds were studied on FR 900. The procedure was more complicated. A bird was placed in the box and reinforced at, on the average, every 50th peck until four reinforcements had been made. It was then removed, injected with saline or a drug, and then replaced in the darkened box. Fifteen minutes later the key light came on, and the 900th peck made thereafter was reinforced. After reinforcement, the key was dark for 5 minutes after which the key light came on and again the 900th peck was reinforced. The number of pecks made during the first 15 minutes of illumination of the key following injection of the bird was measured. However, the experiment was not terminated at this time. It was allowed to continue until terminated according to the following scheme. When a 5-minute period without any peck had elapsed, the key light was extinguished for a 5-minute period. The fourth time the light was extinguished on this criterion, it remained out; this was the end of the experiment.

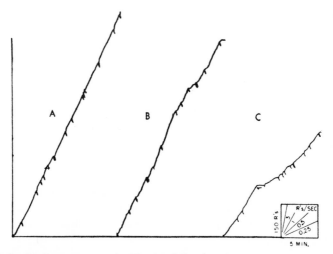

FIGURE 1.   Performance on 1' VI. A: following 0.5 ml. of normal saline. B: following 0.3 mgm. of methamphetamine. C: following 1 mgm. of methamphetamine. The short diagonal lines show the occurrence of rewards. Scale as shown, "R's" mean pecks.

Measurement of drug effects.   The drug effects on performances on 1' VI, FR 50, and 15' FI are all expressed as the ratio of the number of pecks made in 15 minutes of operation of the schedule starting 15 minutes after drug administration to the number of pecks made in 15 minutes of operation of the schedule before drug administration on the same day. This ratio is the output ratio previously defined (Dews, 1955b).

It was not feasible to make control observations on the same day prior to drug administration when the pigeons were working on FR 900, so the drug effects are expressed as the ratio of the number of pecks made after a drug to the average number made after an injection of 0.5 ml. of saline. Separate indices were obtained for 15-minute periods after injection (as for the other schedules) and also for the total number of pecks made until the experiment terminated.

All points on the dose effect curves represent the average of at least duplicate determinations in at least three birds, except as noted in the figure legends.

Drugs.[3]   Methamphetamine hydrochloride was dissolved in 0.9 per cent sodium chloride solution and injected intramuscularly. Pipradrol hydrochloride, *d*-amphetamine sulfate, sodium pentobarbital, and scopolamine hydrobromide were given in the same way. Doses are given in terms of these salts and, in all cases, are of the total dose administered to the bird.

RESULTS.   1' VI gave rise to a steady sustained rate of pecking (Fig. 1, A) while FR 50 produced a similarly sustained but much higher rate of pecking (Fig. 2, D). On the other hand, 15' FI produced a much lower average over-all rate of pecking, and also an orderly increase in rate through the interval, from very low rates at the beginning (long periods without a peck) to moderately high sustained rates towards the end (Fig. 3, G). All these findings are in complete agreement with previously published descriptions (Dews, 1955 a, b; Ferster and Skinner, 1957), as is the finding of greater variability of performance on 15' FI than on 1' VI or FR 50 (Table 1).

The performance engendered by FR 900 was unstable in the sense that it changed progressively with time, other than as a consequence of satiation of the bird with food. The approximately 200 pecks required to obtain the first four rewards were usually made at a high rate without hesitation. Following injection, when 900 pecks were necessary to obtain a reward, the bird usually started pecking at a high rate, that was maintained until reward (Fig. 4, J). After the first reward, when the key was re-illuminated, the bird sometimes started pecking again fairly soon; on other occasions,

---

[3] The drugs used in these studies were kindly given by the following companies: methamphetamine (Methedrine) by Burroughs Wellcome & Co., pipradrol (Meratran) by Wm. S. Merrell Co., *d*-amphetamine (Dexedrine) by Smith, Kline & French Laboratories, pentobarbital (Nembutal) by Abbott Laboratories, and scopolamine by Merck-Sharpe & Dohme Inc.

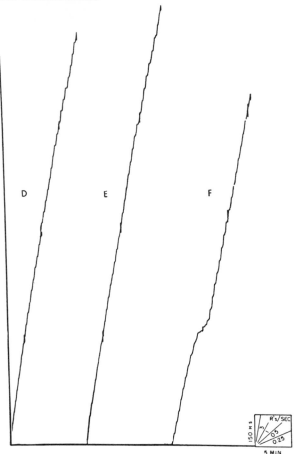

FIGURE 2.   Performance on FR 50. D: following 0.5 ml. of normal saline. E: following 0.25 mgm. of methamphetamine. F: following 1 mgm. of methamphetamine. The occurrence of rewards is not shown on these records.

as in the instance illustrated in Fig. 4, J pecking was resumed only after a long pause. Untreated birds rarely obtained more than two or three rewards before the occurrence of the fourth inter-response time greater than 5 minutes (which terminated the experiment). When only the first 15 minutes was considered, the variability of the performance was about the same as that of the birds on 15′ FI; but, as might be expected, if the entire experiment up to its arbitrary conclusion was considered, the variability was greatly increased (Table 1).

   The effects of drugs on performances on 1′ VI was as previously described (Dews, 1955b); dose-effect curves are given for the sake of comparison (Fig. 5A). Methamphetamine caused no more than slight increase in output of pecks at any of the dose levels studied. Pentobarbital at the

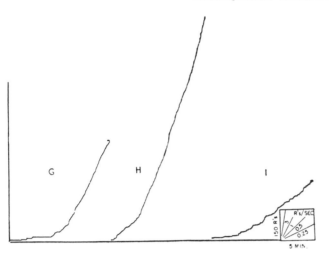

FIGURE 3.   Performance on 15' FI. Single intervals are shown. G: following 0.5 ml. of normal saline. H: following 0.25 mgm. of methamphetamine. I: following 1 mgm. of methamphetamine. A single reward occurred at the end of each part of the record.

1-mgm. dose level caused as great an increase as any found following methamphetamine. Increasing doses of both these drugs caused progressive decrease in output of pecks. The curve for scopolamine has a lower slope than that for pentobarbital and shows the much greater absolute potency of scopolamine.

TABLE 1.   Effects of methamphetamine on output ratios of birds working on various schedules.

Total Dose of Metham- phetamine	Schedule				
	1' VI	FR 50	15' FI	FR 900*	FR 900†
mgm.					
0‡	0.92 (0.20)§	0.96 (0.14)§	0.60 (0.41)§	1.00¶(0.48)§	1.00¶(0.87)§
0.1	1.05	1.01‖	3.56‖	1.29	4.06
0.3	0.87	0.98**	1.42**	1.36	2.69
1.0	0.48	0.69	0.36	0.37	2.59
1.7	0.22			0.04	0.09

* First 15 minutes.
† Total experiment as defined in text.
‡ Five-tenths ml. normal saline injected.
§ Figures in parentheses are standard deviations of saline experiments. These estimates were based on the following numbers of observations: for 1' VI—56, for FR 50—27, for 15' FI—6, and for FR 900—48.
¶ Necessarily 1.00—see text.
‖ Observations made following 0.0625 mgm. of methamphetamine.
** Observations made following 0.25 mgm. of methamphetamine.

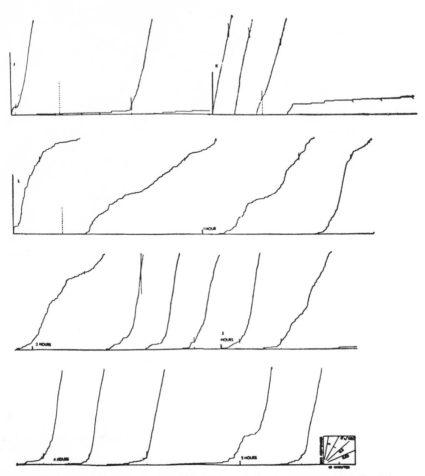

FIGURE 4. Performance on FR 900. Three whole experiments as defined in text are shown, starting at vertical lines just before letters. J: following 0.5 ml. of normal saline. K: following 0.3 mgm. of methamphetamine. L: following 1 mgm. of methamphetamine. The end of 15 minutes' exposure to the schedule is indicated by the vertical dotted line; this permits these records to be compared with Figs. 1–3. In addition, hours are marked off on record L.

The effects of drugs on performances on FR 50 were almost identical with those just described for effects on performances on 1′ VI (Fig. 5B). Again, methamphetamine never caused more than a slight increase in output of pecks relative to saline alone, and doses in excess of 0.3 mgm. caused a progressive decline in output.

The effects of drugs on performances on 15′ FI. In contrast to the effects of methamphetamine just described, the output of pecks by birds working on 15′ FI was greatly increased by appropriate doses of

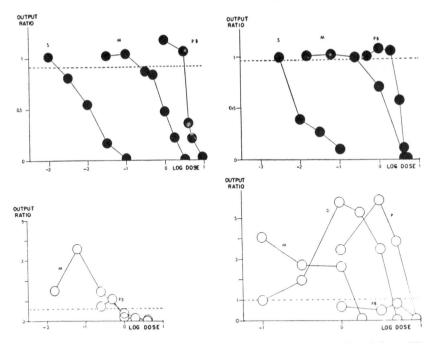

FIGURE 5. Effect of drugs on performance on various schedules. Top left: 1' VI. Top right: FR 50. Bottom left: 15' FI. Bottom right: FR 900. (Output ratios calculated for whole experiments, not just the first 15 minutes.) S: scopolamine. M: methamphetamine. PB: pentobarbital. D: d-ampetamine. P: pipradrol. The filled in circles above and the open circles below are to emphasize the change in scale of the ordinate between the upper pair and the lower pair.

methamphetamine (Fig. 5C). Most of the increase was due to a great increase in the number of pecks made early in the interval; the steady rate in the later part of the interval was not much increased by methamphetamine (Fig. 3). In spite of the high standard deviation of the saline controls, the effect of methamphetamine is highly significant. The output ratio of 0.0625 mgm. of methamphetamine (which is based on six determinations) is more than ten estimated standard errors of groups of six saline experiments from the mean output ratio of the saline experiments. Even taking into account the *post hoc* selection of this dose level as the one at which the significance test would be made, this is a highly significant deviation. The curve for pentobarbital in Fig. 5C is that previously published, and is reproduced here for comparison. Although a slight increase over saline controls, in output of pecks, can be obtained with pentobarbital, an increase of the magnitude obtainable with methamphetamine was never seen.

The effects of drugs on performances on FR 900. A modest increase in output of pecks in the first 15 minutes of operation of this schedule was obtained with methamphetamine (Table 1, Fig. 4). As in the case with

15′ FI, the increase was seen with doses of methamphetamine of 0.3 mgm. or less. A dose of 1 mgm. of methamphetamine usually caused a marked reduction in number of pecks made in the first 15 minutes (Table 1).

When the number of pecks made in the whole experiment, as defined above, was considered, it was found that methamphetamine led to much greater increase in total number of pecks made (Fig. 5D). Even a dose as large as 1 mgm. led to a great increase. The manner in which 1 mgm. of methamphetamine caused a decrease in number of pecks in the first 15 minutes, but increase in the total made in the experiment can be seen from Fig. 4. This dose caused reduction in the sustained rate of pecking at first; but it also led to a greatly reduced tendency to go for long periods without a peck. Since the duration of the experiment depends upon the occurrence of periods of 5 minutes without a peck, this latter action of methamphetamine led to prolongation of the experiment. The average effective length of an experiment when saline alone had been given was about ninety minutes; 0.3 mgm. of methamphetamine caused an increase to about one hundred and fifty minutes and 1.0 mgm. to one hundred and eighty minutes.

Observations were made in single pigeons on the effects of *d*-amphetamine, pipradrol and pentobarbital on performance on FR 900. The effects of *d*-amphetamine and pipradrol were qualitatively quite similar to the effects of methamphetamine. While the increase in output of pecks following these drugs is unquestionably a real effect, the precise position and form of the individual dose-effect curves cannot be regarded as established. That is to say, since the curves for *d*-amphetamine and pipradrol in Fig. 5D were each obtained on a single but different bird, no meaningful estimate can be made of the relative potency of the drugs. Pentobarbital was studied in the third bird. All effective doses of pentobarbital caused a decrease in output of pecks, thus decisively distinguishing this drug from the other three studied.

DISCUSSION.   The studies reported here were made on a free operant —"free" in the sense that the response could be made at any time during the experiment and not only at arbitrary times specified by the experimenter; and "operant" because the behavior studied, the peck, was maintained by its consequences, namely, presentation of food, some of which could be eaten. The dependent variable was occurrences of the response as a function of time, and the object was to seek for relationships between this and the effects of methamphetamine.

When the pecking behavior of the pigeons was maintained by 15′ FI or FR 900, methamphetamine could produce great increases in output of pecks. When the behavior was maintained by 1′ VI or FR 50, only slight increases in output were produced even by optimum doses of methamphetamine. While the absence of a stimulating action of methamphetamine on performance on FR 50 could be attributed to the very high sustained rate of pecking normally engendered by this schedule, making further increase physically impossible, this could not account for the absence of a stimulating action on 1′ VI performance. Comparison of Figs. 1 and 2 shows that the pigeons were capable of pecking at least twice as fast as they did normally when working on 1′ VI; yet the maximum increase obtained following methamphetamine averaged only 5 per cent. The most obvious difference between the performances on 15′ FI and FR 900 and the performances on 1′ VI and FR 50 is that the former pair of schedules gives rise to sustained pecking at a fairly constant rate while the latter pair characteristically gives rise to varying rates and periods with no pecks. This difference seems to be responsible for the differential effect of methamphetamine. Most of the increased output of pecks following methamphetamine is due to an increased number of pecks occurring at times when the control performance shows very low rates of pecking (Figs. 3 and 4). The rate during sustained pecking is only slightly increased by optimum doses of methamphetamine, irrespective of whether the schedule operating is 1′ VI, FR 50, 15′ FI or FR 900. Larger doses of methamphetamine (*ca.* 1 mgm.) cause decrease in rates during sustained pecking, while still increasing the tendency to peck during periods with very low control rates (Fig. 3, I and Fig. 4, L). Still larger doses cause complete cessation of pecking. The lethal dose of methamphetamine has not been determined but several doses of 10 mgm. have been given to pigeons alone in their living cage, without any deaths. Hence, pecking is abolished by doses which are much less than the lethal dose. However, doses greater than 1 mgm. might cause nausea, and thus specifically interfere with the reinforcing power of food presentation. This would limit the generality of the results obtained with the larger doses.

The results can probably be best stated in terms of inter-response times; *i.e.,* the times elapsing between consecutive responses (or from the appearance of the key light to a response). When a control performance contains long inter-response times, administration of low effective doses of methamphetamine tends to reduce their number and length. Higher doses (1 mgm. and greater), in addition to the foregoing, also tend to increase the length of short inter-response times. Inter-response time distributions were not directly observed; it is clearly desirable that this should be done. However, inspection of the cumulative record indicates that in the present context, inter-response times in excess of 5 to 10 seconds may be considered as "long," while those of 1 second or less may be considered "short."

A tendency for long inter-response times to be shortened by amphetamine has been reported for rats working under either avoidance contingencies or under differential reinforcement of a low rate by Sidman (1956). The increase in output of responses during extinction following amphetamine reported by Skinner and Heron (1937) might also be ascribed to a shortening of long inter-response times. A substantial increase in output of lever presses by a rat working on a 1' VI following amphetamine is illustrated by Brady (1956). At first sight this seems to be in conflict with the results presented here. However, the average inter-response time in the illustration appears to be about 6 seconds, in contrast to less than 1 second for the pigeons; the much greater increase in output in the rat experiment may thus be due to the much greater incidence of long inter-response times. Morse and Herrnstein (1956) give clear instances of shortening of long inter-response times by methamphetamine and also lengthening of short inter-response times with higher doses. Finally, the tendency of methamphetamine to cause a breakdown of certain discriminatory performances (Dews, 1955b) might be partly attributable to the selective tendency of methamphetamine to decrease long inter-response times in doses having little or no effect on short inter-response times. It is not suggested that all behavioral effects of methamphetamine can be attributed to differential effects on inter-response times of different length. It doubtless has other effects.

The ease with which decrease in output of behavior was obtained when the dose of methamphetamine was increased confirms the results of Novelli and Tainter (1943); the few observations on the relative activity of *d*-amphetamine are not in conflict with the results obtained by these workers.

For the behavioral effect of methamphetamine to be further analyzed and related to other determinants of behavior (such as type and degree of deprivation, quantity of food or other reinforcer presented, schedule parameters, nature of discriminant stimuli, *etc.*), prior systematic knowledge of the effect of change of all these factors on the behavior is necessary. Such a full account is not yet available. In the meantime, "interpretation" of these results in colloquial language can be made easily—all too easily, since the terms ordinarily used are sufficiently ambiguous to permit many alternative interpretations and to preclude definitive choice between them. The effect of small doses of methamphetamine on 15' FI performance could be described as making the bird more "impatient." Or it could be described as "making time seem to pass more quickly." Or it could be described as making the bird "forget it had just had a food presentation." Similarly the effects on FR 100 could be described as making the bird more "ambitious," or less easily "discouraged" or even "more desirous of getting the food." None of these "interpretations" adds anything to an understanding of the drug effect, and they may interfere with recognition of a relatively simple and consistent effect of the drug. Finally, no useful interpretation can be given in terms of the concepts of the general theories of behavior, such as reaction potential, properties of the phase sequence, or anxiety, since these concepts have not, so far, been able to account for even the control performances on the schedules studied.

SUMMARY. The number of responses made by pigeons in a fixed period of time is greatly increased by methamphetamine, when the birds are working under certain schedules (15' FI and FR 900); but is only slightly increased when they are working under other schedules (1' VI and FR 50). It is suggested that, in appropriate doses, methamphetamine tends to reduce the number and length of inter-response times in excess of 5 seconds but that rather larger doses also tend to prolong inter-response times shorter than 1 second. Some similar effects were obtained with d-amphetamine and pipradrol.

REFERENCES

Brady, J. V.: *Ann. N.Y. Acad. Sci.,* **64**:632, 1956.

Dews, P. B.: *Brit. J. Pharmacol.,* **8**:46, 1953.

Dews, P. B.: *J. Pharmacol. exp. Ther.,* **113**:393, 1955a.

Dews, P. B.: *J. Pharmacol. exp. Ther.,* **115**:380, 1955b.

Ferster, C. B.: *Psychol. Bull.,* **50**:263, 1953.

Ferster, C. B., and Skinner, B. F.: *Schedules of reinforcement,* Appleton-Century-Crofts, New York, 1957.

Ivy, A. C., and Krasno, L. R.: *War Medicine,* **1**:15, 1941.

Morse, W. H., and Herrnstein, R. J.: *Ann. N.Y. Acad. Sci.,* **65**:303, 1956.

Novelli, A. N., and Tainter, M. L.: *J. Pharmacol. exp. Ther.,* **77**:324, 1943.

Sidman, M.: *Ann. N.Y Acad. Sci.,* **65**:282, 1956.

Skinner, B. F.: *The behavior of organisms,* p. 19, Appleton-Century-Crofts, New York, 1938.

Skinner, B. F., and Heron, W. T.: *Psychol. Record.,* **1**:340, 1937.

Wentink, E. A.: *J. Exper Psychol.,* **22**:150, 1938.

46

The influence of *dl-*, *d-*, and *l*-amphetamine and *d*-methamphetamine on a fixed-ratio schedule

JOHN E. OWEN, JR.

In 1910, a systematic pharmacological investigation of a series of aliphatic and aromatic amines (Barger and Dale, 1910) revealed a number of compounds that had properties similar to those of epinephrine. These compounds elicited physiological responses of varying degree similar to functional stimulation of the sympathetic nervous system. From this work the term sympathomimetic amine was coined. Prior to this (in the 1880's), ephedrine, the active principle of the Chinese herb Ma Huang, had been studied and was discarded as being too toxic. Upon reinvestigation by Chen and Schmidt (1924), the pharmacological importance of ephedrine as a sympathomimetic was recognized. Publication of this work stimulated new interest in these amine compounds, especially the phenylethylamines and the phenylisopropylamines, the chemical nucleus structures of epinephrine and ephedrine, respectively.

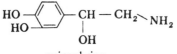

phenylethylamine

phenylisopropylamine
(amphetamine)

epinephrine

ephedrine

desoxyephedrine
(methamphetamine)

Amphetamine was first described (Pines *et al.*, 1930) as inducing a marked rise in blood pressure in man and dogs with drying of their mouths. Another report (Alles, 1933) noted that the compound increased

From *Journal of the Experimental Analysis of Behavior*, 1960, 3, 293–310. Copyright 1960 by the Society for the Experimental Analysis of Behavior, Inc., Bloomington, Ind.

respiration and caused awakening of lightly anesthetized animals. These effects were considered to be a result of stimulation of the central nervous system rather than of increased blood circulation. Subsequently, other investigators (Ehrich and Krumbhaar, 1937) reported that with the administration of large doses of amphetamine, normal growth of young rats was retarded by decreasing food intake. Clinically, Nathanson (1937) observed that patients taking this drug for other purposes showed a "loss of appetite" (inferred from reduced food consumption), with definite reduction in body weight. Another study, comparing amphetamine with ephedrine (Bahnsen *et al.*, 1938), showed that amphetamine produced marked "appetite loss" (derived from subjective reports), whereas ephedrine appeared to have little of this effect.

Physically, amphetamine is a mixture of equal parts of optically active isomers, *d*-amphetamine and *l*-amphetamine. The mixture is referred to as *dl*-amphetamine.

Pharmacologically, these three compounds have been found qualitatively similar in their actions but different in potency. For example, *d*-amphetamine was reported (Prinzmetal and Alles, 1940) to be 1.5–2 times as potent as the *dl*-amphetamine and 3–4 times as potent as the *l*-isomer on the central nervous system (verbal reports). Otherwise, the three compounds were about equipotent in peripheral effects (blood pressure and heart rate) in human subjects. Another investigator (Rosenberg, 1940), using *dl*-amphetamine and *d*-amphetamine in obese patients, observed that the chief advantage of the latter compound was its greater central activity: ". . . it overcomes both the depression and the craving for food which are so typical of obstinate cases of obesity," without increase in other untoward side actions.

The compound *d*-methamphetamine was described as having activity similar to that of amphetamine (Hauschild, 1938), with an enhanced effect on the central nervous system, i.e., wakefulness and euphoria with less intense undesirable side effects. Subjective studies in man (Jacobsen, 1938, 1939), comparing a series of sympathomimetic amines, found *dl*-methamphetamine somewhat less active than *dl*-amphetamine in "appetite depression" and about equal in other effects. However, Jacobsen reported that in small animals the *dl*-methamphetamine appeared to be the more active compound.

The drug action which facilitates the weight loss has been attributed to a variety of mechanisms (Harris *et al.*, 1947), e.g., delayed stomach-empting time, suppression of gastric secretions, diuresis, increased metabolic rate, increased motor activity, or decrease of "the desire or appetite for food." A comprehensive study by Harris *et al.* (1947) of *dl*-amphetamine- and *d*-amphetamine-induced weight losses indicated that these agents act primarily on the central nervous system on either a cerebral or hypothalamic level to induce a decrease in food intake. Other mechanisms which might be influenced by the drugs were considered as secondary factors which could contribute to the phenomena.

An appeal to "increased motor activity" or a "decrease in appetite" as possible explanations for the observed weight losses correlated with the administration of these compounds can be justified only on the basis of behavioral data. Whereas the appeal to increased motor activity" refers to an easily observed datum, any explanation in terms of loss of appetite, hunger, or desire for food is inferred from the observation that the subjects ate less.

The first series of experiments to go beyond simple observations of food intake were the studies of Skinner and Heron (1937) and of Wentink (1938). Wentink showed that 15 minutes after doses of *dl*-amphetamine, rats on a fixed-interval (FI) schedule increased their lever-pressing behavior but decreased their food consumption. Skinner and Heron demonstrated that rats trained on FI schedules showed typical depressed curves after daily sessions of extinction runs. On the fourth day of extinction, caffeine, and on the eleventh day *dl*-amphetamine, induced responding rates almost equal to pre-extinction rates. These drugs therefore were thought to cause an organism to release energy at a higher rate than normal whether or not eating behavior was inhibited.

Dews (1956) reported that methamphetamine and pentobarbital more readily disturbed the fixed-interval (FI) than the fixed-ratio (FR) performance on multiple FI FR schedules. Morse and Herrnstein (1956) have shown that with appropriate low ratios on FR schedules, pigeons maintained stable base lines of performance over extended experimental sessions. However, as the value of the ratio was increased, pausing after reinforcement occurred more frequently; and the duration of these pauses increased until at high enough ratios, responding ceased altogether. Lower response rates often occurred between the end of the pause and the resumption of the bird's regular high terminal rate before reinforcement. This phenomenon has been termed ratio strain (Morse and Herrnstein, 1956; Ferster and Skinner, 1957). Low doses (0.5 milligram) of methamphetamine decreased the duration of the pauses without appreciably affecting the response rate. A dose of 2 milligrams appeared virtually to eliminate the long pauses after reinforcement and to depress the running rate markedly. Dews (1958) has further shown that at optimal doses, methamphetamine, *d*-amphetamine, and pipradol increased the rate of responding of pigeons under schedules that require longer periods of time between reinforcements, e.g., FI 15 minutes or FR 900. With shorter schedules, VI 1 minute or FR 50, the rate increased only slightly. Recently, Kelleher and Cook (1959) reported that a wide range of doses of *d*-amphetamine depressed response rates of rats on an FR 50 schedule of food reinforcement.

The above data have shown that these compounds affect many different aspects of free-operant performance in different ways. Some of the effects depend on the kind of schedule used and the parameters specific to it (the length of an FI or the size of an FR). Furthermore, the performances in such procedures have been shown to be functions of the quality and quantity of reinforcement (Hutt, 1954).

The purpose of this study was to examine further the influence of dl-amphetamine sulfate, d-amphetamine sulfate, l-amphetamine phosphate, and d-methamphetamine hydrochloride in rats trained to obtain milk on a moderate FR schedule (30:1) which produced minimal or no straining.

METHOD. The subjects were eight male albino rats of a Wistar-derived strain, initially weighing 400–450 grams and deprived to 65–75% of their original body weight. They were trained on an FR 30. Each reinforcement consisted of 0.5 milliliter of a mixture of sweetened condensed milk, water, and Homicebrin (homogenized multiple vitamins, Eli Lilly and Company) in proportions of 1:1:0.01.

Two identical experimental cages were used in this study, each measuring 9 by 9 by 7.5 inches. The lever, a specially modified Switchcraft Lev-R No. 3002 (Verhave, 1958), was mounted 2 inches from the floor on one wall. It was adjusted to operate at approximately 10 grams of pressure through an excursion of approximately 0.25 millimeter. The reinforcement was delivered by a motor-driven dipper with a cup capacity of 0.5 milliliter. Illumination inside the cage was provided during a session by a single pilot light located in the wall above the lever. During the 8-second interval that the reinforcement was available to the rat, the light in the wall was switched off, and another pilot light illuminated the cup. At the end of a session the light over the lever was extinguished and a house light came on below the floor of the experimental cage. The cages were contained in light-proof, sound-resistent, ventilated boxes isolated from the control equipment.

The procedure was programmed on appropriate electrical and electronic timers and relay circuitry. The data were recorded on electrical impulse counters, running-time meters, and cumulative recorders.

The rats were given daily sessions of 40 reinforcements per session except on those days when drugs were tested. At the completion of each session, each rat was given sufficient dry food to maintain the deprivation weight level. The drugs were dissolved in distilled water and administered subcutaneously. On days when drugs were given, each rat was run for 9–11 reinforcements prior to injection as a normal control period for that day. Following drug administration the rat was placed in a small observation cage for 30 minutes to allow the drug to be absorbed and take effect. (With d-methamphetamine, however, this time period was 20 minutes.) The animal was then returned to the experimental cage and permitted to obtain 40 reinforcements or until no responding had occurred for at least 60 minutes.

In addition to drug sessions, each rat was run several sessions with physiological saline. Other sessions were run in the same manner without drug to show changes in the curves when an unlimited number of reinforcements was available and satiation occurred.

RESULTS.   Rat 82 (Fig. 1) showed an occasional pause following reinforcement and a response rate of 2.50 responses per second during regular 40-reinforcement control sessions. As this rat neared satiation, the rate slowed irregularly (Fig. 2), and the pauses between and after reinforcements lengthened. The three amphetamine drugs caused a general depression of the response rate. This depression appeared on the curves both as smooth, even slopes and as erratic, irregular slopes which were frequently interrupted by very brief pauses. These pauses even further depressed the over-all character of the curves. (See Fig. 2B for a detailed segment of such a curve.) At the two highest doses of *d*- and *l*-amphet-

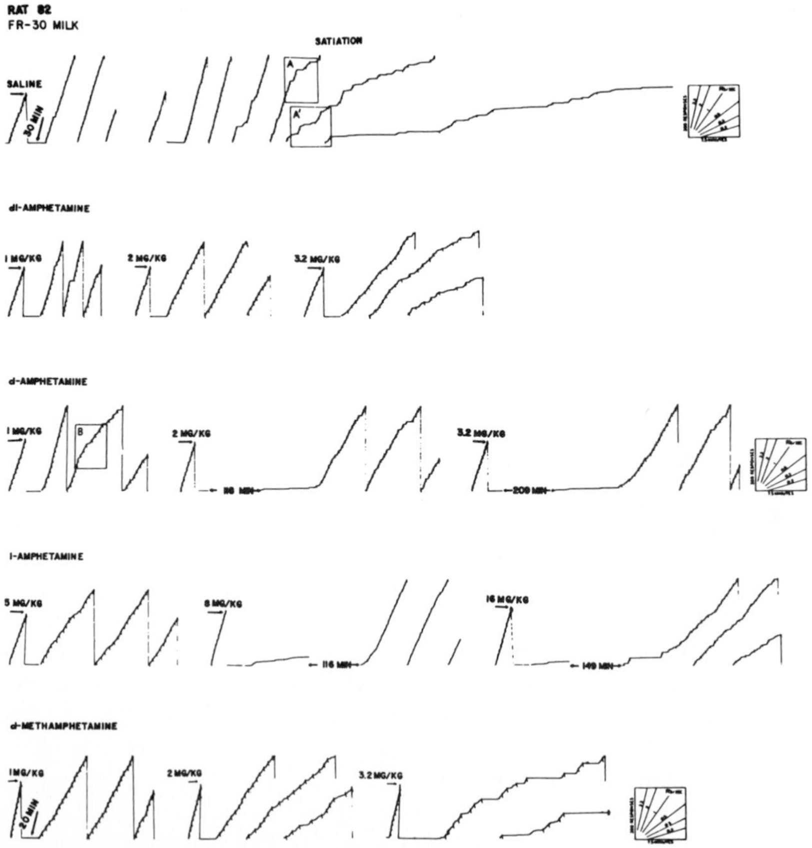

FIGURE 1.   Cumulative records for Rat 82 under conditions noted.

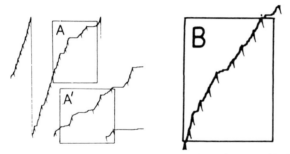

FIGURE 2.   Segments taken from cumulative records for Rat 82. Parts A and A′ show an atypical approach to satiation. Part B shows a detail of irregular slowing of response rate after administration of 1 milligram per kilogram of d-amphetamine.

amine, lever pressing temporarily stopped when the rat was returned to the cage after drug administration.

With d-methamphetamine at all three doses the rate declined. At 1 milligram per kilogram the decline in rate was even, with infrequent irregular segments. With the two higher doses, the rate was irregularly slowed, with definite pauses appearing during responding between reinforcements. At 3.2 milligrams per kilogram the rat completely ceased responding after 21 reinforcements.

Rat 84 (Fig. 3) had a normal rate [1] of about 2.55 responses per second and showed frequent very brief pauses after reinforcement. It approached satiation with a marked lengthening of every second or third pause with little or no slowing of the running rate. (See the segment of the satiation curve including the last 14 reinforcements.) The administration of the amphetamines induced only a slight depression of the response rate. The main effects were to increase the number and length of the pauses following reinforcement as well as to induce complete cessation of lever pressing for varying lengths of time prior to the return of responding. The size of the dose did not necessarily influence the duration of this initial pause. (See both the d- and the l-amphetamine data.) With d-methamphetamine the curves were the same as those with d- and l-amphetamine, except that the short pauses following reinforcement were not so apparent or frequent. Again, at the two higher doses the long delay before resumption of lever pressing appeared after drug administration. Also, with dl-amphetamine at 2 and 3.2 milligrams per kilogram and d-amphetamine and d-methamphetamine at 1 milligram per kilogram, this rat produced long pauses (7.5–10 minutes) after the first 14–26 reinforcements.

Rat 86 (Fig. 4), with a normal rate of about 3.2 responses per second,

---

[1] Normal rate, hereafter in this report, refers to base-line performance determined as the mean response rate of 10 randomly selected daily sessions excluding immediate postdrug-day sessions.

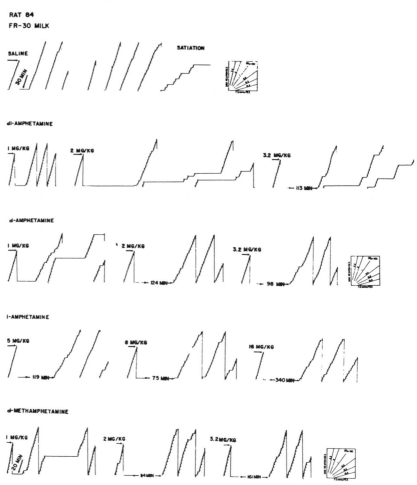

FIGURE 3. Cumulative records for Rat 84 under conditions noted.

showed a 25-to-50-second pause after every fourth to eighth reinforcement. These pauses lengthened noticeably when the animal approached
satiation, and the rate then became slightly irregular. With *dl*-amphet-
amine, the rate was irregularly slowed, with marked pauses following reinforcement. (See Fig. 5B for detailed segment of curve showing irregular
responding.) These two effects became accentuated with the higher doses
used. At doses of 1 and 2 milligrams per kilogram of *d*-amphetamine the
effects on rate and pausing were similar to those seen with *dl*-amphetamine.
Complete suppression of bar pressing occurred for 103 and 214 minutes,
respectively, on doses of 2 and 3.2 milligrams per kilogram of *d*-amphet-
amine. The return of responding on the higher dose was characterized by
an almost normal rate for 25 reinforcements, when it abruptly became

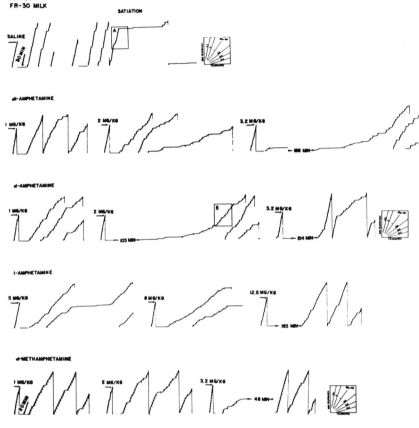

FIGURE 4.   Cumulative records for Rat 86 under conditions noted.

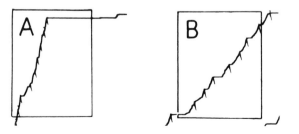

FIGURE 5.   Segments taken from cumulative records for Rat 86. Part A shows the approach of satiation. Part B shows a detail or irregular slowing response rate after 2 milligrams per kilogram of *d*-amphetamine.

slowed with the appearance of distinct pauses. At 5 and 8 milligrams per kilogram, *l*-amphetamine produced a regular slowed rate. At 12.5 milligrams per kilogram the lever pressing was suppressed for 193 minutes, and then resumed at a slightly slowed, even rate with short distinguishable pauses following reinforcement.

At doses of 1 and 2 milligrams per kilogram of *d*-methamphetamine, the over-all running rate of Rat 86 was slowed. Short pauses following reinforcement appeared regularly, in addition to other slightly longer pauses which appeared similar to those seen with the saline and satiation curves. At 3.2 milligrams per kilogram, the rat worked erratically for four reinforcements and then paused for 48 minutes. After this period of no responding, lever pressing resumed at an almost normal rate. Toward the end of the run, distinct pausing again appeared, without changes in the running rate.

Rat 88 (Fig. 6) normally produced a stable response rate of about 2.60

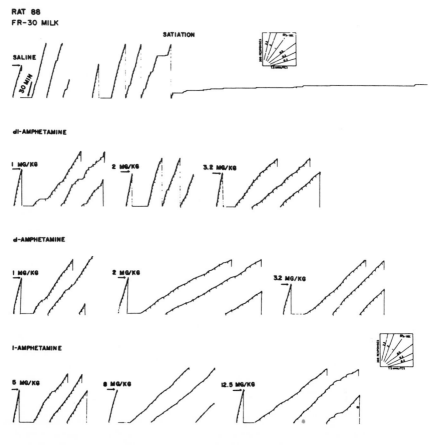

FIGURE 6.   Cumulative records for Rat 88 under conditions noted.

responses per second. With approaching satiation, the rate slowed very slightly, with increasingly longer pauses. The last several pauses showed occasional short bursts of from 4 to 10 lever presses per burst. Under the influence of the drugs at the doses used, the rate of responding became regularly slowed, with very few discernible pauses. Occasionally at the higher doses, especially with 12.5 milligrams per kilogram of *l*-amphetamine, the rate immediately following reinforcement was somewhat higher than it was toward the end of the ratio run. This effect showed up as negatively accelerated rate segments between reinforcements.

Rat 182 (Fig. 7) produced a normal lever-pressing rate of about 3.40 responses per second. As the animal became satiated the rate appeared to be unaffected; however, as the pauses became longer, short bursts of 5–10

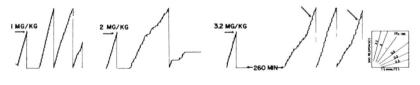

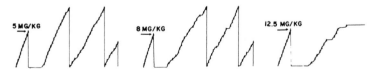

FIGURE 7.   Cumulative records for Rat 182 under conditions noted.

responses appeared. The drugs induced marked irregularities in the response rate. In some instances at the low doses of these drugs the rate was initially slightly accelerated and then became slowed toward the end of the session. The higher doses showed random mixing of both slowed and increased rates. At 3.2 milligrams per kilogram of *d*-amphetamine the rat frequently continued responding during the 8-second interval that the dipper was available for reinforcement (indicated by the arrows in Fig. 7).

Rat 183 (Fig. 8) exhibited a consistent normal rate of about 3.13 responses per second. The effect of approaching satiation was characterized by pauses of varying length after reinforcement without alteration of the rate. With *dl*-amphetamine at all three doses, the rat resumed lever pressing at an almost normal rate. However, at the midpoints of the sessions the rates declined irregularly, with distinct pausing; and at doses of 3.2 milligrams per kilogram, responding completely ceased. All three doses of *d*-amphetamine produced a somewhat irregular resumption of lever pressing. After 1 milligram per kilogram, at about the midpoint of the session, the rate again appeared to be about normal, although brief pauses occurred after reinforcement. At 2 milligrams per kilogram, after 9 reinforcements, responding completely stopped for 116 minutes. At 3.2 milligrams per kilo-

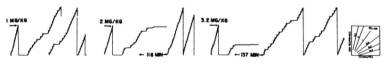

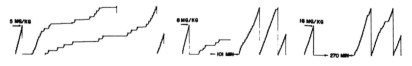

FIGURE 8.   Cumulative records for Rat 183 under conditions noted.

gram, responding stopped for 137 minutes after 3 reinforcements. With *l*-amphetamine at 5 milligrams per kilogram, the rate after drug administration appeared almost normal; but after about 6 reinforcements, pausing became quite marked and lengthened progressively. At the 26th reinforcement the running rate returned almost to normal. The cumulative curve at 8 milligrams per kilogram appeared much the same as the curve for 2 milligrams per kilogram of *d*-amphetamine. A dose of 16 milligrams per kilogram completely suppressed responding for 270 minutes following drug administration; at this point responding resumed at almost the normal rate.

Rat 184 (Fig. 9), with a high normal rate of 3.50 responses per second, initially showed little or no pausing. As satiation approached, the pausing

RAT 184
FR-30 MILK

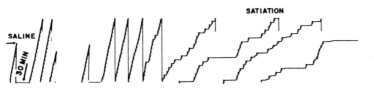

dl-AMPHETAMINE

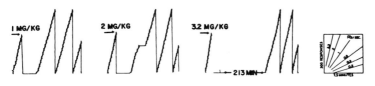

d-AMPHETAMINE

I-AMPHETAMINE

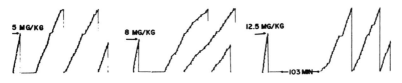

FIGURE 9.   Cumulative records for Rat 184 under conditions noted.

became frequent and quite pronounced. In several of these pauses, occasional short bursts of lever pressing were apparent. The *dl-* and *d-*amphetamine doses created little effect on the response rate. Their main effect appeared to be that of inducing complete suppression of pressing after drug administration at the higher doses. At all three doses, *l-*amphetamine induced a somewhat irregular decline in the rate; and at doses of 8 and 12.5 milligrams per kilogram, no responding occurred for 2.5 and 103 minutes before the return of lever-pressing behavior.

Rat 186 (Fig. 10), with a normal rate of 2.9 responses per second, showed the approach of satiation by frequent very short pauses with an occasional long one, with little or no change in rate. At the doses used, the amphetamine drugs produced a pronounced slowing of the rate, with frequent pausing both after reinforcement and between reinforcements. Some extremely long pauses were seen at various points during the drug sessions, especially with *d-*amphetamine at 2 milligrams per kilogram and *l-*amphetamine at 5 and 12.5 milligrams per kilogram. With *dl-*amphetamine at 2 and 3.2 milligrams per kilogram, *d-*amphetamine at 2 milligrams per kilogram, and *l-*amphetamine at 8 milligrams per kilogram, responding

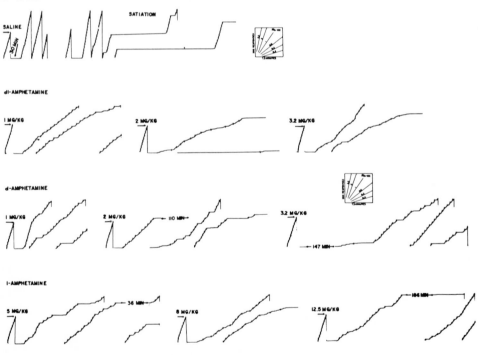

FIGURE 10.   Cumulative records for Rat 186 under conditions noted.

completely stopped before the ends of the sessions. At 3.2 milligrams per kilogram, *d*-amphetamine caused complete suppression of responding for 147 minutes following drug administration.

Table 1 summarizes the relationship of drug and dosage to the various effects on behavior. Table 2A gives a more detailed summarization of the influence of *dl*-, *d*-, and *l*-amphetamine on the individual rats. The alteration of response rate is expressed as the ratio of the rate with drug to the normal rate. The time spent pausing, expressed in minutes, includes all pauses of 5 seconds or greater and the time spent not responding immediately following the return to the box after drug administration. The number of pauses includes only those pauses of 5 seconds or more. Table 2B presents the means of 10 nondrug sessions for each rat showing normal response rates, times spent pausing, and numbers of pauses. Saline control data are also shown in this Table.

DISCUSSION.   As the cumulative curves indicate, the amphetamine compounds and *d*-methamphetamine influenced the FR 30 performance in three ways: (*a*) the response rate was altered; (*b*) the frequency and duration of pausing increased (straining); (*c*) the rats failed to resume pressing the lever when returned to the box after the 20- or 30-minute waiting period which immediately followed drug administration.

In general, the effects of the drugs in each rat were manifested by combinations of at least two of these three alterations of the lever-pressing behavior. In some rats, e.g., Rats 84, 183, and 184, there was predominantly little alteration in response rate but there were marked changes in the number of pauses following reinforcement. Other animals, Rats 82 and 88, for the most part, showed a slowing of rate with a minimum of pausing. Rats 86, 182, and 186 produced curves which showed both a slowing of rate and the appearance of definite pausing. The delayed resumption of responding occurred at least once in all the rats except 88. In Rat 182, this effect was seen only at the high dose of *d*-amphetamine. At the other extreme, Rat 84 exhibited this in all instances except at the low dose of *dl*- and *d*-amphetamine and *d*-methamphetamine. Rat 183 showed this delay only at 16 milligrams per kilogram of *l*-amphetamine; however, with the two high doses of *d*-amphetamine and the dose of 8 milligrams per kilogram of *l*-amphetamine after 3–8 reinforcements, extremely long pauses of 100 minutes or more occurred.

In spite of the variability of effects among animals, the general types of drug effects varied little from one compound to another in the individual rats. The chief variant appeared to be an enhancement of the particular type of influence of the drug. However, the actions of one compound in a rat did not always present a typical dose-response sequence, e.g., Rats 88 and 186. (See Table 2A for these and other examples.)

The *dl*- and *d*-amphetamine and *d*-methamphetamine were all given at

TABLE 1. Summary of effects on drug-dose relationships in individual rats.

Rat 82

Effect	a			b			c		
Dose	L	M	H	L	M	H	L	M	H
dl-amphetamine	0	+	+	-	-	+	-	-	-
d-amphetamine	+	+	+	+	+	+	-	+	+
l-amphetamine	+	+	+	-	-	+	-	+	+
d-methamphetamine	+	+	+	-	-	+	-	-	+
satiation	+								

Rat 84

Effect	a			b			c		
Dose	L	M	H	L	M	H	L	M	H
dl-amphetamine	-	-	-	-	+	+	-	+	+
d-amphetamine	-	-	0	+	+	+	-	+	+
l-amphetamine	-	-	0	+	+	+	+	+	+
d-methamphetamine	0	0	0	+	+	+	-	+	+

Rat 86

Effect	a			b			c		
Dose	L	M	H	L	M	H	L	M	H
dl-amphetamine	0	+	+	+	+	+	-	-	+
d-amphetamine	+	+	+	+	+	+	-	+	+
l-amphetamine	+	+	+	+	+	+	-	+	+
d-methamphetamine	+	+	+	+	+	+	-	-	+
satiation	0								

Rat 88

Effect	a			b			c		
Dose	L	M	H	L	M	H	L	M	H
dl-amphetamine	+	+	+	+	0	0	-	-	-
d-amphetamine	+	+	+	0	0	-	-	-	-
l-amphetamine	+	+	+	0	-	-	-	-	-
satiation	0								

Rat 182

Effect	a			b			c		
Dose	L	M	H	L	M	H	L	M	H
dl-amphetamine	-	+	+	-	+	+	-	-	-
d-amphetamine	-	+	+	-	+	+	-	-	0
l-amphetamine	0	+	+	-	+	+	-	-	+
satiation	0								

Rat 183

Effect	a			b			c		
Dose	L	M	H	L	M	H	L	M	H
dl-amphetamine	0	0	-	+	+	+	-	-	-
d-amphetamine	0	0	-	+	+	+	-	+	+
l-amphetamine	-	-	-	+	+	+	-	+	+
satiation	-								

Rat 184

Effect	a			b			c		
Dose	L	M	H	L	M	H	L	M	H
dl-amphetamine	-	-	-	-	-	-	-	+	+
d-amphetamine	-	-	-	-	+	-	-	+	+
l-amphetamine	+	+	+	+	+	+	-	+	+
satiation	0								

Rat 186

Effect	a			b			c		
Dose	L	M	H	L	M	H	L	M	H
dl-amphetamine	+	+	+	+	+	+	-	-	-
d-amphetamine	+	+	+	+	+	+	-	-	+
l-amphetamine	+	+	+	+	+	+	-	-	-
satiation	-								

Key: L M H low, medium, high doses

Effect: *a* alteration of response rate
b pausing after reinforcement
c long pause following drug administration

+ change from normal
- no change from normal
0 mixed or questionable change

490

TABLE 2A. Effects of *dl*, *d*, and *l*-amphetamine on rate of responding (ratio of rate with drug to normal rate), total time spent pausing, and number of pauses.

Rat No.	*dl*-Amphetamine				*d*-Amphetamine				*l*-Amphetamine			
	Dose (mg/kg)	Rate Ratio	Time (min)	No. of Pauses	Dose (mg/kg)	Rate Ratio	Time (min)	No. of Pauses	Dose (mg/kg)	Rate Ratio	Time (min)	No. of Pauses
82	1	0.92	0.88	7	1	0.66	2.30	24	5	0.48	1.12	31
	2	0.44	0.99	17	2	0.64	129.16	48	8	0.56	137.90	16
	3.2	0.44	12.96	106	3.2	0.62	213.70	55	16	0.40	156.71	73
84	1	0.93	0.18	3	1	0.88	16.17	34	5	0.93	124.00	32
	2	0.73	45.08	25	2	1.19	130.20	41	8	0.92	62.20	37
	3.2	0.76	139.36	24	3.2	1.14	87.11	26	16	0.87	235.00	34
86	1	0.86	9.00	39	1	0.35	10.20	28	5	0.27	16.79	57
	2	0.44	30.06	82	2	0.37	127.50	65	8	0.23	36.00[a]	53
	3.2	0.38	102.00	68	3.2	0.72	220.40	21	12.5	0.87	233.20	83
88	1	0.43	5.53	38	1	0.40	1.26	15	5	0.39	1.60	15
	2	0.73	1.41	5	2	0.20	5.24	98	8	0.26	0.63	33
	3.2	0.23	2.24	50	3.2	0.45	1.19	13	12.5	0.25	4.00	58
182	1	0.73	0.08	1	1	0.67	0.06	1	5	0.99	2.05	38
	2	0.53	1.36	10	2	0.43	14.50	18	8	0.76	2.48	26
	3.2	0.42	19.00[h]	22	3.2	0.64	211.80	42	12.5	0.45	11.00[d]	—
183	1	0.67	1.17	22	1	0.80	7.67	47	5	1.06	46.87	55
	2	0.59	9.04	54	2	0.65	122.07	17	8	0.82	109.28	40
	3.2	0.68	13.00[c]	21	3.2	0.83	150.63	50	16	0.48	247.40	20
184	1	0.76	0.30	5	1	0.66	0.10	1	5	0.72	3.46	38
	2	0.73	55.00	2	2	0.71	1.34	3	8	0.55	4.55	38
	3.2	0.84	97.00	1	3.2	0.91	213.00	0	12.5	0.33	106.10	25
186	1	0.33	17.14	93	1	0.43	13.74	56	5	0.50	64.34	84
	2	0.22	55.86	72	2	0.50	148.00	58	8	0.27	31.00[h]	87
	3.2	0.29	34.64[e]	92	3.2	0.46	151.00	63	12.5	0.50	204.80	81

[a] 23 reinforcements   [b] 18 reinforcements   [c] 20 reinforcements   [d] 11 reinforcements

[e] 22 reinforcements   [f] 12 reinforcements   [g] 29 reinforcements   [h] 25 reinforcements

491

TABLE 2B. Normal and saline control data for Table 2A.

Rat No.	Normal Means			Saline		
	Rate (response per sec)	Time (minutes)	No. of Pauses	Rate Ratio	Time (minutes)	No. of Pauses
82	2.50	0.63	14.1	0.99	0.49	6
84	2.55	0.86	20.0	0.99	0.46	19
86	3.22	1.68	6.4	1.00	1.57	6
88	2.60	1.20	3.5	1.00	0.87	6
182	3.40	1.19	31.3	0.94	1.13	14
183	3.13	1.16	24.3	0.98	0.84	26
184	3.47	0.15	2.0	1.10	0.02	1
186	2.91	4.06	35.8	1.09	---	18

the same doses: 1, 2, and 3.2 milligrams per kilogram. Considering the three general effects of these drugs, the cumulative curves indicated that d-amphetamine was the most potent of these three componuds. In two of the three rats, d-methamphetamine appeared to be the next most active compound. Except for Rats 86 and 186, dl-amphetamine appeared next in the order of potency. In Rat 186 the dl- componud was more potent than its d- isomer. Rat 86 showed greater effect with dl-amphetamine than with d-methamphetamine. Also, l-amphetamine, which was given in a higher range of doses, presented the same general picture as the other drugs in their lower range.

With the notable exception of Rat 82, these rats showed satiation curves typical of those described by Sidman and Stebbins (1954); i.e., as satiation approached, the response rate was maintained, but the pauses after reinforcement became more frequent and of greater length. Toward the completion of the satiation sessions, Rats 86, 88, 182, and 184 began to show short bursts of lever pressing between reinforcements. These appeared as "knees," in both nominal pausing and, occasionally, in the middle of protracted pauses of several minutes or more. With a few rare exceptions, these bursts appeared to occur at the individual rat's normal rate. Rat 82, whose satiation curve became very irregular toward the end of the session, showed a variety of intermittent bursts of lever pressing. Some of these appeared almost normal, while other small segments were quite definitely slowed. In many respects, segments of this rat's satiation curve were similar to the effects of the drugs both in declination and irregularity of responding rate. Rats 84, 86, and 183 also showed similarities in their approach to satiation and the effects of these drugs on this FR schedule. Rats 186 and 88 differed from the other rats inasmuch as in approaching satiation the rates remained normal or almost normal; but with drugs the running rates were clearly depressed and/or irregular.

In some respects, the slowed irregular segments that occurred in some of the rats' drug curves appeared as aberrant forms of ratio straining in which very brief bursts of lever pressing were followed by extremely short (on the order of 2–5 seconds) pauses (Fig. 2 and 5), which are not normally seen in sessions without drugs. This type of alteration of the response curves appeared similar to the "responses at a lower rate" seen between the long pause and high rate just before reinforcement described by Morse and Herrnstein (1956). They also noted an increase in occurrence of the "low and intermediate rates" with methamphetamine.

The effects of slowed and/or irregular response rates and of the increased frequency and duration of pausing in rats with these sympathomimetic amines could be described in terms of "a lowering of the threshold for fixed-ratio straining." However, in respect to the pausing alone, these drugs appeared to have an influence that mimics, in exaggerated form, the effects of a high number of accumulated reinforcements.

The delay in the return of responding appeared as the peak effect of the drug in those instances in which it occurred. Likewise, extremely long pauses in the middle of a session or the complete cessation of lever pressing before the maximum number of reinforcements were obtained appeared as manifestations of peak effects.

SUMMARY.   Eight rats, trained on an FR 30 schedule for milk reinforcement, were given *dl-, d-,* and *l*-amphetamine and *d*-methamphetamine in appropriate dose ranges. The resulting cumulative curves were examined for alteration of the FR behavior.

In this study the drugs influenced the performance in three broad ways: (*a*) the response rate was altered, generally slowed either smoothly or irregularly; (*b*) the frequency and duration of pausing following reinforcement increased; (*c*) the rat temporarily failed to resume responding when returned to the cage after drug administration.

The effects of the drugs varied among animals. However, in the individual rats the general types of effects varied little among drugs.

A discussion of the results is presented, comparing normal (control) FR curves and satiation curves with the general types of behavioral effects obtained with the drugs.

REFERENCES

Alles, G. A. The comparative physiological actions of *dl*-β-phenylisopropylamines. *J. Pharmacol. & Exper. Therap.,* 1933, 47, 339–354.

Bahnsen, P., Jacobsen, E., and Thesleff, H. Studien über die Wirkung von β-Phenylisopropylaminsulfat (Mecodrin) auf normale Menschen. *Klin. Wchnschr.,* 1938, 17, 1074–1078.

Barger, G., and Dale, H. H. Chemical structure and sympathomimetic action of amines. *J. Psysiol.,* 1910, **41**, 19–59.

Chen, K. K., and Schmidt, C. F. The action of ephedrine, the active principle of the Chinese herb Ma Huang. *J. Pharmacol. & Exper. Therap.,* 1924, **24**, 339–357.

Dews, P. B. Modification by drugs of performance on simple schedules of positive reinforcement. *Ann. N.Y. Acad. Sci.,* 1956, **65**, 268–281.

Dews, P. B. Studies on behavior. IV. Stimulant actions of methamphetamine. *J. Pharmacol. & Exper. Therap.,* 1958, **122**, 137–147.

Ehrich, W. E., and Krumbhaar, E. B. Effects of large doses of Benzedrine sulfate on the albino rat: Functional and tissue changes. *Ann. Int. Med.,* 1937, **10**, 1874.

Ferster, C. B., and Skinner, B. F. *Schedules of reinforcement.* New York: Appleton-Century-Crofts, 1957.

Harris, S. C., Ivy, A. C., and Searle, L. M. The mechanism of amphetamine-induced loss of weight. *J.A.M.A.,* 1947, **134**, 1468–1475.

Hauschild, F. Tierexperimentelles über eine peroral wirksame zentralanaleptische Substanz mit peripherer Kreislaufwirkung. *Klin. Wchnschr.,* 1938, **17**, 1257–1258.

Hutt, P. J. Rate of bar pressing as a function of quality and quantity of food reward. *J. comp. & physiol. Psychol.,* 1954, **47**, 235–239.

Jacobsen, E., Wollstein, A., and Christensen, J. T. Die Wirkung einiger Amine auf das zentrale Nervensystem. *Klin. Wchnschr.,* 1938, **17**, 1580–1583.

Jacobsen, E. Studies on the subjective effects of the cephalotropic amines in man. *Acta Med. Scand.,* 1939, **100**, 188–202.

Kelleher, R. T., and Cook, L. Effects of *d*-amphetamine, meprobamate, phenobarbital, mephenesin, or chlorpromazine on DRL and FR schedules of reinforcement with rats. *J. exp. anal. Behav.,* 1959, **2**, 267 (Abstract).

Morse, W. H., and Herrnstein, R. J. Effects of drugs on characteristics of behavior maintained by complex schedules of positive intermittent reinforcement. *Ann. N.Y. Acad. Sci.,* 1965, **65**, 303–317.

Nathanson, M. H. The central action of beta-aminopropylbenzene (Benzedrine). *J.A.M.A.,* 1937, **108**, 528.

Pines, G., Miller, H., and Alles, G. A. Clinical observations on phenylaminoethanol sulfate. *J.A.M.A.,* 1930, **94**, 790–791.

Prinzmetal, M., and Alles, G. A. The central nervous system stimulant effects of dextrol-amphetamine sulphate. *Am. J. med. Sci.,* 1940, **200**, 665–673.

Rosenberg, P. The further use of amphetamine (Benzedrine) sulfate and dextroamphetamine in the treatment of obesity. *Med. World,* 1942, **60**, 210–212 and 227.

Sidman, M., and Stebbins, W. D. Satiation effects under fixed ratio schedules of reinforcement. *J. comp. & physiol. Psychol.,* 1954, **47**, 114–116.

Skinner, B. F., and Heron, W. T. Effects of caffeine and Benzedrine upon conditioning and extinction. *Psychol. Rec.,* 1937, **1**, 340–346.

Verhave, T. A sensitive lever for operant-conditioning experiments. *J. exp. anal. Behav.,* 1958, **1**, 220.

Wentink, E. A. The effects of certain drugs and hormones upon conditioning. *J. exp. Psychol.,* 1938, **22**, 150–163.

47

Action of chlordiazepoxide on two types of temporal conditioning in rats

M. RICHELLE, B. XHENSEVAL, O. FONTAINE, and L. THONE

INTRODUCTION.   Chlordiazepoxide [1] is a now widely used tranquilizer. A number of effects have been described, both experimentally and clinically, including anxiety reducing effects in human patients, taming of aggressive animals, appetite stimulation, muscle relaxation, anticonvulsant action, and others. Animal activity studies gave evidence of its depressive properties (Randall, 1961). However, it has been shown in previous experiments, that, unexpectedly enough, chlordiazepoxide increases the rate of conditioned activity in cats (Richelle, 1962). The drug had also a disruptive effect on the temporal discrimination generated by the experimental situation used.

The question arises whether this paradoxical effect is specific to cats, or could also be observed in other species, and, secondly, whether it could be obtained in other situations than the one used in our experiment. The aim of the present study is to replicate the experiment with rats and to show the action of the drug on another kind of temporal conditioning.

METHODS.   a. Apparatus.   The experimental cage is a classical Skinner-box, equipped with a small lever and an electromagnetic tap through which a controlled amount of sweet condensed milk is delivered as reinforcement. The cage is isolated in a relatively soundproof compartment, the noise of a ventilator providing for additional masking of the auditory stimuli in the surroundings.

The method of operant conditioning is based on the control of behaviour by its consequences. A reinforcement, here a small amount of food, is made contingent on a well defined response, here pressing the lever.

The experiment is automatically programmed by means of relays and timers located outside the experimental room. Results are automatically recorded on a cumulative pen recorder and on a series of digital counters.

b. Subjects.   Eight white albino rats (Large Wistar strain) were used, the weights of the animals ranging from 150 to 200 g. The rats, about four months old at the beginning of the experiment, were living in individual

From *International Journal of Neuropharmacology*, 1962, 1, 381–391. Copyright 1962 by Pergamon Press, Inc., New York, New York.

[1] Kindly supplied by Roche, under the trade name Librium.

home cages in the animal room, and spending 1 hr a day, 5 days per week, in the experimental cage. They usually take their food for the day during the experimental session. When not so, they are given a supplement in order to be kept at about eighty five per cents of their ad libitum feeding weight.

Three female rats, numbered 018, 040 and 045, were the subjects in Experiment I. Five rats, numbered 024, 025, 033, 034 and 036, all females except for 025, were the subjects in Experiment II.

c. Schedules of reinforcement. The expression *schedule of reinforcement* refers to the relation between the response and the reinforcement, as operationally defined by the experimenter. Experiments I and II differ with respect to the schedule of reinforcement.

Experiment I: The responses are reinforced on a Fixed Interval schedule (interval = 2 min) or FI 2. A reinforcement is delivered following the first response emitted after a 2 min interval has elapsed since the last reinforcement. The animal is free to respond in the interval, though its responses are not reinforced.

The distribution of responses in the interval is recorded by dividing the total interval of 2 min into eight 15-sec periods. By means of a stepper, a given response is recorded by that of eight digital counters which corresponds to the 15 sec period during which it is emitted.

The schedule used in Experiment I is exactly the same as the one used in our previous study with cats.

Experiment II: The schedule used here is referred to as Differential Reinforcement of Low Rates of responding, or DRL (Ferster and Skinner, 1957). A response is reinforced only if it is emitted after a minimal interval of time has elapsed since the previous response. The interval used is 34 sec. Thus responses spaced by less than 34 sec will never be reinforced. The temporal discrimination is the condition for reinforcement.

d. Experimental programme. Experiment I. After the subjects had learned the operant response, they were trained on the FI schedule until their behaviour showed a stable pattern from one day to another. The pharmacological tests were then started. As a rule, no drug was administered unless the behaviour had returned to its baseline value, defined by the total number of responses and their distribution in the interval. The total number of experimental sessions on the FI schedule was about fifty for each animal.

Chloridiazepoxide was injected intraperitoneally 1 hr before the experimental session. The solution was 2 mg chlordiazepoxide in 1 ml saline. The following doses were administered to each subject: 1.2 mg, 2, 3, 4, 5, 6, and 7 and 8 mg. These are absolute doses and should be multiplied by five to six to obtain an approximation of doses kg of body weight.

After the standard procedure had been completed with all three animals, Rats 040 and 045 were injected with 8 mg of the drug for 22 and 13 consecutive days, respectively. The same experimental procedure was continued during that period.

Experiment II: As in Experiment I, the subjects were trained on the particular schedule before the pharmacological tests began. The baseline was simply defined as a regular pattern of behaviour, as it will be seen clearly on the curves below, not necessarily representing the optimal performance that the animal might be able to accomplish, were it run on a few more sessions for training. This provides for a possible modification of behaviour in both directions, plus and minus, under drug action.

The total number of sessions on the DRL schedule was about fifty for Rats 024, 025 and 033, about thirty for Rats 034 and 036. These last two animals died in the course of the experiment, one from an accident when injected, the other from undefined disease.

The conditions of administration of the drug were the same as in Experiment I, except for doses. Plans were made to test doses as high as 13 mg, by steps of 1 mg: Rat 034 died after the dose of 9 mg and Rat 036 after the dose of 7 mg; Rat 024 did not receive the doses of 1.2, 2 and 3 mg, Rat 025 the doses of 3 mg.[2]

RESULTS.   *Experiment I.*   Under normal conditions, the Fixed Interval schedule generates a very typical pattern of behaviour, characterized by long pausing after each reinforcement. The subject starts responding towards the end of the interval, thus maximizing its chances of obtaining the reinforcement as soon as it is available. A temporal discrimination is clearly developed, though it is not imposed to the animal as a condition for reinforcement. We will refer to this discrimination as *spontaneous,* meaning that it shows an optimal adjustment of the organism to the conditions of the environment, without these conditions making such an adjustment necessary. A sample of that normal behaviour is given in Fig. 1, curve A, obtained from Rat 045. Similar patterns were recorded for the other two animals. The abscissa is time and corresponds to 1 hr. Responses are cumulated on the ordinate as they are emitted. Each deflection of the pen on the cumulative curve indicates a reinforcement. The pen tracing the horizontal line is deflected when the two minutes delay is completed; it remains in the down position until the reinforced response occurs.

All the subjects return to the pre-drug level of responding, both qualitatively and quantitatively, on the first day following a pharmacological test. This is illustrated by curve B, in Fig. 1.

Chlordiazepoxide has two main effects, unequivocally present in all three animals: it induces an increased conditioned activity and a disruption of the temporal discrimination.

---

[2] The reasons for this are accidental and related to a change introduced in the experimental programme. With the intention of keeping our conditions as similar as possible to those used with cats, we started by administering the drug orally, but were not satisfied with the poor control this procedure gave us on this variable.

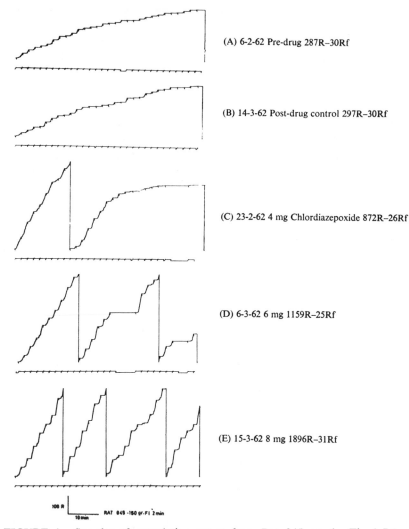

(A) 6-2-62 Pre-drug 287R–30Rf

(B) 14-3-62 Post-drug control 297R–30Rf

(C) 23-2-62 4 mg Chlordiazepoxide 872R–26Rf

(D) 6-3-62 6 mg 1159R–25Rf

(E) 15-3-62 8 mg 1896R–31Rf

100 R
10 min
RAT 045 -160 gr.-FI 2 min

FIGURE 1.   Samples of cumulative curves from Rat 045 on the Fixed Interval schedule of reinforcement. Responses are cumulated on the ordinate as the paper unrolls from left to right. The pen resets automatically to its origin on the ordinate after 500 responses. Oblique pips on the cumulative curves indicate the reinforcements. The pen tracing the horizontal line at the lower part of each graph is kept in the down position when the 2 min interval is over and comes up again as soon as the reinforced response is emitted. R: responses; Rf: reinforcements.

The first effect is easily measured by the number of responses emitted. Table 1 gives the values for each subject, under normal pre-drug and post-drug conditions, and for each dose of chlordiazepoxide. The figures correspond to the mean numbers per reinforcement, i.e., the mean number of

TABLE 1. Mean numbers of responses emitted per interval in the fixed interval schedule.

Dose of chlordiazepoxide	Rat 018	Rat 040	Rat 045
Pre-drug control	18·02	7·66	11·58
Post-drug control	17·38	6·49	12·21
1·2 mg	37·05	6·17	19·70
2 mg	27·63	9·23	24·71
3 mg	31·10	11·75	15·45
4 mg	44·14	9·69	35·08
5 mg	37·31	13·60	28·63
6 mg	11·41	16·61	48·56
7 mg	30·55	25·61	70·58
8 mg	28·87	31·99	65·61

responses emitted during one interval of 2 min including the reinforced response. Values for normal conditions, pre-drug and post-drug control, are averaged from a minimum of six experimental sessions.

Except for one atypical result in Rat 018 with the dose of 6 mg, we never observed decreased activity under the drug. The relation *amount of activity/doses* is not rigorous, but the general trend is clear. A maximum is reached for different doses by each individual animal. This maximum represents 2.5 times the base line number for Rat 018, 4 times for Rat 040 and 6 times for Rat 045.

These data are illustrated by the examples of cumulative curves obtained from Rat 045 and shown in Fig. 1, C, D and E.

The disruption of the temporal discrimination was measured by computing the proportion of responses emitted in each 15-sec class composing the total interval of 2 min. This proportion is expressed in percentages of the total number of responses in the interval. These results are presented in the form of histograms in Fig. 2. Each histogram corresponds to a given session with the indicated dose for an individual subject. Pre-drug and post-drug controls are averaged from a minimum of six sessions. The higher the proportion of responses in the last parts of the interval (represented by the blocks at the right end of the distribution), the better the temporal discrimination. Obviously, the quality of the discrimination is altered for doses as low as 1.2 mg (Rats 018 and 045) or 2 mg (Rat 040). The disruption does not necessarily reach its maximal value for the highest dose of 8 mg. This might indicate that the animal is able to readjust, at least to some extent, to the environmental conditions in spite of the drug. It might also be interpreted as the behavioural aspect of a simple phenomenon of tolerance.

Rats 040 and 045 remained at the same level of performance, both qualitatively and quantitatively, during the whole period of chronic administration of 8 mg per day. This part of the experiment, which is only exploratory,

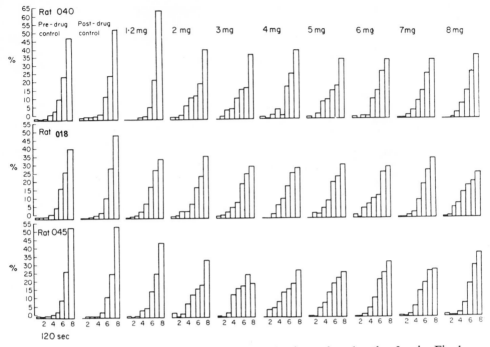

FIGURE 2. Distribution of responses in the interval under the 2 min Fixed-Interval schedule of reinforcement, for Rats 040, 018 and 045. Each histogram is divided into eight blocks, corresponding to eight fifteen seconds periods. The height of a block corresponds to the proportion of responses emitted during that 15 sec period, expressed as a percentage of the total number of responses. The larger percentage of responses massed toward the end of the interval, i.e., in the block at the right end of a histogram, the better the *spontaneous* temporal discrimination. Results with drug are for one session with the indicated dose of chlordiazepoxide. Pre-drug and post-drug controls are averaged from a minimum of six sessions.

shows also that the behavioural action of chlordiazepoxide never lasts as long as 24 hr: when no drug is injected prior to the experimental session, or when saline solution only is injected, the behaviour returns to its normal baseline.

Experiment II.   The best information regarding the results of Experiment II may be obtained from Figs. 3 and 4, taken as representative examples (Rat 025 and 034). Particularly, the graph corresponding to the first animal performance has been selected because the effects of the drug are especially conclusive. The curves can be read in the same manner as those in Fig. 1. The pen tracing the horizontal line is deflected and kept in the down position whenever the 34 sec delay has elapsed without a response. The reinforced response brings it back to its original position, recycling the timer.

Under normal conditions, the DRL schedule generates a very regular

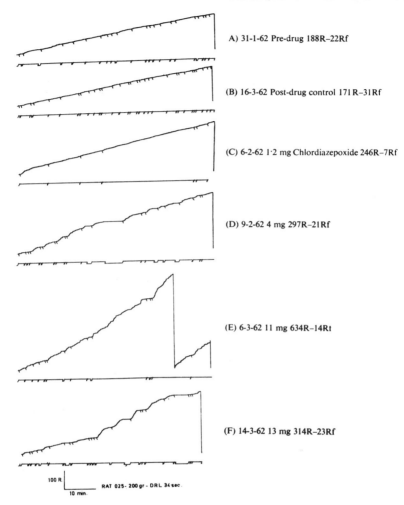

A) 31-1-62 Pre-drug 188R–22Rf

(B) 16-3-62 Post-drug control 171R–31Rf

(C) 6-2-62 1·2 mg Chlordiazepoxide 246R–7Rf

(D) 9-2-62 4 mg 297R–21Rf

(E) 6-3-62 11 mg 634R–14Rt

(F) 14-3-62 13 mg 314R–23Rf

100 R

RAT 025- 200 gr - DRL 34 sec

10 min.

FIGURE 3. Samples of cumulative curves from Rat 025 on the schedule of Differential Reinforcement of Low Rates. See Fig. 1 for key to reading. The fixed pen tracing the horizontal line at the lower part of each graph is kept in the down position whenever the 34 sec delay has elapsed; the reinforced response brings it back to its original position.

pattern of responding as shown by curves A in Figs. 3 and 4. Timing is not always accurate, so that a certain proportion of responses only are reinforced. However, the pause between responses is never considerably long as compared to the required delay: as can be seen, the pen is kept in down position for a generally negligible length of time.

During sessions without drug, the animals return to the pre-drug behaviour (see curves B in Figs. 3 and 4). In some subjects, timing behaviour appears somewhat improved, resulting in a larger proportion of reinforced

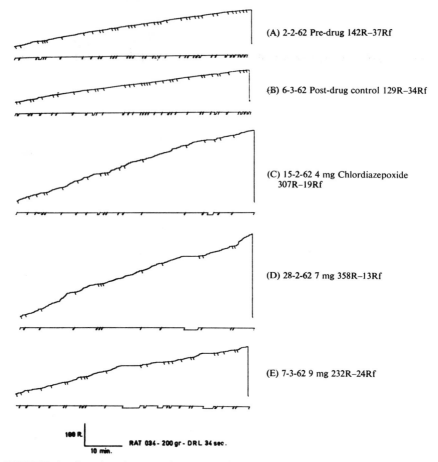

(A) 2-2-62 Pre-drug 142R–37Rf

(B) 6-3-62 Post-drug control 129R–34Rf

(C) 15-2-62 4 mg Chlordiazepoxide
    307R–19Rf

(D) 28-2-62 7 mg 358R–13Rf

(E) 7-3-62 9 mg 232R–24Rf

RAT 034 - 200 gr - DRL 34 sec.

FIGURE 4.   Samples of cumulative curves from Rat 034 on the schedule of Differential Reinforcement of Low Rates. See Figs. 1 and 3 for key reading.

responses (Rat 025). It should be remembered that the pharmacological tests were started when the subjects had not necessarily reached their best performance on the schedule. Longer training is probably responsible for the improvement observed in post-drug controls, rather than some hypothetical after-effect of the drug.

The action of chlordiazepoxide is qualitatively similar, if not quantitatively, to that observed in Experiment I, i.e. increased conditioned activity and disruption of the temporal discrimination.

The increase of activity is evidenced by the number of responses presented in Table 2. It is far less dramatic than in Experiment I. The maximum number of responses represents 1.5 to 3.4 times the control numbers, according to the subject being considered. The critical dose inducing this effect unequivocally is usually higher than for animals trained on the FI

TABLE 2. Number of responses emitted during the one hour session in the DRL schedule, under control and different dosage conditions. In brackets: number of reinforcements.

Rat Dose	024	025	033	034	036
Pre-drug control	125 (30)	188 (22)	128 (34)	142 (37)	205 (20)
Post-drug control	145 (41)	171 (31)	129 (39)	129 (34)	193 (21)
1·2 mg	—	246 (7)	132 (34)	170 (23)	—
2 mg	—	—	180 (20)	246 (15)	302 (13)
3 mg	—	—	169 (25)	201 (21)	231 (18)
4 mg	119 (34)	297 (21)	167 (19)	307 (19)	199 (17)
5 mg	176 (47)	293 (6)	172 (14)	222 (21)	294 (12)
6 mg	120 (26)	247 (15)	196 (15)	331 (17)	315 (18)
7 mg	140 (28)	249 (15)	271 (8)	358 (13)	109 (34)
8 mg	105 (47)	365 (14)	252 (17)	341 (19)	—
9 mg	102 (30)	317 (11)	241 (23)	232 (24)	—
10 mg	320 (16)	506 (11)	171 (28)	—	—
11 mg	232 (21)	634 (14)	313 (8)	—	—
12 mg	221 (21)	622 (10)	188 (27)	—	—
13 mg	213 (23)	314 (23)	252 (16)	—	—

schedule. The interpretation of these results will be discussed in the last section of this paper.

An increased number of responses, compared with the regular rate observed under normal conditions, goes together with an impairment of timing behaviour. If more responses are emitted within the one hour session, they are likely to be spaced by too short intervals to have the possibility of being reinforced.

The shortening of interresponse time is already observable with small doses of the drug and results in fewer reinforcements. However, the rate of responding is still fairly regular, as it is evidenced by the smoothness of curve C in Fig. 3. With higher doses, the subjects respond more erratically, fast bursts of responses alternating with unusually long pauses. Curves E and D in Figs. 3 and 4 illustrate this effect. The slope is irregular, with very steep portions indicating high rates. It should be observed that such irregular pattern of responding, particularly evident for high doses, can produce more reinforcements. These are clearly not due to a better timing, but to the fact that any response following a long pause will necessarily be reinforced. This effect could be avoided by using a DRL schedule with limited hold in which the reinforcement is available for only a short period after the delay is completed.

The modifications of operant behaviour in Rats 024 and 025 persisted through the series of chronic administration of chlordiazepoxide. The same observations were made as in Experiment I as to the recovery of predrug performance when nothing or saline only was injected.

DISCUSSION.   The present study confirms the results previously obtained with cats in the same experimental conditions as those used in Experiment I

(Richelle, 1962). The only difference is in the way of administration of the drug: the cats were given chlordiazepoxide per os. Increased activity and disruption of the temporal discrimination were found in both cats and rats. However, rats always returned to the normal behaviour in the first control session following by 24 hr a session with drug. For cats, three to fifteen daily sessions were necessary for the recovery of a normal behaviour after administration of high doses—corresponding to 4 and 8 mg in the rat study if expressed proportionally to the animal's body weight. This difference might be related to a difference in the rate of metabolization. Rats were found to metabolize chlordiazepoxide significantly faster than men or dogs (Schwartz and Koechlin, 1961), but data are lacking for a comparison with cats in this respect. At this point, a purely behavioural explanation is still tenable: for some unknown reasons, the baseline behaviour, once disrupted, is to be *reacquired* by cats, while the behavioural effects of the drug would not outlast its pharmacological effects in rats.

The comparison of the effect of chlordiazepoxide in the FI and in the DRL schedule makes clear two points. First, the increased activity and the disruption of the temporal discrimination are not specifically bound to the FI conditions, since they are also present in the DRL program. Secondly, the increase of activity appears very different in the two experiments, both in terms of degree, as shown by the number of responses and in terms of the dose which produces a clear-cut modification. It will be remembered that, under the DRL schedule, sufficiently large spacing of responses is the condition for reinforcement. One might expect the performance in such conditions to be more resistant to the action of the drug than the performance in the FI program, where the number of reinforcements is unrelated to the rate of responding. By responding at a higher rate in the DRL schedule, the animal practically puts itself in a situation where no reinforcement may be obtained as long as the high rate is maintained. This is equivalent to experimental extinction, in which the probability of responding is progressively reduced to zero as a consequence of withdrawing the reinforcement. Thus the increased activity leads to temporary extinction, which leads itself to decreased activity, which in turn makes reinforcement more probable. Contrariwise, there is no unfavourable counterpart to increased activity in the FI schedule.

The comparison between the two experimental programs provides a very typical instance of drug-behaviour interaction (Sidman, 1959). It is irrelevant to qualify a psychotropic drug as a depressant or a stimulant of activity unless the situational context in which activity has been measured is specified. In our study the modifications of activity induced by the drug are clearly a function of the schedule of reinforcement. Still more striking is the opposition between the effects observed in the two experiments described above and studies which showed the depressant action of chlordiazepoxide on general activity (Frommel *et al.*, 1960). The conditioned operant behaviour is modified by the drug in a direction and to an extent which are fully unpredictable from the modifications observed in the general behaviour of the animals. With larger doses (generally above 8 mg), the subjects are somnolent, show marked muscular hypotony, can be handled like animals unable to manifest any aggressive reaction; they keep sitting quietly in the cage and show a seriously impaired coordination when they move. All these observations are in the line of a depressing effect on activity. But once in the experimental cage, as was seen, the picture is different.

If the notion of activity has any usefulness at all in characterizing a tranquilizing drug, which kind of activity, general or conditioned, is to be given more attention? And what is the relevance of each kind to human behaviour?

Our results leave important problems open to further investigations, in order to explain the paradoxical action of chlordiazepoxide. The main question is whether the increased activity and the disruption of the temporal discrimination are causally related, and, if so, which of these two aspects is the cause of the other. One might suggest to interpret, hypothetically, the disruption of timing behaviour as being the primary effect, with the increased activity being the consequence. The muscle relaxant action of chlordiazepoxide would be responsible for the impairment of the temporal discrimination. This interpretation is based on the hypothesis that timing behaviour is related to proprioceptive cues from muscular tonus. A first experimental step toward the solution of this problem would be a comparison between the action of chlordiazepoxide on two schedules of reinforcement, one involving a temporal regulation of behaviour, the other providing for a measure of activity alone.

SUMMARY.   The action of chlordiazepoxide on two kinds of behaviour involving a temporal component is studied. Rats were trained, in an operant conditioning situation to press a lever for food either on a fixed interval schedule of reinforcement or on a schedule of differential reinforcement of low rates of responding. In both cases, a temporal discrimination develops; in the first case it is *spontaneous,* while it is the condition for reinforcement in the second case. Chlordiazepoxide increases the conditioned activity, as measured by the number of responses, and produces a disruption of timing behaviour. Both effects are more pronounced, and can be observed for smaller doses of the drug, under the fixed interval schedule, where the temporal discrimination *is not* the condition for reinforcement. Results are discussed in terms of drug-behaviour interaction. The muscle relaxant action of chlordiazepoxide is hypothetically suggested as an explanation of its effects on timing behaviour.

REFERENCES

Ferster, C., and Skinner, B. F. (1957). *Schedules of reinforcement,* Appleton-Century-Crofts, New York, pp. 741.

Frommel, Ed., Fleury, C., Schmidt-Ginzkey, J., and Beguin, M. (1960). De l'action pharmacodynamique d'un nouveau tranquillisant: le methaminodiazepoxide ou Librium. Etude expérimentale. *Thérapie,* **15**:1233–1244.

Randall, L. O. (1961). Pharmacology of chlordiazepoxide (Librium). *Diseases of the Nervous System.* Suppl. Vol. **22**: No. 7.

Richelle, M. (1962). Action du chlordiazepoxide sur les régulations temporelles dans un comportement conditionné chez le chat. *Arch. intr. Pharmacodyn.* **140**:434–449.

Schwartz, M. A., and Koechlin, B. A. (1961). The metabolic fate of chlordiazepoxide (Librium). *Fed. Proc.* **20**:171.

Sidman, M. (1959). Behavioral pharmacology, *Psychopharmacologia,* **1**:1–19.

48

Effects of chlorpromazine and *d*-amphetamine on escape and avoidance behavior under a temporally defined schedule of negative reinforcement [1]

NORMAN A. SIDLEY and WILLIAM N. SCHOENFELD

Sidley (1962) has demonstrated that both "escape-like and "avoidance-like" behavior may be obtained within a single temporally defined schedule of negative reinforcement. It seemed worth ascertaining whether the behaviors generated by that schedule would be affected in a similar way by the same variables that affect customary "escape" and "avoidance" behavior. Among these latter variables are several drugs, including chlorpromazine hydrochloride and *d*-amphetamine sulphate. The present study examined the effects of these two drugs on the behavior of two animals previously exposed to such a temporal schedule.

APPARATUS AND PROCEDURE.   The apparatus used in the present experiment has been described in detail by Sidley. On the response side, a force of 11 gms was required to depress a stainless steel bar which closed a microswitch activating a system of programming and recording equipment. When scheduled, a 1-milliamp polarity-scrambled shock was delivered to the feet of the animal through 16 stainless steel rods composing the grid floor. The animals used were two male albino Wistar strain rats approximately 170 days old when the experiment began. They were maintained on *ad libitum* food and water throughout. These animals had been used in Sidley's experiment (from which their identification numbers of 6c and 7c have been continued here), finishing their service there some five days before the start of the present study.

Briefly, the conditioning schedule involved three temporal variables: (1) $t_A{}^D$, a period during which an aversive stimulus is scheduled to occur, (2) $t_A{}^\triangle$, a period, alternating with $t_A{}^D$, during which an aversive stimulus is not scheduled, and, (3) *TO* (Time Out), a response-produced period of time during which any aversive stimulus scheduled to occur is withheld. During *TO*, responding has no effect upon the length of that *TO*. For the present study, the schedule was defined by $t_A{}^D = 0.5$ sec, $t_A{}^\triangle = 59.5$ sec, and

From *Journal of the Experimental Analysis of Behavior*, 1963, 6, 293–295. Copyright 1963 by the Society for the Experimental Analysis of Behavior, Inc., Bloomington, Ind.

[1] This research was supported by the National Science Foundation under grant G18633.

TO = 10 sec. This schedule provides that a 0.5 sec shock will occur every 59.5 sec if the animal does not respond at all. Every response not occurring during a *TO* will initiate a *TO* lasting 10 sec. Thus, a response during a shock will terminate that shock, and any response not in a *TO* which occurs within 10 sec before a scheduled shock will have the effect of canceling that shock.

The drugs were administered intra-peritoneally, always 30 min before an experimental session. Sessions lasted either 100 or 150 min, and were conducted daily, seven days per week. The sequence of drug dosages, identical for both animals, was: drug day 1–1.0 milligram of chlorpromazine per kilogram of body weight; drug day 2–2.0 mg/kg chlorpromazine; drug day 3–4 mg/kg chlorpromazine; drug day 4–0.5 mg/kg *d*-amphetamine; drug day 5–1 mg/kg *d*-amphetamine; drug day 6–0.8 mg/kg *d*-amphetamine. Three 50-min control (no drug) days were interspersed between any two drug administrations to counteract the cumulative effect, if any, of the drugs on the baseline behavior.

RESULTS AND DISCUSSION.   Figure 1 exhibits the cumulative response records of each animal for the entire drug session at each of the dosages. The "pips" on the curves represent shock occurrences. A control (no drug) day's record, taken from one of the three days between the last chlorpromazine dose (4 mg/kg on drug day 3) and the first *d*-amphetamine dose (0.5 mg/kg on drug day 4), is inserted for comparison. Cumulative records for control days showed no effects of the drugs, and the two control records shown may be taken as typical of the "baseline" performance of the two animals.

Chlorpromazine has the effect in our data of slowing the overall rate of responding, and the resulting greater number of shocks gives the appearance of a decrease in "avoidance" efficiency. If this drug is not simply a general activity depressant, but rather is specific to behavior maintained by "avoidance" contingencies, then the foregoing may be evidence that the temporal schedule in the present study does produce "avoidance" behavior. Verhave, Owen and Slater (1958) have shown that chlorpromazine at some doses can selectively reduce the number of "avoidance" responses by rats while having relatively little effect on "escape" responses. In any event, the relationship between dosage and response rate appears here to be an inverse monotonic one, and this is what Weissman (1959) has reported for a customary non-cued avoidance schedule.

Figure 1 also shows that the effect of *d*-amphetamine is to increase the rate of response, and thereby to decrease the number of shocks delivered. In addition, the cumulative records are marked by periods of sporadic rapid responding, especially at the 1 mg/kg dose. Sidman (1956) has shown similar effects in rats with amphetamine on a usual non-schedule; and Weissman (1959) has confirmed this finding for a non-component of a

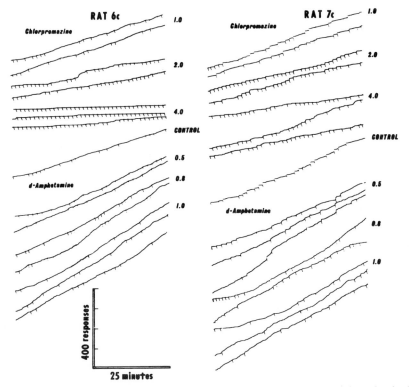

FIGURE 1.   Complete cumulative response curves for entire drug sessions for both animals in the experiment. Shock occurrences are indicated by "pips." Dosages in mg/kg are shown to the right of their respective records. Each record segment represents 50 min of a session, with total session length being either 100 or 150 min. The uppermost segment of each session's record is the first 50 min, and so on. Control sessions were 50 min long (see text for schedule of control sessions).

multiple schedule, observing also, that at doses below 1 mg/kg the effect of raising response rate was felt throughout the multiple schedule and was not specific to the avoidance component. The heightened "avoidance" effected by the amphetamines must be cautiously interpreted since it may be only an artifactual by-product of the general rise in response rate produced by this family of drugs. It may perhaps be noted in this connection that Owen (1960) has found with rats that d-amphetamine in dosages from 1 to 3.2 mg/kg has the effect of decreasing the rate of response with behavior maintained by a positive reinforcement schedule.

SUMMARY.   Chlorpromazine hydrochloride and d-amphetamine sulphate were administered to two rats responding on a baseline temporally defined schedule of negative reinforcement which produced both "escape-like" and "avoidance-like" behavior. The effects of these drugs appeared similar to those expected on the more customary sort of non-cued avoidance schedule.

REFERENCES

Owen, J. E., Jr., The influence of *dl-, d-,* and *l*-amphetamine and *d*-methamphetamine on a fixed ratio schedule. *J. exp. Anal. Behav.,* 1960, 3, 293–309.

Sidley, N. A., Two parameters of a temporally defined schedule of negative reinforcement. Unpublished doctoral dissertation, Columbia University, 1962.

Sidman, M., Behavioral pharmacology. *Psychopharmacologia,* 1959, 1, 1–19.

Verhave, T., Owen, J. E., Jr., and Slater, O. H., Effects of various drugs on escape and avoidance behavior. *Progr. Neurobiol.,* 1958, 3, 267–301.

Weissman, A., Differential drug effects on a three-ply multiple schedule of reinforcement. *J. exp. Anal. Behav.,* 1959, 2, 271–287.

49

Technique for assessing the effects of drugs on timing behavior

Murray Sidman

Before a drug can safely be recommended for relief of a specific physiological malfunction it must be checked for possible deleterious effects upon other systems. Careful consideration must also be given to the possibility of "toxic" effects upon normal adaptive behavior, particularly in the case of those drugs that are known to produce behavioral changes. In view of the importance of temporal orientation in normal behavioral functions, the effect of drugs upon timing would appear to constitute a primary area of investigation. The purpose of this report is to describe a method, based on earlier work by Skinner (1), for producing and measuring timing behavior in experimental animals, and to present some data resulting from the administration of amphetamine and alcohol (2).

White rats, deprived of water for 22.5 hours, were placed in a small chamber containing a lever and a mechanism for automatic delivery of a small drop of water. In the first session every depression of the lever by the animal produced the water reinforcement. In all following sessions, each 2 hours long, reinforcement was contingent on lever presses spaced at least 21 seconds apart. That is, a response produced the water only if it followed the preceding lever depression by at least 21 seconds. Programming and recording were accomplished automatically by timers, magnetic counters, and associated relay circuits.

Using this procedure, Wilson and Keller have demonstrated that the rate of lever pressing is inversely related to the length of the required delay between responses (3). Since drug-produced general excitatory or depressive effects might themselves alter the rate of lever pressing (4), a more useful measurement of the timing is the relative frequency distribution of interresponse times (intervals between successive responses). This distribution, which displays no consistent trend after the animals have been exposed to the experimental procedure for 30 to 60 hours, is illustrated by the "saline" control records of Fig. 1. The large proportion of responses that are spaced less than 3 seconds apart is typical and unexplained, but the remainder of the distribution provides a clear description of the timing behavior. The relative frequencies of interresponse times rise to a peak between 18 and 21 seconds and then display a gradual decline.

The center sections of Fig. 1 illustrate the effects of two relatively large

From *Science*, 1955, **122**, 925.

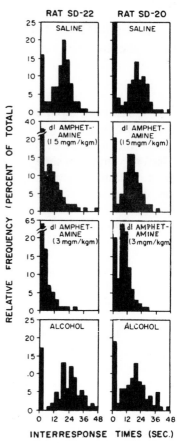

FIGURE 1. Relative frequency distributions of the time intervals between successive lever presses. Each distribution represents one animal's performance in a single 2-hour session.

doses of *dl*-amphetamine sulfate administered subcutaneously, 5 minutes prior to the experimental session, in a solution of 1 mg/ml of physiological saline. Increasing doses of this drug tend to move the peak of the distribution progressively toward the short interresponse times. That is, the animals press the lever more frequently before the required interval has elapsed.

In addition to the shifts in the relative frequency distribution, large increases in the total response output occurred (Table 1). In contrast, intra-

TABLE 1.   Total number of lever presses emitted during each 2-hour session.

| Rat | Saline | *dl*-Amphetamine | | Alcohol |
		1.5 mg/kg	3.0 mg/kg	
SD-20	471	534	854	201
SD-22	433	820	1816	176

peritoneal injection of 3 ml of a 10-percent ethyl alcohol solution, representing a dose of 1 mg/kg, produced a decline of more than 50 percent in the rate of lever pressing. The relative interresponse time frequencies, however, as shown in the lower section of Fig. 1, displayed little change except for a slight leveling of the total distribution. Although alcohol, in the dose administered, produced a general depression of lever-pressing behavior, there was relatively little effect upon the timing.

This technique for generating and measuring timing behavior is applicable to the minimally restrained individual organism, produces stable behavior over long periods of time, has procedural simplicity, and permits automatic programming and recording. The orderly response to drugs, illustrated by this data, indicates the feasibility of including this method in programs designed to screen drugs for their behavioral effects.

REFERENCES AND NOTES

1. B. F. Skinner, *The behavior of organisms* (Appleton-Century-Crofts, New York, 1938), p. 306.
2. The author gratefully acknowledges the technical assistance of Irving Geller and George Susla in the conduct of these experiments.
3. M. P. Wilson and F. S. Keller, *J. Comp. Physiol. Psychol.* 46, 190 (1953).
4. B. F. Skinner and W. T. Heron, *Psychol. Rec.* 1, 340 (1937).

50

Modification by drugs of performance on simple schedules of positive reinforcement *

PETER B. DEWS

The basic elements of technique for the use of the free operant are by now quite well-known.[3] The purpose of this paper is to illustrate the use of the technique for drug studies by showing how one particular procedure has been used to start the analysis of the behavioral effects of some drugs. The work described here has been done on pigeons kept close to a constant weight of between 80 and 90 per cent of the weight at which they stabilized when fed *ad libitum*. The pigeons were trained to work as previously described, the arrangement being shown in Fig. 1.[1, 3] They pecked at a translucent plastic disk that had variously colored lights behind it. Each peck broke a circuit that enabled it to be recorded and counted. According to a schedule, the pigeon was rewarded ("reinforced") for pecking with food

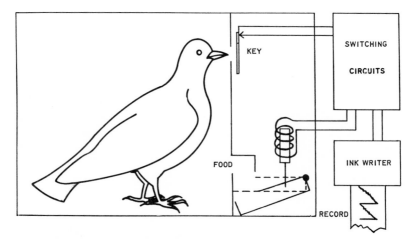

FIGURE 1. Diagram of apparatus. The "key" is a translucent plastic disk with variously colored lights (not shown) behind it. The food is normally out of reach of the pigeon, but it can be made available by the activation of a solenoid.[1]

From *Annals of the New York Academy of Sciences*, 1956, **65**, 268–281. Copyright 1956 by The New York Academy of Sciences, New York.

* This work was supported by funds received from the William F. Milton Fund of Harvard University, Cambridge, Mass.; the Roche Anniversary Foundation of Hoffman-La Roche, Inc., Nutley, N.J.; and a grant (No. M 1226) from the National Institute of Mental Health, National Institutes of Health, Public Health Service, Department of Health, Education, and Welfare, Bethesda, Md.

from a tray that rose so that the food was accessible to the bird for 5 seconds.

The distribution of pecks in time, that is, the rate of pecking from time to time, is extremely sensitive to the precise contingencies relating pecks to rewards. For example, if every sixtieth peck is rewarded under the conditions of our experiments, the pigeon comes to peck at high sustained rates. This is a fixed ratio schedule; there is a fixed ratio of reinforcements to pecks. Henceforth this performance will be referred to as "ratio performance." On the other hand, if a single peck is rewarded when, and only when, a constant interval of time (for example, 15 minutes) has elapsed, there is a period at the beginning of the interval when the bird does not peck at all, and then there is a fairly smoothly accelerating rate of pecking until the rewarded peck. This is a fixed interval schedule; a fixed interval of time must elapse before a reward can be obtained, and the pattern of pecking engendered by it will be referred to as "interval performance." It can be arranged that when a light of one color is on, the schedule is fixed ratio, and when a light of a different color is on, the schedule is fixed interval. The bird comes to perform appropriately to each of the schedules according to which light is on. Thus the bird's performance can be observed on more than one schedule during a short period of time without disturbing the animal in any way. This is a "multiple schedule" in the terminology of Ferster and Skinner.

Pigeons have some advantages for this type of work.[3] They stay adult and in their prime for many years without apparent change. They very rarely show signs of disease and they stand food deprivation for long periods without obvious ill effects. Their food, grain, is very convenient both for use in an automatic magazine and for daily weighing to maintain the birds close to constant weight. Their excellent vision makes use of colored lights as discriminant stimuli possible. These lights are very convenient and make it easy to employ many different stimuli in a single experiment. Perhaps the most important advantage is the relative "pureness" of the behavioral "response" used; that is, the peck. The pigeon can operate the key only with its beak, and although the precise topography of the peck undoubtedly varies from time to time, the variation is necessarily within fairly narrow limits. This is not always true for most other species and it is perhaps the main reason why, by and large, experiments on pigeons seem to progress faster than those performed with other species— a by no means unimportant consideration in a new branch of science. The main disadvantage of the use of pigeons is the great phylogenetic gap between birds and humans. All that one can say is that the general laws of operant behavior seem to show remarkable constancy from species to species, and that so far we have not found drug effects in pigeons that outrageously contradict the known effects of the same drugs in humans. On the contrary, the effects seem quite analogous.

A specific multiple schedule used extensively is illustrated in Fig. 2. When there was a red light behind the key the bird was rewarded on the sixtieth peck made (fixed ratio), and when there was a blue light behind the key the bird was rewarded for the first peck made when 15 minutes had elapsed since the preceding reward (fixed interval). The standard "run" consisted of the following sequence: fixed ratio, fixed interval, fixed ratio, 2 fixed intervals, 10 fixed ratios, 2 fixed intervals and 3 fixed ratios. It can

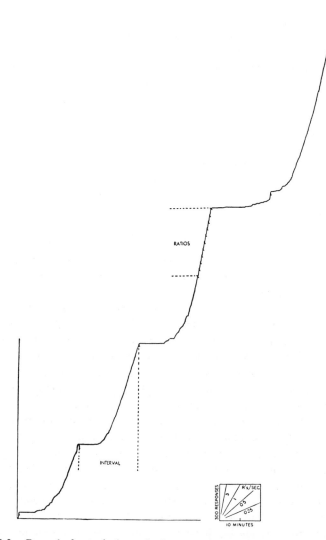

FIGURE 2.   Record of a typical standard run on the multiple schedule used in most studies. Abscissa = time, ordinate = cumulative number of pecks. The scales are as shown. The short diagonal lines on the record show the occurrence of rewards.

be seen that as soon as the red light came on, for example, as at the beginning of the series labelled "ratios" in Fig. 2, the bird immediately started to peck at a high rate that was maintained until reinforcement. On the other hand, when the blue light came on, as at the beginning of the period labelled "interval" in Fig. 2, the bird waited several minutes before pecking and then showed a gradual increase in rate up to reinforcement.

When the birds were given this standard run daily, the whole performance became stable and reproducible, and it remained so indefinitely or, at least, over a period of many months.

Eight birds were given 30 mg. of phenobarbital sodium intramuscularly,* and then put through the standard run at various times after injection. To minimize reduction in photographic reproduction, only selected parts of each run for a single bird are shown in Fig. 3 and those following, and the

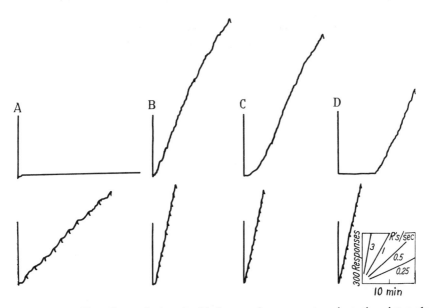

FIGURE 3. The effects of phenobarbital on performance at various time intervals after injection. The upper series shows the selected interval, and the lower series shows the 10 ratios. The interval above each sequence of ratios is from the same standard run. Symbols: A = 18 hours, B = 24 hours, C = 36 hours, and D = 48 hours after injection.

* In all of the work described in this paper, the birds were given a constant dosage of the drug, irrespective of the weights of the different birds. This is because, in general, we were concerned with the comparison of drug effects in the same bird or birds. In fact, the birds differed so little in weight (about plus or minus five per cent of the mean weight of the birds used in this series of experiments) that the doses were almost constant in terms of dosage per kilogram. Since the mean weight of the birds was 435 gm. the dosages per kilogram are rather more than twice the dosages shown in the text and in Table 1.

parts chosen are the single interval and the 10 consecutive ratios labelled in Fig. 2. At 3 hours after injection (Record A, Fig. 3) interval performance was almost abolished and ratio performance much disturbed. At 24 hours, ratio performance was almost normal, while interval performance was still profoundly disturbed (Record B, Fig. 3). The initial pause was lost and the bird pecked irregularly through the whole interval. The rate was constantly changing although the changes were quite smooth, so the cumulative record shows a succession of rounded convexities and concavities. Recovery proceeded progressively and essentially normal interval performance had returned by 50 hours (Record D, Fig. 3).

Similar experiments were conducted following injection of 3 mg. of methamphetamine. This dose of drug did not appreciably affect ratio performance (Fig. 4), while interval performance was greatly changed. As was the case following phenobarbital, the initial pause was lost, but the rate of pecking showed abrupt changes from high rates to zero, giving a steplike appearance to the cumulative record. This phenomenon is best seen in Record C of Fig. 4, but can also be seen in Records B and D. As might be expected, administration of the central nervous system stimulant meth-

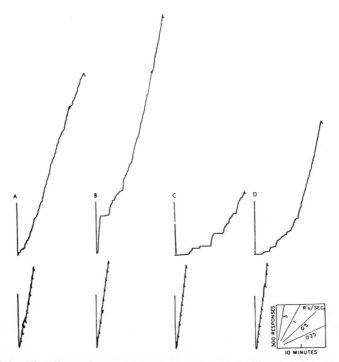

FIGURE 4.   The effects of methamphetamine. The schedule and arrangement is the same as that in Fig. 3. Symbols: A = 4 hours, B = 20 hours, C = 38 hours, and D = 44 hours after injection.

amphetamine leads to an increase in the total number of pecks made (Records A and B, Fig. 4) in contrast to the early decrease caused by the depressant phenobarbital. A final point of interest is that the pigeon ignores one of the food presentations in the ratio series (Fig. 4). This is indicated by a discontinuity of the record (third reward presentation, Record B ratios, Fig. 4) caused by the pigeon continuing to peck the key straight through the period of food presentation.

Similar changes due to phenobarbital and to methamphetamine have been found in a series of experiments on birds working on a multiple schedule with different parameter values, that is, ratios of 30 and intervals of 5 minutes, and with a different sequence of ratios and intervals in the standard run. The effects of the drugs described do not seem to be crucially dependent on these arbitrarily chosen factors. Furthermore, in these experiments the birds were studied at a fixed time interval of 15 minutes following injection of branded doses of the drugs. The results confirmed that the sequence of changes at various time intervals following a single large dose of drug shown in Records A through D in Figs. 3 and 4 are equivalent to those caused by graded doses of the drugs at a constant time interval (Figs. 5 and 6).

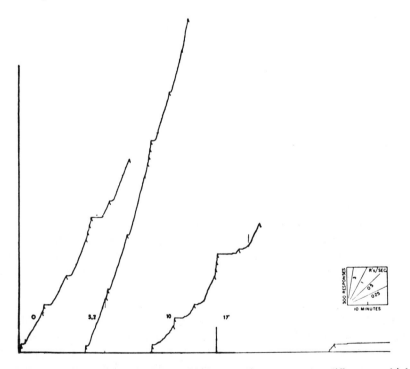

FIGURE 5. The effects of phenobarbital on performance on a different multiple schedule. Complete standard runs are shown, all starting 15 minutes after injection of the indicated dose (in milligrams). Symbol: 0 = injection of saline alone.

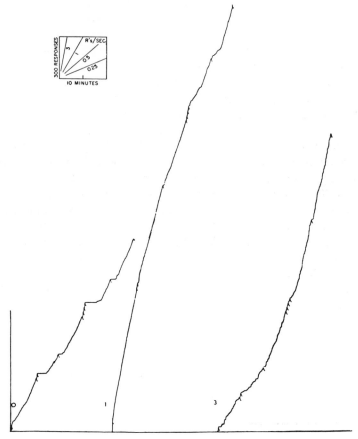

FIGURE 6.   The effects of methamphetamine. The arrangement is the same as that in Fig. 5.

Interval performance was more readily disturbed by both drugs than was ratio performance. Similar findings have been reported previously for pentobarbital.[1] This seems to be a rather general phenomenon. Interval performance is more readily disturbed by all significant variables than is ratio performance. On the other hand, the effects of phenobarbital and of methamphetamine on interval performance differ, as can be seen by inspection of Figs. 3 and 4.

How may the behavioral effects of these drugs be analyzed?

Traditionally, behavioral effects of drugs are attributed to effects of the drugs on emotions such as fear and anxiety, and on ambitions, inhibitions, drives, and other hypothetical or arbitrarily defined "states." The system of experimentation under discussion leads logically to a different approach; it leads to an analysis in operationally defined terms. The pecking performance of the pigeons in these experiments in the absence of a drug depends on a number of explicitly defined variables, many of which are under direct experimental control. The state of food deprivation of the animal can be changed by simply changing the amount of food given. The size of the ratio and the length of the interval are under direct experimental control. The presentation of colored lights, correlated with schedule, comes to have an important effect on performance, and these stimuli can be changed. That rewards are contingent upon pecking has, of course, extreme importance in determining pecking performance. It is easy to arrange that pecks will no longer be rewarded (extinction). These are examples of some of the independent variables under the control of the experimenter that influence the dependent variable; that is, the rate of pecking. In analyzing the effects of a drug, the logical first step is to search for simple interactions between such factors and the effects of the drug; in other words, to determine to what extent the drug effects are "like" in the sense of having the same effect on behavior, the effect of change of level of deprivation, the change of size of ratio, extinction, and so on. Needless to say, this will only be the *first* step in the analysis of the effect of the drug, as will be pointed out later in this paper and in subsequent papers in this monograph.

First, are any of the effects of the drugs described above like the effects of changing the level of deprivation of the animal? Presumably, a drug effect of this kind would be like a sudden reduction in deprivation. Accordingly, experiments were done in which the birds were given free access to food for 15 minutes. The birds ate rapidly at first, but had stopped eating before the end of the 15 minutes. At various time intervals later, they were given the standard run. The bird whose performance is illustrated in Fig. 7 gained 70 gm. in the 15 minutes of free feeding. In spite of this, the bird gave an essentially normal ratio performance 4 hours later (Record A, Fig. 7) although some of the rewards were ignored. At much the same time, the interval performance was much disturbed, illustrating again the relative insensitivity of ratio performance. Of more interest is the nature of the disturbance of interval performance at 10 and 29 hours after free feeding. The sudden changes in rate are strongly reminiscent of the effects of methamphetamine and quite different from the effects of phenobarbital. On the other hand, feeding did not lead to a reduction in the initial pause, nor did it lead to an increase in total output of pecks except perhaps after 36 hours. Hence part, but only part, of the effects of methamphetamine are like the effects of sudden reduction in deprivation. This is interesting in view of the well known "appetite-reducing" effect of methamphetamine in humans. The analogy cannot be sustained at the present time, however, since the effect of methamphetamine has not been shown to be specific to behavior maintained through food deprivation in the pigeons.

The effect of the drugs might mimic the effect of discontinuing rewards, that is, putting the birds on an extinction program. Accordingly, it was arranged that the food tray rose at the usual time called for by the schedule

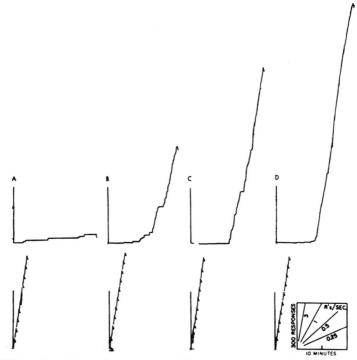

FIGURE 7.   The effects of a period of *ad libitum* feeding on performance at various times later. Symbols: A = 4 hours, B = 10 hours, C = 29 hours, and D = 36 hours after feeding.

but the bird was prevented from eating by blocking the entrance to the tray. By the time the bird came to the 10 ratio, that is, when 5 rewards had been missed, the bird continued to peck straight through the (blocked) presentation of food (Fig. 8). Also the initial pause at the beginning of the interval tended to be reduced, often more strikingly than in this example, with a consequent general straightening out of the interval pattern also characteristic of drug effects. We may therefore tentatively suggest that a part of the effect of both methamphetamine and phenobarbital is due to a weakening of the behavioral control of the stimuli associated with reinforcement, similar to that obtained in extinction.

Other environmental factors whose modification might simulate the effects of drugs are the parameters of the schedule. As a matter of fact, for this *particular schedule,* change in the parameter value of the interval within wide limits causes only an orderly progressive change in the behavior, quite unlike the drug effects. Even considerable changes in the ratio value had no obvious acute effect on either the rate or pattern of pecking (Fig. 9).

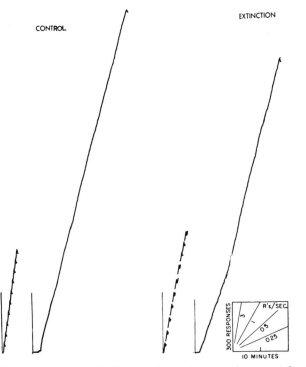

FIGURE 8.   Selected interval and 10 ratios from the control run and from the run in which no rewards were given. Note the discontinuities in the record in ratio series in extinction caused by the bird continuing to peck through the period of the presentation of the "reward."

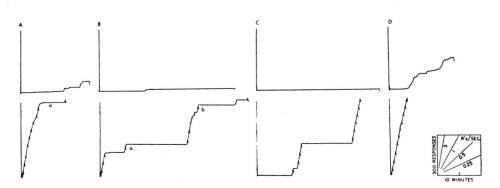

FIGURE 9.   The effects of reserpine on performance at various time intervals after injection. The arrangement is the same as that in Fig. 3. Symbols: $A = 23$ hours, $B = 30$ hours, $C = 40$ hours, and $D = 48$ hours after injection.

A final external control that will be considered is the effect of the two different key lights. Drugs might make the bird behave as though "it could not longer tell red from blue," to use loose phraseology. A study of this possible type of drug effect has already been completed on a different system and is in the literature.[2] In fact, a simple pair of stimuli like the red and blue lights used here seem to retain control even when the birds are under the effect of large doses of all the drugs studied to date. This phenomenon is evidenced by the normal ratio behavior in Figs. 3, 4, 5, and 6 when the bird was definitely under the influence of the drugs. This finding is prima facie evidence for continued control by the red light. It seems that the drugs studied so far just do not have this kind of effect.

In conclusion, it has been possible tentatively to segregate out some of the effects of phenobarbital and methamphetamine as being like the effects of change of some of the external controlling variables.

This discussion has been illustrative rather than exhaustive and conclusive. While it is suggested that this sort of simple analysis should be the first step in the analysis of the effect of a given drug, it is not suggested that all the effects of any drug will be expressible in terms of simple interactions with individual environmental variables. After all, most drugs affecting behavior act on the brain, and there is no reason why their effects there should coincide with the effects of any combination of external physical stimuli. Fortunately, the use of the free-operant technique for analysis of drug effects is not limited to analysis along the lines just discussed, as will be apparent below and in later papers in this monograph. The discussion has been limited to one type of schedule performance, purely in order to keep within reasonable bounds, but it is not a recommended procedure. Part of the extraordinary power of the free-operant technique results from the fact that it permits performances to be "tailor-made" in order to obtain optimum circumstances for manifestation of any specific aspect of a drug effect on which one wishes to focus attention.

The effects of reserpine on performance on the multiple schedule are instructive. Birds were given 100 μg. of reserpine intramuscularly. The drug effect developed slowly, reaching a maximum in about 1 hour. With this dose, pecking was abolished for about 18 hours. Recovery then proceeded progressively, as shown in Fig. 10. The striking thing about these records are the long pauses in the ratios. The bird was physically capable of pecking at a high rate. The pecking started at a high rate, stopped abruptly, often for many minutes, and then it started again at the same rate. This effect was not peculiar to this particular pigeon, for it was seen in 5 of 6 pigeons given this dose, but has not been seen under any circumstances except following a drug. Increasing the size of the ratio, that is, the number of pecks required for a reward, from 60 to 250 or even more in the absence of a drug, does not engender a pause (Fig. 9). In other experiments, it has been shown that if a ratio is increased to 500–1000, then pauses do

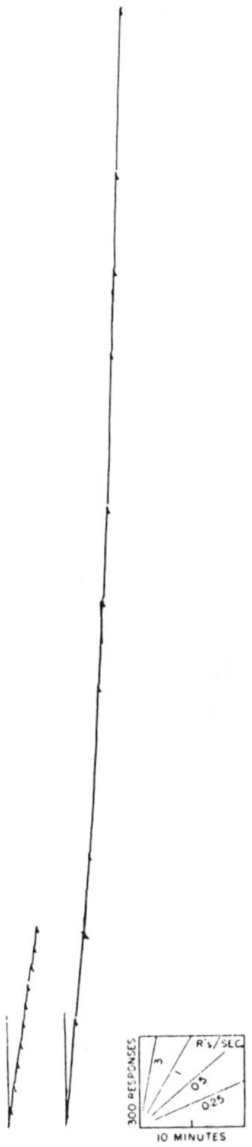

FIGURE 10.   The effect of changing the size of the ratio on the ratio performance. Even though the number of pecks required for reward has been increased suddenly as much as tenfold, the pigeon maintains a high standard rate without pausing at any time during the series of 10 ratios.

develop, but they occur characteristically directly following reinforcement before pecking has restarted. Once the bird had started pecking, it continued to do so, sometimes at an increasing rate, right on to reinforcement. This is quite different from the reserpine effect, in which the pauses come in the middle of the ratio as often as at the beginning. Again we may loosely compare this effect with the effects of reserpine described in humans. Reserpine liberates the pigeon from the normally powerful stimulus control of the red light just as it may liberate people from "tension" by reducing "obsessive-compulsive drives." [4]

In addition to the use of these procedures for analysis of drug effects, some exploration has been performed of their potential usefulness for screening purposes. For this use, it is necessary to be able to summarize the information contained in the cumulative record into a few simple numbers that will characterize as far as possible the different types of drug effect. The ratio performances have been used mainly as an indicator of the physical capabilities of the animal. While the ratio performance remains relatively normal it is safe to conclude that any changes seen in the interval performance are not due to the effects of a drug on the physical ability of the pigeon to peck. The obvious characteristics of the interval that are modified by drugs are (1) the total number of pecks made, and (2) the amount of pausing. Therefore, the pecks were counted on digital counters, and the total duration of pauses was recorded on clocks. The length of a pause was defined as the time beyond 10 seconds until the next peck. When performance is severely disturbed, the bird sometimes fails to pause even at the beginning of the interval. In order to detect this effect, the pecks that occurred in the interval, before any pause of 10 seconds or more had occurred, were counted separately. The value of 10 seconds was chosen as being considerably shorter than the normal initial pause in the interval and longer than the interresponse times once the animal had started pecking.

Some results are shown in Table 1. The "total pecks" column permits the central nervous system stimulants (methamphetamine, pipradol, and methyl phenidylacetate) that led to more than the control number of pecks being made, to be distinguished immediately from the depressants (phenobarbital, glutethimide, and methyprylon) that led to fewer than the control number of pecks being made. There are many simpler methods available which will do this too, however. In general, as would be expected, the total time spent pausing increased as the decrease in total number of pecks

TABLE 1.   Effect of drugs * on interval performance.

Drug	Dose (mg.)	No. of birds	Total pecks†	Pausing†	Prop. of pecks before pause
Methamphetamine.	1	6	1.22	.74	0
Methamphetamine.	3	2	1.53	1.68	.26
Pipradol.	3	2	2.08	.36	.16
Methyl phenidylacetate.	1	2	1.18	.62	.01
Methyl phenidylacetate.	1.7	2	1.31	.77	.01
Methyl phenidylacetate.	3	2	1.62	.66	.12
Phenobarbital.	10	8	.97	1.01	0
Phenobarbital.	17	7	.57	1.66	0
Glutethimide.	30	2	.24	2.00	0
Methyprylon.	17	5	.90	1.75	0
Methyprylon.	30	2	.92	.53	.02
Chlorpromazine.	3	3	1.42	.82	.13
Chlorpromazine.	10	3	.52	1.03	.03
Chlorpromazine.	17	7	.43	1.70	.01

* The drugs used in these studies were kindly supplied as follows:
   Methamphetamine as Methedrine by Burroughs, Wellcome & Co., Tuckahoe, N. Y.; pipradol as Meratran by Wm. S. Merrell Co., Cincinnati, Ohio; methyl phenidylacetate as Ritalin by CIBA Pharmaceutical Products, Inc., Summit, N. J.; glutethimide as Doriden by CIBA Pharmaceutical Products, Inc., Summit, N. J.; methyprylon as Noludar by Hoffman-La Roche, Inc., Nutley, N. J.; and chlorpromazine as Thorazine by Smith, Kline & French Laboratories, Philadelphia, Pa.
   † As proportion of control.

made. The increase both in total pecks and in time pausing following administration of 3 mg. of methamphetamine necessarily means that the general rate of pecking between pauses must have been higher than normal. This phenomenon is a reflection of the sudden changes in rate described above. This dose of methamphetamine caused marked disturbance of normal behavior patterns, as is evidenced by 26 per cent of pecks occurring before a pause (control values are uniformly 0). A useful measure of the potency of stimulant drugs would be in terms of how much "pure" stimulation, that is, increased total output of behavior, can be obtained before the normal patterns are disturbed.

On the average, phenobarbital tended to cause reduction in total pecks and increase in pausing, although in many individual intervals there was virtually no pausing. This effect is even more marked with methyprylon. Following a dose of 30 mg. the effect was sufficiently consistent to cause a decrease in average pausing. The 3-mg. dose of chlorpromazine caused a decrease in pausing, but it also caused an increase in total pecks and in pecks before a pause, just as a stimulant does. Higher doses caused changes like those caused by phenobarbital. The effects are obviously complex.

In short, the screening procedure shows indications of having considerable power to discriminate between different kinds of drugs affecting the central nervous system.

Before concluding, two criticisms of the general method will be mentioned. The first is that it is not always easy to translate the results into the traditional language used in the description of behavioral effects of drugs, the language of emotions, inhibitions, and so on. This limitation may, in fact, be an advantage. The traditional terms are notoriously ill-defined, and have led to a tendency to speculate rather than to design new experiments to obtain more facts.

The second criticism is that the dependent variable, the rate of pecking, is only a tiny fragment of the total behavior of the animal. Whatever validity this criticism may have from the immediately practical standpoint of discovering new drugs, it seems to be quite invalid from the standpoint of basic research. We do not accuse biochemists of triviality when they attempt to isolate pure enzyme systems, although any one such system is only a tiny fragment of the total biochemical machinery of the cell. A detailed analysis is a prerequisite of a worthwhile scientific synthesis.

REFERENCES

1. Dews, P. B. 1955. Studies on behavior. I. Differential sensitivity to pentobarbital of pecking performance in pigeons depending on schedule of reward. *J. Pharmacol.* 113:393.

2. Dews, P. B. 1956. Studies on behavior. II. The effects of pentobarbital, metham-phetamine and scopolamine on performances in pigeons involving discriminations. *J. Pharmacol.* **115**:380.
3. Ferster, C. B. 1953. The use of the free operant in the analysis of behavior. *Psychol. Bull.* **50**:263.
4. Kline, N. S. 1954. The use of *Rauwolfia serpentina* Benth. in neuropsychiatric conditions. *Ann. N.Y. Acad. Sci.* **59**(1):107.

51

Effects of chlorpromazine and promazine on performance on a mixed schedule of reinforcement [1]

PETER B. DEWS

An important way in which drugs affect behavior is to change the frequency with which an easily repeatable response is made (4, 2). Such effects are probably best studied as effects on the final stable pattern of responding engendered by a schedule of reinforcement (1). A schedule of reinforcement is a formal statement of deliberately arranged relations between a response and the occurrence of a particular kind of stimulus, called a reinforcer, which influences the future frequency of emission of that response under similar environmental circumstances. The term schedule is extended to refer to the actual programmed arrangement of the contingencies between response and reinforcement. In addition to the nature of the response and the reinforcing stimulus, and the state of deprivation of the animal and related factors, the schedule of reinforcement is an extremely important determinant of the frequency and temporal pattern of occurrence of responses. With many schedules, if an animal is given repeated exposures to the schedule (e.g., in daily experimental sessions), a stable day-to-day performance develops. Further, an animal may be subjected to more than one type of reinforcement schedule during each session. For example, during a single session, reinforcement may occur sometimes at the 50th response made from the onset of a stimulus (FR 50) and sometimes at the first response after 15 minutes has elapsed from the onset of a stimulus (FI 15). If the stimuli present during the FR and FI components are different (e.g., different colored lights on the response key for the pigeon), eventually the performance in the presence of each of the two stimuli comes to be appropriate to whichever schedule component is in operation. In this example, a high constant rate of responding occurs when the fixed-ratio component is current (similar to that seen during continuous operation of a simple fixed-ratio schedule), and a lower, progressively increasing rate of responding occurs during the fixed-interval component (similar to that seen during continuous operation of a simple fixed-

From *Journal of the Experimental Analysis of Behavior,* 1958, 1, 73–82. Copyright 1958 by the Society for the Experimental Analysis of Behavior, Inc., Bloomington, Ind.

[1] This work was supported by a grant from the U.S. Public Health Service (M-1226). The author wishes to thank Miss Beverly Meeker for meticulous assistance with the experiments. Chlorpromazine was kindly supplied by Smith, Kline, and French Laboratories as Thorazine, and promazine by Wyeth Laboratories as Sparine.

interval schedule). This type of compound schedule is called a multiple schedule (4, p. 503). While there is undoubtedly some interaction between the behaviors on the component schedule, the performances during the individual components retain most of the features of the performance of animals working on that schedule alone (4, p. 503; 2).

If the different components of a compound schedule are not correlated with specific environmental stimuli—if the key color, etc., remain constant irrespective of which schedule component is current—the compound schedule is called a mixed schedule. A variety of such schedules has been described by Ferster and Skinner (4). The interaction between schedule components is much greater with a mixed schedule than with the corresponding multiple schedule. For example, on a mixed schedule with components of FI 15 and FR 50 (i.e., similar to the multiple schedule described above), the FI 15 components start with a period of fast responding, in contrast with the very low initial rates in the FI 15 components of the multiple schedule; FR 50 components produce similar behavior on the two schedules (4). The differences in the behavior of the animal in the different components of a mixed schedule cannot be based on a discrimination of exteroceptive environmental stimuli, since, apart from the time of occurrence of the reinforcement, all such stimuli are constant throughout the session. It has been suggested that such discriminatory performances are more sensitive to modification by drugs than are discriminations based on explicit environmental stimuli (1, 6).

In the present experiments, the mixed schedule with fixed-interval and fixed-ratio components (mix FI 15 FR 50) described above has been used to generate a base line for studies on the effects of two drugs, chlorpromazine and promazine. These drugs differ only in that chlorpromazine has chlorine and promazine has hydrogen at position 2 on the phenothiazine nucleus. They are used clinically for similar purposes.

MATERIALS AND METHODS. The subjects were four mature, male Carneaux pigeons, maintained at 80 per cent of their weight when given free access to food. Their previous histories differed widely; all had had considerable experience on other schedules. They were studied in experimental spaces arranged in the form of a "turntable" (5). A standard pigeon key and food magazine were used. The response was a peck of the key which tripped a relay, and the reinforcing stimulus was the operation of the food magazine giving the pigeon access to food for 4 seconds. The schedule was programmed with electromagnetic relays and counters, and with electric timers.

The sequence of components (of the mix FI 15 FR 50) was kept constant through all the experiments; the sequence was (R equals fixed ratio, I equals fixed interval):RRRIRIIRRRRRRRRRRIIR. For purposes of description the five interval components will be referred to as first through fifth according to their order in this sequence in the individual sessions. Each bird was exposed to this routine for 5 days per week (Monday through Friday). Although the performance on Mondays did not differ noticeably from that on other days, drug observations were not made on Monday. When inspection of the cumulative records indicated a stable day-to-day performance had developed (see Fig. 1), drug injections were made occasionally on days of the week other than Monday. The hydrochlorides of the drugs were dissolved in 0.9 per cent sodium chloride solution and injected intramuscularly. Doses are given in terms of the total dose to the bird. (The weights of these birds varied from 400 to 430 grams.) The injections were made between 4 and 7 hours prior to the experimental session. Each day on which a drug was given was paired with another day (usually the preceding day) on which no drug was given. The results on the latter days have been used for analysis of the "control" performance. On some of these days, saline was injected; but since the observations were made at least 4 hours after the injection, the saline injection was found to be entirely without discernible effect, and, for most purposes, information from saline-injection and no-injection days has been pooled. For the four birds, an aggregate of 59 control sessions have been analyzed. Most of the drug observations were made in duplicate on each bird. The results are presented in the form of a representative series of cumulative records (Fig. 3 and 4), obtained on the same bird (Pigeon 55), showing each dose level

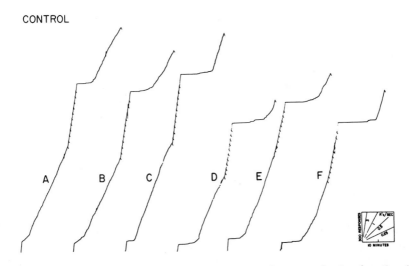

FIGURE 1. Pigeon 55. Cumulative responses vs. time records showing the development of a stable performance on mix FI 15 FR 50. Each segment of Records A-F shows the 3rd fixed interval, the 10 consecutive fixed ratios, and the 4th fixed interval. A, Oct. 17, 1956; B, Oct. 18, 1956; C, Jan. 28, 1957; D, May 28, 1957; E, June 6, 1957; and F, June 11, 1957. Short diagonal lines show occurrences of reinforcements. Faint vertical lines occur where recorder "reset"; these are of no significance.

of drug studied; and also in the form of averaged data taken from all four birds. Almost all the drug effects described in RESULTS can be clearly seen both in the behavior of the individual birds and also in the averaged data.

RESULTS.   The stable performance was in accord with the description given by Ferster and Skinner (4, p. 620). Following a reinforcement, the bird would respond at a high rate until either a response was reinforced (if the component was FR 50) or a number of responses greater than 50 had been emitted (if the component was FI 15). In the latter case, the initial period of fast responding was followed by a pause and then the resumption of a pattern resembling that developed on a fixed-interval schedule (4, p. 133). Figure 1 has cumulative records showing the consecutive sequence of 10 fixed ratios and the preceding and succeeding fixed intervals. These samples are taken from records obtained during an 8-month period and are chronologically arranged from left to right. There is a progressive increase in the length of the pause following the initial period of fast responding on the fixed-interval components through Records A to D; but Records D, E, and F show an essentially stable performance. This figure also indicates that the length of the pause was greater in the 4th fixed interval (following the 10 consecutive fixed ratios) than in the 3rd fixed interval (which directly followed the 2nd fixed interval). This was a consistent finding. The 4th interval uniformly had a longer pause and fewer responses, under control conditions, than did any of the other fixed intervals. This is illustrated in Fig. 2, which shows the isolated fixed intervals from three representative daily sessions. Even when the over-all rate of responding fell considerably (as in the middle row, Fig. 2), this relationship between the numbers of responses in the 4th fixed interval to the numbers in the others persisted. The phenomenon was studied quantitatively in the following way. The numbers of responses in the five individual fixed intervals of a session were expressed as a proportion of the total numbers of responses in all the fixed intervals of that session, and these proportions averaged over the 69 control sessions. The proportions were: 0.21, 0.21, 0.24, 0.12, and 0.23 for the 1st through the 5th intervals, respectively. It will be noted that in addition to the small number of responses in the 4th fixed interval, fixed intervals 1 and 2 tended to have fewer responses than fixed intervals 3 and 5. Fixed intervals 1 and 2 followed fixed-ratio components, while fixed intervals 3 and 5 followed a fixed interval. In short, then, there was clearly a second-order effect in the sense that the behavior of the animal during a fixed-interval component was influenced by the nature of the preceding schedule components. While this sort of phenomenon has long been recognized, it has never been systematically studied.

Doses of either promazine or chlorpromazine of 0.1 milligram had no recognizable effects on the behavior. Even following a dose of 0.3 milli-

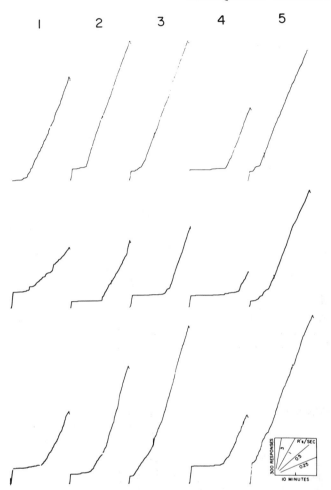

FIGURE 2.   Pigeon 55. Examples of performance in "fixed-interval" components of mix FI 15 FR 50. The five records in each row show the "fixed intervals" of a single day. Top row, May 21, 1957; middle row, April 10, 1957; and bottom row, Jan. 25, 1957.

gram, the effects were confined to a slight increase in the periodic irregularities of rate during the fixed-interval components. (See Fig. 3 and 4, which show the same section of the daily session as that in Fig. 1.) Following 1.0- and 3.0-milligram doses, the length of the pause is reduced following the initial high rate in the fixed-interval components. This is particularly marked in the 3rd fixed intervals in the illustrated records, although it also occurred in the 4th fixed intervals, as in the illustrated record following 3.0 milligrams of chlorpromazine. In all these effects, the two drugs were indistinguishable. Following 10-milligram doses, there is a clear difference in the effects of the two drugs. Chlorpromazine caused an intensification

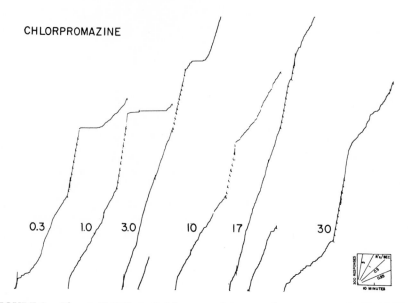

FIGURE 3.   Pigeon 55. Effect of chlorpromazine on performance on mix FI 15 FR 50. Samples of records as in Fig. 1. The numbers give the dosage of drug, in milligrams, administered between 4 and 7 hours previously.

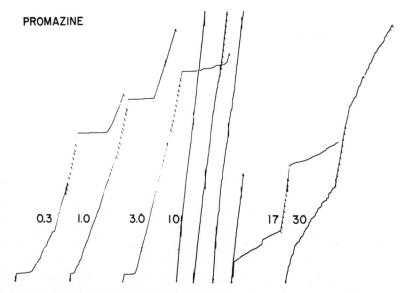

FIGURE 4.   Pigeon 55. Effect of promazine on performance on mix FI 15 FR 50. Samples of records as in Fig. 1. The numbers give the dosage of drug, in milligrams, administered between 4 and 7 hours previously.

of the effects seen with smaller doses; with doses of 10 milligrams or higher, the abrupt pause is completely abolished, although there is still evidence of a discrimination of the "number" in the fixed ratio since the rate falls from its initial high level. With promazine at a dose of 10 milligrams, in addition to the changes seen with chlorpromazine, three out of the four birds showed sustained responding at a high rate. The example shown in Fig. 4 is the most dramatic; this bird emitted a total of more than 14,500 responses in the five 15-minute fixed intervals, in contrast with the control average of about 4000. Higher doses had much less tendency to cause prolonged responding at high rates, and chlorpromazine in all doses had much less tendency to do so. (See, however, the effect of 17 milligrams of chlorpromazine in Fig. 3.)

All these effects are summarized in the dose-effect curve in Fig. 5. The horizontal line designated "saline" was actually obtained from all the control days, including days when no saline was injected. (As previously mentioned, an injection of saline 4 or more hours before the session had no effect on the performance.) The mean number of responses in the five fixed intervals of control sessions was 3659 responses, with a standard deviation of 950 responses. Since most of the points on the drug curves are the means of eight observations (duplicate determinations on four birds), the expected standard error of such means is 336 responses. At doses up to 3.0 milligrams, the drugs are similar in their effect on total output of responses; with doses greater than 3.0 milligrams, promazine has a clear tendency to cause

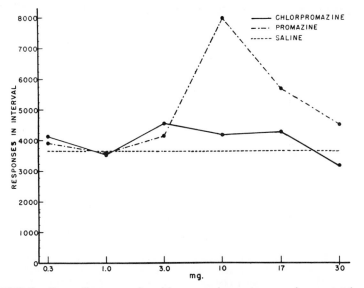

FIGURE 5.   Dose-effect curve for chlorpromazine and promazine on total number of responses in fixed-interval components. Each point is the mean of (usually duplicate) determinations on all four birds (55, 62, 166, 175).

a much greater output of responses than chlorpromazine. The figures for promazine are far outside the range which could reasonably be attributed to sampling errors. The individual points for chlorpromazine all fall within the range expected from sampling errors; however, the persistent elevation of the curve for doses between 3.0 and 17 milligrams may be indicative of a real effect of the drug.

Following large doses (greater than 3.0 milligrams) of either drug, the number of responses in fixed interval 4 became much more nearly equal to the number in the other fixed intervals than under control conditions. The ratio of the number of responses in fixed interval 4 to those in fixed interval 5 was used as a measure of the second-order effect previously described. In the 69 control sessions this ratio averaged 0.53. Following increasing doses of either drug, the value of the ratio increased, until following 17-milligram doses, it averaged greater than 1.0 (i.e., actually more responses were made in the 4th fixed interval—following the 10 fixed ratios—than in the 5th fixed interval—directly following the 4th fixed interval). This phenomenon is illustrated in the dose-effect curve of Fig. 6. The horizontal dotted line shows the average for the control sessions, while the solid line shows the pooled results from experiments with both chlorpromazine and promazine. (Hence, most points are the average of 16 observations.) From the variability of the control observations the expected standard error of means of 16 observations is 0.07; so the effects of the drugs shown in Fig. 6 are clearly far greater than the expected sampling error.

Finally, high rates of responding were maintained in the fixed-ratio components following all doses of the drugs studied, so even the highest doses could not have caused serious motor incapacity. There is one abnormal

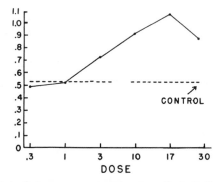

FIGURE 6.   Effect of drugs on a second-order effect. Ordinate: means of ratios of numbers of responses in the 4th fixed interval to numbers in the 5th fixed interval. The solid line shows the pooled results from experiments with chlorpromazine and promazine, while the horizontal dotted line shows the mean of the control experiments.

period in the fixed ratios shown in Fig. 3 following 17 milligrams of chlor-promazine. Since this was an isolated example, an accidental environmental influence is suspected in this particular instance.

DISCUSSION.   Both chlorpromazine and promazine had marked effects on the frequency of occurrence of the response. Probably the most readily affected aspect of the performance was the pause following the initial period of fast responding in the fixed-interval components of the schedule. This finding is in agreement with the suggestion made in the introduction that discriminatory behavior not based on exteroceptive stimuli is more readily disrupted by drugs than discriminatory behavior based on explicit environmental stimuli. However, it has not yet been established whether this is a qualitative difference, or whether it depends on the greater consistency and grossness of the environmental stimuli ordinarily used (1, 6). The effect on the pause in the fixed-interval components is not a specific effect of these drugs; it has been seen following suitable doses of sodium pentobarbital (4, p. 627) and methamphetamine (unpublished observations).

The variation in numbers of responses in fixed-interval components has been attributed to the influence of the immediately preceding schedule components. From the point of view of formal experimental design, these effects are confounded with the over-all order of the components, since this was kept constant. Thus, the 4th fixed interval was always the 4th fixed interval, as well as being the fixed interval following the 10 consecutive fixed ratios. Inspection of Fig. 2 and the figures given in the text for the proportionate numbers of responses in the fixed intervals gives no indication of any important influence of the order of the fixed interval per se on the performance in the component. There seems to be little doubt that the preceding schedule components are of predominant importance in the second-order effect described.

The considerable difference in the effects of promazine and chlorpromazine in large doses on the output of responses shows that the general experimental procedure is competent to detect differences in the effects of very closely related drugs. The difference between the effects of the drugs may be only at very high dose levels; on the other hand, recognition of differences in the effects of the drugs in clinical doses may only await methods adequate for their detection.

Finally, the progressive abolition of the second-order effect on fixed-interval responding by both drugs is also in keeping with the suggestion that an important action of the drugs is to reduce the behavioral control exerted by very subtle (perhaps particularly endogenous) stimuli, while leaving the control of more gross stimuli—such as the key lights and magazine stimuli in this situation—virtually unimpaired.

SUMMARY. 1. Chlorpromazine and promazine tend to abolish the pauses in the fixed-interval components of pigeons working under mix FI 15 FR 50 schedule of reinforcement.

2. Large doses of both drugs also modified the control over performance in fixed-interval components exerted by the nature of the preceding schedule components.

3. At the higher doses studied, promazine had a much more pronounced tendency to cause prolonged responding at high rates than did chlorpromazine.

REFERENCES

1. Dews, P. B. Studies on behavior. I. Differential sensitivity to pentobarbital of pecking performance in pigeons depending on the schedule of reward. *J. Pharmacol. & Exper. Therap.,* 1955, **113**, 393–401.
2. Dews, P. B. Modification by drugs of performance on simple schedules of positive reinforcement. *Ann. N.Y. Acad. Sci.,* 1956, **65**, 268–281.
3. Dews, P. B. Studies on behavior. III. Effects of scopolamine on reversal of a discriminatory performance in pigeons. *J. Pharmacol. & Exper. Therap.,* 1957, **119**, 343–353.
4. Ferster, C. B., and Skinner, B. F. *Schedules of reinforcement.* New York: Appleton-Century-Crofts, 1957.
5. Herrnstein, R. J., and Morse, W. H. Some effects of response-independent positive reinforcement on a maintained operant. *J. comp. physiol. Psychol.,* 1957, **50**, 461–467.
6. Morse, W. H., and Herrnstein, R. J. Effects of drugs on characteristics of behavior maintained by complex schedules of intermittent positive reinforcement. *Ann. N.Y. Acad. Sci.,* 1956, **65**, 303–317.

52

Behavioral variables affecting the development of amphetamine tolerance *

CHARLES R. SCHUSTER, WILLIAM S. DOCKENS, and
JAMES H. WOODS

Amphetamine administration produces a disruption of timing behavior in subjects who are reinforced for responding at a low rate (Sidman, 1956; Dews and Morse, 1958). With continued daily administration of amphetamines, performance changes progressively toward that observed under saline control conditions (Schuster and Zimmermann, 1961; Zimmerman and Schuster, 1962). General activity measures taken from the same subjects are consistently elevated over the course of the chronic-drug period. The evidence suggests a certain specificity in what behaviors will show the development of tolerance to chronically administered amphetamines. The present report deals with a series of experiments designed to analyze the role of reinforcement contingencies as one class of variables that influence the development of behavioral tolerance to amphetamines.

EXPERIMENT I

MATERIALS AND METHODS. *Subjects.* Three Sprague-Dawley male rats were used that ranged in weight from 300–320 g. The subjects were gradually reduced to 70% of their original body weight and maintained at this level by adjusted feedings after each experimental session.

Apparatus. The experimental chamber was a standard Gerbrands rat box containing a lever operandum, a Gerbrands pellet dispenser that delivered 45 mg Noyes rat pellets and two 5 watt bulbs to provide visual stimuli. The experimental chamber was enclosed in a modified picnic chest which was enclosed in a large sound-attenuating chamber. Programming of stimulus events and response recording was accomplished by switching and timing circuits, a cumulative recorder, and electrical impulse counters.

Procedure. The animals were initially conditioned to press a response lever for a pellet of food. After one session in which every response was reinforced with food, the subjects were placed under the contingencies

From *Psychopharmacologia* (Berl.), 1966, 9, 170–182. Copyright 1966 by Springer-Verlag, Heidelberg, Germany.

* This research was supported by grant no. USPHS MH-08506-02 from the National Institute of Mental Health.

of a 2-ply multiple schedule of reinforcement. The multiple schedule consisted of fixed-interval (FI) and differential reinforcement of low rate (DRL) components. In the FI component the subject was reinforced with a presentation of food for the first lever response occurring after 30″ had elapsed from the previously reinforced response. Responses occurring before the 30″ had elapsed were recorded but had no other programmed consequences. The house lights were illuminated continuously during the FI. After 10 minutes on the FI schedule a 30″ black-out period occurred during which all lights in the experimental chamber were turned off. Lever responses during the 30″ black-out period had no experimentally specified consequences and were not recorded. Following the black-out period, the DRL schedule was presented for 10 minutes. During this period the subject was reinforced with food for those responses which occurred a minimum of 30″ after the preceding response. Responses occurring prior to the 30″ minimum time interval reset the 30″ timer and therefore postponed reinforcement opportunity by 30″. During the DRL component the house lights flashed in an irregular pattern with an average of 2 per second. The total session length of 62.5 minutes was comprised of three 10 minute FI periods alternated with three 10 minute DRL periods. The 30″ black-out period occurred after each schedule change. The subject's performance stabilized in both schedules after 75 consecutive daily sessions.

The total number of lever-pressing responses and food reinforcements were recorded separately for the FI and DRL components. In addition, the subject's lever-pressing responses in the FI component were recorded separately in each of the 6 consecutive 5″ periods covering the 30″ FI length. The sixth counter cumulated all responses occurring from 25″ on. This method of recording allows the analysis of the temporal distribution of FI responses. A convenient way of summarizing these data is to determine the average length of time expired before 25 and 75% of the total number of responses had occurred.

The subject's DRL lever-pressing responses were recorded in an 11–5″ compartment inter-response time (IRT) distribution (Sidman, 1956). For example, a response occurring between 30–35″ from the previous response was recorded in counter 7. Counter 11, the final counter, recorded all responses occurring 50″ or more from the previous response. To present the large amount of data accrued in the present report the IRT data was simplified using a method described by Hodos (1963). In this method the mode of the IRT distribution is selected by visual inspection exclusive of the first compartment. The variability of responses around the mode is quantified by computing the interquartile range disregarding the first compartment. The first IRT compartment is not used in this computation or in the selection of the mode since the large number of responses occurring here reflect a response "burst" rather than temporally spaced responses.

Drug administration. d-Amphetamine SO_4 was dissolved in physiological saline in a concentration of 1.0 mg/cc. This solution was diluted appropriately so that a constant volume (.1 cc/100 g of body weight) was given for all dosages. Drug solutions were freshly prepared every 5 days. The drug was administered subcutaneously along the flank of the animal 30 muintes prior to the experimental session. Control injections of physiological saline were administered in the same manner.

Pre-chronic drug.   A dose-response curve for *d*-amphetamine was obtained spacing the drug administration so that 4 non-drug sessions intervened between each drug session. Dosages of .125, .25, .50 and 1.0 mg/kg of *d*-amphetamine SO$_4$ were tested in a random order in addition to six saline control sessions.

Chronic drug.   The subjects were placed on a chronic-drug regimen in which 1.0 mg/kg of *d*-amphetamine was administered 30 minutes prior to each experimental session, for 30 consecutive days. Following this chronic-drug regimen the subjects performed daily for approximately one month (26–32 days) under saline control conditions.

Post-chronic drug.   A post-chronic drug dose-response curve for *d*-amphetamine was obtained using the same procedure and dosages as above (pre-chronic drug).

For the saline control periods and the chronic-drug regimen the FI-DRL data were analyzed in 6 session averages. For the averages the standard error of the mean was computed as a measure of variability.

RESULTS.   Under saline control conditions the subjects' performance in the FI components showed the typical "scallop" shaped temporal distribution of lever-pressing responses. The low rates of lever responding and the frequency of reinforcement in the DRL component approximate that observed in previous experiments using DRL schedule alone (Zimmerman and Schuster, 1962).

Figure 1 (pre-chronic drug) shows the effects of various dosages of *d*-amphetamine on the total number of lever-pressing responses in the FI and DRL components. As can be seen for subject R-2 the total responses in the FI and DRL show a marked increment as a function of *d*-amphetamine dosage. Subject R-5 shows a slight increase in the total number of responses in the FI and a marked increase in the total number of responses in the DRL. Subject R-4, on the other hand, shows a marked decrement in total FI responses and negligible change in total DRL responses at the dosages tested.

Figure 1 (chronic drug) shows the average responses for the FI and DRL components under saline control conditions and over the course of the chronic-drug regimen. For subject R-2 the total number of FI responses shows a marked and sustained increase throughout the 30-day drug period. The total number of responses in the DRL component, however, shows, after an initial increment, a gradual decline over the course of the

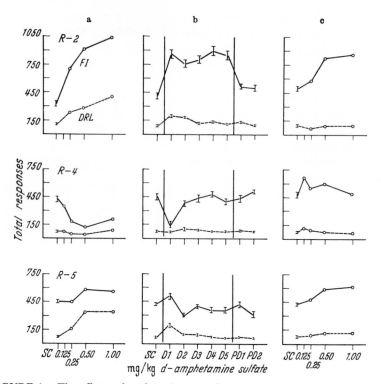

FIGURE 1. The effects of various dosages of *d*-amphetamine on total responses in the FI and DRL schedules of reinforcement prior to the chronic-drug regimen (a). Average number of responses in the FI and DRL under saline control conditions (SC, PD, and PD₂) and during the chronic-drug regimen (D1–D5). Each point represents an average of 6 sessions (b). Repetition of dose-response function after the chronic-drug regimen (c). Solid line: FI; dashed line: DRL.

drug period. The total number of responses in the FI for subject R-4 shows a marked decrement in the initial period of the chronic-drug regimen followed by a return to the normal number of responses throughout the last 24 days of the chronic-drug period. The total number of responses in the DRL component for this subject was unaffected by this dosage of *d*-amphetamine. Subject R-5 shows no consistent change in the total responses in the FI over the chronic-drug period. The total number of responses for subject R-5 in the DRL component, however, shows a marked increment in the first 6 days of the chronic-drug regimen followed by a gradual return to the rate observed under saline control conditions.

A more refined analysis of the subjects' DRL performance under saline control and chronic-drug conditions is given in Table 1. The mode, Q_1, and Q_3 values of the IRT distributions are shown in this table. For all three subjects the mode of the IRT distribution under the pre-drug saline control condition closely approximates the 30 second minimum interval by

TABLE 1. The mode and interquartile range (Q_1-Q_3) for DRL inter-response times under saline control and chronic d-amphetamine administration. Values are six session averages.

Drug Treatment condition	Subjects					
	R 2		R 4		R 5	
	Mode	Q_1-Q_3	Mode	Q_1-Q_3	Mode	Q_1-Q_3
Saline Control	33.0	20.5—36.0	27.5	24.0—37.0	35.0	26.0—40.0
Drug Periods D1	7.5	9.0—22.0	12.5	19.0—41.0	12.0	13.0—31.5
D2	7.5	8.0—28.0	17.5	16.5—29.0	17.5	17.5—30.0
D3	17.5	13.0—34.0	22.5	19.0—31.5	22.5	17.5—29.0
D4	18.5	12.5—32.0	22.5	22.0—33.0	27.5	21.0—40.0
D5	23.0	16.5—36.0	27.5	22.5—40.0	32.5	27.5—45.0
Post Drug Saline Control PDSC1	15.5	12.5—31.0	27.0	21.0—47.0	30.5	23.0—38.5
PDSC2	26.0	16.5—31.0	32.0	23.0—42.0	32.5	26.0—41.5

which responses were required to be separated for reinforcement. In the initial portion of the chronic-drug regimen (D1) the mode shows a marked decrement indicative of more frequent short inter-response times. With continued administration of the drug, however, (D2–D5) the mode and the Q_1 and Q_3 values show a progressive increment ultimately reaching a value closely approximating that observed under the pre-drug saline control condition.

Table 2 presents Q_1 and Q_3 values for the FI response time distributions under saline control and chronic-drug conditions. These measures show no change as a function of the chronic-drug regimen for any of the subjects. This is particularly impressive in the case of subjects R-2 and

TABLE 2. Time elapsed before 25% (Q_1) and 75% (Q_3) of the total FI responses are emitted under saline control and chronic d-amphetamine administration. Values are six session averages.

Drug Treatment condition	Subjects		
	R 2	R 4	R 5
	Q_1-Q_3	Q_1-Q_3	Q_1-Q_3
Saline Control	22.5—28.5	22.0—28.0	24.0—28.5
Drug Periods D1	20.5—29.0	23.5—27.0	23.5—28.5
D2	20.5—28.0	22.0—27.5	22.5—28.0
D3	21.0—28.0	23.5—28.5	24.5—28.5
D4	21.0—28.0	24.0—29.0	23.5—28.5
D5	21.0—28.5	24.5—28.0	24.0—29.0
Post-Drug Saline Control PDSC1	24.0—28.5	22.5—28.5	22.0—27.5
PDSC2	23.0—28.5	23.0—27.5	23.5—28.0

TABLE 3. Average number of total reinforcements for the FI and DRL components under saline control conditions and chronic *d*-amphetamine administration. Values are six session averages and variability is expressed as the standard error of the mean.

Drug Treatment condition		R 2		R 4		R 5	
		FI	DRL	FI	DRL	FI	DRL
Saline Control		55.0 ± 1.0	29.0 ± 2.1	55.0 ± 1.1	26.0 ± 1.5	55.0 ± 1.0	31.0 ± 1.1
Drug Periods	D 1	54.0 ± 1.0	9.0 ± 2.4	41.0 ± 2.4	19.0 ± 1.1	55.0 ± 1.0	16.0 ± 3.9
	D 2	52.5 ± 1.3	16.0 ± 2.3	49.0 ± 1.8	15.0 ± 1.6	52.0 ± 1.1	16.5 ± 2.1
	D 3	54.5 ± 1.1	14.5 ± 1.8	51.0 ± 2.0	17.5 ± 1.3	55.0 ± 1.0	14.5 ± 1.3
	D 4	53.0 ± 1.0	13.0 ± 2.1	52.5 ± 1.1	21.0 ± 2.1	50.0 ± 2.3	24.0 ± 1.8
	D 5	54.0 ± 1.5	19.5 ± 1.7	54.0 ± 1.3	23.0 ± 2.6	53.5 ± 1.0	30.0 ± 2.0
Post-Drug Saline Control	PDSC 1	54.5 ± 1.3	12.5 ± 1.8	54.0 ± 2.1	27.0 ± 1.6	53.0 ± 1.0	28.0 ± 1.5
	PDSC 2	55.0 ± 1.1	15.5 ± 2.4	55.0 ± 1.3	29.5 ± 1.8	52.5 ± 1.0	32.0 ± 2.0

R-4, who showed marked and opposite changes in the total number of responses.

Table 3 shows the average number of reinforcements received in the FI and DRL components under saline control and chronic-drug conditions. Total number of FI reinforcements for subjects R-2 and R-5 was unaffected by the chronic-drug regimen. In contrast, the total number of DRL reinforcements is lower at the beginning of the chronic-drug regimen (D1) than at the end (D5). Subject R-5 has an average number of DRL reinforcements as great at the end of the chronic-drug regimen (D5) as ever observed under saline control conditions. Subject R-4 shows an initial decrement in average FI and DRL reinforcements in the first 6 sessions of the chronic-drug regimen (D1) followed by a gradual trend towards saline control values.

Figure 1 (post-chronic drug) shows the dose response function obtained one month after the chronic-drug regimen. The total number of FI responses of subjects R-2 and R-5 shows an increment as a function of dosage comparable to that observed in the pre-chronic drug dose-response curve. The total responses in the DRL for these subjects, however, do not show an increment at any dosage comparable to that seen in the pre-chronic drug dose-response curve. In the post-chronic drug dose-response curve for R-4 the total number of responses in the FI shows an increment at the lower dosages. This is in contrast to the marked decrement observed at these dosages in the pre-chronic drug dose-response function. The total number of DRL responses for R-4 shows an increase only at the lowest dosage tested in the post-chronic drug-response curve.

DISCUSSION.   The disrupting effects of amphetamines on the accuracy of timing behavior generated by a DRL schedule of reinforcement are by now well confirmed (Sidman, 1956; Dews and Morse, 1958; Schuster and Zimmerman, 1961; Zimmerman and Schuster, 1962). The gradual diminution in the drug's effect observed in the present experiment with continued daily administration of d-amphetamine, corroborates the previously noted development of behavioral tolerance using simple or multiple DRL schedules (Schuster and Zimmerman, 1961; Zimmerman and Schuster, 1962). We do not imply a mechanism by suggesting that the term behavioral tolerance be applied to this phenomenon, rather that the term can be used with operational clarity when we observe a gradual decrease in a behavioral effect of amphetamines with repeated administration.

The dose-response curves for amphetamine reveal marked individual differences in our subjects. It has been our experience that this occurs frequently with amphetamines particularly with complex schedules of reinforcement. We have attempted to utilize this variability in the present experiment. In this regard subjects R-2 and R-4 are of particular interest. Subject R-2 showed a marked increment in the total number of FI responses which was sustained throughout the entire chronic-drug regimen. The stimulating effects of amphetamine in the FI performance showed no diminution with repeated administration. Therefore, by definition, this subject's FI performance did not show the development of tolerance. The post-chronic drug dose-response function of this subject showed comparable stimulation in the total FI responses to that observed in the pre-chronic drug dose-response function. Subject R-4, in contrast, showed an initial depression in total FI responses followed by a progressive decrement in the effect of the drug with repeated administration. This gradual diminution with repeated administration of the depressant effect of the drug on the subject's FI performance fits our conception of behavioral tolerance.

For both the DRL and FI performance tolerance was observed in the post-chronic drug dose-effect curves. That is, those subjects who developed tolerance during the chronic-drug regimen remained resistant to the actions of amphetamine 30 days after the cessation of chronic administration of the drug. Further parametric experimentation is needed to determine the variables controlling the permanence of amphetamine tolerance.

We are now faced with the question of what common variables may account for the observed behavioral tolerance to repeated administration of d-amphetamine in DRL performance while tolerance is observed in FI performance only when the rate of response is decreased by the action of the drug. Clearly the common physiological mechanisms responsible for drug tolerance cannot be appealed to as an explanation. If the tolerance observed was attributable to changes in absorption or metabolism, there would be no explanation for the differential development of tolerance in the different behaviors. Table 3 which shows the average number of FI and DRL reinforcements under saline control and chronic-drug conditions may hold the key to this problem. Where the initial effect of the drug on either DRL or FI performance was such that the reinforcement frequency fell, we have observed the development of behavioral tolerance. We shall delay a more explicit statement of our hypothesis regarding this relationship between reinforcement frequency and amphetamine tolerance until our discussion following the next experiment.

EXPERIMENT II

SHOCK-AVOIDANCE.   The second experiment in this series was undertaken to determine whether or not behavioral tolerance would develop to chronically administered d-amphetamine where the drug enhances conditions of reinforcement through changes in behavioral output. A second question which this experiment was designed to answer was whether or not the facilitating effects of amphetamines would transfer after long-term chronic administration to the non-drug condition. Previous reports have shown that amphetamines have a facilitating effect upon avoidance behavior generated by a Sidman avoidance schedule (Verhave, 1958). This effect is particularly pronounced in subjects whose avoidance is below optimum (Hearst and Whalen, 1963). We selected, therefore, for our investigation "poor avoidance" animals trained in a modified Sidman-avoidance procedure (Sidman, 1953).

METHOD AND APPARATUS.   *Subjects.*   The subjects were four Sprague-Dawley rats approximately 350–375 g in body weight. Subjects were given ad-lib food and water in their home cages.

Apparatus.   The experimental chamber was a standard Gerbrands rat box containing a lever operandum for the rat to depress, with a grid floor wired for the delivery of electric shock. A single 5 watt bulb provided illumination during the experimental session. The experimental chamber was enclosed in a modified picnic chest which in turn was located in a sound-attenuating chamber. Programming of the onset, duration, and intensity of the electric shock was controlled by timers and a Grason-Stadler shock source and grid-scrambler. The shock intensity was set at 2.0 ma. throughout the experiment. The subjects' lever-pressing performance was recorded on electrical impulse counters, running time meters, and a Gerbrands Model C cumulative recorder.

Procedure.   The subjects were exposed daily to a 90 minute session of shock avoidance. In this schedule failure to make a lever-pressing response for a period of 30 seconds resulted in the onset of shock which continued until the lever was depressed or for a maximum of 10 seconds. It should be noted that in this procedure there is no exteroceptive warning stimulus prior to the shock. The total number of lever responses, shocks, and escape latencies were recorded.

After 125 hours of training four subjects were selected from a larger group of animals because of their "poor" but stable avoidance performance. Following 7 saline control sessions they were started on a 35 day chronic-drug regimen in which 1.0 mg/kg of *d*-amphetamine was administered subcutaneously 30 minutes prior to each daily session. This condition will be referred to as chronic drug I.

After 20 saline control sessions two of the subjects were again placed on a chronic-drug regimen for 20 days. In the second chronic-drug period the dosage of the drug was begun at 1.0 mg/kg and reduced daily by .05 mg/kg. An additional 7 saline control sessions were run at the end of this second chronic-drug regimen.

RESULTS.   Figure 2 shows the total number of lever responses and shocks for the 4 subjects under saline control (SC and PDSC) and chronic-drug (D1–D5) conditions. The total number of responses was increased for all subjects throughout the entire course of the chronic-drug regimen. Subjects AV-1, AV-4, AV-5, showed a large increment in number of responses at this dosage of *d*-amphetamine and the number of shocks received was

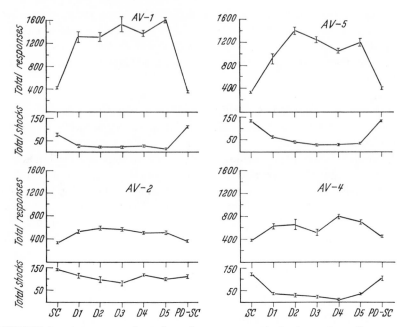

FIGURE 2.   Average number of total responses and shocks under saline control conditions (SC, PDSC) and during the chronic-drug regimen (D1–D5). Each point represents an average of 7 sessions and the brackets indicate the standard error of the mean.

markedly decreased over the course of the chronic-drug regimen. AV-2 showed a smaller increment in response rate and did not show a clear decrease in number of shocks received. The drug regimen did not affect the approximate .6 second escape latencies for any subject. When the subjects were returned to the saline control condition their performance immediately returned to that observed prior to the chronic-drug regimen.

Figure 3 illustrates the effects of the gradual withdrawal of amphetamines on the avoidance performance of AV-1 and AV-5. The subjects' total number of responses shows an orderly decline, and total number of shocks increases as a function of diminishing dosage of the drug. The drug regimen did not affect the subjects' escape latencies. Again the animals' saline control performance following this second chronic-drug regimen shows no change from the pre-chronic drug avoidance performance.

DISCUSSION.   The administration of 1.0 mg/kg d-amphetamine to "poor" Sidman avoidance subjects resulted in a clear-cut facilitation in 3 of the 4 subjects. This dosage was fixed in order to make relevant comparisons to the first experiment in this series. Facilitation of the avoidance performance might have been obtained with a higher dosage in the case of subject AV-2 (Hearst and Whalen, 1963). The important consideration here is the fact that the increased total number of responses and the decre-

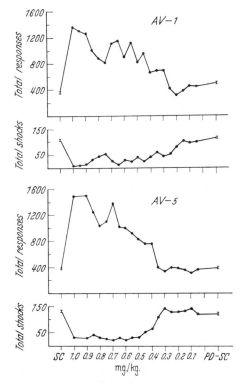

FIGURE 3. Total responses and shocks under saline control conditions (SC and PDSC) and as a function of daily decreasing dosages of *d*-amphetamine.

ment in shock frequency showed no tendency to diminish with prolonged daily administration of this dosage of *d*-amphetamine. Clearly these subjects' avoidance performance did not reflect the development of behavioral tolerance to this dosage of *d*-amphetamine.

It is also of some importance to note that despite the subjects' prolonged experience with higher response rates leading to diminished shock frequency there was no permanent improvement following the chronic-drug regimen. This was true whether the drug was abruptly withdrawn (chronic drug I) or gradually diminished in dosage (chronic drug II). Despite the more favorable reinforcement conditions under the drug, the subjects did not transfer any improved performance from the drugged to the non-drugged states.

GENERAL DISCUSSION: EXPERIMENT I AND II

On the basis of this preliminary evidence we have evolved the following working hypothesis concerning the role of reinforcement contingencies in determining what aspect of an organism's behavioral repertoire will show the development of tolerance to amphetamines.

Behavioral tolerance will develop in those aspects of the organism's behavioral repertoire where the action of the drug is such that it disrupts the organism's behavior in meeting the environmental requirement for reinforcements. Conversely, where the actions of the drug enhance or do not affect the organism's behavior in meeting reinforcements requirements we do not expect the development of behavioral tolerance.

This hypothesis is not intended as a replacement for the classical physiological theories of drug tolerance (Eddy, 1941; Sollman, 1948). Rather this hypothesis is put forth as an additional variable which may be operative in those behavioral situations where tolerance develops in a manner not predictable from the classical conceptions.

SUMMARY

The behavioral effects of chronic administration of d-amphetamine in rats at a dosage of 1 mg/kg were studied with baselines involving either food or shock reinforcement. Food reinforcement was assigned according to a fixed interval or on the basis of differential reinforcement of low rate in a multiple schedule of reinforcement. Behavioral tolerance was observed in response to chronic administration of d-amphetamine when the action of the drug led to a decrease in frequency of food reinforcement regardless of the schedule of reinforcement. In the second experiment, a shock avoidance situation was employed in which each avoidance response postponed the onset of grid shock. An escape contingency was provided for occasions on which an avoidance response did not occur. The chronic administration of d-amphetamine led to a uniform increase in response rate throughout the drug regimen with the consequence of decreasing rate of shock reinforcement. An hypothesis was put forward on the basis of these results which considers the development of behavioral tolerance to amphetamine administration to be a function of the drug's action in relation to its effects on the organism's behavior in meeting reinforcement requirements.

REFERENCES

Dews, P. B., and Morse, W. H.: Some observations on an operant in human subjects and its modification by dextro-amphetamine. *J. exp. Anal. Behav.* 1, 359–364 (1958).

Eddy, N. B.: The pharmacology of the opium alkaloids: Part 1. *Public Health Reports Suppl.* 165, 687 (1941).

Hearst, E., and Whalen, R. E.: Facilitating effects of *d*-amphetamine on discriminated avoidance performance. *J. comp. physiol. Psychol.* **56**, 124–128 (1963).

Hodos, W.: A simple method for the description of inter-response time distributions. *J. exp. Anal. Behav.* **6**, 90 (1963).

Schuster, C. R., and Zimmerman, J.: Timing behavior during prolonged treatment with *dl*-amphetamine. *J. exp. Anal. Behav.* **4**, 327–330 (1961).

Sidman, M.: Avoidance conditioning with brief shock and no exteroceptive warning stimulus. *Science* **118**, 157–158 (1953).

Sidman, M.: Time discrimination and behavioral interaction in a free operant situation. *J. comp. physiol. Psychol.* **49**, 469–473 (1956).

Sollman, T. A.: *A manual of pharmacology and its applications to therapeutics and toxicology.* Philadelphia: W. B. Saunders Co. 1948.

Verhave, T.: The effect of methamphetamine on operant level and avoidance behavior. *J. exp. Anal. Behav.* **1**, 207–218 (1958).

Zimmerman, J., and Schuster, C. R.: Spaced responding in multiple DRL schedules. *J. exp. Anal. Behav.* **5**, 497–504 (1962).

53

Effects of *dl*-amphetamine under concurrent VI DRL reinforcement

EVALYN F. SEGAL [1]

Several reviews of psychopharmacological research on the amphetamines have appeared within recent years (Brady, 1957; Dews and Morse, 1961; Owen, 1960; Sidman, 1959). From these reviews and the supporting data, some principles of amphetamine action are gradually emerging that promise to unify the vast and paradoxical body of amphetamine findings. The following are among the principles with the best experimental support. (1) Amphetamine reduces food and water consumption (Dews and Morse, 1961) and possibly some vague entity called "appetite" (Owen, 1960). (2) In carefully circumscribed conditions, amphetamine increases the total amount of "spontaneous activity" (Dews and Morse, 1961). (3) Amphetamine enhances "conditioned emotionality," [2] especially aversively aroused emotionality (Brady, 1957; Teitelbaum and Derks, 1958) and "post-drug depression" (Verhave, 1958), but perhaps also "euphoric" types of emotion (Dews and Morse, 1961; Miller, 1956, 1957). (4) Amphetamine differentially affects behavior maintained by different reinforcement schedules (Dews and Morse, 1961) and by different parameters of a given schedule (Dews, 1960). (5) Amphetamine influences rates of responding both by shortening long (5 sec or more) IRT's and lengthening short (less than 1 sec) IRT's (Dews, 1958; Dews and Morse, 1961; Morse and Herrnstein, 1956).

Another finding, which is not so well confirmed as those above but yet is mentioned in the experimental literature, is that appropriate doses of amphetamine affect discriminative behavior. Apparently, simple discriminations are not affected (Dews, 1955; Sidman, 1956a, 1956b), but complex

From *Journal of the Experimental Analysis of Behavior,* 1962, **5**, 105–112. Copyright 1962 by the Society for the Experimental Analysis of Behavior, Inc., Bloomington, Ind.

[1] This research was completed during the writer's tenure of a Postdoctoral Research Fellowship from the National Institute of Neurological Diseases and Blindness, under the sponsorship of Dr. J. V. Brady. Thanks are due to the Laboratory of Psychopharmacology of the University of Maryland for provision of some of the research facilities under Grant No. MY-1604 from the National Institute of Mental Health, and to Mr. C. R. Schuster for advice and assistance in the conduct of the experiment.

[2] Dews and Morse (1961) think that the evidence on this point is no more than suggestive; nonetheless, it has sufficient experimental support to qualify as a promising integrative principle.

"conditional" discriminations are (Dews, 1955). Moreover, impairment of "sensory responsiveness" or "attentiveness" is suggested by failure to respond to stimuli signalling the brief availability of food (Teitelbaum and Derks, 1958; Weissman, 1959). The failure of food consumption may, of course, be interpreted simply as a consequence of reduced "hunger." However, as Teitelbaum and Derks (1958) contend, and this writer concurs, animals under amphetamine often show a quality of "obliviousness"; they may work at very high response rates, yet fail to respond to food signals.

One area of conflicting data concerns the nature of amphetamine effect on *rate* of responding. Dews and Morse (1961) have noted that amphetamine sometimes increases rates of reinforced responding (*e.g.,* Brady, 1957; Dews and Morse, 1958; Miller, 1956; Morse and Herrnstein, 1956; Sidman, 1955, 1956a, 1956b; Skinner and Heron, 1937; Verhave, 1958; Weissman, 1959; Wentink, 1938) and rates of extinction responding (*e.g.,* Miller, 1956; Skinner and Heron, 1937; Weissman, 1959); amphetamine sometimes decreases response rates (*e.g.,* Dews, 1955, 1958, Miller, 1956; Owen, 1960; Verhave, 1958; Weissman, 1959); and sometimes, as in operant level (Verhave, 1958) and some variable-interval schedules (Dews, 1955, 1958), amphetamine has no appreciable effect on rate of responding. Dews and Morse (1961) explain these disparities by the principle that amphetamine reduces long IRT's (hence tending to increase rate) but lengthens short IRT's (hence tending to decrease rate). To account for Verhave's operant-level data, they add the qualification that the response must at some minimum strength before any amphetamine effect occurs.

This IRT principle of amphetamine action brings some coherency to the confusing welter of contradictory data. Thus, Dews and Morse are able to explain the dependency of amphetamine effects on reinforcement schedule in terms of the type of IRT distribution generated by the schedule. Among other implications, their position makes dubious the view that amphetamine-induced changes in DRL performance are due to a specific disruption of timing mechanisms. Dews and Morse interpret the DRL result as simply one among many similar effects on IRT's common to many reinforcement schedules and not specifically related to temporal factors.

Possibly amphetamine, like many other independent variables, may selectively and differentially affect various dimensions of a single response class, or various components of an organism's response repertoire. Several authors have lately argued, in other contexts, for the examination of other dimensions of response besides rate (*e.g.,* Herrnstein, 1961; Millenson and Hurwitz, 1961; Notterman, 1959), and for the consideration of larger portions of the response repertoire (Bindra, 1961) and the interrelations among components of the repertoire having differing probabilities of emission (Premack, 1959, 1961). Segal (1959) has suggested that food- and water-deprivation might differentially affect responses which are already at high strength; and this suggestion is equally relevant to other experimental variables. It is reminiscent of Dews and Morse's (1961) explanation for the lack of amphetamine effect on operant level. The converse is equally likely, namely, that some independent variables may differentially affect responses which are at low strength. Premack (1961) and Premack and Collier (1961) have made a similar proposal in differentiating between "recurrent" and "nonrecurrent" responses; they suggest that many experimental variables may have differential effects upon these two classes of behavior. Dews (1960) has presented supporting evidence, in the form of inverse functional relations between pentobarbitial- and amphetamine-induced rate increases, and control response rate. Finally, there may be complex interactions, such that responses at high strength are altered in one direction and responses at low strength are altered in the opposite direction, by one and the same experimental treatment.[3] This is closely related to Dews and Morse's description of amphetamine effects on IRT, but the principle may extend to other independent variables besides amphetamine.

In the present experiment, I examined the effects of amphetamine on characteristic IRT distributions generated by the two components of a concurrent schedule. The experiment was designed around the following facts. (a) Food-motivated, variable-interval responding is characterized by a monotonically decreasing IRT distribution (Anger, 1956). (b) Variable-interval responding increases or decreases under amphetamine, presumably as a function of the proportion of long and short IRT's in the control (saline or nondrug) sessions (Dews, 1958). (c) Food-motivated DRL schedules of reinforcement generate a characteristic bimodal IRT distribution, with one mode at the shortest recorded IRT interval, and a second mode at or near the minimum reinforceable IRT interval (Sidman, 1955, 1959). (d) Amphetamine causes an increase in over-all DRL response rate, accompanied by a shift in the second IRT mode toward shorter IRT's (Sidman, 1955, 1959).

In spite of the shifts toward shorter IRT's, DRL behavior under amphetamine shows evidence that *some* temporal discrimination is retained: The IRT distribution remains bimodal (Sidman, 1959). This is in line with Dews and Morse's (1961) argument; the disruption of timing behavior caused by amphetamine may be the simple result of shortening in long IRT's, or "motor excitation," and not a specific derangement of temporal discrimination.

The present experiment tests this notion under conditions of concurrent VI DRL reinforcement on two levers. If amphetamine similarly affects the IRT distributions of both response classes, it will confirm Dews and Morse's position.

METHOD.   The subjects were three adult, male, albino rats, deprived to 80% of free-feeding weight. The apparatus was a two-lever Foringer en-

---

[3] Dr. Ardie Lubin (personal communication) has given the name "disordinal interaction" to such cases.

closure, located in an air-conditioned, sound-resistant experimental room, and isolated from programming and recording equipment. The reinforcer was diluted condensed milk, delivered *via* a dipper which rested in the *down* position when not energized. A buzzer sounded throughout the dipper-operation, up-down cycle.

Following a day of magazine training, the animals were placed on a DRL 16-sec reinforcement schedule on one lever, and kept on this procedure for 54 daily sessions. The second lever was inoperative at this time. Beginning with the 25th session, *dl*-amphetamine sulfate ("Benzedrine") was administered intraperitoneally in physiological saline from time to time. At least two nondrug days intervened between drug administrations, and drug was never given oftener than twice in 1 week. Five saline sessions preceded the first drug session. Thereafter, a day of saline always preceded a day of amphetamine, and served as a control for drug observations. On all injection days, the animals were placed in the experimental apparatus and the session begun immediately following injection.

Drug dosages from 0.5 mg/kg to 2.5 mg/kg were given in mixed order during this stage of the experiment. Finally, a single dosage was selected for each animal which produced easily observable, but not extreme, behavioral effects. For Rats No. 1 and No. 3, this dosage was 1.0 mg/kg; and for Rat No. 2, it was 1.5 mg/kg. Only this "moderate" dosage was used thereafter, in this and succeeding stages of the experiment.

Following the 54th session on DRL 16, a concurrent, 3-min, variable-interval schedule of food reinforcement was introduced on the second lever. Amphetamine was administered twice during concurrent VI 3 DRL 16, on the 24th and 28th daily sessions of the new procedure.

After the 28th session on concurrent VI 3 DRL 16, the schedule on the second lever was changed to VI 1 min, and amphetamine was administered twice, on the 30th and 35th sessions of this final procedure.

Saline and noninjection sessions were run until 150 food reinforcements had been given; drug sessions were run either to 150 reinforcements or until 100 min had elapsed, whichever occurred first.

RESULTS. Figure 1 shows saline and drug IRT distributions under the DRL schedule, for each stage of the experiment. The distributions were computed from the data of complete sessions. No systematic differences in the IRT distributions as a function of pairing with a concurrent VI schedule were apparent in these sessions.[4]

In all cases, the effect of drug was to shift the IRT distributions toward shorter intervals. Temporal patterning of DRL responses was not completely lost, however. In most of the drug IRT distributions in Fig. 1, the responses tended to be spaced farther apart than the minimum (0–4 sec)

[4] Interactions between the components of a concurrent VI DRL schedule occur early in exposure to the schedule (Segal, 1961), but disappear after prolonged exposure.

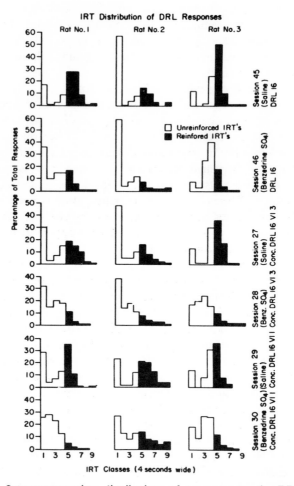

FIGURE 1. Inter-response-time distributions of responses on the DRL lever for selected saline and drug sessions.

recorded interval. In fact, the proportion of DRL responses spaced less than 4 sec apart was not markedly affected by drug. Rather, the primary effect was on the proportion of responses spaced far enough apart to earn reinforcement, that is, 16 sec or more. These data support Dews and Morse (1961), who set the critical limits for amphetamine effects at IRT's longer than about 5 sec or shorter than about 1 sec.

Figure 2 shows saline and drug IRT distributions on the VI lever under concurrent VI 3 DRL 16 and concurrent VI 1 DRL 16. Again, the distributions were computed from data for complete sessions, and represent stabilized behavior after extended exposure to the experimental conditions.

The variable-interval reinforcement contingencies generated moderately

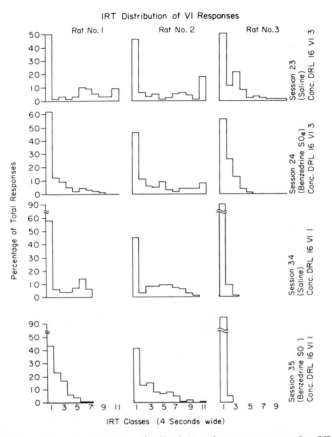

FIGURE 2. Inter-response-time distributions of responses on the VI lever for selected saline and drug sessions.

high rates of responding. This is reflected in the unimodal character of the IRT distributions, with the single mode at the shortest recorded IRT interval. The effect of amphetamine was a very slight shift to the left in the distributions. The proportion of responses at the shortest IRT interval was not markedly changed, but the proportion of responses spaced 4–12 sec apart was increased, relative to the proportion of still longer IRT's. These effects occurred for all animals, in spite of marked disparities between the characteristic forms of their respective IRT distributions. Again, the result confirms Dews and Morse's (1961) description of amphetamine action on VI responding.

Figure 3 shows frequency distributions of the number of responses occurring on the VI lever between each two consecutive responses on the DRL lever. These plots reflect patterning of switches *between* the two levers. The modes at zero VI responses between two consecutive DRL responses are the consequence of fast "bursts" of DRL responses.

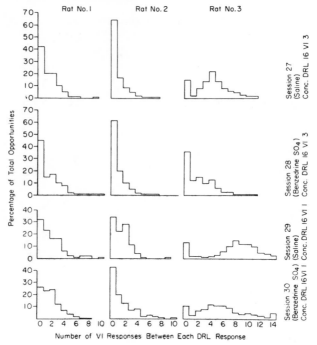

FIGURE 3. Frequency distributions showing number of responses on the VI lever between each two consecutive responses on the DRL lever, for selected saline and drug sessions.

Whatever the pattern of responding between the two levers for individual animals, it was relatively unaffected by amphetamine. The records for Rats No. 1 and No. 2 show no marked differences between saline and drug days. However, Rat No. 3 shifted slightly toward fewer VI responses between DRL responses under drug.

Table 1 shows the changes in rate of bar pressing on each lever as a result of amphetamine, expressed as a ratio of the rate on the drug day to the rate on the preceding saline day [what Dews (1955) has called the "output ratio"]. The rates in the computations were not corrected for eating time. Ratios above 1.00 indicate drug-induced increases in response rate, and ratios below 1.00 indicate drug-induced decreases. For the first stage of the experiment, simple DRL on one lever, only the results for the reinforced, DRL lever are shown.

Of the 27 ratios computed, 22 reflect drug-induced rate increases of at least 22%; 3 reflect increases of 7–9%; and 2 reflect rate decreases of 4–6%. Rate changes under 10% may reasonably be dismissed as insignificant, leaving the conclusion that at the dosages given, amphetamine either increased over-all response rates or left them unaffected. The drug produced no significant decreases in rate.

TABLE 1. Ratio of bar-pressing rate under *dl*-amphetamine to bar-pressing rate on the preceding physiological saline session ("output ratio").

Procedure	Rat No. 1		Rat No. 2		Rat No. 3	
	DRL Lever	VI Lever	DRL Lever	VI Lever	DRL Lever	VI Lever
DRL 16: Drug, Session 46 / Saline, Session 45	1.96	—	1.27	—	1.29	—
VI 3 DRL 16: Drug, Session 24 / Saline, Session 23	1.51	2.57	1.33	1.42	1.22	1.52
Drug, Session 28 / Saline, Session 27	1.60	1.83	1.07	1.07	1.50	0.94
VI 1 DRL 16: Drug, Session 30 / Saline, Session 29	1.71	1.72	1.27	1.29	1.37	1.09
Drug, Session 35 / Saline, Session 34	1.38	1.34	1.40	1.23	1.40	0.96

There was no systematic interaction of the drug effect with the schedule of reinforcement. For the most part, drug increased rates of bar pressing about as much or as little under simple DRL and concurrent VI DRL.

Incidental observation of the animals during drug sessions indicated that they did not always drink the milk reinforcer on these days. Yet, responding continued unabated throughout drug sessions. No failures to consume the milk on nondrug days were noted. These observations confirm the many previous reports of reduced consumption of freely available food (Dews and Morse, 1961), as well as reports of failures to consume liquid food reinforcers in a bar-pressing apparatus under amphetamine (Teitelbaum and Derks, 1958; Weissman, 1959).

DISCUSSION. The data confirm previous findings that some temporal discrimination is retained under amphetamine. Even under drug, the temporal patterning of responses on the two levers continued to be markedly different. The VI responding, which showed no temporal spacing under saline, *a fortiori* showed none under drug. The DRL responding, which did show temporal patterning under saline, continued to show it under drug, although the efficiency of temporal spacing with respect to the reinforcement contingencies was impaired.

The finding that amphetamine affected response rates on the two components of the concurrent schedule about equally indicates that the main effect of the drug was apparently a motor excitatory one, and not a specific disruption of some *internal* timing mechanism. This is completely consistent with Dews and Morse's (1961) contention that amphetamine simply reduces the long IRT's of DRL (and other) reinforcement schedules.

The precise mediating factors in temporal discrimination are not well understood. The present findings support the interpretation that other overt behavior, consisting of some regular cycle performance, may intervene between DRL responses and mediate the temporal spacing of DRL responding. The fact that the pattern of responding *between* the two levers was relatively unaffected by amphetamine is consistent with such an interpretation: The cycle of behavior on the two levers, including switching between them, was simply run off faster under drug. To the extent that *overt* behavior mediates timing behavior, then amphetamine may be said to disrupt temporal discrimination. But this is a secondary effect, produced not by interference with an internal timing mechanism, but rather by increasing the rate of emission of all overt behavior.

Of course, internal timing mechanisms still may exist. Brady and Conrad (1960) have demonstrated that intracranial self-stimulation (ICS) of the globus pallidus causes an interference with timing behavior similar to that produced by amphetamine. Moreover, their data strongly suggest a precisely localized neural timing mechanism, because ICS in the medial forebrain bundle (MFB) or the thalamus did not share the disruptive effect of globus pallidus stimulation on DRL performance.

The fact that DRL behavior is similarly disrupted by amphetamine and by ICS in the globus pallidus does not argue that the mode or site of action of these two treatments is necessarily the same. On the contrary, several lines of evidence make such a conclusion dubious. Miller (1957) has reported that amphetamine increases the speed of bar pressing to turn on ICS of the MFB, at the same time decreasing speed of bar pressing to turn off the stimulation. Two investigators (reviewed in Dews and Morse, 1961) have found that amphetamine-induced suppression of feeding is exaggerated in hypothalamic hyperphagics. Finally, Brady and Conrad (1960) report that the rate of VI (*but not DRL*) responding is higher when the reinforcement is MFB stimulation that when it is sugar pellets. Taken together, these findings suggest that amphetamine's neural action may be upon motivational mechanisms located in the hypothalamus. They offer no evidence of an amphetamine effect directly on the globus pallidus, where Brady and Conrad have localized a timing mechanism. These data do not strictly rule out the possibility that amphetamine may act upon the hypothalamus *via* the basal ganglia, but neither do they provide any support for such a contention. On present evidence, then, amphetamine action and timing mechanism appear to be neurally independent.

The failure of food consumption in the apparatus on drug days may be interpreted either as a reduction in "hunger motivation," or as a result of the motor excitation induced by amphetamine: The animals may have been "too busy" pressing the levers to respond promptly and efficiently to the sound of the buzzer associated with the brief availability of the milk dipper in the *up* position. As mentioned earlier, it is not likely that the effect is on simple discriminative capacity, but it might represent a derangement in "attention."

SUMMARY. Three adult, food-deprived rats were given IP injections of *dl*-amphetamine sulfate under DRL and concurrent VI DRL reinforcement schedules. The drug results were as follows.

(1) The IRT distributions of DRL responses shifted to the left, but some temporal discrimination remained. (2) The IRT distributions of VI responses shifted slightly to the left. (3) The distinguishing characteristics of VI and DRL IRT distributions were preserved. (4) The frequency distribution of number of VI responses between two consecutive DRL responses was relatively unaffected. (5) Over-all response rates on the two components of the concurrent schedules increased more or less proportionately.

These findings imply that the primary behavioral effect of *dl*-amphetamine was a motor excitatory one. The drug's disruption of timing behavior was not due to a derangement of internal timing mechanisms, nor to interference with the topography or pattern of behavior. Rather, it might be a secondary result of the accelerated emission of overt behavior patterns mediating the temporal spacing of DRL bar presses.

REFERENCES

Anger, D. The dependence of inter-response-times upon the relative reinforcement of different inter-response-times. *J. exp. Psychol,* 1956, **52**, 145–161.

Bindra, D. Components of general activity and the analysis of behavior. *Psychol. Rev.* 1961, **68**, 205–215.

Brady, J. V. A review of comparative behavioral pharmacology. *Ann. N.Y. Acad. Sci.,* 1957, **66**, 719–732.

Brady, J. V., and Conrad, D. G. Some effects of brain stimulation on timing behavior. *J. exp. Anal. Behav.* 1960, 3, 93–106.

Dews, P. B. Studies on behavior. II. The effects of pentobarbital, methamphetamine and scopolamine on performances in pigeons involving discriminations. *J. pharmacol. exp. Therap.* 1955, **115**, 380–389.

Dews, P. B. Studies on behavior. IV. Stimulant actions of methamphetamine. *J. pharmacol. exp. Therap.* 1958, **122**, 137–147.

Dews, P. B. Free-operant behavior under conditions of delayed reinforcement. I. CRF-type schedules. *J. exp. Anal. Behav.,* 1960, 3, 221–234.

Dews, P. B., and Morse, W. H. Some observations on an operant in human subjects and its modification by dextroamphetamine. *J. exp. Anal. Behav.,* 1958, 1, 359–364.

Dews, P. B., and Morse, W. H. Behavioral pharmacology. *Ann. Rev. Pharmacol.,* 1961, 1, 145–174.

Herrnstein, R. J. Stereotypy and intermittent reinforcement. *Science,* 1961, **133**, 2067–2069.

Millenson, J. R., and Hurwitz, H. M. B. Some temporal and sequential properties of behavior during conditioning and extinction. *J. exp. Anal. Behav.*, 1961, **4**, 97–106.

Miller, N. E. Effects of drugs on motivation: The value of using a variety of measures. *Ann. N.Y. Acad. Sci.*, 1956, **65**, 318–333.

Miller, N. E. Experiments on motivation. *Science*, 1957, **126**, 1271–1278.

Morse, W. H., and Herrnstein, R. J. Effects of drugs on characteristics of behavior maintained by complex schedules of intermittent positive reinforcement. *Ann. N.Y. Acad. Sci.*, 1956, **65**, 303–317.

Notterman, J. M. Force emission during bar pressing. *J. exp. Psychol.*, 1959, **58**, 341–347.

Owen, J. E., Jr. The influence of *dl-*, *d-*, and *l*-amphetamine and *d*-methamphetamine on a fixed-ratio schedule. *J. exp. Anal. Behav.*, 1960, **3**, 293–310.

Premack, D. Toward empirical behavior laws. I. Positive reinforcement. *Psychol. Rev.*, 1959, **66**, 219–233.

Premack, D. Predicting instrumental performance from the independent rate of the contingent response. *J. exp. Psychol.*, 1961, **61**, 163–171.

Premack, D., and Collier, G. Analysis of nonreinforcement variables affecting response probability. *Psychol. Monogr.*, 1962, **76**, Whole No. 524.

Segal, Evalyn F. Confirmation of a positive relation between deprivation and number of responses emitted for light reinforcement. *J. exp. Anal. Behav.*, 1959, **2**, 165–169.

Segal, Evalyn F. Behavioral interaction under concurrent spaced-responding, variable-interval schedules of reinforcement. *J. exp. Anal. Behav.*, 1961, **4**, 263–266.

Sidman, M. Technique for assessing the effects of drugs on timing behavior. *Science*, 1955, **122**, 925.

Sidman, M. Time discrimination and behavioral interaction in a free operant situation. *J. comp. physiol. Psychol.*, 1956, **49**, 469–473. (a)

Sidman, M. Drug-behavior interaction. *Ann. N.Y. Acad. Sci.*, 1956, **65**, 282–302. (b)

Sidman, M. Behavioral pharmacology. *Psychopharmacologia*, 1959, **1**, 1–19

Skinner, B. F., and Heron, W. T. Effects of caffeine and Benzedrine upon conditioning and extinction. *Psychol. Rec.*, 1937, **1**, 340–346.

Teitelbaum, P., and Derks, P. The effect of amphetamine on forced drinking in the rat. *J. comp. physiol. Psychol.*, 1958, **51**, 801–810.

Verhave, T. The effect of methamphetamine on operant level and avoidance behavior. *J. exp. Anal. Behav.*, 1958, **1**, 207–219.

Weissman, A. Differential drug effects upon a three-ply multiple schedule of reinforcement. *J. exp. Anal. Behav.*, 1959, **2**, 271–287.

Wentink, E. The effects of certain drugs and hormones upon conditioning. *J. exp. Psychol.*, 1938, **22**, 150–163.

54

Some observations on an operant in human subjects
and its modification by *d*-amphetamine [1]

PETER B. DEWS and WILLIAM H. MORSE

This paper describes an experiment in which the response of pressing a telegraph key by normal human subjects led to the delivery of nickels under contingencies which combined features of both fixed-ratio and DRL [2] schedules of reinforcement. In this schedule the reinforcing stimuli (delivery of nickels) are presented each *nth* time a response occurs which follows the immediately preceding response by at least *x* seconds. Responses which occur within less than *x* seconds since the preceding response merely start a new inter-response time, and do not count toward the completion of the *n* responses. The schedule stands in the same relation to a simple DRL as does FR to *crf*.[3]

Studies with animals (Dews, 1958; Morse and Herrnstein, 1956; Sidman, 1955) have suggested that the effects of the amphetamines are likely to be seen best when responses occur relatively infrequently. The above schedule would be expected to, and in fact did, give a low rate of responding. It was therefore used in an exploratory experiment to determine whether this operant behavior of normal subjects would be consistently modified by small doses (5 milligrams) of *d*-amphetamine sulfate.

METHOD. A telegraph key was mounted on a wooden base. Immediately behind the key was a box (12 by 12 by 24 inches) which enclosed a coin vending machine. The coin machine was a modified "change maker" such as used in soft-drink dispensers, and was set to deliver four nickels when pulsed. The apparatus was set on a bench so that a subject could sit with his arm resting comfortably on the bench and his hand on or near the

From *Journal of the Expermiental Analysis of Behavior,* 1958, 1, 359–364. Copyright 1958 by the Society for the Experimental Analysis of Behavior, Inc., Bloomington, Ind.

[1] This research was supported by grants from the U.S. Public Health Service (M 1226) and from Burroughs-Wellcome & Co. The *d*-amphetamine and placebo tablets were kindly supplied by Smith, Kline & French laboratories.

[2] Following contemporary usage, we modify Ferster and Skinner's (1957) terminology by using the term DRL in place of *crf drl*.

[3] This schedule may be alternatively described as fixed-ratio reinforcement of responses, each of which concludes an inter-response time exceeding a minimum value (i.e., a fixed ratio of responses meeting a "DRL contingency," or as a tandem DRL DRL DRL . . . DRL.

key. The nickels were ejected towards the subject through an orifice in the front of the box. Also in the front of the box were two 6-watt pilot lamps, one lighted for the duration of the experimental session, and the other lighted only during the delivery of nickels.

The basic schedule has been described already. Two pairs of values for the schedule parameters n and x were used. In one pair, n was 100 and x seconds was 2.5 seconds; for the other pair, n was 10 and x seconds was 25 seconds. The distribution of inter-response times was recorded automatically, with class intervals of 0.5 second or 5 seconds depending upon whether the required delay was 2.5 seconds or 25 seconds, respectively.

Subjects were seven male medical students. Each subject was alone in the experimental room during the session. The programming equipment was in a different room, separated from the experimental room by an intervening room, and its operation was inaudible to the subject. The subject was introduced into the experimental room, and then a tape recording of the following message was played:

The experiment begins when the light on the left comes on and finishes when it goes off, one hour later. During the experiment you are to push the telegraph key. Your object is to obtain as many nickels as possible. The light on the right will come on and nickels will be delivered to you when you have pressed the key a minimum of 100 times. However, presses made within two and one-half seconds of a previous press will *not* count. On the other hand, any time you wait beyond two and one-half seconds is wasted time. To obtain as many nickels as possible you should therefore press the key regularly at intervals as little as possible in excess of two and one-half seconds. The following sequence of clicks occur at intervals of two and one-half seconds. [Then followed 8 clicks at 2.5-second intervals.] Start pressing the key as soon as the light on the left comes on.

When the other pair of parameter values was in operation, a similar message was played, except that the references to 100 responses and 2.5 seconds were changed to 10 responses and 25 seconds, respectively.

Five subjects were studied at each of the two pairs of values for the parameters. (Although seven subjects were studied, only three were observed at both parameter values.) The results to be presented are for a "control" day and a "drug" day. Observations were made during a period of 1 hour and were at weekly intervals for individual subjects. On the "drug" days (which sometimes preceded and sometimes succeeded the "control" days), the subject was given a small orange tablet containing 5 milligrams of d-amphetamine. He swallowed it under direct observation and then drank 150 milliliters of water. One-half hour later the experimental session was started. On control days, an identical routine was followed except that the tablet swallowed contained no pharmacologically active ingredients. All subjects had been exposed to the schedule for at least one session before either the control or drug day. Preliminary experimentation suggested that there was no consistent trend in the performance after the initial session on each procedure.

RESULTS.   Figure 1 shows mean inter-response-time distributions for five subjects at both parameter values. The unbroken lines give the average distribution for "control" days and the dotted lines are for the "drug" days. Sample cumulative records of daily sessions for individual subjects are shown in Fig. 2 and 3. For each pair of parameter values, a control and a drug session are shown for two subjects.

Control performance.   The form of the distribution of inter-response times (i.e., the population of intervals between consecutive responses) was similar for all subjects and at both parameter values. The distributions were skewed to the right, with a peak in the class interval just in excess of the minimum "effective" delay value. For individual subjects, the mode was in the class interval 2.5 to 3.0 seconds on all but one occasion, when the "required" delay was 2.5 seconds; and in the class interval 25 to 30 seconds, on all but one occasion, when the "required" delay was 25 seconds.

The subjects performed "more efficiently" when the delay was 25 seconds than when it was 2.5 seconds in that they (a) obtained more nickel

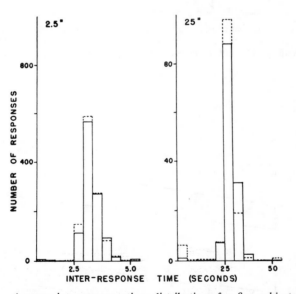

FIGURE 1.   Average inter-response-time distributions for five subjects. In the portion of the figure labeled 2.5″, the 100th response which followed the immediately preceding response by at least 2.5 seconds was reinforced. In the portion labeled 25″, the 10th response which followed the immediately preceding response by at least 25 seconds was reinforced. The solid lines show the average distributions following a placebo; the dotted lines show the average distributions following 5 milligrams of *d*-amphetamine.

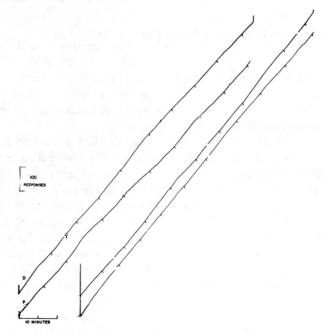

FIGURE 2. Cumulative-response records for two human subjects. The 100th response which follows the immediately preceding response by at least 2.5 seconds is reinforced. A drug (D) and a placebo (P) record is shown for each subject.

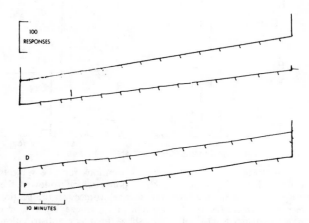

FIGURE 3. Cumulative-response records for two human subjects. The 10th response which follows the immediately preceding response by at least 25 seconds is reinforced. A drug (D) and a placebo (P) record is shown for each subject.

deliveries on the average (11.8 vs. 9.0); (b) the proportion of responses in the class interval just in excess of the minimum delay was greater (0.67 vs. 0.54); and (c) the coefficient of variation [4] of the inter-response times was less (0.10 vs. 0.20), i.e., they were "steadier." The latter effect is best seen in the sample cumulative records. In contrast to the steady rate maintained when the parameter values were 10 responses and 25 seconds, the prevailing rate fluctuated gradually up and down during the session when the values were 100 responses and 2.5 seconds.

Effect of d-*amphetamine.*   On days when 5 milligrams of *d*-amphetamine had been given, the inter-response times tended to be shorter than when placebo had been given. Although the mean number of responses emitted during the session increased slightly following the drug (an increase from 1067 to 1120 responses during the hour session on the 2.5-second delay, and an increase from 130 to 135 responses during the hour session on the 25-second delay), the effect is better seen in the distributions of inter-response times. That is, the form of the distribution was changed more consistently than the total number of responses. In Fig. 1, the average distributions based on the drug sessions are shifted to the left for both sets of parameter values. The changes in both distributions are statistically significant by x^2, and all but one subject showed the effect. The average number of reinforcements was not changed at all by the drug (an average of 10.4 reinforcements under both conditions on control days and 10.5 reinforcements on drug days), nor was the variability in the inter-response-time distributions, as measured by the coefficient of variation.

DISCUSSION AND SUMMARY.   The subjects in this experiment obtained between 80 and 90% of the number of nickels that were theoretically possible in the time available, which is a higher percentage of "effective" responses than is ordinarily obtained using a DRL schedule in animals. Compared with other published distributions of inter-response times from DRL schedules, the peaks in these distributions at the class interval just exceeding the DRL requirement are more pronounced. In animals working on a DRL schedule, a considerable proportion of responses occur following very short inter-response times (Sidman, 1955). Holland (1958) has seen this phenomenon, commonly called "bursts," in human subjects. In our subjects, however, bursts were uncommon, although by no means absent. (See Fig. 1.)

There are several possible reasons for the differences between these inter-response-time distributions and those ordinarily obtained with animals.

1. The subjects were verbally informed as to the nature of the schedule,

[4] Means and standard deviations of the distributions in Fig. 1. were obtained by multiplying the number of responses in each class interval by the mid-point of the class interval. However, since interresponse times are not interdependent observations, these statistics should be used only for descriptive purposes.

and, further, were given samples of the interval they were to "aim for" before each session. They were not discouraged from "counting to themselves," and, in fact, all subjects developed a counting sequence which led up to the response.

2. Although our subjects could earn about $2.00 in the hour session, it is by no means clear to what extent the delivery of four nickels to a medical student is comparable with the delivery of food or water to a severely deprived animal.

3. The change from DRL to a schedule requiring a number of minimum inter-response times per reinforcement may have increased the control of the contingencies of the schedule, but this is unlikely as an explanation since pigeons working on comparable schedules show bursts just as they do on a simple DRL schedule (unpublished).

The effects of d-amphetamine were consistent with the results obtained with experiments on animals (Dews, 1958; Sidman, 1955). The inter-response-time distributions were shifted in the direction of shorter inter-response times. It should be noted, however, that the number of reinforcements obtained was not different for the control days and the drug days.

REFERENCES

Dews, P. B. Studies on behavior. IV. Stimulant actions of methamphetamine. *J. Pharmacol. Exptl. Therap.*, 1958, **122**, 137–147.

Ferster, C. B., and Skinner, B. F. *Schedules of reinforcement.* New York: Appleton-Century-Crofts, 1957.

Holland, J. G. Human vigilance. *Science,* 1958, **128**, 61–67.

Morse, W. H., and Herrnstein, R. J. Effects of drugs on characteristics of behavior maintained by complex schedules of intermittent positive reinforcement. *Ann. N.Y. Acad. Sci.,* 1956, **65**, 303–317.

Sidman, M. Technique for assessing the effects of drugs on timing behavior. *Science,* 1955, **122**, 925.

55

Adjusting fixed-ratio schedules in the squirrel monkey

ROGER T. KELLEHER,[1] WILLIAM FRY, and LEONARD COOK

On fixed-ratio (FR) schedules of reinforcement, the animal is reinforced whenever it completes a specified number of responses (the response requirement). Performance on FR schedules is characterized by an initial pause followed by an abrupt change to a high response rate maintained until reinforcement; the average duration of the initial pause is directly related to the FR response requirement (Ferster and Skinner, 1957). The phenomenon of long initial pauses at large response requirements is called ratio strain.

On an adjusting FR schedule of reinforcement, the response requirement is varied as a function of the animal's performance. For example, Ferster and Skinner (1957) described an adjusting FR schedule in which the response requirement was varied as a function of the initial pause in each ratio. During the initial pause, the response requirement slowly decreased; the first response increased the requirement by five responses. If initial pauses were long, the FR response requirement would be low; however, the frequency of reinforcement would be limited by the duration of the initial pauses. If the animal continuously responded at a high rate, the frequency of reinforcement would be high at a given response requirement; however, the response requirement would be continually increasing. The birds did not go to either of these extremes. Each pigeon adjusted to FR response requirements of about 400 responses without developing prolonged initial pauses.

An adjusting schedule can be considered as comprising two component schedules. For example, an adjusting FR schedule comprises both the basic FR schedule of primary reinforcement and the schedule that varies some parameter of the FR schedule. Ferster and Skinner (1957) noted that in their adjusting FR schedule, the schedule that varied the FR value had some of the characteristics of an interval schedule; *i.e.,* the probability of reinforcement increased as a function of time since the previous reinforcement.

From *Journal of the Experimental Analysis of Behavior,* 1964, 7, 69–77. Copyright 1964 by the Society for the Experimental Analysis of Behavior, Inc., Bloomington, Ind.

[1] Preparation of this article by the first author was supported in part by Research Grants M-2094 and MY-2645 from the Institute of Mental Health of the National Institutes of Health, U.S. Public Health Service. The work described was supported and carried out at Smith Kline and French Laboratories.

The purpose of the present experiments was to analyze adjusting FR schedules of the type described by Ferster and Skinner (1957) in terms of their component schedules. The results suggest that this type of adjusting schedule can be considered as a second-order schedule in which FR performance is reinforced according to a DRL schedule.

METHOD

SUBJECTS. Three male squirrel monkeys (Ss) were maintained at 75 to 80 per cent of their free-feeding weights, which ranged from 603 to 648 g. The Ss had previously been trained on ratio schedules ranging up to FR 200.

APPARATUS. The 9 by 9 by 7.5 in. experimental chamber was enclosed in a picnic icebox; the icebox was enclosed in a large ventilated chamber that almost completely attenuated extraneous sounds (Gill, Fry, and Kelleher, 1962). An aluminum lever [2] was mounted in the wall of the experimental chamber. When S pressed the lever with a force of 14 g or more, a response was recorded. During experimental sessions, two 6-w lamps provided general illumination, and each response produced the audible click of a relay. The reinforcement was 8-sec access to 0.5 cc of liquid food (Herndon, Greenberg, Van Loon, Kelleher, Cook, and Davidson, 1958). A solenoid operated dipper delivered the food to a small recessed cubicle below and to the right of the lever. During reinforcement, the experimental chamber was dark, while the recessed cubicle was illuminated by a 6-w lamp.

GENERAL PROCEDURE. Experimental sessions were conducted daily from Monday through Friday. On weekends, supplementary feedings maintained Ss at appropriate body weights. Water was continuously available in the home cage and in the experimental chamber. Durations of the daily sessions were 3 hr for Monkeys K38 and K14 and 5 hr for Monkey K12.

EXPERIMENT I. The purpose of this experiment was to determine the FR value to which Ss would adjust as a function of the specified duration of the initial pause.

Procedure. The FR response requirement could range from a minimum of 10 to a maximum of 1,000, taking the following arbitrarily chosen intermediate values: 50, 100, 110, 130, 160, 200, 250, 310, 380, 460, 550, 650, 750, and 870. The response requirement increased whenever two successive initial pauses were shorter than the specified duration. The re-

---

[2] The lever was manufactured by Lehigh Valley Electronics, Allentown, Pa. (LVE 1352 rat lever).

TABLE 1.   Sessions in which different required pause times (min.) were in effect in Experiment I.

Sessions	Required Pause	Sessions	Required Pause
1-17	2	42-78	4
18-27	1	79-87	2
28-33	4	88-104	1
34-41	8	105-127	15

sponse requirement remained constant if initial pauses shorter than the specified duration alternated with initial pauses longer than the specified duration. The response requirement decreased whenever two successive initial pauses were longer than the specified duration; however, at FR 1,000 a single pause longer than the specified duration decreased the response requirement to FR 870. Each session started at FR 10. Required initial pause durations (required pauses) of 1, 2, 4, 8, and 15 min were studied. The number of sessions at each required pause are shown in Table 1.

Results.   The cumulative response records in Fig. 1 show representative performances for Monkey K38 at various required pauses. The required

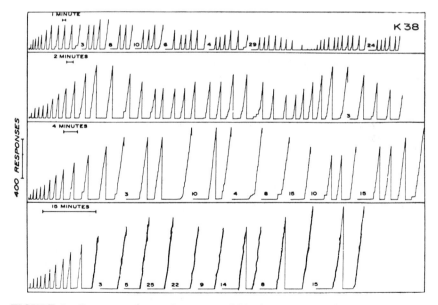

FIGURE 1.   Representative performances of Monkey K38 at various required pause times; the required pause times are indicated in each frame of the figure. The ratio values could range from FR 10 to FR 1,000; each session started at FR 10. Where the records are broken, the numbers indicate the minutes of pausing that have been omitted from the record. The recording pen reset to the bottom of the record following each reinforcement; the recorder did not run during reinforcement.

pause for each record is indicated by the scale at the upper left of each frame of the figure. For example, in the upper frame of Fig. 1, the required pause was 1 min. Each of the first eight reinforcements in the session shown in this frame were obtained before an initial pause exceeded 1 min. Thus, the response requirement increased from FR 10 for the first reinforcement to FR 250 for the eighth reinforcement. Then, the response requirement remained at FR 250 for several reinforcements because initial pauses of more than 1 min alternated with initial pauses of less than 1 min. In a later part of this record, successive initial pauses of more than 1 min reduced the response requirement to FR 10 again.

As shown in Fig. 1, at the start of each session the response requirements increased rapidly until a relatively large response requirement was in effect. For the remainder of each session, there were cycles of decreasing and increasing response requirements. As the required pause was increased, however, higher maximum response requirements were reached early in each session, and fewer pauses exceeded the required pause. Note that many of the record segments have a step-like appearance.

Figure 2 shows representative performances for Monkey K12. In general, these records are similar to those of Monkey K38. In the records of Monkey K12, however, the step-like appearance of many ratio segments is more apparent (as at *a, b, c,* and *d*). This resulted from runs of responses at a very high rate alternating with brief pauses.

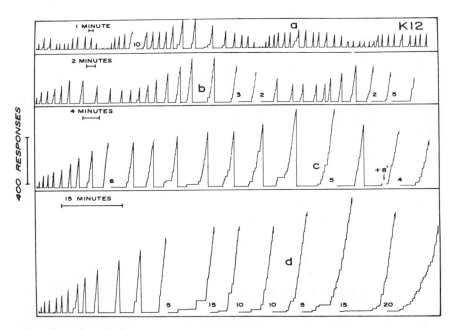

FIGURE 2.   Representative performances of Monkey K12 at required pause times ranging from 1 to 15 min.

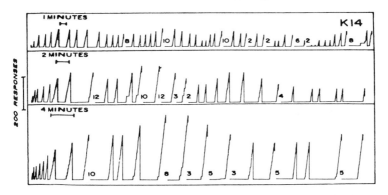

FIGURE 3.   Representative performances of Monkey K14 at required pause times ranging from 1 to 4 min.

Figures 3 and 4 show representative performances for Monkey K14. At required pauses ranging from 1 min to 15 min, the performances of Monkey K14 were similar to those of other animals. At the required pause of 15 min, however, Monkey K14 characteristically paused briefly following reinforcement and then responded at a stable rate of about 40 responses per min. Because of this response pattern, Monkey K14 maintained FR 1,000 throughout most of each session.

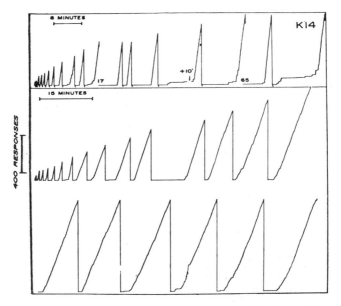

FIGURE 4.   Representative performances of Monkey K14 at required pause times of 8 and 15 min.

Procedure. The ratio value was held constant in each session. When the initial pause was longer than a required pause, the ratio terminated with reinforcement. When the initial pause was shorter than the required pause, the ratio terminated with a 0.5 sec time-out (dark experimental chamber). Required pauses of 1 min and 2 min were studied at FR 200; ratio values of FR 100, FR 200, and FR 300 were studied at a 2 min required pause. The procedure is summarized in Table 3.

Meprobamate was orally administered to Monkeys K38 and K14 just before Session 34 and to Monkey K12 just before Session 42. Previous results had shown that a dose of 50 mg/kg would increase the response rates of monkeys on simple DRL schedules. The drug was suspended in a 0.5 per cent gum tragacanth solution. The volume of solution administered was always less than 1 ml. Comparable volumes of gum tragacanth solution were administered just before the preceding session (control).

Results. The results for Monkey K38 are presented in detail to show both transitional effects and final performances. Figure 6 shows performance on FR 200 with required pauses of 1 min and 2 min. The recording pen reset to the bottom of the record at the completion of each ratio. The small solid circles at the top of some record segments indicate reinforcements. Beginning in Session 4, the duration of the initial pause in each ratio was recorded, and pause time distributions were computed for each session.

The relative frequencies of different pause times are shown in the histograms at the left of each cumulative response record. In the upper frame of Fig. 6, the first 10 bars of the histogram represent 6-sec class intervals (6″ CI). The eleventh bar indicates the relative frequency of initial pauses of more than 1-min and corresponds to the relative frequency of reinforced ratios. In Session 4, only about 35 per cent of the ratios have initial pauses of more than 1 min. By Session 7, however, more than 80 per cent of the initial pauses were longer than 1 min. Although the histogram does not indicate the actual durations of the pauses of more than 1 min, inspection of cumulative response records from Session 7 indicated that they ranged up to 2 min.

In Sessions 8 to 17, FR 200 was still in effect but the required pause was increased to 2 min. In the lower frame of Fig. 6 each of the first 10 bars of

TABLE 3.   Sessions in which different required pause times and FR values were in effect in Experiment II.

Session	Required Pause (Min.)	FR
1-7	1	200
8-17	2	200
18-23	2	300
24-42	2	100

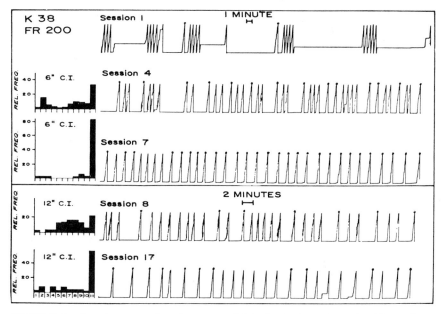

FIGURE 6.   Development of performance of Monkey K38 at FR 200 with required pauses of 1 min (upper frame) and 2 min (lower frame). The solid circles indicate ratios that were reinforced; the other ratios were terminated by a 0.5-sec time-out. The recorder did not run during time-outs or reinforcements. The relative frequencies of different initial pause times are shown in the histogram at left. The class intervals are shown above each histogram.

the histogram represent 12-sec class intervals; the eleventh bar shows the relative frequency of pauses of more than 2 min. The relative frequency distribution for Session 8 is bi-modal. The mode between 1 and 2 min suggests persistence of the response pattern that had developed at the 1-min required pause. The mode at more than 2 min indicates that the response pattern was changing, probably because the frequency of reinforcement in Session 8 was lower than in Session 7. In Session 17 about 58 per cent of the pauses were longer than 2 min; inspection of the cumulative response records indicated that pauses ranged up to 2.5 min.

In Sessions 18 to 23 the required pause was held at 2 min; however, the response requirement was increased to FR 300. Results from Sessions 18 and 23 are shown in the upper frame of Fig. 7. An increase in the relative frequency of pauses longer than 2 min occurred in Session 18. By Session 23 almost all initial pauses exceeded 2 min; inspection of the cumulative response records indicated that these pauses actually ranged up to 3 min.

In Sessions 24 to 42 the required pause was held at 2 min, and the response requirement was decreased to FR 100. The results are shown in the lower frame of Fig. 7. In Sessions 24 and 25 the S frequently completed two or three ratios in rapid succession. By Session 40, the ratios were more

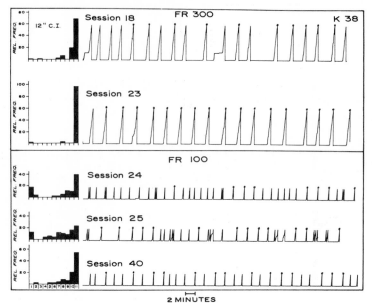

FIGURE 7.   Development of performance of Monkey 38 with a required pause of 2 min at FR 300 (upper frame) and FR 100 (lower frame).

evenly spaced; however, many initial pauses ranged from 72 sec to 119 sec. The relative frequency of reinforced ratios ranged from 25 to 60 per cent in different sessions. Results obtained with Monkeys K12 and K14 were generally comparable; however, Monkey K14 occasionally responded at intermediate rates (see control records in Fig. 9 and 10).

Figures 8, 9, and 10 show the effects of meprobamate on the performance of each S. In each figure, a comparison of the cumulative response records and pause time distributions in the upper and lower frames shows that meprobamate increased average response rates by decreasing the durations of initial pauses.

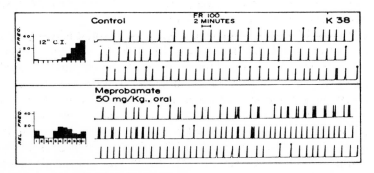

FIGURE 8.   The effects of meprobamate on the performance of Monkey K38 at FR 100 with a required pause of 2 min.

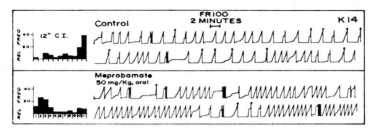

FIGURE 9.   The effects of meprobamate on the performance of Monkey K14.

Discussion.   On DRL schedules there is a required pause between single responses; the relative frequency of pauses longer than the required pause is inversely related to the length of the required pause. Although there is no required pause on FR schedules, the average durations of initial pauses are directly related to the size of the ratio. On the adjusting FR schedule used in Exp. II there was a required pause between ratios; *i.e.,* the FR was treated as a unit of behavior that was reinforced according to a DRL schedule. When the required pause was increased from 1 min to 2 min at FR 200, and when the ratio was increased from FR 200 to FR 300, the average duration of initial pauses increased. The opposite effect occurred when the ratio was decreased from FR 300 to FR 100.

The results of Exp. II support the notion that the adjusting FR schedule is a type of second-order schedule involving a combination of DRL and FR schedules. The characteristics of FR and DRL schedules suggest that, as the ratio value is increased at a given required pause, performances should be increasingly similar to performances on an FR schedule; as the ratio value is decreased, performances should be increasingly similar to those on

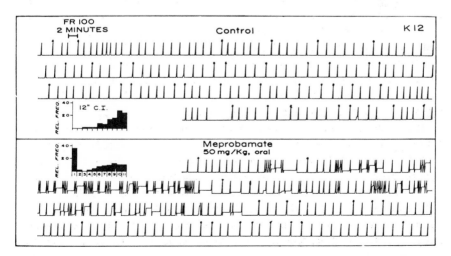

FIGURE 10.   The effects of meprobamate on the performance of Monkey K12.

a DRL schedule. (Of course, at the extreme value of FR 1, the adjusting FR schedule is identical with the DRL schedule.)

At FR 300 with a 2-min required pause, almost all initial pauses were longer than 2 min; however, at FR 100 with a 2-min required pause, there was a relatively high frequency of initial pauses shorter than 2 min. Presumably, as the ratio is decreased, the results are less influenced by ratio strain and more influenced by the required pause.

The results of Exp. II show, that as the ratio was decreased from FR 300 to FR 100, the relative frequency distributions of initial pause times became more similar to the distributions of interresponse times on DRL schedules. Nevertheless, the results suggest that the required pause was having an effect even at FR 300. It is characteristic of FR strain that the durations of the individual initial pauses are highly variable. In Exp. II, the initial pauses at FR 300 were relatively stable.

Meprobamate consistently decreased the durations of the initial pauses. This effect is qualitatively similar to the effects of meprobamate in increasing the relative frequency of short interresponse times in DRL schedules (Kelleher, Fry, Deegan, and Cook, 1961). The results obtained with meprobamate are consistent with the notion that the adjusting FR schedule is a second-order schedule in which the FR is a unit of behavior that is reinforced according to a DRL; however, there are no reported studies on the effects of meprobamate on initial pauses in ratios as large as FR 100. Thus, meprobamate might decrease pausing on both DRL and FR schedules.

There are many different types of adjusting schedule (*e.g.,* Lindsley, 1957; Weiss and Laties, 1959; Boren and Malis, 1961; Stein and Ray, 1959, 1960); they have the common characteristic that some parameter of a basic schedule of reinforcement is varied as a function of the animal's performance. Although performances on adjusting schedules are sometimes discussed in terms of thresholds, it is usually found that the threshold value depends upon the parameter values of the adjusting schedule. (Weiss and Laties, 1959; Boren and Malis, 1961.) Also, most adjusting schedules can be considered as combinations of other schedules. The present results suggest that the characteristics of these component schedules may be critical, especially when the effects of drugs are being studied with an adjusting schedule (*cf.* Boren and Malis, 1961).

The notion that adjusting schedules are combinations of other schedules also suggests new techniques for the analysis of basic schedules of reinforcement. In Exp. II, for example, we can consider the FR schedule as a unit of behavior that is itself on a DRL schedule of reinforcement. The functional relationships obtained with FR 100 as the unit of behavior are similar to those obtained when a single response is the unit of behavior. The size of the ratio does affect the results; this effect may be similar to changing the amount of effort required for a single response. Further studies with the type of second-order schedule used in Exp. II should advance understanding of both DRL and FR schedules.

It is apparent that there are many possible ways in which schedule performances, as units of behavior, can be scheduled. In a recent monograph Findley (1962) describes several experiments on the scheduling of complex sequences of behavior. The results of the present investigation, as well as the experiments by Findley (1962), indicate that these second-order schedules provide a powerful technique for the analysis of behavior.

SUMMARY

On an adjusting schedule of reinforcement, a parameter of the schedule is varied as a function of some characteristic of the animal's performance. In Experiment I, the fixed-ratio response requirement was varied as a function of the time that elapsed before the animal started responding in each fixed-ratio (initial pause). When initial pauses were shorter than a specified duration, the response requirement was increased; when they were longer than the specified duration, the response requirement was decreased. Specified durations of 1, 2, 4, 8, and 15 min were studied. The average response requirement maintained by each monkey was directly related to the length of the specified duration of initial pause. In Experiment II, the fixed-ratio response requirement was constant, but reinforcement occurred only when the initial pause was longer than a specified duration. The average durations of initial pauses were directly related to the length of the specified duration and to the response requirement. Meprobamate consistently decreased the average durations of initial pauses.

REFERENCES

Boren, J. J., and Malis, J. L. Determining thresholds of aversive brain stimulation. *Am. J. Physiol.*, 1961, **201**, 429–433.

Ferster, C. B., and Skinner, B. F. *Schedules of reinforcement.* New York: Appleton-Century-Crofts, 1957.

Findley, J. D. An experimental outline for building and exploring multi-operant behavior repertoires. *J. exp. Anal. Behav.*, 1962, **5**, 113–166.

Gill, C. A, Fry, W., and Kelleher, R. T. Sound-resistant housing for experimental chambers. *J. exp. Anal. Behav.*, 1962, **5**, 32.

Herndon, J. F., Greenberg, S. M., Van Loon, E. J., Kelleher, R. T., Cook, L., and Davidson, A. A liquid diet for animals in behavioral studies. *J. exp. Anal. Behav.*, 1958, **1**, 291–292.

Kelleher, R. T., Fry, W., Deegan, J., and Cook, L. Effects of meprobamate on operant behavior in rats. *J. Pharmacol.*, 1961, **133**, 271–280.

Lindsley, O. R. Operant behavior during sleep: A measure of depth of sleep. *Science,* 1957, **126,** 1290–1291.

Skinner, B. F., and Morse, W. H. Sustained performance during very long experimental sessions. *J. exp. Anal. Behav.,* 1958, **1,** 235–244.

Stein, L., and Ray, O. S. Self-regulation of brain-stimulating current intensity in the rat. *Science,* 1959, **130,** 570–572.

Stein, L., and Ray, O. S. Brain stimulation reward "thresholds" self-determined in rat. *Psychopharmacologia,* 1960, **1,** 251–256.

Weiss, B., and Laties, V. G. Titration behavior on various fractional escape programs. *J. exp. Anal. Behav.,* 1959, **2,** 227–248.

56

The effects of pentobarbital on performance
maintained by an interlocking fixed-ratio fixed-interval
reinforcement schedule [1]

ROBERT GROVE and TRAVIS THOMPSON

An important determinant of the behavioral action of drugs is the reinforcement schedule (Sidman, 1956; Thompson and Schuster, 1968). Dews
(1955) demonstrated that barbiturates differently affect behavior maintained by simple fixed-ratio (FR) schedules and those maintained by simple
fixed-interval (FI) schedules. Dews (1955) found that low doses of pentobarbital (1–2 mg) in the pigeon decreased response rate and disrupted the
patterning on the fixed-interval schedule while slightly increasing or not
affecting response rates and patterning on a fixed-ratio schedule. Morse
(1962) replicated this effect in the pigeon with both pentobarbital and another barbiturate, amobarbital, using a multiple schedule in which the FR
and FI components were signaled by discriminative stimuli. Herrnstein and
Morse (1956) also demonstrated that pentobarbital (3 mg) differentially
affected fixed-interval and fixed-ratio components in a tandem schedule
(*tand* FI 10 FR 13) in which no exteroceptive stimuli signaled the change
from the FI to the FR component.

Another schedule sharing features of both ratio and interval schedules is
called an interlocking schedule (*interlock*) (Ferster and Skinner, 1957).
In an interlocking reinforcement schedule a response is reinforced on the
basis of the number of responses emitted since the occurrence of the previous reinforcement; however, the absolute number of responses required for
reinforcement changes as a function of time since the last reinforcement. In
the simplest case, the number of responses required for reinforcement
decreases as the interval following reinforcement increases, and may alternatively be described as a time-dependent, progressively decreasing ratio schedule. The designation *"interlock"* is used to emphasize that this particular
schedule combines in a complex manner some of the features of both a
fixed-ratio and a fixed-interval schedule: like the FR, reinforcement is contingent upon the number of responses emitted, but like the FI, reinforcement is also dependent upon elapsed time since the previous reinforcement
(Berryman and Nevin, 1962).

Interlocking FR/FI schedules are defined by two parameters, response-
base and time-base. The response-base designates the maximum number

[1] This research was supported in part by Research Grants MH-11135 and MH-
14112, to the University of Minnesota.

of responses required for reinforcement if elapsed time were to have had no effect on the schedule; the time-base designates the minimum elapsed time necessary for reinforcement if only the first response following completion of the time-base interval were reinforced. However, since the response requirement decreases with elapsed time in an *interlock* schedule, response-base and time-base refer to the extreme values defining the slope of a particular *interlock* FR/FI schedule (Skinner, 1958).

Berryman and Nevin (1962) have shown that the most important determinant of the response pattern generated by interlocking FR/FI schedules was the relation between the response-base (FR) and time-base (FI) values. At certain schedule values, the response pattern was unlike those found under simple FR or FI schedules. Instead, the schedule generated performance which shared characteristics of both FR and FI performance. As in FR schedules, overall response rate was relatively high and periods of pausing occurred following reinforcement. However, interval-like effects were also apparent. The post-reinforcement pause was longer than in most FR schedules, and responding often resumed in a positively accelerated fashion, exhibiting the "scalloped" pattern typical of FI performance. Furthermore, when the response-base (FR) value was increased, the overall response rate fell and interval-like "scalloping" predominated. Conversely, when the time-base (FI) was lengthened, overall rate increased, pausing decreased, and the "scalloping" dropped out, shifting the pattern to that of ratio-like performance. Berryman and Nevin (1962) concluded that interlocking FR/FI schedules in general generate performance that shares characteristics of both ratio and interval performance.

The present study examined the effects of pentobarbital on an interlocking FR/FI schedule with a response-base (FR) of 120 responses and a time-base (FI) of 90 seconds (*interlock* 120/90″), wherein the number of responses required for reinforcement decreased in a linear fashion from 120 to 1 (one) over a 90 second period from the previous reinforcement. Pentobarbital has been shown to affect performance maintained by FR schedules in a fashion different from performance maintained by FI schedules under conditions where the FR and FI components were presented singly (i.e., simple schedules; Dews, 1955) or successively (i.e., the "multiple" and "tandem" schedules; Morse, 1962; Herrnstein and Morse, 1956). The purpose of this study was to determine if pentobarbital would have similar differential effects on performance maintained by a complex schedule in which the FR and FI contingencies were presented simultaneously and conjointly in an interlocking FR/FI schedule. Because interlocking performance is maintained by a combination of the variables controlling both simple ratio and interval schedules, the drug effect should reflect such drug-schedule interaction, depending on the dose administered and the time elapsed following injection.

This experiment examined the effects of pentobarbital on three reinforcement schedules: (1) FR 120, (2) FI 90 seconds, and (3) *interlock* 120/90″. Thus the parametric values for FR and FI were used as the values in the *interlock* FR/FI schedule. One animal was tested on FR 120, one animal on FI 90″, and three animals on *interlock* 120/90″. Rat 263, which was run on the *interlock* schedule in a pilot study and later on FI 90″, was run on an FR schedule in the present experiment.

METHOD.   *Subjects.*   Rat 263 had a past history of both *interlock* and FI performance. Four other experimentally naive male albino rats from the same strain were also used. These animals were approximately eight months old at the beginning of the experiment. All rats were maintained at approximately 80 percent free-feeding weight.

Between sessions all animals were housed in separate cages in a room isolated from the programming apparatus.

Apparatus.   Five experimental chambers were used. Two Gerbrands rat levers, positioned 4 inches above the bottom of each cage, were mounted on one wall of a 9 by 8 by 7 inch high plexiglass and aluminum experimental chamber. The chamber was enclosed in a sound-attenuating box. One stimulus light was located above each lever. The feeder magazine was placed in a recess between the two levers at the level of the cage floor. During each session a light above the right lever was illuminated, and bar presses on the right operandum were recorded and fed into the programming apparatus located in an adjoining room. Pressing the left lever had no programmed consequence. When reinforcement was scheduled a lever press operated a pellet dispenser which delivered one 45 mg Noyes standard laboratory rat-food pellet into the magazine.

Procedure.   Each session lasted 3 hours and 15 minutes. Following three consecutive extinction sessions, Rat 263, which had previously been run under *interlock* 120/90″ and FI 90″ conditions, was exposed to an FR 30 schedule for one session, then to an FR 60 for the next two sessions, and finally to the terminal value of FR 120. All other rats were first maintained on a continuous food-reinforcement schedule for three sessions and the first 50 responses of the fourth session, after which the schedule was changed without interruption to either *interlock* 120/90″ or FI 90. All animals were maintained on their respective schedules for a minimum of thirty sessions before the injection schedule began. Responding was not recorded for the first 15 minutes of each session. They were injected in the middle of the recorded session, 90 minutes later. This procedure enhanced the reliability of the drug data by partially correcting for day-to-day variability in baseline. Pre- and post-injection data could then be analyzed for the same subject in the same session, with the pre-injection data serving as an additional control procedure (Dews, 1955; Boren, 1966).

The injection schedule began with two consecutive saline administrations separated by a minimum of one non-injection session. The first response following injection was always reinforced. Three doses of pentobarbital, 5, 10, and 20 mg/kg, were administered, and each dose was given twice to the same animal. The order of pentobarbital administration was random. A minimum of four days intervened between drug injections, to minimize the development of tolerance (Shideman, 1958).

RESULTS.   Drug-schedule interactions were similar for all three *interlock* animals; for clarity only the performance of Rat 264 will be presented.

1. *FR 120: pre-injection baseline.*   Four representative pre-injection baseline cumulative records of the performance of Rat 263 on FR 120 are shown on the left half of Fig. 1. The animal paused after each reinforcement for periods of a few seconds to more than a minute; the rate then shifted, usually abruptly or following a short burst of responses, to about 120 responses per minute, which was maintained until the completion of the ratio (except for two FR segments, A and B, in row 3 of Fig. 1, where there was a small pause immediately preceding completion of the ratio). The overall rate of responding was constant at about 80 responses per minute throughout the pre-injection segments. Rat 263 emitted the char-

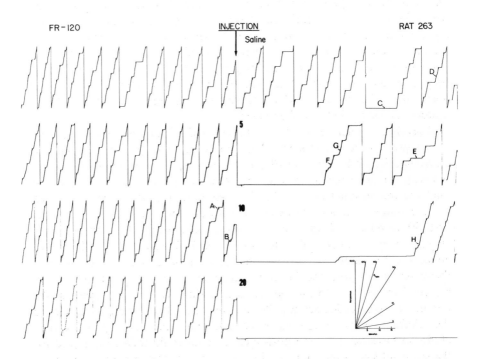

FIGURE 1.   Cumulative records illustrating the effects of saline, 5.0, 10.0, and 20.0 mg/kg i.p. of pentobarbital on food-reinforced FR 120 schedule performance. The primary effect of pentobarbital on FR performance was to exaggerate pausing, with minimal effects on running rate.

acteristic "break-and-run" pattern which distinguishes typical FR performance from that of other schedules (Ferster and Skinner, 1957).

2. *FR 120: post-injection.*   Post-injection FR performance is shown in the right half of Fig. 1. The baseline behavior was altered following saline administration, with pausing and intermediate rates appearing midway through the session (C and D). These effects accounted for the decline in overall rate of responding from a pre-injection rate of 80 responses per minute to a post-injection rate of about 55 responses per minute. The "output ratio," the ratio of the total number of responses emitted in the last 90 minutes of a session to responses emitted in the first 90 minutes (Dews, 1955), was compared for both the eight non-injection and the two saline-injection sessions. The mean output ratio for the saline sessions was 0.73 (i.e., 73 percent of the responses emitted in the first half of the session were emitted in the second half of the session), ranging from 0.63 to 0.83. The mean output ratio for the eight non-injection sessions was 0.80, ranging from 0.67 to 1.03. The increase in pausing observed here is occasionally observed on high-valued FR performance in extended sessions (Ferster and Skinner, 1957, p. 77).

At all doses of pentobarbital the FR baseline was severely disrupted (Fig. 1). In general, the drug suppressed the overall rate by successively increasing pausing following injection as the dose was increased. At 5 mg/kg, the drug increased pausing immediately after reinforcement; in addition, a second pause or series of pauses and bursts of responding often occurred in the early segments of some ratios (e.g., at E, Fig. 1). Although some curvature appeared in the second and third ratios following 5 mg/kg (F and G), responding tended to occur at a high steady rate typical of the characteristic FR baseline running rate. At 10 mg/kg the rat paused for 45 minutes following the first reinforcement and then completed about 50 responses at an intermediate rate of about 30 responses per minute in a negatively accelerating fashion to a near-zero overall rate. Toward the end of the session approximately normal ratio performance was maintained except for a short pause (H). Responding was almost completely suppressed at the high dose. Gross observations of this and other animals following injection revealed no obvious signs of hypnosis or ataxia at any point following administration of the low and intermediate doses. Hypnosis was, however, observed for approximately 20 minutes and slight ataxia for the next 15 to 20 minutes following the high dose.

3. *FI 90": pre-injection baseline.*   Four representative baseline records of Rat 310's FI 90" performance are similarly shown on the left half of Fig. 2. In general, the animal paused from about 60 to 80 seconds following reinforcement; a transition then occurred to an intermediate terminal rate of about 50 responses per minute, either abruptly or following a short period of positive acceleration in rate, giving the curvature ("scalloping") typical of FI performance (Ferster and Skinner, 1957, p. 135; Cummings

and Schoenfeld, 1958). The overall rate (three to six responses per minute) and degree of scalloping remained fairly constant across these four pre-injection periods. In a few instances, however, the terminal rate was assumed early in the interval (as at A) or immediately followed reinforcement and continued through until the next reinforcement (as at B). The latter effect has occasionally been observed in FI schedules and has been described as a "second-order effect," where two intervals together form one single positively accelerated unit (Ferster and Skinner, 1957, p. 159).

4. *FI 90": post-injection.* Post-injection FI performance for Rat 310 is shown on the right half of Fig. 2. Saline had no apparent effect on FI behavior. However, the overall rate following the low dose was slightly increased, but began to decline at the end of the session. Terminal rates did not appear to change from the pre-injection period; however, the duration of the post-reinforcement pause decreased. At the intermediate dose, overall rate increased and was maintained for a longer period, so the negative curvature appeared later in the session. Again the terminal rate remained fairly constant and pause duration decreased. At the high dose responding was completely suppressed for about 40 minutes following completion of

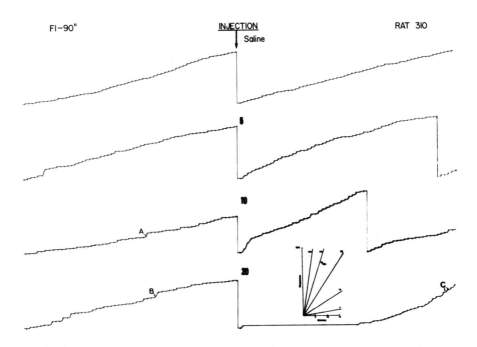

FIGURE 2. Cumulative records illustrating the effects of saline, 5.0, 10.0, and 20.0 mg/kg i.p. of pentobarbital on food-reinforced FI 90" schedule performance. At 5.0 and 10.0 mg/kg doses, there was an initial rate increase during the first part of the session due to reduced pausing and increased terminal rates. At all doses, pentobarbital affects responding throughout each reinforcement cycle.

the first interval, after which responding resumed with a definite overall positive curvature.

5. *"Interlock" 120/90": pre-injection baseline.*   Figure 3 shows representative cumulative records of Rat 264 responding on *interlock* 120/90". The overall response rate during the pre-injection periods was constant. The most consistent pattern involves a 30 to 40 second period of no responding followed by an intermediate or high rate terminated by the reinforced response (e.g., at A). Other segments occasionally exhibit response patterns characteristic of the typical FI schedule, i.e., a long pause followed by a positive acceleration in the rate of responding (i.e., at B) or characteristic of typical low-valued FR performance, i.e., a short pause followed by an abrupt shift to an intermediate or high steady rate (e.g., at C).

In general the *interlock* pre-injection pattern in Fig. 3 exhibits characteristics intermediate between those of pre-injection FR 120 and FI 90" schedule patterns in Figs. 1 and 2. This is consistent with the suggestion that the behavior generated by *interlock* is controlled by a combination of contingencies which usually control simple FR and FI schedules (Berryman and Nevin, 1962). The higher overall rate suggests that the ratio con-

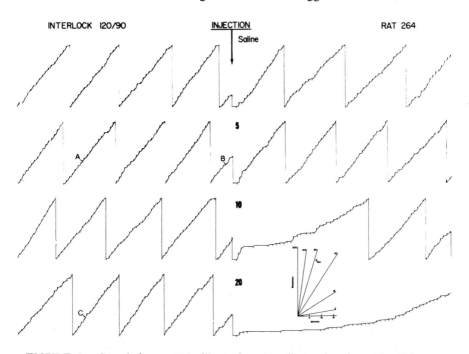

FIGURE 3.   Cumulative records illustrating the effects of saline, 5.0, 10.0, and 20.0 mg/kg i.p. of pentobarbital on food-reinforced interlocking FR 120/FI 90 schedule performance. The effects on overall rate reflect the combination of influences on individual schedule components, including increased pausing at 10.0 and 20.0 mg/kg doses (similar to FR 120 alone) and increased terminal rates at 5.0 and 10.0 mg/kg doses (similar to FI 90 alone).

tingency exercises more control over the *interlock* performance than the interval contingency.

6. *"Interlock" 120/90": post-injection.* Saline administration had no apparent effect on post-injection *interlock* responding (Fig. 3). Likewise there was little disruption following 5 mg/kg, although short pauses and high running rates appeared in the first two post-injection segments. Again at 10 mg/kg, high rates appeared in the first two post-injection segments, suggesting a brief initial increment in rate induced by pentobarbital during absorption. Upon completion of these first two segments at the intermediate dose, however, responding was suppressed to a near-zero overall rate. There was an overall positive curvature in the record for approximately the next 50 minutes, after which responding returned to baseline levels. At the high dose normal responding was suppressed after the first segment was completed. An overall positive curvature was also observed on this record, but it did not return to baseline by the end of the session. For about the first 40 minutes no consistent responding occurred, and the frequency of reinforcement dropped sharply. Responding then resumed in a manner similar to that during the period of positive curvature at 10 mg/kg.

DISCUSSION.   The role of schedules in drug-behavior interaction cannot be considered independently of other behavioral variables. In addition to establishing the specified contingency for reinforcement (e.g., FR, FI, *interlock* FR/FI), the schedule interacts with the ongoing behavioral processes to generate specific response patterns characteristic of so-called "schedule-controlled behaviors," and the contingency, the parameter value of the schedule, and the ongoing behavior in turn combine to determine the frequency of reinforcement for a specific schedule. Therefore the analysis of drug-schedule interactions involve a second-order relationship between the conditions maintaining schedule-controlled behavior and the effects of drugs on that behavior. Non-monotonic dose-schedule interactions further complicate this relationship by suggesting that different behavioral mechanisms are altered at different doses, or that the same behavioral process is affected biphasically.

In view of the above considerations, the primary generalization that can be made from previous demonstrations of differential sensitivity of FR and FI schedules to pentobarbital is that all classes of behavior are not altered in a unitary manner by this drug. Differential dose-schedule interactions have been confounded in these studies by failing to equate other variables such as baseline frequency of reinforcement. Because reinforcement frequencies differed markedly under these conditions, differential "schedule" sensitivity may have been an artifact of, or at least a less important variable than, high vs. low frequencies of reinforcement generated by these schedules in determining the drug effect.

In this experiment the FR 120 schedule generated approximately 18 reinforcements per half hour on the pre-injection baseline while the FI 90″ schedule generated 19 reinforcements. Nevertheless, marked differences in dose-schedule sensitivity were found, suggesting that the contingencies established by FR and FI schedules equated for reinforcement frequency are indeed important variables determining differential drug effects. Frequency of reinforcement was slightly but consistently high under baseline *interlock* contingencies (approximately 23 reinforcements per half hour); this difference did not appear to make the performance more or less sensitive to the drug effects because drugged performance changes were consistently intermediate between those of FR and FI subject.

It should also be apparent that the parameter value of a schedule (e.g., number of responses on FR or time interval on FI) is a potentially important variable determining the behavioral effect of drugs.

Berryman and Nevin (1962) had previously shown that *interlock* schedules tend to generate ratio-like and interval-like performance in various proportions as the relation between the response-base (FR) and time-base (FI) was shifted. Data from several studies suggest that as the FR or FI value increases, the behavior becomes more susceptible to the suppressant action of pentobarbital (Kornetsky, 1963; Hearst, 1960; Waller and Morse, 1963; Dews, 1955; Dews, 1958; Morse, 1962). If the differential sensitivity generalization was valid for *interlock* schedule-controlled performance, a functional relation should be demonstrable between the predominating baseline ratio-like (or interval-like) response pattern and its sensitivity to alteration by pentobarbital. The results of this experiment were consistent with this suggestion. The predominant response pattern generated by *interlock* 120/90″ schedule was "break-and-run," a characteristic of typical ratio performance. Interval-like effects were also apparent but these occurred less frequently. Low doses had no appreciable effect, but intermediate and high doses produced a transitory suppression of rate which returned to baseline through a series of interval-like "scallops."

Although consistent with the differential sensitivity generalization, the effect could also be due to conditions such as a decrement in deprivation conditions, interference with the required response topography, and/or a non-specific "sedative" effect. Rat 263, trained on FR 120, showed marked suppression at all doses and nearly complete suppression at the high dose (Fig. 1), an effect which was much more pronounced than the degree of suppression observed when this animal was trained on *interlock* 120/90″ in a pilot study. FI 90″ performance, on the other hand, increased immediately at low and medium doses, and also increased following an initial period of suppression at the high dose (Fig. 2). Baseline *interlock* 120/90″ performance for Rat 264 was more ratio-like (Fig. 3). At medium and high doses, a "scalloping" pattern consistently occurred during the recovery period.

Comparing FR, FI, and *interlock* dose-schedule effects (Figs. 1, 2, and

3), this investigation demonstrated that it is possible to generate a behavioral baseline which shares properties of both FR and FI schedules, which are revealed by various doses and times since administration of pentobarbital. The postulated dominant ratio-like contingencies in the *interlock* behavioral baseline of Rat 264 (Fig. 3) appear to have been suppressed by pentobarbital, revealing the previously less apparent interval-like contingencies, which temporarily exercised greater control. At each dose level it appears that some combination of the dominant drug effects over the session for FR 120 and FI 90″ could account for much of the prevailing drug-behavior interaction found in the *interlock* animals (refer to Figs. 1, 2, and 3).

Berryman and Nevin (1962) found that shifts in interlocking FR/FI performance to ratio-like responding were produced by increasing *interval* value (time-base), while shifts to interval-like performance were produced by increasing the *ratio* size (response-base). This suggests that the behavioral mechanism of the pentobarbital effect on schedules equated for frequency of reinforcement may lie in changes in effective values of controlling ratio or interval schedule contingencies. In FR schedules the time-base is infinitely long; in FI schedules the response-base is immeasurably high. Both parameters are limited by the *interlock* contingency. Therefore FR effects may be comparable to increasing ratio size (response-base), and FI effects to increasing interval length (time-base). The primary interlocking FR/FI effect observed here was a transitory shift from baseline ratio-like to drug-induced interval-like performance. This is comparable to concurrently increasing the dominant baseline contingency (ratio size), which would increase the probability of low-rate interval-like behavior, and secondarily increasing the recessive interval-like contingency (time-base), which would increase the probability of higher ratio-like rates. Thus by a successive fading of the dominant drug-induced ratio-size effect and recessive time-base effect over time, performance returns to baseline levels through a series of progressively increasing interval-like, then ratio-like components.

REFERENCES

Berryman, R., and Nevin J. A. Interlocking schedules of reinforcement. *J. exp. Anal. Behav.,* 1962, 5, 213–223.

Boren, J. J. The study of drugs with operant techniques. In *Operant behavior: Areas of research and application,* W. K. Honig (Ed.). New York: Appleton-Century-Crofts, 1966.

Cummings, W. W., and Schoenfeld, W. N. Behavior under extended exposure to a high-value fixed interval reinforcement schedule. *J. exp. Anal. Behav.,* 1958, 1, 245–263.

Dews, P. B. Studies in behavior. I. Differential sensitivity to pentobarbital of pecking performance in pigeons depending on schedule of reward. *J. Pharm. exp. Ther.*, 1955, 113, 393–401.

Dews, P. B. Studies in behavior. IV. Stimulant actions of methamphetamine. *J. Pharm. exp. Ther.*, 1958, 122, 137–147.

Ferster, C. B., and Skinner, B. F. *Schedules of reinforcement.* New York: Appleton-Century-Crofts, 1957.

Hearst, E. Multiple schedules of time-correlated reinforcement. *J. exp. Anal. Behav.*, 1960, 3, 49–62.

Herrnstein, R. J., and Morse, W. H. Selective action of pentobarbital on component behaviors of a reinforcement schedule. *Science,* 1956, 124, 367–368.

Kornetsky, C., Dawsen, J., and Pelikin, E. Individual animal variation in the effects of pentobarbital and dextro-amphetamine. In *Specific and non-specific factors in psychopharmacology,* Max Rinkel (Ed.). New York: Philosophical Library, 1963, pp. 161–171.

Morse, W. H. Use of operant conditioning techniques for evaluating effects of barbiturates on behavior. In *First Hahnemann Symposium on Psychosomatic Medicine,* J. H. Nodine and J. H. Moyer (Eds.). Philadelphia: Lea and Febiger, 1962.

Shideman, F. E. Sedatives and hypnotics, II: Barbiturates. In *Pharmacology in medicine,* V. A. Drill (ed.), New York: The Macmillan Co., 1958.

Sidman, M. Drug-behavior interaction. *Ann. N.Y. Acad. Sci.,* 1956, 65, 282–292.

Skinner, B. F. Programming schedules of reinforcement. *J. exp. Anal. Behav.,* 1958, 1, 67–68.

Thompson, T., and Schuster, C. R. *Behavioral pharmacology.* Englewood Cliffs, N.J.: Prentice-Hall, Inc., 1968.

Waller, M. B., and Morse, W. H. Effects of pentobarbital on fixed ratio performance. *J. exp. Anal. Behav.,* 1963, 6, 125–130.

57

Drug-behavior interaction

MURRAY SIDMAN

It is a common clinical observation that a given drug will display great variability in its behavioral effects not only from individual to individual but in the same individual at different times. Such variability often can be traced to the cumulative effects of the drug itself; that is, repeated doses sometimes result in greater tolerance, and sometimes they result in greater susceptibility to the drug. When such factors are not demonstrable, the usual recourse is to ascribe the observed variability to unidentified physiological fluctuations.

In recent years, however, it has become evident that a hitherto-neglected set of variables contributes powerfully to the uncertain behavioral consequences of drug administration. These variables, broadly described, are the relations between behavior and its controlling environment. Drug effects are dependent not only on the physiological state of the organism, but also on the environmental contingencies that are maintaining its behavior at the time.[1] Such contingencies vary tremendously, both qualitatively and quantitatively, among individuals and for a given individual at different times.

With the development of techniques that permit a high degree of experimental control over the behavior of the individual it has become possible to identify and explore many of the contingencies that generate behavioral processes.[2-4] The techniques developed independently of pharmacologic applications have yielded, in their recent extension to this area, a wealth of data on interrelations between drugs and behavior. In fact, a new kind of problem has arisen. Having made the point that drugs and behavior are interactive, the young science of psychopharmacology (or pharmacopsychology, depending upon in which of the two fields one's major interest lies) faces the formidable task of systematizing the observed relations into an empirically sound and rational classification. While the present paper does not pretend to offer any such classificatory scheme, it is hoped that the data to be presented will emphasize the need for such an undertaking and will perhaps supply some useful leads.

DIFFERENTIAL REINFORCEMENT OF LOW RATES: AMPHETAMINE, ALCOHOL, AND SODIUM PENTOBARBITAL.   One relatively simple contingency that is sensitive to pharmacologic manipulation generates a form of behavior

From *Annals of the New York Academy of Sciences,* 1956, **65,** 282–302. Copyright 1956 by The New York Academy of Sciences, New York.

that has been termed "spaced responding," [5] or "timing." [6] "Differential reinforcement of low rates" (DRL), more descriptive of the actual contingency, is a term adopted at the Harvard Psychological Laboratories, Cambridge, Mass., and will be used here.

The subjects, albino rats in this case, are first placed on a water-deprivation schedule on which water is available to them for 1 half-hour at the same time each day. Dry food is always available except during experimental sessions. These sessions run for 2 hours just prior to the normal watering time. After the drinking rhythm has been established, the animals are placed in a chamber containing a lever and an apparatus that delivers a small drop of water each time the animal presses the lever. Lever pressing may be "shaped up" according to the procedure described by Skinner,[2] or the animal may be left to his own devices. In either case, the DRL contingency is introduced after the animal has pressed the lever 100 times and has received 100 water rewards (reinforcements).

In the DRL procedure, the animal must space his responses in time if he is to secure a drop of water. For example, on a 20-second DRL, used throughout these experiments, a lever press produces a reinforcement only if 20 seconds or more have elapsed since the preceding response. If a response occurs too soon, the DRL timer is reset and the timing interval begins anew.

A direct measure of the behavioral adaptation to this contingency is provided by the relative-frequency distribution of time intervals between successive responses (interresponse times). These interresponse times are shown in Fig. 1, which illustrates the development of spaced responding by three rats. In the first session the distributions are roughly similar to those expected on the basis of "random" responding.[7] During the second session the DRL contingency shows a clear effect upon response spacing. The behavior gradually becomes more efficient, and the distributions reach their final form at least by session 25 (after 50 hours). The high proportion of "bursts" of responses, as indicated by the large number of interresponse times of less than 2 seconds, is typical of this procedure, and it has not yet received a satisfactory explanation. With the exception of these bursts, the peak frequency is usually located between 18 and 20 seconds, just short of the required interval, although an occasional animal displays a more appropriate peak between 20 and 22 seconds.

Some effects of amphetamine and alcohol upon the DRL interresponse time distribution have been reported elsewhere.[6] Amphetamine moves the peak of the distribution toward shorter interresponse times. That is, the animals tend to respond too soon under the influence of this drug. Alcohol does not affect the location of the peak, but it flattens the distribution slightly because of a small increase in the frequency of very long pauses between responses.

The relative-frequency distribution of interresponse times does not pro-

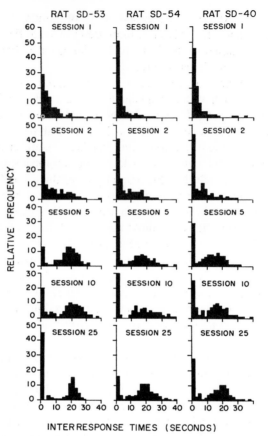

FIGURE 1. Differential reinforcement of low rates (DRL). Development of the temporal discrimination.

vide us with any information about the time course of the drug action or about the total behavioral output. Such information is contained in the cumulative response curves "drawn" by the animals. Figure 2 illustrates a normal DRL curve and another curve produced following an intraperitoneal injection of amphetamine (approximately 3 mg./kg.). The upper curve demonstrates the over-all stability of the DRL base line, while the lower curve shows the behavioral output gradually reaching a maximum level under the influence of amphetamine and beginning to fall toward the end of the session as the drug wears off.

In Fig. 3, a 1 gm./kg. dose of 10 per cent ethyl alcohol is seen to produce a decline in output, with relatively long periods of no responding interspersed among periods of normal rates. Again, a continuous picture of the drug's time course is provided by the cumulative record.

In Figs. 2 and 3 we have seen two drugs, alcohol and amphetamine, dis-

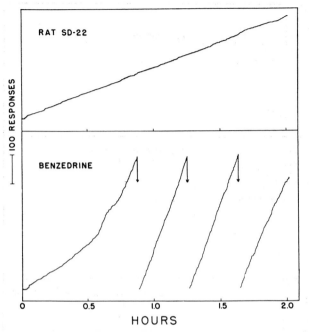

FIGURE 2. Cumulative lever-pressing curves illustrating the normal rate and the effect of amphetamine on DRL response.

playing nearly opposite effects upon the same type of behavior. It is not necessary, however, that all effective drugs fall into one or the other of these two categories. Sodium pentobarbital, for example, in the proper dosage, depresses the total output, but does so in a quantitatively and qualitatively different fashion than does alcohol. An experiment was performed in which doses of 2, 4, 6, and 8 mg./kg. of sodium pentobarbital were injected. An effect was observed only with the highest of these doses, as illustrated in Fig. 4. Here the interresponse-time distributions are presented together with

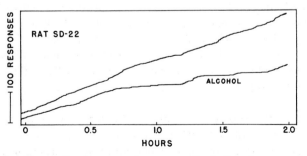

FIGURE 3. Cumulative lever-pressing curves illustrating the normal rate and the effect of alcohol upon DRL response.

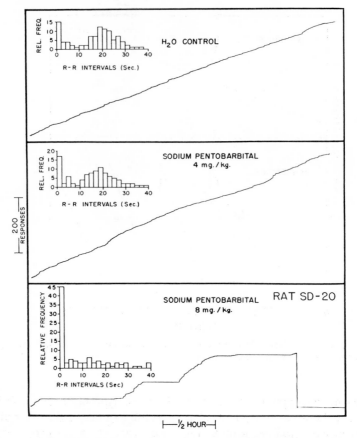

FIGURE 4. Cumulative lever-pressing curves and interresponse time distributions illustrating the effect of phenobarbital upon DRL response.

their corresponding cumulative curves. The 8 mg./kg. dose produced behavior characterized by alternating pauses and bursts of rapid responding. The bursts possibly correspond to the clinical observation of an excitatory state in the early stages of anesthesia. The interresponse-time distribution is markedly different from that observed after alcohol administration.[6] While the latter drug showed only a slight effect upon the distribution, sodium pentobarbital almost completely does away with all evidence of timing behavior. The distribution of interresponse times is nearly flat, with the exception of the increased proportion of rapid bursts of responses.

COMBINED DRL AND SIMPLE DISCRIMINATION: AMPHETAMINE AND RESERPINE.   In some of our DRL experiments, two levers are available to the animal. On one lever, the animal is reinforced according to the DRL contingency. That is, a response on the DRL lever produces a drop of water every time that 20 seconds or more have elapsed since the last response on that lever. The other lever produces a reinforcement only if it is pressed during the presence of an auditory stimulus. A reinforced response on this lever also terminates the stimulus, so that only one reinforcement per stimulus presentation is possible. Every 4 minutes the programming apparatus is "conditioned" in such a way that the next 3-second pause after a response on the DRL lever will produce the stimulus. Thus the stimulus, when it appears, always follows a DRL response by 3 seconds. This program was arranged to minimize interaction effects between the two levers.[8]

With this procedure, simultaneous auditory and temporal discriminations are built into the animal's behavioral repertoire. Under such conditions the DRL behavior is typical of that already described. When the auditory stimulus is presented there is usually a quick response on the second lever, with few "extra" responses on this lever in the absence of the stimulus. The frequency of such extra responses, along with the latency of the appropriate response in the presence of the stimulus, form the two principal measures of the auditory-stimulus discrimination.

When amphetamine is administered to animals working under the dual contingency, the usual effect upon DRL responding is observed; that is, the response rate increases, and the modal interresponse time shifts to a lower value. The amphetamine effect, however, is not confined to the timing behavior. The animals also display a substantial increase in output on the stimulus-discrimination lever. Although there is no decrement in the latency of response to the auditory stimulus, the animals press the second lever more frequently when the appropriate stimulus is absent. This indicates that the effect of amphetamine is not confined to temporal discriminations alone. There is evidently a more general effect upon several classes of discriminations.

A relation of a different order has been found between reserpine and behavior controlled by these contingencies. Two rats working on the combined DRL-stimulus discrimination procedure were given daily intraperitoneal injections of reserpine in doses of 0.2 mg./kg. The injections were given within 1 to 4 hours *after* each experimental session. One animal showed no effects of the drug treatment. The data for the second animal may be seen in Fig. 5, in which no striking effect appears until the animal has been on the drug regimen for 2 weeks. At this point the temporal discrimination displays marked deterioration. Unsystematic observation of the animal's normal activity and his reactions to handling did not reveal any changes. The stimulus discrimination also appeared relatively unaffected with respect to the frequency of extra responses on the stimulus lever and the latency of responses to the stimulus. The latency measure is actually reflected in the distributions of Fig. 5. These distributions include not only response-response (R-R) intervals, but also response-reinforcement (R-S^R) intervals, regardless of which lever produced the reinforcement.

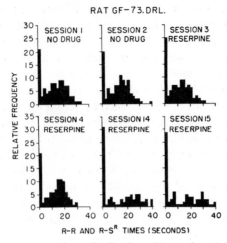

FIGURE 5. Interresponse time distributions illustrating the differential effect of reserpine upon temporal and stimulus discriminations.

Since the stimulus occurred 3 seconds after a response on the DRL lever, short-latency responses on the stimulus lever recorded an R-S^R time of 3 to 6 seconds. These responses usually show up in the control and early drug sessions as a minor peak in the distribution between 4 and 6 seconds. This peak is especially prominent during sessions 14 and 15, when the virtual elimination of short DRL interresponse times makes the R-S^R intervals stand out. Thus we see reserpine, unlike amphetamine, producing a differential effect upon time and stimulus discriminations. The different result observed in the two animals is probably a matter of dosage, as will be indicated in data presented below.

AVOIDANCE BEHAVIOR: AMPHETAMINE AND RESERPINE.   We have seen some effects of several drugs upon behavior controlled by a specific reinforcement contingency. The type of behavior generated by this contingency was labeled "timing." One drug, amphetamine, acted similarly upon behavior under temporal control and behavior controlled by an auditory stimulus. Another drug, reserpine, showed a differential interaction with the two contingencies. Both forms of behavior were under appetitive control. That is, the programmed contingencies set up the conditions under which thirsty animals could secure water. The question arises as to whether drug-behavior interactions may be classified along the lines of appetitive versus aversive techniques of behavioral maintenance. This question becomes especially important with respect to the new "tranquilizing" drugs.

One technique of aversive control that we have employed generates a stable rate of avoidance behavior and, at the same time, permits the investigation of temporal discrimination. As with the appetitive techniques, the

animals are placed in a chamber containing a lever. Brief shocks are delivered to the animal through the grid floor of the cage. Both the lever and
the walls of the cage must be included in the shock circuit, or else many
animals will develop avoidance behavior of a different topography than the
pattern that our apparatus will record. The shocks are delivered at regular
intervals; that is, every 20 seconds, unless the animal presses the lever.
Every lever depression postpones the shock for another 20 seconds. Only
the initial lever depression delays the shocks, and continued holding of the
lever by the animal has no effect upon the time of shock delivery. If the
animals do not acquire the avoidance response under these conditions,
they may be helped along by decreasing the time interval between shocks
whenever they fail to respond. That is, the "shock-shock" interval may be
made considerably briefer than the "response-shock" interval.[9] A "shaping"
process similar to that used with positive reinforcement may also be employed. That is, the class of behavior that will postpone the shock may be
restricted gradually by the experimenter until the behavior finally includes
only movements that succeed in depressing the lever.

Figure 6 depicts an example of relatively rapid acquisition of the lever-
pressing response under conditions in which the shock-shock and response-
shock intervals are both 20 seconds. The rate is relatively stable and ready
for use as a base line by the twelfth session (after 72 hours). Typical stable
states are shown for three animals in Fig. 7. The number of hours required

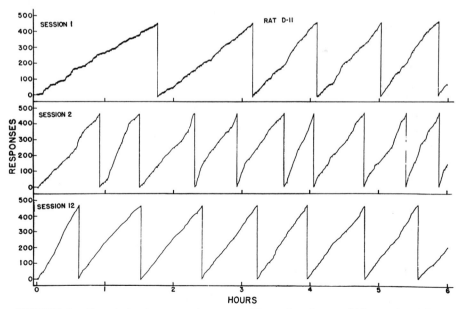

FIGURE 6.   Cumulative lever-pressing curves illustrating the acquisition and steady
state of avoidance behavior. The oblique "pips" on the record indicate shocks.

to achieve stability, and the rates of responding in the final state, may vary considerably from animal to animal, but a given subject may be depended upon to produce consistent behavior from session to session.

As with the DRL procedure, we may also record relative frequency distributions of time intervals between successive avoidance responses. Although we have shown elsewhere that the avoidance responses need not be temporally spaced in a manner indicating time discrimination, such spacing does occur to a greater or lesser extent with continued training,[10] and the process may be facilitated by special procedures.[11] Distributions indicating a timing process were utilized in the experiments described below.

In the upper frame of Fig. 8 is an interresponse time distribution fairly typical of those observed after a time discrimination has become well-established. The only atypical feature of this distribution is the absence of the usual high frequency of rapid bursts. It will be noted that the interresponse times gradually rise to a maximum frequency shortly before a shock is due.

When this animal was given a 3 mg./kg. dose of amphetamine, the rate of avoidance responding increased and the time discrimination was affected in much the same way as in the DRL procedure. The intervals between responses became shorter, with the maximal effect showing up within the first hour (Fig. 8). The effect diminished slightly during the second hour, and the behavior returned to an approximately normal state after 3 hours. We

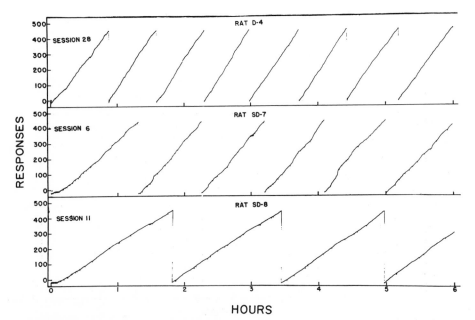

FIGURE 7.   Cumulative lever-pressing curves illustrating avoidance behavior in the steady state. The oblique "pips" on the record indicate shocks.

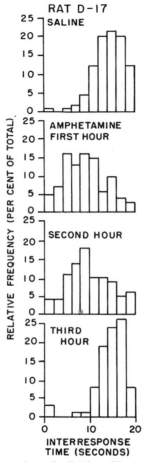

FIGURE 8.   Interresponse time distributions illustrating the effects of amphetamine upon avoidance behavior.

observe, then, that the effect of amphetamine on timing is not confined to behavior under appetitive control but extends also to the avoidance situation. Similar results have been reported by Milner,[12] who used a somewhat different avoidance technique.

In the experiments in which reserpine was used, the avoidance procedure was slightly modified in that an intermittent-shock schedule was employed. The "100 per cent shock" schedule was the same as that described above. Each time the animal waited 20 seconds without pressing the lever, a shock was administered. In the "20 per cent shock" schedule, however, the animal did not receive a shock *every* time 20 seconds elapsed without a response. Instead, the shock occurred only on 20 per cent of the occasions on which it was "due." That is, for every 5 times, on the average, that the animal waited 20 seconds, it received one shock. With the animals employed in these studies, it had previously been found that a 20 per cent shock schedule, with no drug, produced about the same response rate and interresponse-time distribution as did the 100 per cent shock schedule.[13]

Two rats were given 0.2 mg./kg. doses of reserpine following each 6-hour avoidance session. The response rates declined rapidly in both cases, but as one of the animals became ill and subsequently died, we present only one set of data in Fig. 9. It may be seen that the rate declined steadily on the 20 per cent shock schedule, but that the peak interresponse time was relatively unaffected until the rate became so low that the distribution could not be considered reliable. In session 6, when the shock schedule was changed to 100 per cent, we see a hint of an interesting drug-behavior interaction. The more demanding schedule seemed to produce a slight amelioration of the reserpine effect, in that there was an increase in rate and some indication of a return of the timing behavior.

This effect was followed up more systematically with two animals and with a reserpine dose of 0.1 mg./kg., one half of the dose used previously. In Fig. 10 are presented the rate data for one of these animals. Here again may be seen a steady decline in rate of avoidance responding on the 20 per cent shock schedule during the period of drug administration. Each time the 100 per cent shock procedure was introduced, however, the rate of responding rose to its normal level. Changing the shock contingency eradicated the drug effect even though, in the *untreated* animal, the two shock schedules showed no differential effects.

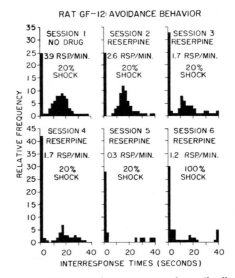

FIGURE 9. Response rates and interresponse time distributions illustrating the effects upon avoidance behavior of a 0.2 mg./kg. daily maintenance dose of reserpine.

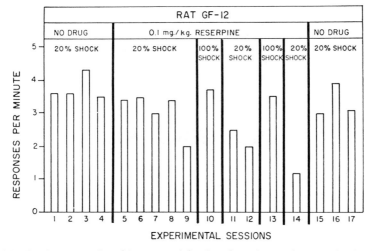

FIGURE 10.   Rate of avoidance as a joint function of reserpine and shock schedule.

In the case of the second animal, there was an even more intriguing effect. Fig. 11 again demonstrates a difference in rate of avoidance behavior between the 20 and 100 per cent shock schedules, but in this case there actually appears to be a gradual recovery even on the 20 per cent shock contingency. Here we have the possibility, which deserves more complete exploration, of a "therapeutic" effect extending from behavior governed by one contingency to behavior governed by another.

Interresponse time distributions corresponding to the rates shown in Fig. 11 may be seen in Fig. 12. Although the 20 per cent shock distributions under reserpine are somewhat more irregular than the controls be-

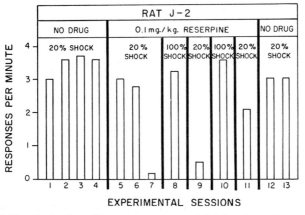

FIGURE 11.   Rate of avoidance response as a joint function of reserpine and shock schedule.

means of the multiple-schedule technique developed by Ferster and Skinner.[18] In the multiple-schedule situation the animal works under two or more reinforcement schedules. Each schedule, however, is under stimulus control; that is, there is a different stimulus correlated with each reinforcement schedule. The animal learns to behave in accordance with the current schedule that is identified by the stimulus present at any moment.

The multiple schedule employed in this experiment involved three reinforcement contingencies. In the presence of a steady tone, the DRL contingency was in effect. Responses were reinforced only when 30 seconds or more had elapsed since the preceding response. When a clicking noise was presented, a fixed-ratio schedule was programmed. On this schedule, 10 lever presses were required for each reinforcement. When neither the tone nor the clicker was in operation, a variable-interval schedule was in effect in which responses were reinforced at irregular intervals, with a mean interval of approximately 30 seconds. The three schedules were programmed in a mixed order, and the duration of each stimulus was variable.

While the behavior at the time of reserpine administration was not as stable as might be desired, stimulus control of the behavior appropriate to each schedule was clearly evident, as may be seen in the left-hand curve of Fig. 14. The letters refer to the schedule in effect in each portion of the curve. The variable-interval schedule is indicated by a, the DRL by b, and the fixed ratio by c.

A large reserpine dose of 1 mg./kg. almost completely depressed all lever-pressing behavior regardless of the reinforcement contingency. Subsequent reduction of the daily maintenance dose did not bring back the behavior that is depicted in its depressed state in the "reserpine" curve of Fig. 14. When the animal began to show other generalized effects of the drug, such as loss of weight, flaccidity, and sluggishness, a 2 mg./kg. dose

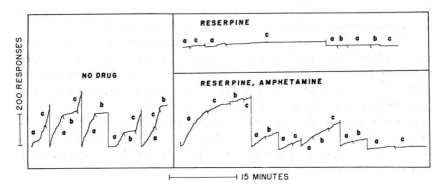

FIGURE 14. Cumulative lever-pressing curves illustrating the normal multiple-schedule performance, the effect of a large dose of reserpine, and the effect of reserpine-plus-amphetamine. Behavior on the variable-interval schedule is indicated by a, DRL behavior by b, and fixed-ratio behavior by c. The recorder pen was reset at the start of each variable-interval period.

of amphetamine was administered just prior to the next experimental session. As shown in Fig. 14 (lower right), amphetamine succeeded in bringing back lever-pressing behavior for a short time. There was, however, no differential behavior as a function of the reinforcement contingency. This may indicate that the reserpine had eliminated either the stimulus control, the schedule control, or both. On the other hand, this effect may be a consequence of the amphetamine, although a similar dose has been shown to sharpen, rather than to eliminate, stimulus control in the conditioned-suppression procedure.[17]

A more direct example of differential reserpine effects upon positive-reinforcement schedules was obtained by administering a lower dose, 0.1 mg./kg., in the multiple-schedule procedure. With this dose there was a clear depression of the fixed-ratio and variable-interval rates, while the DRL displayed a greater resistance consistent with the data presented above. The response rates on each of the three schedules are plotted session by session in Fig. 15. The drug was administered daily, following each experimental run, after sessions 2 through 13. Not only is there a differential sensitivity of the behavior under the three schedules, but there is also a marked difference in the time course of action of the drug, depending upon the reinforcement contingency. Depression of the fixed-ratio behavior begins immediately, and the variable-interval behavior begins somewhat later,

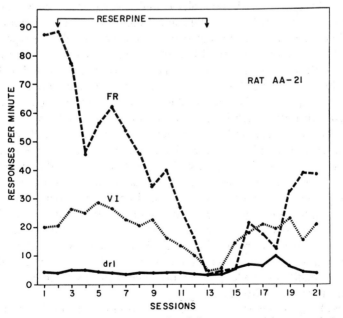

FIGURE 15. Response rates under each reinforcement contingency of the multiple schedule, illustrating the time course of action of a daily maintenance dose of reserpine of 0.1 mg/kg.

while the DRL behavior remained relatively stable throughout the drug treatments. This intimate relation between drug and reinforcement contingency continues into the recovery period where the variable-interval behavior returns to its base level well before the fixed-ratio behavior. The slight rise in the DRL rate following withdrawal of the drug had not been observed in the previous DRL-reserpine experiments. The temporary increase in the variable-interval rate during the early drug sessions, however, has been observed consistently in conditioned suppression-reserpine experiments that employed a variable-interval base line.[19] It may be noted that the differential time course of reserpine action as a function of the reinforcement-maintaining schedule suggests that the effect of the drug is on the schedule control rather than on the stimulus control. Although the evidence is not conclusive, there seems to be no a priori reason to believe that the two auditory stimuli (fixed-ratio and DRL) would display such markedly different sensitivity with respect to each other and to the condition in which both stimuli were absent (variable interval).

SUMMARY.   The data presented in this paper serve to emphasize the interdependence of pharmacologic and behavioral variables. It is clear that the relations between drugs and behavior are a function not only of the drug but also of the conditions under which the behavior is generated. The evidence also suggests that while drugs and behavior interact differentially, it will be difficult if not impossible to find a drug whose effects are confined to one specific behavior-environment contingency. The common-sense distinctions that we are accustomed to make between different types of behavior do not suffice to establish a classificatory scheme. We have seen reserpine affecting both positively and aversively maintained behavior. Within this classification, we have seen differential interactions as a function of more specific behavior variables such as shock frequency and reinforcement schedules. Such behavioral variables not only help to determine the drug effect, but also influence the temporal course of the effect.

In the case of amphetamine we have found an effect upon timing behavior in both appetitive and aversive situations, yet evidence presented here and elsewhere [20] indicates that amphetamine has a more general effect than simply upon timing behavior. Alcohol and sodium pentobarbital also affect timing behavior, but they do so in a fashion different from each other and from amphetamine. Behavior is not only differentially affected by drugs, but it also may respond to drugs in qualitatively and quantitatively different ways. Avoidance behavior is suppressed by reserpine under appropriate conditions while presumably related behavior in an "anxiety" situation increases in frequency.

The techniques reported in this paper and elsewhere in this monograph that permit the elucidation of such interactions between drugs and behavior reveal simultaneously both their strengths and their weaknesses. As techniques, their strength is made evident by the multiplicity of relations whose existence they have revealed and by the many untapped areas that it is now possible to explore. It is difficult for the behavioral scientist to restrain himself from probing these areas where one can hardly fail to observe striking behavioral changes as a consequence of injecting some mysterious subsubstance into the gut of an experimental animal. This fact points up the weakness of the techniques. In their present form, and with our current state of understanding of the behavioral phenomena generated by the techniques, the result of such probing will be little more than a bewildering array of highly interesting but completely unsystematic data. A small amount of restraint in the form of systematic behavioral investigation *prior* to drug investigation cannot fail to bring some order into the accumulated facts of drug-behavior interaction. A search for relations, rather than differences, among reinforcement contingencies; the unification of principles of aversive and positive control; a more precise delineation and classification of behavioral variables; and the discovery of relations between behavior and other biological phenomena will lead inevitably to the elimination of a great deal of psychopharmacologic investigation that now seems exciting but is actually little more than aimless wandering when compared to future potentialities in this field.

REFERENCES

1. Dews, P. B. 1955. Studies on behavior. I. Differential sensitivity to pentobarbital of pecking performance in pigeons depending on the schedule of reward. *J. Pharmacol. Exptl. Therap.* 113:393–401.
2. Skinner, B. F. 1938. *The behavior of organisms.* Appleton-Century-Crofts. New York, N.Y.
3. Skinner, B. F. 1953. Some contributions of an experimental analysis of behavior to psychology as a whole. *Am. Psychol.* 8:69–78.
4. Sidman, M. 1953. Avoidance conditioning with brief shock and no exteroceptive warning signal. *Science.* 118:157–158.
5. Wilson, M. P., and Keller, F. S. 1953. On the selective reinforcement of spaced responses. *J. Comp. and Physiol. Psychol.* 46:190–193.
6. Sidman, M. 1955. Technique for assessing the effects of drugs on timing behavior. *Science.* 122:925.
7. Mueller, C. G. 1950. Theoretical relationships among some measures of conditioning. *Proc. Natl. Acad. Sci. U.S.* 36:123–130.
8. Sidman, M. 1956. Time discrimination and behavioral interaction in a free operant situation. *J. Comp. and Physiol. Psychol.* 49: 469–473.
9. Sidman, M. 1953. Two temporal parameters of the maintenance of avoidance behavior by the white rat. *J. Comp. and Physiol. Psychol.* 46:253–261.
10. Sidman, M. 1954. The temporal distribution of avoidance responses. *J. Comp. and Physiol. Psychol.* 47:399–402.
11. Sidman, M. 1955. Some properties of the warning stimulus in avoidance behavior. *J. Comp. and Physiol. Psychol.* 48:444–450.

12. Milner, P. M. 1954. The effect of benzedrine on time estimation in the rat. *Am. Psychol.* 9:581.
13. Boren, J. J., and Sidman, M. 1956. *Maintenance and extinction of avoidance behavior as a function of intermittent shocks.* Eastern Psychol. Assoc. Atlantic City, N.J.
14. Estes, W. K., and Skinner, B. F. 1941. Some quantitative properties of anxiety. *J. Exptl. Psychol.* 29:390–400.
15. Brady, J. V., and Hunt, H. F. 1955. An experimental approach to the analysis of emotional behavior. *J. Psychol.* 40:313–324.
16. Azrin, N. 1956. Some effects of two intermittent schedules of immediate and non-immediate punishment. *J. Psychol.* 42:3–21.
17. Brady, J. V. 1956. Assessment of drug effects on emotional behavior. *Science.* 123:1033–1034.
18. Ferster, C. B., and Skinner, B. F. 1957. *Schedules of reinforcement.* Appleton-Century-Crofts. New York, N.Y.
19. Brady, J. V. 1956. A comparative approach to the evaluation of drug effects upon affective behavior. *Ann. N.Y. Acad. Sci.* 66(3):632–643.
20. Skinner, B. F., and Heron, W. T. 1937. Effects of caffeine and benzedrine upon conditioning and extinction. *Psychol. Rec.* 1:340–346.

58

Escape behavior and punished behavior [1]

Roger T. Kelleher and William H. Morse [2]

Drugs that are thought to be clinically useful in reducing fear and anxiety are of particular interest in behavioral pharmacology, and many researchers have been predisposed to look for specific effects of these drugs on behavior controlled by aversive stimuli. The two main ways in which aversive stimuli have been used to affect behavior are as negative reinforcers and as punishers. A negative reinforcer is a stimulus which can sustain behavior that precedes its cessation. Behavior that is sustained by the termination of a negative reinforcer will be called escape behavior. A punisher is a stimulus which can suppress behavior that precedes its presentation.[3] Behavior that is suppressed by the presentation of an aversive stimulus will be called punished behavior. In the present paper, we shall analyze the specificity of the effects of drugs on escape behavior and punished behavior.

Much of the interest in the effects of drugs on behavior controlled by aversive stimuli derives from motivational interpretations of the clinical uses of these drugs. It is assumed that aversive stimuli control behavior by engendering a generalized state of fear or anxiety, and that drugs act by modifying these underlying emotional states. The strength of this motivational analysis is its plausible generality. Explanations of drug effects in terms of fear and anxiety have been applied to the effects of drugs on both escape behavior and punished behavior (relevant evidence will be discussed in the section on punished behavior). A similar attempt has been made to apply motivational interpretations to the effects of drugs on behavior maintained by positive reinforcers. Changes in performance after drug have been explained as changes in hunger, thirst, etc., but experiments using patterns

From *Federation Proceedings,* 1964, **23**, 808–817. Copyright 1964 by the Federation of American Societies for Experimental Biology, Bethesda, Md.

[1] Some of the work described in this paper was supported by Research Grants MH 02094 and MH 07658 from the Institute of Mental Health of the National Institutes of Health, U.S. Public Health Service. We wish to thank Mrs. Catherine Jackson for meticulous assistance with the punishment experiments.

[2] This work was supported in part by a Public Health Service research career program award, 5-K3-GM-15,530, from the Institute of Mental Health.

[3] We do not suggest that the suppression of behavior is an invariant effect of presenting an aversive stimulus. In contrast to this empirical definition, punishment is sometimes defined formally as the presentation of a negative reinforcer. The formal definition of punishment circumvents considering the complex and paradoxical effects of punishment, and emphasizes the usual contrasting effects of presenting and terminating a particular reinforcer. Unfortunately, there is not always a reciprocal behavioral effect between presenting and terminating a negative reinforcer.

of behavior maintained by schedules of positive reinforcement show that these motivational interpretations of drug effects are inadequate and frequently misleading.

The behavioral effects of drugs are markedly influenced by the temporal and sequential relations between stimuli presented to the subject, responses of the subject, and further stimuli consequent on these responses. These sequential relations between responses and consequent stimuli are, of course, what we call a schedule (13, 17). There are many reports of how the effects of drugs depend upon schedule-maintained patterns of behavior. For example, the effect of a particular dose of pentobarbital can be changed from a decrease in responding to an increase by varying the type and the parameter value of the schedule of positive reinforcement (9, 36). This dependence of drug effect upon the schedule has been shown in the pigeon under a multiple schedule comprising two component schedules, each associated with a visual stimulus. In the presence of a blue light, the reinforcer (food) was presented every 30th response (key peck); this schedule is called a 30-response fixed ratio. In the presence of a red light, the reinforcer was presented following the first response after 5 min; this schedule is called a 5-min fixed interval.

Figure 1 shows performance of a food-deprived pigeon on this multiple schedule. Under the fixed-ratio component, responding occurred at a high steady rate. Under the fixed-interval component, an initial pause was fol-

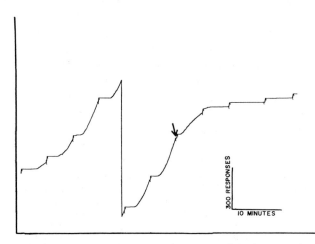

FIGURE 1. Effect of pentobarbital on performance of a pigeon under a multiple fixed-interval, fixed-ratio schedule. Ordinate: cumulative number of responses; abscissa: time. Food deliveries are marked by short diagonal strokes. At the beginning of the record, a 30-response fixed ratio was in effect; following food delivery, a 5-min fixed-interval schedule was in effect. These schedules alternated throughout each session. Sodium pentobarbital (3 mg) was administered intramuscularly at the point indicated by the arrow (body weight, 430 g). From Morse (36). Courtesy of Lea and Febiger.

lowed by positively accelerated responding. After an intramuscular injection of 3 mg of pentobarbital (at the arrow), responding was markedly reduced in the fixed-interval component but not in the fixed-ratio component (36). Since the degree of food deprivation is the same in both schedule components, the drug obviously did not have its main effect by modifying motivation. This type of drug effect should lead one to question the usefulness of motivational interpretations of the effects of drugs on escape behavior and punished behavior.

ESCAPE BEHAVIOR. Many investigators have attempted to study the motivational specificity of drugs by comparing their effects on behavior maintained by positive reinforcement with their effects on behavior maintained by negative reinforcement. Although this appears to be a straightforward experimental problem, the difficulties involved in making such comparisons are formidable. For example, it is difficult to equate the schedules used with each type of reinforcer to prevent the introduction of confounding schedule effects. It has been reported that chlorpromazine has more marked effects on negatively reinforced responding than on positively reinforced responding, but opposite effects have also been reported (7, 13, 17, 41). It seems likely that either result can be obtained consistently, depending on the type and the parameter of the schedule controlling each of these patterns of responding. One could select pairs of schedules that would seem to show that chlorpromazine specifically affected behavior maintained under either type of reinforcer. It is unreasonable to presume that any one arbitrarily chosen schedule of negative reinforcement is comparable to any one arbitrarily chosen schedule of positive reinforcement (13, 48, 50).

The most satisfactory way to attack these many problems is to establish dose-effect relations for a variety of drugs on a variety of patterns of behavior maintained by schedules of positive and negative reinforcement. The functional relations between drugs and schedules of positive reinforcement can then be compared to the functional relations between drugs and schedules of negative reinforcement. Such a program obviously requires a prodigious amount of experimental work, but there is no suitable alternative at present. Fortunately, consistent generalities relating the effects of drugs to schedule-controlled patterns of responding have emerged from the substantial number of dose-effect relations already established with schedules of positive reinforcement. What is most needed at the present time is comparable information about schedules of negative reinforcement.

We have established schedules of negative reinforcement that are formally comparable to useful schedules of positive reinforcement, comparable not only with respect to the specific schedules, but also with respect to the patterns of responding these schedules generate. The following experiments illustrate this approach. Three food-deprived squirrel monkeys were trained on a multiple fixed-interval, fixed-ratio schedule of positive (food) reinforcement similar to that prescribed previously for the pigeon. These monkeys were studied individually in a conventional experimental chamber; on one wall were mounted a response key, a food dispenser, and a translucent panel which could be transilluminated by visual stimuli. In the presence of a red stimulus light, a 30-response fixed-ratio schedule was in effect. In the presence of a white stimulus light, a 10-min fixed-interval schedule was in effect. When the stimulus panel was transilluminated with a pattern of horizontal bars, food was never delivered, and responses had no programmed consequences.

Another three monkeys were studied individually while restrained in a primate chair (Fig. 2), making it possible to deliver electric shocks to the

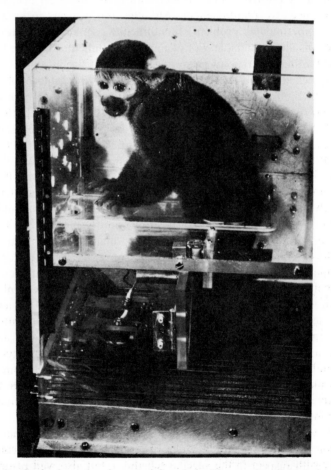

FIGURE 2.   Squirrel monkey in restraining chair. The monkey is restrained in the seated position by a waist lock; its tail is held motionless by a small stock. Electric shock is delivered through two hinged metal plates that rest lightly on a shaved portion of the tail; electrode paste insures electrical contact. The response lever, which is mounted in the metal wall, is shown just to the right of the monkey. The rectangular area above the lever can be transilluminated by stimulus lights and patterns.

animal's tail (25). A response key and stimulus panel were mounted on a wall in front of the monkey. These animals were trained on a multiple fixed-interval, fixed-ratio schedule of negative reinforcement in which responses terminated visual stimuli correlated with the periodic delivery of brief (50-msec) electric shocks according to the schedule in operation. In the presence of a pattern of horizontal bars, shocks were never delivered, and responding had no programmed consequences. In the presence of a red stimulus light, shocks were scheduled to occur at 30-sec intervals; the 30th response terminated the red stimulus and produced the pattern of horizontal bars. This is a 30-response fixed-ratio schedule of escape. In the presence of a white stimulus light, shocks were scheduled to occur at 1-sec intervals starting after 10 min; the first response after 10 min terminated the white stimulus light and produced the pattern of horizontal bars. This is a 10-min fixed-interval schedule of escape. This multiple fixed-interval, fixed-ratio schedule of negative reinforcement is formally comparable to the multiple fixed-interval, fixed-ratio schedule of positive reinforcement described above.

Performances under these multiple schedules of positive and negative reinforcement are shown in Fig. 3. Under both fixed-interval and fixed-ratio schedules of positive and negative reinforcement, characteristic patterns of responding are maintained. Performance on a 10-min fixed interval is characterized by a pause (period of no responding) followed by positively accelerated responding. Performance on a 30-response fixed ratio is characterized by a steady high rate of responding. The upper records in Fig. 3 show the performance of a squirrel monkey responding under a procedure in which fixed-interval and fixed-ratio schedules of food reinforcement alternate throughout each experimental session. The lower records in Fig. 3 show the performance of another squirrel monkey responding under fixed-interval and fixed-ratio escape schedules. Although the performances in the upper and lower parts of the figure are maintained by completely different types of reinforcing stimuli (presentation of food, and termination of shocks) the patterns of responding are remarkably similar.

The effects of d-amphetamine and chlorpromazine on rates of responding under each of the component schedules of positive and negative reinforcement are shown in Fig. 4. d-Amphetamine increased rates of responding on both fixed-interval schedules, except at the highest dose level, but decreased the rates of responding on both fixed-ratio schedules. Note that 0.3 mg/kg of d-amphetamine, which produced the maximum increase in rates of responding on both fixed intervals (relatively low control rates), decreased rates of responding on both fixed ratios (relatively high control rates). Many investigators have found that amphetamines tend to increase response output on schedules of positive reinforcement that maintain low rates of responding, but tend to decrease response output on schedules of positive reinforcement that maintain high rates of responding (10, 11, 31, 38, 51). The present results indicate further that the effects of d-amphet-

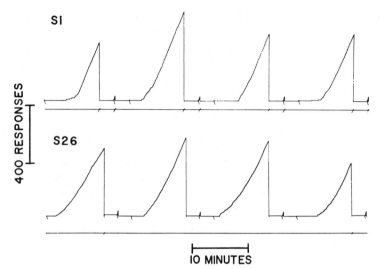

FIGURE 3. Performance maintained by a positive reinforcer (food) compared to performance maintained by a negative reinforcer (electric shock) under multiple fixed-interval, fixed-ratio schedules in the squirrel monkey. Ordinate: cumulative number of responses; abscissa: time. Upper records: a sample of the performance of monkey S1 on the multiple schedule of positive reinforcement. At the beginning of the records, the 10-min fixed-interval schedule was in effect in the presence of a white stimulus. At reinforcement, the cumulative recording pen resets to the bottom of the record and a short diagonal stroke appears on the event record. Following reinforcement, a pattern of horizontal bars was presented on the stimulus panel for 2.5 min; in the presence of this pattern, responses had no specific consequences and reinforcements never occurred. The next short diagonal stroke on the cumulative record indicates that the 30-response fixed-ratio schedule was in effect in the presence of a red stimulus. Again, the cumulative recording pen reset to the bottom of the record at reinforcement, a short diagonal stroke appears on the event record, and the pattern of horizontal bars was presented for 2.5 min. This cycle was repeated throughout each session. Lower records: a sample of the performance of monkey S26 on the multiple schedule of negative reinforcement. The sequence of visual stimuli and corresponding schedules is the same as in the upper records. The cumulative recording pen reset to the bottom of the record when a response terminated the white or red stimulus light. The short diagonal stroke on the event record indicate shock deliveries. Note the similarities of the patterns of responding under these multiple schedules of positive and negative reinforcement.

amine depend upon the nature of the schedules maintaining the behavior. Comparable schedules produce comparable dependencies whether the schedule is maintained by positive or negative reinforcers.

With respect to the motivational specificity of amphetamine, the descending portions of the dose-effect curves in Fig. 4 are significant. Graded doses of amphetamines may produce dose-effect curves with both increases and decreases in responding (fixed-interval curves), or simply decreases in responding (fixed-ratio curves). Despite the general occurrence of decreases in responding after high doses of amphetamine, many investigators presume that decreases in responding maintained by food reinforcement

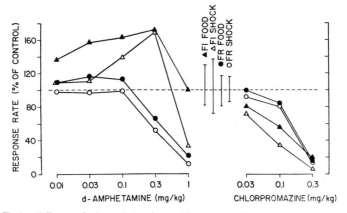

FIGURE 4. Effects of *d*-amphetamine sulfate and chlorpromazine hydrochloride on rates of responding under multiple fixed-interval, fixed-ratio schedules of positive and negative reinforcement. Three monkeys were studied on each multiple schedule. Each drug was given intramuscularly immediately before the beginning of a 2½-hr session. At least duplicate observations were made in each monkey at each dose level. Summary dose-effect curves for the four component schedules were obtained by computing the means of the percentage changes in average response rates from control to drug sessions. The dashed line at 100% indicates the mean control level for each component. The vertical lines in the middle of the figure indicate the ranges of control observations, including saline injections, expressed as a percentage of the mean control value. Note the general similarity of the pairs of dose-effect curves for fixed-interval and for fixed-ratio components.

are caused by anorexic effects of amphetamine. The similarity of the pairs of dose-effect curves in the present experiment suggests that such interpretations are specious. Although amphetamine may have special effects on food-maintained behavior, a mere decrease in responding after amphetamine is not sufficient evidence of anorexia.

Chlorpromazine produced graded decreases in rates of responding under both fixed-interval and both fixed-ratio schedules. The rates of responding on the fixed-ratio schedules were relatively less affected at the lower doses. Cook and Kelleher (7) show a similar selective effect of chlorpromazine on the fixed-interval and fixed-ratio components of a multiple schedule of food reinforcement in the squirrel monkey. The present results are also consistent with the findings of Waller and Waller (48) that comparable patterns of responding maintained by positive and negative reinforcers are affected similarly by chlorpromazine. These investigators trained dogs on a multiple schedule in which responses in the presence of one stimulus produced food on a variable-interval schedule; responses in the presence of another stimulus postponed electric shocks. Each of these schedules maintained steady intermediate rates of responding (about 0.8 response/sec). As the dose of chlorpromazine was increased, rates of responding decreased comparably on both schedules.

These experiments with chlorpromazine and *d*-amphetamine show the type of results found when dose-effect relations are established with comparable schedules of positive and negative reinforcement. Many other drugs and many other schedules of positive and negative reinforcement should be compared in this way. Some differences in the effects of drugs on behavior maintained by positive and negative reinforcers may eventually be found. But certainly in these experiments the effects of drugs depend more upon schedule-controlled patterns of responding than upon the nature of the reinforcer maintaining the behavior. In addition, these results show that specific dependencies of the effects of drugs on schedule-controlled behavior, previously reported for schedules of positive reinforcement, can be generalized to schedules of negative reinforcement.

PUNISHED BEHAVIOR.   Not only can a negative reinforcer sustain behavior that leads to its cessation (escape), but it can also suppress behavior that leads to its presentation (punishment). The use of electric shock to suppress responding has been a popular method in behavioral pharmacology. The most widely used procedure for studying suppressed behavior was developed originally by Estes and Skinner (15). They showed that a stimulus which repeatedly preceded an unavoidable electric shock (preshock stimulus) suppressed ongoing responding maintained under a schedule of food reinforcement in the rat. Subsequent studies have shown that a preshock stimulus can suppress responding of various other species on various schedules of positive reinforcement, the degree of suppression depending on the conditions (e.g., 1, 5, 46). The general procedure of superimposing a stimulus terminating with electric shock on a baseline of ongoing behavior is called the Estes-Skinner procedure.

The Estes-Skinner procedure initially attracted the interest of behavioral pharmacologists because it seemed analogous to clinical anxiety; that is, ongoing behavior is disrupted by an impending aversive event. Many studies have been conducted to determine whether drugs, particularly tranquilizing drugs, would restore suppressed behavior (e.g., 6, 8, 18, 27–29, 34, 35, 41, 46, 52). The results of these drug studies have been confusing and disappointing. Studies reporting that reserpine restored responding in a preshock stimulus (6, 41) have not been confirmed by others (34, 52); similarly, a report that morphine restored responding (27) has not been confirmed (35). There has been general agreement that chlorpromazine, meprobamate, and amphetamine do not attentuate suppression (6, 18, 34, 41); however, one recent study does suggest that meprobamate, as well as some barbiturates and chlordiazepoxide, can restore responding in a preshock stimulus (35). Some investigators have simply concluded that the Estes-Skinner procedure is not a useful technique for studying the effects of drugs (34).

Although the Estes-Skinner procedure has been widely used for studying the effects of drugs, the interactions among variables inherent in this procedure are still poorly understood. Several experiments have shown that the degree of suppression of responding is dependent upon a number of procedural variables. Using the ongoing behavior of rats maintained on a variable-interval schedule of water reinforcement, Stein, Sidman, and Brady (45) found that the degree of suppression depended upon the relative durations of the presence and absence of a preshock stimulus; the degree of suppression was greatest when the preshock stimulus was present for relatively short periods of time. Other investigators have shown that the degree of suppression is dependent upon the schedule of reinforcement that is used to maintain responding and upon the experimental history of the animal (5, 26, 33, 43, 49). Under some conditions, responding is facilitated rather than suppressed during the presentation of the preshock stimulus. When the Estes-Skinner procedure is considered in the light of these behavioral conditions rather than in terms of anxiety, it seems perfectly reasonable that drug effects would be extremely variable.

The Estes-Skinner procedure does not give a sufficient specification of a schedule of punishment. It specifies a temporal relation between a stimulus (preshock stimulus) and shock; but because shocks are independent of responses, temporal relations between responses and shocks will depend on ongoing patterns of responding. Azrin (1) directly compared the Estes-Skinner procedure, in which shocks are adventitiously related to responses, with a similar procedure, in which responses produced shocks. He found a greater degree of suppression when responses immediately produced shocks (immediate punishment) than when shocks followed responses after unspecified delays (adventitious punishment).

In recent years, Geller and his co-workers, as well as a number of other investigators, have studied the effects of drugs on behavior that is suppressed by immediate punishment (19–23, 30, 37, 40, 42). Note that the schedule of punishment is specified under the immediate punishment procedure! In contrast to the results obtained with the Estes-Skinner procedure (adventitious punishment), the results with immediate punishment procedures have shown that the suppression of responding is attenuated by pentobarbital, amobarbital, phenobarbital, meprobamate, and chlordiazepoxide; but not by trifluoperazine, chlorpromazine, promazine, morphine, or amphetamine. Although the various studies included different species (rats, pigeons, and monkeys) and different types of ongoing behavior (learned and unlearned), the results for each drug with immediate punishment procedures have been characteristically consistent (cf. 8).

The following experiment with pentobarbital illustrates the effect of a drug on punished behavior. Pigeons were trained to peck a transilluminated response key under a fixed-ratio schedule of food reinforcement. Following some responses, electric shocks were administered to the birds through gold wire electrodes that were implanted around bone in the tail region according to the method described by Azrin (1, 2). In the presence of an orange key-light, a 30-response fixed-ratio schedule was in effect; this will be called the nonpunishment component. In the presence of a white key-light, the 30-response fixed-ratio schedule was still in effect, but each of the first 10 responses in the fixed ratio produced a 25-msec electric shock; this will be called the punishment component. The nonpunishment and punishment components alternated throughout each experimental session. Nonpunishment components terminated after five reinforcements; punishment components terminated after five reinforcements or after 3 min had elapsed. Continuous high rates of responding prevailed in nonpunishment components (2 to 4 responses/sec), but responding seldom occurred in punishment components. The effects of pentobarbital on this performance are shown in the upper frame of Fig. 5. The drug increased rates of responding in the punishment components to about the same level as in the nonpunishment components.

Most schedules used in studying the effects of drugs on punished behavior have been multiple schedules comprising punishment and nonpunishment components designated by stimuli. Such multiple schedules permit the

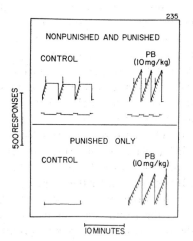

FIGURE 5.   Effects of pentobarbital (PB) on responding suppressed by punishment. Each frame shows a complete control session followed by a complete drug session for bird 235. The drug was given intramuscularly 15 min before the beginning of drug sessions. Upper frame: in nonpunishment components (event record displaced upward) a 30-response fixed-ratio schedule of positive reinforcement was in effect in the presence of an orange stimulus. The termination of each nonpunishment component is indicated by a small arrow. In punishment components (event record displaced downward), a 30-response fixed-ratio schedule was in effect in the presence of a white stimulus; each of the first 10 responses of each ratio produced a brief (35-msec) electric shock of 6 ma. The termination of each punishment component is indicated by the resetting of the pen to the bottom of the record. Lower frame: the punishment procedure was in effect throughout each session in the presence of a white stimulus. Note that pentobarbital attenuates the suppression of responding by punishment under both procedures.

simultaneous observation of the effects of drugs on punished and nonpunished behavior. Multiple schedules may, however, produce interactions between punished and nonpunished behavior. Reports in the literature discuss the possibility that drugs restore responding in punishment components of a multiple schedule by affecting the interaction between punished and nonpunished responding (e.g., 21). That the effect of pentobarbital on punished responding is not dependent upon such an interaction is shown by another experiment in which the punishment procedure alone was in effect throughout each session. Rates of responding were near zero. Nevertheless, as shown in the lower frame of Fig. 5, pentobarbital produced dramatic increases in rates of responding.

Are the effects of drugs on punished behavior specific? Drugs differ in their tendencies to increase or decrease rates of responding, and the rate-increasing effects of drugs are usually greater in situations in which control rates of responding are low (as they usually are in punishment components). Barbiturates, meprobamate, and chlordiazepoxide have been shown to increase rates of responding, especially under schedules of reinforcement that engender low rates of responding. Chlorpromazine and morphine usually decrease rates of responding in most species (7, 31, 36). Perhaps it could be argued that the tendency of a drug such as chlorpromazine to decrease responding might mask an underlying tendency to attentuate suppression of responding. Yet there are species, such as the dog and the pigeon, in which chlorpromazine can increase rates of responding over a wide range of doses (10, 12, 16, 32, 47). We studied the effects of chlorpromazine on the performance of pigeons on the 30-response fixed-ratio schedule in which nonpunishment and punishment components alternate. The results shown in Fig. 6 indicate that chlorpromazine increased the already high rate of responding in the nonpunishment component, but did not affect responding in the punishment component. Chlorpromazine does not restore behavior that has been suppressed by punishment even under conditions in which it has a general tendency to increase rates of responding. Further, it has been shown that amphetamine, which has a general tendency to increase rates of responding, does not restore responding that has been suppressed by punishment. Thus, the general rate-increasing or rate-decreasing properties of drugs are not sufficient to account for the effects of these drugs on punished responding. Rather, it appears that some durgs have specific effects on some punished behaviors.

Another illustration of the need for analysis is provided by the effects of morphine on punished behavior. Morphine has been reported to be effective in alleviating fear and anxiety associated with pain in human subjects (24). As mentioned previously, a report that morphine was effective in the rat in restoring behavior that was suppressed by adventitious punishment (27) was not confirmed (35). Morphine did not restore responding suppressed by immediate punishment (20). It may seem puzzling that morphine,

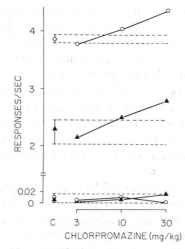

FIGURE 6. Effects of chlorpromazine on rates of responding under the 30-response fixed-ratio procedure in which nonpunishment and punishment components alternate. The points at the left of each record are means of control determinations; the solid vertical lines and dashed horizontal lines indicate the ranges of control observations. The ordinate has been broken to expand the scale at the lower values. The two curves above the break show the rates of responding for two pigeons in the non-punishment component. The circles are for bird 234, which had a control rate of 3.9 responses/sec, and the triangles are for bird 235, which had a control rate of only 2.3 responses/sec. The two curves below the break show rates of responding on the punishment components for the same birds. Note that chlorpromazine produced graded increases in rates of responding in nonpunishment components, but had no effect on responding in punishment components.

a drug with both tranquilizing and analgesic actions, has no significant tendency to attenuate suppression of responding by punishment. There is no more reason to expect morphine to restore punished responding through its tranquilizing action than there is to expect chlorpromazine to do so. As we have already suggested, the analysis of the effects of drugs in terms of changes in motivational states such as fear or anxiety has not been fruitful in predicting the effects of drugs on behavior.

In attempting to reconcile the analgesic properties of morphine with its lack of effects on punished responding, there are two important considerations. First, in the absence of punishment, morphine decreases rates of responding maintained under various schedules of reinforcement at dose levels that are well below those reported to show analgesic effects (14). It is improbable, therefore, that morphine would restore punished responding in a manner analogous to decreasing the shock intensity or omitting shocks.

In the second place, the effects of an abrupt cessation or reduction in intensity of the punisher need to be considered. This is a most important point, yet people who are puzzled that morpine does not restore punished responding seldom ask whether punished responding is attenuated immediately after a reduction in the intensity of the punisher. As Azrin (3) has shown, the answer is complex. If each response is punished with electric shock, even a considerable decrease in the intensity of the electric shock does not immediately increase the rate of responding; the new level of punished responding increases gradually over several daily sessions. If each response is punished, and the shock intensity is low enough so that some responding is still maintained, the abrupt omission of the punishment will produce a dramatic increase in responding. If, however, the punishment has been intense enough to produce an almost complete suppression of responding, or if the punishment has been intermittent, then even the abrupt omission of all punishment does not immediately increase previously punished responding (3, 4). In addition, after responding has been suppressed by punishment, it may remain suppressed for other reasons when punishment is discontinued. The suppression of responding by punishment can result in a decrease in the frequency of reinforcement in the punishment component of a multiple schedule. And, as Morse and Skinner (39) have shown, responding may be suppressed in the presence of a discriminative stimulus adventitiously correlated with a reduced frequency of reinforcement.

We analyzed the effects of omitting scheduled shocks in the 30-response fixed-ratio procedure with punishment and nonpunishment components. At the beginning or in the middle of some daily sessions, scheduled shocks were omitted from the punishment component. Neither bird started to respond immediately when scheduled shocks were first omitted at the beginning of the session. As we repeatedly performed the experiment, the restoration of responding upon the omission of scheduled shocks became faster. Frame A of Fig. 7 shows the effect of omitting scheduled shocks in the middle of a session; high rates of responding typical of the fixed-ratio pattern occurred almost immediately. Frame B shows the following session in which the first 10 responses of each fixed ratio in the punishment components were again followed by shock; no responses occurred in the first punishment component despite the high rates that had prevailed on the previous day, and only 8 responses occurred in the other five punishment components. The tendency for responding to be suppressed by punishment is clearly greater at the beginning of the session than later in the session. Scheduled shocks were again omitted at the beginning of the session shown in Frame C. No responses occurred during the first three punishment components. Since there were no responses, it is not surprising that there was no effect of removing the shock. Some punishment procedures do completely suppress responding. Certain drugs will attenuate this complete suppression; morphine will not. That morphine does not attenuate punished responding does not impugn its efficacy as an analgesic. Morphine cannot produce through its analgesic action any greater reduction in shock intensity than the complete removal of shocks, yet an immediate increase in the level

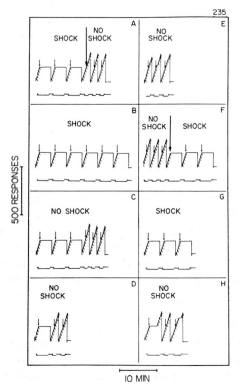

FIGURE 7. Effects of omitting and reinstating scheduled electric shocks on be-havior suppressed by punishment. In nonpunishment components, a 30-response fixed-ratio schedule of food reinforcement was in effect in the presence of an orange stimulus; nonpunishment components terminated after five reinforcements as indi-cated by small arrows. In punishment components, a 30-response fixed-ratio schedule was in effect in the presence of a white stimulus; each of the first 10 responses of each ratio produced a brief electric shock. Punishment components terminated after 5 reinforcements or 3 min, as indicated by the resetting of the pen to the bottom of the record. The frames show successive daily sessions except between B and C, where one session is omitted, and between F and G, where two sessions are omitted. The periods during which scheduled shocks were omitted are indicated. Note the records (Frames C, D, and H), showing suppression of responding at the beginning of sessions in which scheduled shocks were omitted (spontaneous retrogression).

of responding previously suppressed by punishment does not regularly occur when punishment is discontinued.

In Frame C, during the fourth presentation of the punishment compo-nent, responding began abruptly and continued for the remainder of the ses-sion. Yet, on the following day (Frame D), with scheduled shocks still omitted, there was a pause throughout the first punishment component, followed by normal responding for the remainder of the session. The tem-porary suppression at the beginning of the session on the second day with all scheduled shocks omitted (Frame D) further indicates that the suppressant effects of punishment are greatest at the beginning of a session. These results confirm those of Azrin *et al.* (2–4). Thus, the reinstatement of the suppression of responding obtained when shocks are omitted following punishment (*spontaneous retrogression*) occurs under the same conditions as the restoration of responding obtained during extinction following reinforcement (spontaneous recovery).

After scheduled shocks had been omitted for 3 days (Frame E), the fixed-ratio pattern of responding was maintained throughout each session. When, in the middle of the following session, shocks were again presented, responding was completely suppressed after a single response was punished (Frame F). Frame G shows a subsequent day with punishment, and Frame H shows the effects of again omitting the scheduled shocks. Although a high rate of responding in the punishment components developed more quickly than in Frames C and D, there was still some suppression, especially during the first punishment component. Omitting all scheduled shocks is only sometimes effective in increasing suppressed responding, whereas in this situation pentobarbital is always effective in attenuating punished responding even though responses still produce shocks. This analysis simply emphasizes what a powerful drug effect this is!

An example of the effects of morphine on punished responding is shown in Fig. 8. The top record shows control performance. The next record shows the effect of an intramuscular injection of morphine (1 mg/kg) 15 min before the session. This is the highest dose of morphine that does not decrease rates of responding in the nonpunishment component. Seven responses occurred during the first three punishment components (within the control range). Then scheduled shocks were omitted for the remainder of the session; following a response in the fourth component, there was an abrupt increase in responding in punishment components. The next record shows the effect of 3 mg/kg of morphine. This dose did not attenuate suppression of responding by punishment, but did reduce the rate of responding in nonpunishment components (as indicated by the slightly longer session duration). After 10 mg/kg of morphine, almost all responding was eliminated, although the pigeon would still eat when food was presented.

The bottom record of Fig. 8 shows effects of 1 mg/kg of morphine with another pigeon. At the beginning of the session, scheduled shocks were omitted. Responding occurred in punishment components, but when scheduled shocks were reinstated in the fourth punishment component, responding was immediately suppressed. This dose of morphine neither renders the shock ineffective nor prevents the reestablishment of suppression following punishment by electric shock. These results show clearly that morphine lacks the type of effect on punished responding that pentobarbital has.

These results provide a new perspective on the ways in which drugs affect negatively reinforced behavior. Some drugs (for example, chlorpromazine) that are effective in eliminating behavior maintained by the

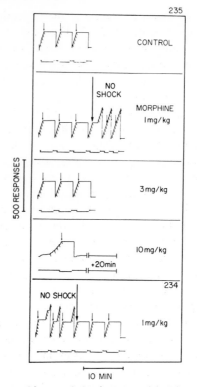

FIGURE 8.   Effect of morphine on behavior suppressed by punishment. The first four frames show performance of bird 235 on the fixed-ratio procedure in which nonpunishment and punishment components alternated. Shocks were scheduled in punishment components except where indicated. The first record shows control performance. The start of the second record shows performance on the same procedure following the intramuscular injection of morphine (1 mg/kg); at the large arrow, scheduled shocks were omitted. The third and fourth records show the effects of larger doses of morphine; 20 min in which no responses occurred have been omitted from the 10 mg/kg record. The lower frame shows the effect of morphine on the performance of bird 234. Scheduled shocks were omitted at the beginning of the record and then reinstated at the large arrow. Note that morphine did not prevent the almost immediate return of suppression by punishment with electric shocks.

termination of a negative reinforcer are ineffective in restoring behavior suppressed by immediate punishment. Other drugs (for example, meprobamate) that are relatively ineffective in eliminating behavior maintained by negative reinforcement are effective in restoring behavior suppressed by immediate punishment. Similar dependencies of drug effects on schedule have, of course, been shown previously with schedules of positive reinforcement.

Motivational interpretations of drug effects on negatively reinforced behavior and on punished behavior assume that both maintenance and suppression of behavior by electric shocks are controlled by fear and anxiety. This assumption has a plausible generality because it accounts for both increases and decreases of behavior with a single concept. Recently there has been a resurgence of interest in explaining all the effects of negative reinforcers with a unitary concept. In a recent review, for example, Solomon (44) suggests that "what holds for punishment and its action on behavior should hold also for escape and avoidance training, and vice versa." However, drugs have different effects on escape responding and punished responding. Despite the cogency of psychological theories, the same drugs that affect punished behavior do not affect escape behavior, and vice versa. This pharmacological separation of escape behavior and punished behavior is an important contribution of behavioral pharmacology to psychology.

It has frequently been assumed that an ideal tranquilizing drug would be effective in modifying all types of negatively reinforced behavior without affecting other types of behavior. It should be remembered, however, that much useful behavior is controlled by negative reinforcers. People who are insensitive to pain can harm themselves; people who are not affected by the suppressive influences in society may end up in jail. There is no more reason to assume that negative reinforcers are necessarily bad than there is to assume that positive reinforcers are necessarily good. Children who have indulgent parents can become spoiled; people who enjoy food too much may become obese.

Motivational interpretations simply fail to provide a consistent account of behavioral effects of drugs. Nevertheless, in our studies, consistent generalizations about the effects of drugs on schedule-controlled behavior did emerge. When the schedule-controlled patterns of escape-maintained and food-maintained behavior were similar, the effects of drugs on these patterns were similar. The results discussed in this paper indicate that the specific behavior that will be present to be affected by a drug is determined by the temporal and sequential relations between responses and stimuli (the schedule of reinforcement). To develop a better understanding of the ways in which drugs interact with schedule-controlled patterns of behavior is the major task currently facing behavioral pharmacology.

REFERENCES

1. Azrin, N. H. *J. Psychol.* **42**:3, 1956.
2. Azrin, N. H. *J. Exptl. Anal. Behavior* **2**:161, 1959.
3. Azrin, N. H. *J. Exptl. Anal. Behavior* **3**:123, 1960.
4. Azrin, N. H. Holz, W. C., and Hake, D. F. *J. Exptl. Anal. Behavior* **6**:141, 1963.
5. Brady, J. V. *J. Psychol.* **40**:25, 1955.
6. Brady, J. V. *Science* **123**:1033, 1956.

7. Cook, L., and Kelleher, R. T. *Ann. N.Y. Acad. Sci.* 96:315, 1962.

8. Cook, L., and Kelleher, R. T. *Ann. Rev. Pharmacol.* 3:205, 1963.

9. Dews, P. B. *J. Pharmacol. Exptl. Therap.* 113:393, 1955.

10. Dews, P. B. *Federation Proc.* 17:1024, 1958.

11. Dews, P. B. *J. Pharmacol. Exptl. Therap.* 122:137, 1958.

12. Dews, P. B., and Morse, W. H. *J. Exptl. Anal. Behavior* 1:359, 1958.

13. Dews, P. B., and Morse, W. H. *Ann. Rev. Pharmacol.* 1:145, 1961.

14. Edwards, R. E. *Federation Proc.* 20:397, 1961.

15. Estes, W. K., and Skinner, B. F. *J. Exptl. Psychol.* 29:390, 1941.

16. Ferster, C. B., Appel, J. B., and Hiss, R. A. *J. Exptl. Anal. Behavior* 5:73, 1962.

17. Ferster, C. B., and Skinner, B. F. *Schedules of reinforcement.* New York: Appleton-Century-Crofts, 1957.

18. Gatti, G. L. In: *Psychotropic drugs,* ed. by S. Garattini and V. Ghetti. Amsterdam: Elsevier Publ. Co., 1957, p. 125.

19. Geller, I. In: *Psychosomatic medicine,* ed. by J. H. Nodine and J. H. Moyer. Philadelphia: Lea and Febiger, 1962, p. 267.

20. Geller, I., Bachman, E., and Seifter, J. *Life Sci.* 4:226, 1963.

21. Geller, I., Kulak, J. T., Jr., and Seifter, J. *Psychopharmacologia* 3:374, 1962.

22. Geller, I., and Seifter, J. *Psychopharmacologia* 1:482, 1960.

23. Geller, I., and Seifter, J. *J. Pharmacol. Exptl. Therap.* 136:284, 1962.

24. Goodman, L. S., and Gilman, A. *The pharmacological basis of therapeutics,* Ed. 2. New York: Macmillan Co., 1955.

25. Hake, D. F., and Azrin, N. H. *J. Exptl. Anal. Behavior* 6:297, 1963.

26. Herrnstein, R. J, and Sidman, M. *J. Comp. Physiol. Psychol.* 51:380, 1958.

27. Hill, H. E., Pescor, F. T., Belleville, R. E., and Wikler, A. *J. Pharmacol. Exptl.* 120:388, 1957.

28. Hunt, H. F. *Ann. N.Y. Acad. Sci.* 65:253, 1956.

29. Hunt, H. F. *Ann. N.Y. Acad. Sci.* 67:712, 1957.

30. Jacobsen, E. In: *Psychotropic drugs,* ed. by S. Garattini and V. Ghetti. Amsterdam: Elsevier Publ. Co., 1957, p. 119.

31. Kelleher, R. T., Fry, W., Deegan, J., and Cook, L. *J. Pharmacol. Exptl. Therap.* 133:271, 1961.

32. Kelleher, R. T., Riddle, W. C., and Cook, L. *J. Exptl. Anal. Behavior* 5:3, 1962.

33. Kelleher, R. T., Riddle, W. C., and Cook, L. *J. Exptl. Anal. Behavior* 6:507, 1963.

34. Kinnard, W. J., Aceto, M. D. G., and Buckley, J. P. *Psychopharmacologia* 3:227, 1962.

35. Lauener, H. *Psychopharmacologia* 4:311, 1963.

36. Morse, W. H. In: *Psychosomatic medicine,* ed. by J. H. Nodine and J. H. Moyer. Philadelphia: Lea and Febiger, 1962, p. 275.

37. Morse, W. H. *Psychopharmacologia* 6:286, 1964.

38. Morse, W. H., and Herrnstein, R. J. *Ann. N.Y. Acad. Sci.* 65:303, 1956.

39. Morse, W. H., and Skinner, B. F. *Am. J. Psychol.* 70:308, 1957.

40. Naess, K., and Rasmussen, E. W. *Acta Pharmacol. Toxicol.* 15:99, 1958.

41. Ray, O. S. *Psychopharmacologia* 5:136, 1964.

42. Sacra, P., Rice, W. B., and McColl, J. D. *Can. J. Biochem. Physiol.* 35:1151, 1957.

43. Sidman, M., Herrnstein, R. J., and Conrad, D. G. *J. Comp. Physiol. Psychol.* 50:553, 1957.

44. Solomon, R. L. *Am. Psychologist* 19:239, 1964.

45. Stein, L., Sidman, M., and Brady, J. V. *J. Exptl. Anal. Behavior* 1:153, 1958.

46. Valenstein, E. S. *J. Exptl. Anal. Behavior* 2:219, 1959.

47. Waller, M. B. *J. Exptl. Anal. Behavior* **4**:351, 1961.
48. Waller, M. B., and Waller, P. F. *J. Exptl. Anal. Behavior* **5**:259, 1962.
49. Waller, M. B., and Waller, P. F. *J. Exptl. Anal. Behavior* **6**:29, 1963.
50. Weiskrantz, L. In: *Neuropsychopharmacology,* ed. by P. B. Bradley, P. Deniker, and C. Radouco-Thomas. Amsterdam: Elsevier Publ. Co., 1959, p. 53.
51. Weiss, B., and Laties, V. G. *J. Pharmacol. Exptl. Therap.* **140**:1, 1963.
52. Yamahiro, R. S., Bell, E. C., and Hill, H. E. *Psychopharmacologia* **2**:197, 1961.